Culture, Society and Sexuality

There has been rapid development within the field of sexuality research in recent years – both conceptually and methodologically. Advance has sometimes occurred in relatively unsystematic ways, however, and academic research often seems distant from the immediate concerns of day-to-day life.

This second edition of *Culture, Society and Sexuality* consolidates the literature on the construction of sexual life and sexual rights – often published in relatively obscure places – and makes it accessible, not only to students, but also to those working on the front lines of activism. Topics discussed include:

- the historical construction of sexual meanings – desires and practices across different periods of history
- the ways in which social theory and research have approached the investigation of things sexual – 'cultural influence' versus 'social constructionism'
- the 'gender hierarchy' and the 'sex hierarchy' as central to the construction of a politics not only of gender oppression but also of sexual oppression
- the dominance of heterosexuality, and the frequent exclusion or neglect of lesbians within the women's movement
- social, cultural and economic globalization – the ways in which gay identities and communities have helped to shape the contemporary world
- violence, sexuality, and gender and public health – sexual pleasure, the control of fertility, and risk for sexually transmitted diseases.

This volume builds on the importance of insights into the social, cultural, political and economic dimensions of sexuality and relationships, and emerging discourses around sexual and reproductive rights. It provides essential reading for researchers, activists, health workers and service providers, who daily confront practical and policy issues related to sexuality, sexual health and sexual rights.

Richard Parker is Professor and Chair of the Department of Sociomedical Sciences and Director of the Center for Gender, Sexuality and Health in the Mailman School of Public Health at Columbia University, and Director and President of the Brazilian Interdisciplinary AIDS Association (ABIA) in Rio de Janeiro, Brazil.

Peter Aggleton is Professor in Education at the Institute of Education, University of London, the editor of the journal *Culture, Health and Sexuality* and senior advisor on HIV and sexuality to a wide range of international organizations and agencies.

Sexuality, Culture and Health

Series editors
Peter Aggleton, Institute of Education, University of London, UK
Richard Parker, Columbia University, New York, USA
Sonia Corrêa, ABIA, Rio de Janeiro, Brazil
Gary Dowsett, LaTrobe University, Melbourne, Australia
Shirley Lindenbaum, City University of New York, USA

This new series of books offers cutting-edge analysis, current theoretical perspectives and up-to-the-minute ideas concerning the interface between sexuality, public health, human rights, culture and social development. It adopts a global and interdisciplinary perspective in which the needs of poorer countries are given equal status to those of richer nations. The books are written with a broad range of readers in mind, and will be invaluable to students, academics and those working in policy and practice. The series also aims to serve as a spur to practical action in an increasingly globalised world.

Also available in the series:

Dying to be Men
Youth masculinity and social exclusion
Gary T. Barker

Sex, Drugs and Young People
International perspectives
Edited by
Peter Aggleton, Andrew Ball and Purnima Mane

Promoting Young People's Sexual Health
International perspectives
Edited by
Roger Ingham and Peter Aggleton

Culture, Society and Sexuality

A reader

Second edition

Edited by
Richard Parker and Peter Aggleton

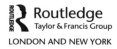

Routledge
Taylor & Francis Group

LONDON AND NEW YORK

First published 1999
by UCL press
Reprinted 2003
by Routledge
This edition published 2007
by Routledge
2 Park Square, Milton Park, Abingdon, Oxon OX14 4RN

Simultaneously published in the USA and Canada
by Routledge
270 Madison Avenue, New York, NY 10016

Routledge is an imprint of the Taylor & Francis Group, an informa business

Typeset in Times New Roman by Bookcraft Ltd, Stroud, Gloucestershire
Printed and bound in Great Britain by The Cromwell Press, Trowbridge, Wiltshire

British Library Cataloguing in Publication Data
A catalogue record for this book is available from the British Library

Library of Congress Cataloging in Publication Data
Culture, society and sexuality: a reader/edited by Richard Parker and Peter Aggleton.–2nd ed.
    p. cm.–(Sexuality, culture and health series)
  Includes bibliographical references and index.
  1. Sex. 2. Sex customs. 3. Heterosexuality. 4. Homosexuality. 5. Sexology.
  6. AIDS (Disease) I. Parker, Richard G. (Richard Guy), 1956– II. Aggleton, Peter.
  HQ21.C846 2007
  306.7–dc22   2006021517

ISBN10: 0-415-40455-X (hbk)
ISBN10: 0-415-40456-8 (pbk)
ISBN10: 0-203-96610-4 (ebk)

ISBN13: 978-0-415-40455-6 (hbk)
ISBN13: 978-0-415-40456-3 (pbk)
ISBN13: 978-0-203-96610-5 (ebk)

For Vavá and Preecha

Contents

viii   *Contents*

Figures

Tables

Editors' note

As in any collection that brings together previously published texts, one of the primary challenges in preparing this book has lain in the task of systematizing often quite different styles, notes and bibliographic references. Throughout the volume, we have sought to preserve the originally published texts. We have tried to adapt notes and references to conform to the style used in the *Sexuality, Culture and Health* series. When possible, we have tried to update references and offer complete bibliographic information, though we regret that we have not always been able to do so successfully. Whenever in doubt, however, we have been guided by the authors' originals, and have attempted, throughout, to stay true to the authors' intentions.

Acknowledgements

The second edition of *Culture, Society and Sexuality* draws on extensive work that went into the first edition, which was carried out over a number of years, and on a number of different continents, with the assistance of a range of different individuals and institutions. We would particularly like to thank Ana Paula Uziel, Juan Carlos de la Concepción, and Rita Rizzo at the Instituto de Medicina Social, Universidade do Estado do Rio de Janeiro, Delia Easton, Charles Klein and Chris White formerly of the HIV Center for Clinical and Behavioral Studies, New York State Psychiatric Institute and Columbia University, and Paul Tyrer, Paula Hassett and Helen Thomas formerly of the Thomas Coram Research Unit, Institute of Education, University of London, for their help in preparing the manuscript. We would also like to thank the Ford Foundation and the John D. and Catherine T. MacArthur Foundation for support to the Program on Gender, Sexuality and Health at the Centro de Pesquisa e Estudos em Saúde Coletiva which made it possible to initiate work on the book. For his extensive contributions to the revised edition, we would like to thank Jonathan Garcia at the Center for Gender, Sexuality and Health in the Department of Sociomedical Sciences of the Mailman School of Public Health at Columbia University.

Special thanks as well to the authors and publishers who gave permission to reprint the essays collected here:

- Robert Padgug and Cambridge University Press, for permission to reprint 'Sexual Matters: On Conceptualizing Sexuality in History', *Radical History Review*, Vol. 20, spring/summer, 1979.
- Transaction Books, for permission to republish William Simon and John Gagnon, 'Sexual Scripts', *Society*, Vol. 22, Issue 1, 1984.
- Carole S. Vance, for permission to republish 'Anthropology Rediscovers Sexuality: A Theoretical Comment', *Social Science and Medicine*, Vol. 33, No. 8, 1991.
- Joan Scott, for permission to republish 'Gender as a Useful Category of Historical Analysis', *American Historical Review*, Vol. 91, No. 5, 1986.
- Donna J. Haraway, for permission to republish '"Gender" for a Marxist Dictionary: The Sexual Politics of a Word', from *Simians, Cyborgs, and Women: The Reinvention of Nature*, New York and London: Routledge, 1991.
- Roger N. Lancaster, for permission to republish '"That We Should All Turn Queer?": Homosexual Stigma in the Making of Manhood and the Breaking of a Revolution in Nicaragua', from *Conceiving Sexuality: Approaches to Sex Research in a Postmodern World*, Richard G. Parker and John H. Gagnon (eds), New York and London: Routledge, 1995.
- Jeffrey Weeks, for permission to republish 'Discourse, Desire and Sexual Deviance: Some Problems in a History of Homosexuality', from *The Making of the Modern Homosexual*, Kenneth Plummer (ed.), London: Hutchinson, 1981.

- Gayle Rubin, for permission to republish 'Thinking Sex: Notes for a Radical Theory of the Politics of Sexuality', from *Pleasure and Danger: Exploring Female Sexuality*, Carole S. Vance (ed.), Routledge and Kegan Paul, 1984.
- R.W. Connell, Gary W. Dowsett, and the Melbourne University Press, for permission to republish '"The Unclean Motion of the Generative Parts": Frameworks in Western Thought on Sexuality', from *Rethinking Sex: Social Theory and Sexuality Research*, R.W. Connell and Gary W. Dowsett (eds), Melbourne: Melbourne University Press, 1992.
- Adrienne Rich, W.W. Norton & Company, and Virago Press, for permission to republish 'Compulsory Heterosexuality and Lesbian Existence', from *Blood, Bread and Poetry: Selected Prose 1979–1985*, New York: W.W. Norton & Company, 1986.
- Serena Nanda and the Haworth Press, for permission to republish 'The *Hijras* of India: Cultural and Individual Dimensions of an Institutionalized Third Gender Role', *Journal of Homosexuality*, Vol. 11, Nos 3/4, pp. 35–54, 1985.
- John D'Emilio and the Monthly Review Press, for permission to republish 'Capitalism and Gay Identity', from *Powers of Desire: The Politics of Sexuality*, Ann Snitow, Christine Stansell and Sharon Thompson (eds), New York: Monthly Review Press, 1983.
- R.W. Connell, for permission to republish 'Masculinities and Globalization' from *The Men And The Boys*, Berkeley: University of California Press, pp. 39–56, 2000.
- Lori L. Heise, for permission to republish 'Violence, Sexuality, and Women's Lives' from *Conceiving Sexuality: Approaches to Sex Research in a Postmodern World*, Richard G. Parker and John H. Gagnon (eds), New York: Routledge, 1995.
- Sonia Corrêa and Rosalind Petchesky, for permission to republish 'Reproductive and Sexual Rights: A Feminist Perspective', from *Population Policies Reconsidered: Health, Empowerment, and Rights*, Gita Sen, Adrienne Germain and Lincoln C. Chen (eds), Boston: Harvard University Press, 1994.
- Elsevier Sciences Ltd., for permission to republish Stephanie Kane, 'HIV, Heroin and Heterosexual Relations', *Social Science and Medicine*, Vol. 32, No. 9, 1991.
- Taylor & Francis, for permission to republish 'An Explosion of Thai Identities: Global Queering and Re-Imagining Queer Theory', *Culture, Health & Sexuality*, Vol. 2, No. 4, pp. 405–24, 2000.
- Taylor & Francis, for permission to republish '*Bhai-Behen*, True Love, Time Pass: Friendships and Sexual Partnerships among Youth in an Indian Metropolis', *Culture, Health & Sexuality*, Vol. 4, No. 3, pp. 337–53, 2002.
- Taylor & Francis, for permission to republish 'Masculinity and Urban Men: Perceived Scripts for Courtship, Romantic, and Sexual Interactions with Women', *Culture, Health & Sexuality*, Vol. 5, No. 4, pp. 295–319, 2003.
- Taylor & Francis, for permission to republish 'Some Traditional Methods Are More Modern Than Others: Rhythm, Withdrawal and the Changing Meanings of Sexual Intimacy in Mexican Companionate Marriage', *Culture, Health & Sexuality*, Vol. 3, No. 4, pp. 295–319, 2001.
- Taylor & Francis, for permission to republish 'Mobility, Sexual Networks and Exchange among *Bodabodamen* in Southwest Uganda', *Culture, Health & Sexuality*, Vol. 6, No. 3, pp. 239–54, 2004.
- Vera Paiva, for permission to republish 'Gendered Scripts and the Sexual Scene: Promoting Sexual Subjects among Brazilian Teenagers' in R. Parker, R.M. Barbosa and P. Aggleton, *Framing The Sexual Subject*, Berkeley: University of California Press, pp. 216–39, 2000.

- Elsevier Science Ltd., for permission to republish 'HIV- and AIDS-Related Stigma and Discrimination: A Conceptual Framework and Implications for Action', *Social Science and Medicine*, Vol. 57, No. 1, pp. 13–24, 2003.
- Ignacio Saiz and the François-Xavier Bagnoud Center for Health and Human Rights, for permission to republish 'Bracketing Sexuality: Human Rights and Sexual Orientation – A Decade of Development and Denial at the UN', *Health and Human Rights*, Vol. 7, No. 2, pp. 49–80, 2004.

1 Introduction

Richard Parker and Peter Aggleton

Until the late twentieth century, human sexuality was largely marginalized as a focus for social enquiry, scholarly reflection and academic activism. Perhaps because the experience of sexuality appears to be so intimately linked to our bodies, it was relatively easy to relegate matters of sexuality to the realms of the biomedical and population sciences. While it had served, through much of the nineteenth century, as the subject matter for obscure medical tomes or arcane psychiatric practices, sexuality seemed to have little to do with the more crucial and immediate problems of social and political life. It was really only during the closing decades of the twentieth century and the early part of the twenty-first century, that this marginalization of sexuality – and its submission to the biomedical gaze – began to give way to more far-reaching social and political analysis. And it is perhaps only over the course of the past two decades, from roughly the late 1980s to the present, that a boom in social sciences research within this field seems to have taken place, transforming the study of sexuality into one of the most active areas of investigation today in both social and cultural studies (see Kimmel and Plante, 2004; Parker, Barbosa and Aggleton, 2000; Seidman, 2003; Williams and Stein, 2002).

The reasons for this explosion of social research on sexuality are complex and diverse. They clearly have much to do with a broad set of changes that have taken place in the social sciences generally, as disciplines such as history, anthropology and sociology have struggled to find new ways of understanding a rapidly changing world. Perhaps more importantly, however, the growing attention to sexuality as a key focus for social analysis has been mandated by a set of movements within society itself. It can be understood, at least in part, as a consequence of the more far-reaching social changes that began to take place during the 1960s and, especially, of the growing feminist and gay and lesbian movements that emerged from the 1960s as among the most powerful and important sources of social change during the 1970s and the 1980s (see Lancaster and Di Leonardo, 1997; Weeks, 2000; Williams and Stein, 2002).

At the same time that social movements have been crucial in calling attention to questions of gender and sexuality, over the course of recent decades growing international concern with issues such as population, women's and men's reproductive health, and perhaps especially the HIV and AIDS pandemic, has in large part intersected with research agendas constructed around feminist and gay and lesbian issues (see Parker and Gagnon, 1995; Parker, Barbosa and Aggleton, 2000). While socially and morally conservative sectors might prefer to dismiss questions related to sexuality as little more than the private concern of perverse minorities, the broader implications of issues such as population, reproductive health and AIDS have in large part guaranteed that the study of sexuality, and of its social and political dimensions, would necessarily emerge as central to many of the most important debates taking place globally in the late twentieth and early twenty-first centuries (see Butler, 2004; Fausto-Sterling, 2000; Kimmel and Plante, 2004; Nagel, 2003; Williams and Stein, 2002). While the intersection of concerns related to sexuality, sexual health and sexual rights has thus increasingly become a central focus of attention for researchers and activists from a range of diverse fields, scientific disciplines and social movements, the challenges that have been faced in seeking to build a more multi-dimensional understanding of sexual life and experience should not be underestimated. As was highlighted by the rapid emergence of the global HIV epidemic, the lack of pre-existing baseline data on human sexuality, and, consequently, the urgent need for data collection on behaviours that may be linked to HIV transmission, has been widely discussed (see, for example, Chouinard and Albert, 1990; Cleland and Ferry, 1996; Laumann *et al.*, 1994; Turner, Miller and Moses, 1989, 1990). Rather less attention has been given, however, to the serious limitations in the dominant theoretical and methodological approaches that have been used in carrying out such research, particularly in relation to public health (see Gagnon, 2004; Parker, 1994, 1996; Parker and Gagnon, 1995). The inadequacies of such approaches are probably most obvious at the theoretical level, precisely because research on sexual behaviour has almost never been driven by a theory of human sexuality or sexual desire. Indeed, in most instances, it has not been driven by any overtly stated theory at all – the emphasis instead has been on the urgent need for descriptive data (such as that likely to be revealed through surveys of HIV- and AIDS-related knowledge, attitudes and reported practices), apparently based upon the hope that theoretical insights will emerge from such data if we only have enough of it (see Parker, 1994). Even when a theoretical framework for conceptualizing sexuality has occasionally been invoked, it has almost always been at best a minimal one – most typically the 'explanation' of behaviours in terms of demographic correlates or the conceptualization of sexual desire as a kind of basic (biologically grounded) human drive which may be shaped somewhat differently in different settings, and which must therefore be described as it manifests itself empirically within these settings (see, for example, Carballo *et al.*, 1989; Cleland and Ferry, 1996; Erens *et al.*, 2003; Laumann *et al.*, 1994; Michael *et al.*, 1994; Wellings *et al.*, 1994; WHO/GPA/SBR, 1989).

This lack of theoretical development is not, of course, unique to population-based studies triggered at least in part by HIV and AIDS – even though it has become rather more visible precisely because of the intensification of research activity in response to the epidemic. On the contrary, it is in many ways the product of a particular tradition of sex research that seems to have been incorporated within the fields of public health and health education more generally – what has been described by Paul Robinson as a kind of 'sex modernism' running from early writers such as Havelock Ellis through Kinsey and his colleagues up to more current sexologists such as Masters and Johnson (see Robinson, 1976). Emerging, in large part, as both an intellectual and a political response to the perceived moral strictures of Victorian society, the primary focus of this tradition has been an attempt to 'demystify' and, in particular, to 'naturalize' human sexual behaviour – and, hence, an attempt to describe, as exhaustively as possible, the forms of sexual expression that exist 'in nature' (Robinson, 1976; see also Gagnon and Simon, 1973; Parker and Gagnon, 1995; Weeks, 1981, 1985, 2000, 2003).

The importance of such a perspective should not be taken lightly – nor should its potential value be underestimated. It is in large part responsible, for example, particularly following the work of Kinsey and his colleagues, for opening up the field of sexual behaviour as an object of scientific investigation rather than as the domain of religion or morality (see Robinson, 1976; Turner, Miller and Moses, 1989). At the same time, its legacy, in particular as it has been incorporated into the field of public health, has clearly been problematic as a kind of extreme empiricism, which, in the absence of a more convincing theory for the explanation of human sexuality and sexual diversity, has focused almost exclusively on documenting behavioural frequencies within a relatively limited range of population groups (see Gagnon, 2004).

This general lack of theoretical development, particularly within the field of public health and in the health sciences, has been directly linked to the poverty that can be identified in the conceptual frameworks of much sexual behaviour research (see Gagnon, 2004). In perhaps the vast majority of research related to sexuality and health, for example, sexual desire has been treated as a kind of given, and the social and cultural factors shaping sexual experience in different settings have largely been ignored – even when a certain degree of lip-service has been paid to their potential importance. In keeping with the dominant tendencies in much health behaviour research, emphasis has been placed largely on the individual determinants of sexual behaviour and behaviour change, and the diverse social, cultural, economic and political factors potentially influencing or even shaping sexual experience have for the most part been ignored (Evans, 1993; Gagnon, 2004; Parker, 1994, 1996, 1999, 2001; Seidman, 2003).

These theoretical limitations in the conceptual frameworks that have been used to examine sexual experience seem to have been linked, in turn, to a series of equally problematic methodological limitations. In much of the mainstream research that has been carried out on sexual experience, the dominant focus has been on the use of survey research methods (once again, an inheritance from Kinsey and his colleagues), and the key question addressed in the design of research has almost inevitably been how to make these methods more effective in the different contexts in which studies of sexual behaviour have been carried out, particularly in the wake of HIV and AIDS – in developing countries, for example, or among problematically defined target populations such as gay and bisexual men or injecting drug users, and so on (see, in particular, Turner, Miller and Moses, 1989, 1990; see also Cleland and Ferry, 1996; Laumann *et al.*, 1994; Michael *et al.*, 1994).

Such approaches have worked reasonably well within the framework of a research agenda defined largely by epidemiological questions, for example, or psychological models of behaviour change. Counting the frequency of sexual acts, if carried out effectively, can clearly offer important insights concerning the course of HIV infection or the risk of unintended pregnancies in specific settings. In much the same way, depending upon one's assumptions, measuring psychosocial indicators may offer insight into the propensity for risk reduction or the likelihood of adopting different contraceptive methods. These frameworks, and the methodological approach stemming from them, have been much weaker, however, as a way of providing a multi-dimensional and, hence, fuller understanding of sexual behaviour more generally – and this, in turn, has had serious consequences, especially in seeking to move from primarily epidemiological questions to the broader issues that must be confronted in intervening through health promotion and education (see Aggleton, 1996, 2004; Laumann and Michael, 2001; Parker, 1994, 1996; Parker and Gagnon, 1995; Parker, Barbosa and Aggleton, 2000), or the kinds of questions that must be addressed in moving from an understanding of epidemiological vulnerability to the crucial tasks of defending the social and political rights of vulnerable groups and communities (Carrillo, 2002; Laumann *et al.*, 2004; Parker, 1999; Parker, Barbosa and Aggleton, 2000).

In spite of the dominant role that a kind of 'naturalistic' understanding of sexual life seems to have played in public health and related fields over the course of a number of decades now, work carried out in a variety of disciplines has therefore challenged this view, focusing instead on what has been described as the 'social and cultural construction' of sexual conduct (see, for example, Gagnon, 1977; Weeks, 1985; see also Parker and Gagnon, 1995; Parker, Barbosa and Aggleton, 2000). In fields such as cultural anthropology, sociology, social psychology and history, attention has increasingly focused on the social, cultural, economic and political forces shaping sexual behaviour in different settings, together with the complex and often contradictory meanings associated with sexual experience on the part of both individuals and social groups (see, for example, Gagnon and Simon, 1973; Herdt and Stoller, 1990; Parker, 1991; Weeks, 1981, 1985, 2003). While this focus on the social and cultural construction of sexual life has passed through a number of different phases, and has taken a variety of different turns, it has nonetheless begun to offer an increasingly important alternative to more naturalist (or 'essentialist') understandings of sexuality in relation to sexual health and wellbeing (see Gagnon, 2004; Laumann *et al.*, 2004; Parker, 1994, 1996; Parker and Gagnon 1995; Parker, Barbosa and Aggleton, 2000). Without in any way unseating or substituting more dominant behavioural approaches within sex research, work informed by social and cultural concerns has become an increasingly strong counter-current within the broader investigation of sexual life.

Developments within the field of sexuality research have often taken place in relatively unsystematic ways, and have frequently seemed quite distant from the immediate understandings of sexual interpretations and categories in our daily lives. Indeed, while it has in fact been heavily influenced by the real-world struggles of social movements focusing on both gender equity and sexual rights, this influence has not been fully appreciated because of the fact that much of the most influential work on the social and cultural construction of sexual life and sexual rights has often been published in relatively obscure places with only limited distribution outside of quite specialized academic settings. Much of the emerging discourse around sexual negotiations and sexual and reproductive rights, for example, has been scattered and fragmented throughout a number of academic journals, often only available by subscription in quite specialized libraries. *Culture, Society and Sexuality* attempts to consolidate some of this literature, which is in large part out of reach for many of those who work in the front lines of activism. The current volume emerged, perhaps above all else, from the editors' sense of potential importance that these insights on the social and cultural dimensions of sexuality and relationships, and the emerging discourse around the concepts of sexual and reproductive health and rights, might potentially have not only for researchers but, equally importantly, for advocates and activists, health workers, service providers, and others involved in the day-to-day response to practical challenges to sexual health and sexual rights in the contemporary world.

In seeking to make some sense of this important body of work, we have tried to organize the book in a way that might offer some idea of the development of the field, first in relation to sexual life in and of itself, and second in relation to more specific instances in which local sexualities and relationships are negotiated and categorized. Of particular importance here is how globalization has brought about international discourses on sexual rights, especially with relation to health. Within each Section and Part, in turn, we have assembled a number of key essays that will offer the reader a sense of major issues that have provided a focus for reflection, theorization and empirical investigation, and that have helped to shape a fuller understanding of the issues raised by notions of sexuality and sexual rights and of ways in which these issues might be reframed and reconsidered.

With these goals in mind, in Section I, 'Culture, society and sexuality', we focus attention on the social and cultural construction of sexuality as an emerging field of enquiry over the course of recent decades, and examine some of the most important theoretical insights and areas of investigation that have emerged as this field has developed. In the first Part,

'Conceptual frameworks', we have included essays from three of the different disciplines that have made some of the most pronounced contributions to work in this area, each of which offers an overview of the kinds of issues that the discipline has begun to struggle with and a sense of the kinds of responses that have begun to emerge. In Chapter 2 'Sexual matters: on conceptualizing sexuality in history', for example, Robert Padgug provides one of the earliest and most influential statements on the historical construction of sexual meanings. He focuses, in particular, on the importance of situating sexual orientation and identity within discrete historical periods and social realities, and highlights the changing meaning of homosexual desires and practices across different periods in the history of Western society. In Chapter 3, 'Sexual scripts', William Simon and John H. Gagnon provide an especially clear and systematic statement of their influential sociological theory of sexual scripts. They distinguish between the broader 'cultural scenarios' that organize sexual meanings in different cultural settings, the 'interpersonal scripts' that are constructed in the ongoing process of social interaction, and the 'intrapsychic scripts' that both cultural meanings and social interaction constitute at the level of individual subjectivity. And in Chapter 4, 'Anthropology rediscovers sexuality: A theoretical comment', Carole Vance provides an especially thorough overview of the ways in which anthropological theory and research have approached the investigation of things sexual. She makes an especially useful distinction between earlier theories of 'cultural influence', which have focused on the ways in which cultural systems shape or mould what are assumed to be underlying biological and psychological realities, and more recent 'social constructionist' work, which has sought to problematize more radically the very notion of such an underlying reality as itself a social and cultural construct.

One of the key areas in which constructionist approaches, from a variety of disciplinary perspectives, have had an especially important impact has been research on gender. In the next Part of the book, 'Gender and power', the focus thus shifts from these different (though often intersecting) disciplinary frames to an examination of the ways in which social constructionist and feminist theory have informed work on gender relations and gender power. In Chapter 5, 'Gender as a useful category of historical analysis', Joan Scott focuses on the development of 'gender' as a category for historical analysis. She emphasizes the extent to which gender has emerged in feminist theory in response to the perceived inadequacy of existing theoretical perspectives for explaining persistent inequalities between men and women, and thus focuses on the complex relationship between gender and power as central to a broader understanding of social relations. In Chapter 6, '"Gender" for a Marxist dictionary: The sexual politics of a word', Donna Haraway examines the recent history of the term 'sex/gender', emphasizing not only the complex textual politics associated with debates about gender as a category in feminist theory, but the importance of historicizing categories such as sex, race, body, biology and nature in order to construct differentiated and located theories of embodiment in society and culture. In Chapter 7, '"That we should all turn queer?":Homosexual stigma in the making of manhood and the breaking of a revolution in Nicaragua', Roger Lancaster pushes many of these same issues further through a detailed examination of gender relations in Nicaraguan culture. He not only emphasizes the relational nature of gender constructs, but highlights not only the ways in which gender power structures relations between men and women, but also the ways in which relations between different kinds of men are used to produce and reproduce normative structures of masculinity (and femininity) as part of a complex 'political economy of the body'.

While research on gender has been centrally important to framing a broader understanding of sex and sexuality, the need to differentiate between gender and sexuality has also been an important area of concern. The third Part of Section I of this volume, 'From gender to sexuality', focuses on this theoretical movement, building on earlier feminist approaches in important ways but focusing more explicitly on the social and historical construction of sexual difference. In Chapter 8, 'Discourse, desire and sexual deviance: Some problems in a history of homosexuality', Jeffrey Weeks develops an early analysis of the historical construction of homosexual identity and community in Western societies. Drawing heavily on Michel Foucault's work, and on the Foucauldian notion of historical ruptures and disconti-nuities, Weeks challenges essentialist interpretations of homosexuality. He argues that homo-sexual behaviours may be present in all societies, but that the organization of a distinct homosexual role in Western societies and cultures can be situated in quite specific ways as part of a broader historical reorganization of sexuality and sexual experience, and suggests that this understanding has important implications for the political project of gay and lesbian liberation. This concern with the interface between analysis and political action is equally important in Chapter 9, 'Thinking sex: Notes for a radical theory of the politics of sexuality', by Gayle Rubin. Rubin had been one of the most influential writers working on gender in the mid-1970s, and had originally introduced the concept of the 'sex/gender system' as a way of framing research on gender power. In this essay, however, she moves beyond this earlier formulation in order to examine gender and sexuality as two separate (though often inter-acting) fields of power: what she describes as the gender hierarchy and the sex hierarchy. She focuses on the need to develop analytic distinctions between these two domains as central to the construction of a politics not only of gender oppression but also of sexual oppression, and examines the ways in which sexual minorities (lesbians and gay men, certainly, but also other sexual minorities involved in S & M, cross-generational relations, and so on) have been both constructed and administered in modern regimes of power and knowledge. In Chapter 10, '"The unclean motion of the generative parts": Frameworks in Western thought on sexuality', R.W. Connell and Gary Dowsett build on these same kinds of insights in pushing the social constructionist framework beyond earlier work. They go so far as to argue that research and theory on the social construction of sexuality must give way to an emerging concern with the sexual construction of society, thus pointing toward the importance of recognizing changing sexual identities and communities as themselves constitutive of the changing order of society, particularly in the post-modern world of the late twentieth century.

This concern with the dynamic and creative potential of sexuality in a range of different cultural settings is clearly evident in the final Part in Section I examining 'Sexual identities/ sexual communities'. In Chapter 11, 'Compulsory heterosexuality and lesbian existence', for example, Adrienne Rich focuses on both the personal and the political bonds among women as central to the constitution of a meaningful women's movement. She examines the dominance of heterosexuality, and the frequent exclusion or neglect of lesbians within the women's move-ment, and develops the notion of a 'lesbian continuum' at the level of political identification as central to the task of uniting women on the basis of their shared gender identity. In Chapter 12, 'The *hijras* of India: Cultural and individual dimensions of an institutionalized third gender role', by Serena Nanda, issues of identity and identification are explored in the very different context of the Indian *hijras*, who are often the objects of stigma and abuse in contemporary Indian society, but who also occupy a particular social space as possessing special spiritual powers. By examining the social and sexual communities formed by the *hijras*, Nanda is able to relativize many of the assumptions that have been associated with the notions of transvestism and transgendered identities in contemporary Western societies, and to suggest some of the ways in which other cultural assumptions may lead to very different readings of the whole notion of sexual difference. Finally, in Chapter 13, 'Capitalism and gay identity', John D'Emilio develops one of the most concise and compelling statements of the ways in which changing social, political and economic structures have been linked to emerging gay identities and communities in the Western world. D'Emilio examines the ways in which a specific pattern of capitalist industrial development, linked to a wide range of social and demographic changes, has opened the way for a new organization of sexual life based on homosexual identity, and suggests some of the ways in which emerging gay identities and communities, in turn, have helped to shape and reshape the contemporary world, at least in the industrialized West. While D'Emilio's discussion focuses largely on the USA and Europe, his arguments point the direction for a new line of research that might well be much further developed in other parts of the world today, as the global capitalist system and the processes of social, cultural and economic globalization extend perhaps more broadly than ever before.

In Section II of this volume, 'Sexual meanings, health and rights', we turn from the social and cultural construction of gender, sexuality and sexual cultures, in and of themselves, to examine the ways in which the conceptual frameworks and insights that have emerged from this work have increasingly come to inform the investigation of sexual experience in relation to sexual health and sexual rights in the contemporary world. In this section, we seek to link the research on the construction of sexuality to a growing body of research about ways in which the construction of identity around gender and sexuality has functioned within social processes such as globalization. The second section also highlights investigations on sexual negotiations and scripted norms that shape sexual interactions and social relationships, and it opens the door to the emerging discourses around sexual and reproductive rights and uses of the human rights frameworks on both local and global levels.

The first Part of Section II, 'Gender, power and rights', focuses on the ways in which gendered identities have been reshaped under conditions of globalization, while at the same time becoming the focus for newly contested meanings within the global system. In Chapter 14, 'Masculinities and globalization', R.W. Connell takes issues of masculinity beyond the local, proving a broader picture and historical framework and thus taking into account the role of the global in understanding the local. Connell addresses the need to take a gender perspective in analysing institutions, such as multinational corporations and the media, and processes, such as imperialism and colonialism, that cut across national boundaries; and he describes how these global processes shape the construction of masculinity. In Chapter 15, 'Violence, sexuality, and women's lives', Lori Heise explores the multiple discourses surrounding the intersection between violence, sexuality, gender, and public health. She pays special attention to the synergistic implications on women's sexual and reproductive lives in domains such as the experience of sexual pleasure, the control of fertility, and risk for sexually transmitted diseases. Heise cautions against reliance on a biomedical model because of the risk of reinforcing the image of women as victims and essentializing male sexuality as biologically prone to inflict violence on women. Finally, in Chapter 16, 'Reproductive and sexual rights: A feminist perspective', Sonia Corrêa and Rosalind Petchesky analyse the concepts of reproductive and sexual rights and the surrounding discourses that permeate both private and public domains. These discourses include, for example, religious fundamentalism, which invokes the language of rights to serve purposes other than the health and empowerment of women. Corrêa and Petchesky define the negotiation of reproductive and sexual rights in terms of power and resources, including domains ranging from fertility and childbearing to sexual activity where women's decisions over their own bodies are being shaped by competing institutions and policies. They trace historically the concepts of reproductive and sexual rights and advocate a contextualized reframing to include the enablement of women's choices as a fundamental dimension to these concepts.

The next Part, 'Sexual categories and classifications', offers ways in which such insights might be applied to understanding how definitions of sexual relationships and sexuality impact on how individual and collective identities have formed within a historical context, and suggests a re-examination of these categories in their application on the local and global levels. In Chapter 17, 'HIV, heroin and heterosexual relations', Stephanie Kane deconstructs homosexual classifications and other, equally questionable, epidemiological categories as they have emerged in HIV and AIDS research. In particular, she explores the complex subcultures organized around drug-injecting practices in the urban USA, and focuses on the questionable status of the female sexual partners of drug-injecting men. Just as behaviourally bisexual and homosexual men fail to constitute a self-conscious or self-identified epidemiological risk group in many cultural settings, Kane argues that the female partners of drug-injecting males share little or no sense of collective identity or social reality, making it virtually impossible not only to effectively map the spread of HIV infection but also to operationalize effective prevention programmes through the use of such artificial and imposed social categories. In Chapter 18, 'An explosion of Thai identities: Global queering and re-imagining queer theory', Peter Jackson discusses recent findings from research on gender and eroticism in Thailand, and the proliferation of Thai gender and sex categories and discourses from the 1960s through to the 1980s. Jackson deconstructs the apparent similarities between new categories and identities in non-Western societies and those of the Western world. He questions the applicability of Foucauldian theoretical frameworks of sexuality in understanding the fluidity of Thai discourses of gender and sexuality; and he calls for a historically and culturally grounded analysis to make better sense of non-Western eroticisms. And in Chapter 19, '*Bhai-behen*, true love, time pass: Friendships and sexual partnerships among youth in an Indian metropolis', Lena Abraham offers an analysis of heterosexual peer networks and partnerships forged between unmarried, low-income, college-attending youth in an urban Indian environment. Abraham looks at youths' experiences with sexuality and the types of relationships that are held in an environment where heterosexuality is a cultural norm. She takes a gender perspective in describing the unequal opportunities for the expression of sexuality and claims that there are differential implications for the health of young men and women.

Next, in Part 7, 'Sexual negotiations and transactions', as in other parts of the book, the goal has been to provide some sense of the range of different concerns that have emerged in seeking to rethink dominant social and behavioural research methods in light of constructionist understandings of gender and sexuality, as well as the special concerns of access to private meanings (and practices) and power dynamics involved in sexual interaction. In Chapter 20, 'Masculinity and urban men: Perceived scripts for courtship, romantic, and sexual interactions with women', David Wyatt Seal and Anke Ehrhardt explore the ways in which heterosexually active men negotiate between emotions and the desire for sexual intimacy by analysing the gender roles and sexual scripts – for courtship and sexual intercourse – revealed in their narratives. These scripts are descriptive of interpersonal and shared expectations, motivations that construct desire and arousal, and they reflect cultural norms and values as they are perceived and internalized by men. This study describes a transition in which emotional elements are becoming more inscribed in the sexual motivations of men. Many of these same concerns are taken up by Jennifer Hirsch and Constance Nathanson in Chapter 21, 'Some traditional methods are more modern than others: Rhythm, withdrawal and the changing meanings of sexual intimacy in Mexican companionate marriage'. Like Seal and Ehrhardt, Hirsch and Nathanson explore the cultural meanings and understandings of heterosexual marriage and partnerships; they examine the use of traditional methods and modern methods of contraception among Mexican women in the USA and in Mexico. Hirsch and Nathanson describe the construction of women's experiences with contraception, looking at the cultural logics and symbolic negotiations invoked by women, such as the effectiveness of certain techniques over others. Women's constructions of birth-control are shaped by migration and by generational change as these processes transform the meanings of intimacy and marriage. Finally, in Chapter 22, 'Mobility, sexual networks and exchange among *bodabodamen* in Southwest Uganda', Stella Nyanzi, Barbara Nyanzi, Bessie Kalina and Robert Pool explore the network of sexual patterns, both occasional and regular, of private motorbike taxi men (*bodabodamen*) in Masaka, Uganda, a highly mobile employment group that practices frequent internal migration. The concentration of employment opportunities around urban areas has created a high demand for the services of the *bodabodamen*, and being a successful *bodabodaman* has often necessitated moving to peri-urban centres sometimes leaving their wives and children while they work during the week. This study highlights the importance of understanding the implications of sexual negotiation and mobility for HIV prevention.

In the final Part of this volume, 'Contemporary and future challenges', the texts included explore different dimensions of emerging frameworks of sexual rights, and their implications for research and action in this field. In Chapter 23, 'Gendered scripts and the sexual scene: Promoting sexual subjects among Brazilian teenagers', for example, Vera Paiva draws on findings derived from a series of safer-sex workshops among night-school students in São Paulo, Brazil: small-group and interactive interventions were used to discover and model sexual communication and negotiation skills. Paiva explores the concept of consciousness-raising through a perspective of Brazilian liberation education by looking at sexual scripts that emerge from negotiated relationships with family and peer groups as well as from the negotiations around sexual culture, expressions and practices. She outlines a new theoretical approach to HIV prevention that promotes what she describes as the sexual 'subject'. In Chapter 24, 'HIV and AIDS-related stigma and discrimination: A conceptual framework and implications for action', Richard Parker and Peter Aggleton provide a theoretical framework to understand and address stigma and discrimination against people living with HIV and AIDS. They argue for a conception that does not treat stigma as an attribute, but instead views it as a social process resulting from relationships and interactions, defining stigma and discrimination as tools of oppression strategically deployed by some groups to dominate others. The article delineates ways in which inequality and social exclusion that result from stigma and discrimination impact the lives of people living with HIV and AIDS, and it ultimately argues that consideration of these social processes should be incorporated into an agenda for research and action around issues of HIV/AIDS. Finally, in Chapter 25, 'Bracketing sexuality: Human rights and sexual orientation – A decade of development and denial at the UN', Ignacio Saiz considers ways in which stigma and discrimination are evident in global alliances and oppositions. Saiz traces the emergence of international discussions about sexuality and sexual orientation and their implications for public health; and the chapter explores ways in which the human rights framework has been employed in discourses and debates about sexual orientation in the United Nations, highlighting the social construction of sexuality and freedom on a global level. He examines the tensions between, on one hand, international political players who use cultural justifications for violating the human right to sexual expression and, on the other hand, advocates who call for the inclusion of sexual orientation within a broader, universal framework of sexual rights and sexual health.

Taken together, the various chapters that make up *Culture, Society and Sexuality* thus offer a broad overview of the wide range of issues that have motivated much recent research about sexuality in general, and about the relationship between sexuality, health and rights in particular. As the essays that are brought together here clearly attest, this understanding of sexuality as being socially constructed has refocused attention on the social and cultural systems that shape not only our sexual experience, but the ways in which we interpret and understand that experience. By directing attention toward the inter-subjective nature of sexual meanings – their shared, collective quality, not as the property of isolated individuals, but of social persons integrated within specific sexual cultures – and by highlighting the complex and often multiple systems and structures of power that play across the sexual field, these alternative paradigms offer the possibility of addressing some of the most complex dilemmas facing those seeking to engage in local and international arenas of contention. These essays speak to us in important ways, as researchers, to be sure, but also as activists, health-care workers, service providers, and others involved in the day-to-day business of responding to the myriad challenges that we currently face in seeking to promote both sexual health and sexual rights in the contemporary world.

References

AGGLETON, P. (1996) 'Global priorities for HIV/ AIDS intervention research', *International Journal of STD & AIDS*, 7 (suppl. 2), pp. 13–16.

—— (2004) 'Sexuality, HIV Prevention, vulnerability and risk', *Journal of Psychology and Human Sexuality*, 16(1), pp. 1–11.

BUTLER, J. (2004) *Undoing Gender*, New York: Routledge.

CARBALLO, M., CLELAND, J., CARAEL, M. and ALBRECHT, G. (1989) 'A cross-national study of patterns of sexual behaviour', *The Journal of Sex Research*, 26, pp. 287–99.

CARRILLO, H. (2002) *The Night is Young: Sexuality in Mexico in the Time of AIDS*, Chicago: The University of Chicago Press.

CHOUINARD, A. and ALBERT, J. (eds) (1990) *Human Sexuality: Research Perspectives in a World Facing AIDS*, Ottawa: International Development Research Centre.

CLELAND, J. and FERRY, B. (eds) (1996) *Sexual Behaviour and AIDS in the Developing World*, London: Taylor & Francis.

ERENS, B., MCMANUS, S., FIELD, J., KOROVESSIS, C., JOHNSON, A.M. and FENTON, K.A. (2003) *National Survey of Sexual Attitudes and Lifestyles II: Technical Report*, London: National Centre for Social Research.

EVANS, D.T. (1993) *Sexual Citizenship: The Material Construction of Sexualities*. London: Routledge.

FAUSTO-STERLING, A. (2000) *Sexing the Body: Gender Politics and the Construction of Sexuality*, New York: Basic Books.

GAGNON, J.H. (1977) *Human Sexualities*, Glenview, IL: Scott Foresman.

—— (2004) *An Interpretation of Desire: Essays in the Study of Sexuality*, Chicago: The University of Chicago Press.

—— and SIMON, W. (1973) *Sexual Conduct: The Social Sources of Human Sexuality*, Chicago: Aldine.

HERDT, G. and STOLLER, R. (1990) *Intimate Communications: Erotics and the Study of Culture*, New York: Columbia University Press.

KIMMEL, M.S. and PLANTE, R.F. (eds) (2004) *Sexualities: Identities, Behaviors, and Society*, New York: Oxford University Press.

LANCASTER, R. and DI LEONARDO, M. (eds) (1997) *The Gender/Sexuality Reader*, New York and London: Routledge.

LAUMANN, E.O. and MICHAEL, R.T. (eds) (2001) *Sex, Love, and Health in America: Private Choices and Public Policies*, Chicago: The University of Chicago Press.

LAUMANN, E.O., GAGNON, J.H., MICHAEL, R.T. and MICHAELS, S. (1994) *The Social Organization of Sexuality: Sexual Practices in the United States*, Chicago: University of Chicago Press.

LAUMANN, E.O., ELLINGTON, S., MAHAY, J., PAIK, A., and YOUM, Y. (eds) (2004) *The Sexual Organization of the City*, Chicago: The University of Chicago Press.

MICHAEL, R.T., GAGNON, J.H., LAUMANN, E.O. and KOLATA, G. (1994) *Sex in America: A Definitive Survey*, Boston, MA: Little, Brown, and Co.

NAGAL, J. (2003) *Race, Ethnicity and Sexuality: Intimate Intersections, Forbidden Frontiers*, New York: Oxford University Press.

PARKER, R.G. (1991) *Bodies, Pleasures and Passions: Sexual Culture in Contemporary Brazil*, Boston, MA: Beacon Press.

—— (1994) 'Sexual cultures, HIV transmission, and AIDS prevention', *AIDS*, 8 (suppl.), pp. S309–S314.

—— (1996) 'Empowerment, community mobilization and social change in the face of HIV/AIDS', *AIDS*, 10 (suppl. 3), pp. S27–S31.

—— (1999) *Beneath the Equator: Cultures of Desire, Male Homosexuality, and Emerging Gay Communities in Brazil*, New York and London: Routledge.

—— (2001) 'Sexuality, culture and power in HIV/AIDS research', *Annual Review of Anthropology*, 30, pp. 163–79.

—— and GAGNON, H. (eds) (1995) *Conceiving Sexuality: Approaches to Sex Research in a Postmodern World*, New York and London: Routledge.

——, AGGLETON, P. and BARBOSA, R.M. (eds) *Framing the Sexual Subject: The Politics of Gender, Sexuality and Power*, Berkeley, Los Angeles and London: University of California Press.

ROBINSON, P. (1976) *The Modernization of Sex*, New York: Harper.

SEIDMAN, S. (2003) *The Social Construction of Sexuality*, New York: W.W. Norton.

TURNER, C.F., MILLER, H.G. and MOSES, L.E. (eds) (1989) *AIDS: Sexual Behavior and Intravenous Drug Use*, Washington, DC: National Academy Press.

—— (1990) *AIDS: The Second Decade*, Washington, DC: National Academy Press.

WEEKS, J. (1981) *Sex, Politics and Society: The Regulation of Sexuality Since 1800*, London and New York: Longman.

—— (1985) *Sexuality and its Discontents: Meanings, Myths and Modern Sexualities*, London: Routledge & Kegan Paul.

—— (2000) *Making Sexual History*, Cambridge: Polity Press.

—— (2003) *Sexuality* (2nd edition), London: Routledge.

WELLINGS, K., FIELD, J., JOHNSON, A. and WADSWORTH, J. (1994) *Sexual Behaviour in Britain*, Harmondsworth: Penguin Books.

WHO/GPA/SBR (1989) *Survey of Partner Relations: Research Package*, Geneva: World Health Organization.

WILLIAMS, C.L. and STEIN, A. (eds) (2002) *Sexuality and Gender*, Oxford: Blackwell.

Section I
Culture, society and sexuality

Part 1
Conceptual frameworks

2   Sexual matters

On conceptualizing sexuality in history

Robert A. Padgug [1979]

Sexuality – the subject matter seems so obvious that it hardly appears to need comment. An immense and ever-increasing number of 'discourses' have been devoted to its exploration and control during the last few centuries, and their very production has, as Foucault points out (Foucault, 1978), been a major characteristic of bourgeois society. Yet, ironically, as soon as we attempt to apply the concept to history, apparently insurmountable problems confront us.

To take a relatively simple example, relevant to one aspect of sexuality only, what are we to make of the ancient Greek historian Alexis' curious description of Polykrates, sixth-century BC ruler of Samos?[1] In the course of his account of the luxurious habits of Polykrates, Alexis stresses his numerous imports of foreign goods, and adds: 'Because of all this there is good reason to marvel at the fact that the tyrant is not mentioned as having sent for women or boys from anywhere, despite his passion for liaisons with males … '. Now, that Polykrates did not 'send for women' would seem to us to be a direct corollary of his passion for liaisons with males. But to Alexis – and we know that his attitude was shared by all of Greek antiquity[2] – sexual passion in any form implied sexual passion in all forms. Sexual categories that seem so obvious to us, those that divide humanity into 'heterosexuals' and 'homosexuals', seem unknown to the ancient Greeks.

A problem thus emerges at the start: the categories that most historians normally use to analyse sexual matters do not seem adequate when we deal with Greek antiquity. We might, of course, simply dismiss the Greeks as peculiar – a procedure as common as it is unenlightening – but we would confront similar problems with respect to most other societies. Or, we might recognize the difference between Greek sexuality and our own, but not admit that it creates a problem in conceptualization. Freud, for example, writes:

> The most striking distinction between the erotic life of antiquity and our own no doubt lies in the fact that the ancients laid the stress upon the instinct itself, whereas we emphasize its object. The ancients glorified the instinct and were prepared on its account to honour even an inferior object; while we despise the instinctual activity in itself, and find excuses for it only in the merit of the object.
>
> (Freud, 1964, p. 38)[3]

Having made this perceptive comment, he lets the subject drop: so striking a contrast is, for him, a curiosity, rather than the starting point for serious critique of the very categories of sexuality.

Most investigators into sexuality in history have in fact treated their subject as so many variations on a single theme, whose contents were already broadly known. This is not only true of those who openly treat the history of sexuality as a species of entertainment, but even of those whose purpose is more serious and whose work is considered more significant from a historical point of view. One example, chosen from the much-admired *The Other Victorians* of Steven Marcus, is typical. Marcus describes a very Victorian flagellation scene that appears in the anonymous *My Secret Life*. After describing its contents, he states categorically:

> But the representation in *My Secret Life* does something which the pornography cannot. It demonstrates how truly and literally childish such behaviour is; it shows us, as nothing else that I know does, the pathos of perversity, how deeply sad, how cheerless a condemnation it really is. It is more than a condemnation; it is – or was – an imprisonment for life. For if it is bad enough that we are all imprisoned within our own sexuality, how much sadder must it be to be still further confined within this foreshortened, abridged and parodically grotesque version of it.
>
> (Marcus, 1974, p. 127)

Marcus already knows the content and meaning of sexuality, Victorian or otherwise. It was not *My Secret Life* that gave him his knowledge, but rather his predetermined and prejudged 'knowledge' that allowed him to use *My Secret Life* to create a catalogue or examples of a generalized and universal sexuality, a sexuality that was not the result but the organizing principle of his study. Given this preknowledge, sexuality in history could hardly become a problem – it was simply a given.

Not surprisingly, for Marcus as well as for many other 'sex researchers' – from Freudians to positivists – the sexuality that is 'given', which is sexuality *tout court*, is what they perceive to be the sexuality of their own century, culture, and class, whether it bears a fundamentally 'popular' stamp or comes decked out in full scientific garb.

In any approach that takes as predetermined and universal the categories of sexuality, real history disappears. Sexual practice becomes a more or less sophisticated selection of curiosities, whose meaning and validity can be gauged by that truth – or rather truths, since there are many competitors – which we, in our enlightened age, have discovered. This procedure is reminiscent of the political economy of the period before, and all too often after, Marx, but it is not a purely bourgeois failing. Many of the chief sinners are Marxists.

A surprising lack of a properly historical approach to the subject of sexuality has allowed a fundamentally bourgeois view of sexuality and its subdivisions to deform twentieth-century Marxism. Marx and Engels themselves tended to neglect the subject, and even Engels' *Origins of the Family, Private Property, and the State* (1884) by no means succeeded in making it a concern central to historical materialism. The Marxism of the Second International, trapped to so great a degree within a narrow economism, mainly dismissed sexuality as merely superstructural. Most later Marxist thought and practice, with a few notable exceptions – Alexandra Kollontai, Wilhelm Reich, the Frankfurt School – has in one way or another accepted this judgement.

In recent years questions concerning the nature of sexuality have been re-placed on the Marxist agenda by the force of events and movements. The women's movement and, to an increasing degree, the gay movement have made it clear that a politics without sexuality is doomed to failure or deformation; the strong offensive of the American right-wing, which combines class and sexual politics, can only re-enforce this view (see Gordon and Hunter, 1977/1978). The feminist insistence that 'the personal is political', itself a product of ongoing struggle, represents an immense step forward in the understanding of social reality, one that must be absorbed as a living part of Marxist attitudes toward sexuality. The important comprehension that sexuality, class, and politics cannot easily be disengaged from one another must serve as the basis of a materialist view of sexuality in historical perspective as well.

Sexuality as ideology

The contemporary view of sexuality that underlies most historical work in this field is the major stumbling block preventing further progress into the nature of sexuality in history. A brief account of it can be provided here, largely in the light of feminist work, which has begun to discredit so much of it. What follows is a composite picture, not meant to apply as a whole or in detail to specific movements and theories. But the general assumptions that inform this view appear at the centre of the dominant ideologies of sexuality in twentieth-century capitalist societies, and it is against these assumptions that alternative theories and practices must be gauged and opposed.

In spite of the elaborate discourses and analyses devoted to it, and the continual stress on its centrality to human reality, this modern concept of sexuality remains difficult to define. Dictionaries and encyclopaedias refer simply to the division of most species into males and females for purposes of reproduction; beyond that, specifically human sexuality is only described, never defined. What the ideologists of sexuality describe, in fact, are only the supposed spheres of its operation: gender; reproduction, the family, and socialization; love and intercourse. To be sure, each of these spheres is thought by them to have its own essence and forms ('the family', for example), but together they are taken to define the arena in which sexuality operates.

Within this arena, sexuality as a general, over-arching category is used to define and delimit a large part of the world in which we exist. The almost perfect congruence between those spheres of existence which are said to be sexual and what is viewed as the 'private sphere' of life is striking. As Caroll Smith-Rosenberg, working partly within this view of sexuality, puts it, 'The most significant and intriguing historical questions relate to the events, the causal patterns, the psychodynamics of private places: the household, the family, the bed, the nursery, and kinship systems' (Smith-Rosenberg, 1976, p. 185). Indeed, a general definition of the most widely accepted notion of sexuality in the later twentieth century might easily be 'that which pertains to the private, to the individual', as opposed to the allegedly 'public' spheres of work, production, and politics.

This broad understanding of sexuality as the 'private' involves other significant dualities, which, while not simple translations of the general division into private and public spheres, do present obvious analogies to it in the minds of those who accept it. Briefly, the sexual sphere is seen as the realm of psychology, while the public sphere is seen as the realm of politics and economics; Marx and Freud are often taken as symbolic of this division. The sexual sphere is considered the realm of consumption, the public sphere that of production; the former is sometimes viewed as the site of use value and the latter as that of exchange value. Sexuality is the realm of 'nature', of the individual, and of biology; the public sphere is the realm of culture, society, and history. Finally, sexuality tends to be identified most closely with the female and the homosexual, while the public sphere is conceived of as male and heterosexual.

The intertwined dualities are not absolute, for those who believe in them are certain that although sexuality properly belongs to an identifiable private sphere, it slips over, legitimately or, more usually, illegitimately, into other spheres as well, spheres that otherwise would be definitely desexualized. Sexuality appears at one and the same time as narrow and limited and as universal and ubiquitous. Its role is both overestimated as the very core of being and underestimated as a merely private reality.

Both views refer sexuality to the individual, whom it is used to define. As Richard Sennett suggests,

> Sexuality we imagine to define a large territory of who we are and what we feel ... Whatever we experience must in some way touch on our sexuality, but sexuality is. We uncover it, we discover it, we come to terms with it, but we do not master it.
>
> (Sennett, 1977, p. 7)

Or, as Foucault rather more succinctly states, 'In the space of a few centuries, a certain inclination has led us to direct the question of what we are to sex' (Foucault, 1978, p. 78). This is, after all, why we write about it, talk about it, worry about it so continuously.

Under the impulse of these assumptions, individuals are encouraged to see themselves in terms of their sexuality. This is most easily seen in such examples of 'popular wisdom' as that one must love people for their inner – that is, sexual – selves, and not for 'mere incidentals', such as class, work, and wealth, and in the apparently wide-spread belief that the 'real me' emerges only in private life, in the supposedly sexual spheres of intercourse and family – that is, outside of class, work, and public life. Sexuality is thereby detached from socio-economic and class realities, which appear, in contrast, as external and imposed.

The location of sexuality as the innermost reality of the individual defines it, in Sennett's phrase, as an 'expressive state', rather than an 'expressive act' (Sennett, 1977, p. 7). For those who accept the foregoing assumptions, it appears as a thing, a fixed essence, which we possess as part of our very being; it simply is. And because sexuality is itself seen as a thing, it can be identified, for certain purposes at least, as inherent in particular objects, such as the sex organs, which are then seen as, in some sense, sexuality itself.

But modern sexual ideologues do not simply argue that sexuality is a single essence; they proclaim, rather, that it is a group of essences. For although they tell us that sexuality as a general category is universally shared by all of humanity, they insist that sub-categories appear within it. There are thus said to be sexual essences appropriate to 'the male', 'the female', 'the child', 'the homosexual', 'the heterosexual' (and indeed to the 'foot-fetishist', 'the child-molester', and on and on). In this view, identifiable and analytically discrete groups emerge, each bearing an appropriate sexual essence, capable of being analysed as a 'case history', and given a normative value. Krafft-Ebing's *Psychopathia Sexualis* of 1886 may still stand as the logical high-point of this type of analysis, but the underlying attitude seems to permeate most of contemporary thought on the subject.

In sum, the most commonly held twentieth-century assumptions about sexuality imply that it is a separate category of existence (like 'the economy', or 'the state', other supposedly independent spheres of reality), almost identical with the sphere of private life. Such a view necessitates the location of sexuality within the individual as a fixed essence, leading to a classic division of individual and society and to a variety of psychological determinisms, and, often enough, to a full-blown biological determinism as well. These in turn involve the enshrinement of contemporary sexual categories as universal, static, and permanent, suitable for the analysis of all human beings and all societies. Finally, the consequences of this view are to restrict class struggle to non-sexual realms, since that which is private, sexual, and static is not a proper arena for public social action and change.

Biology and society

The inadequacies of this dominant ideology require us to look at sexuality from a very different perspective, a perspective that can serve both as an implicit critique of the contemporary view as well as the starting point for a specifically Marxist conceptualization.

If we compare human sexuality with that of other species, we are immediately struck by its richness, its vast scope, and the degree to which its potentialities can seemingly be built upon endlessly, implicating the entire human world. Animal sexuality, by contrast, appears limited, constricted, and pre-defined in a narrow physical sphere.

This is not to deny that human sexuality, like animal sexuality, is deeply involved with physical reproduction and with intercourse and its pleasures. Biological sexuality is the necessary precondition for human sexuality. But biological sexuality is only a precondition, a set of potentialities, which is never unmediated by human reality, and which becomes transformed in qualitatively new ways in human society. The rich and ever-varying nature of such concepts and institutions as marriage, kinship, 'love', 'eroticism' in a variety of physical senses and as a component of fantasy and religious, social, and even economic reality, and the general human ability to extend the range of sexuality far beyond the physical body, all bear witness to this transformation.

Even this bare catalogue of examples demonstrates that sexuality is closely involved in social reality. Marshall Sahlins makes the point clearly, when he argues that sexual reproduction and intercourse must not be

> ... considered *a priori* as a biological fact, characterized as an urge of human nature independent of the relations between social persons ... [and] acting upon society from without (or below). [Uniquely among human beings] the process of 'conception' is always a double entendre, since no satisfaction can occur without the act and the partners as socially defined and contemplated, that is, according to a symbolic code of persons, practices and proprieties.
>
> (Sahlins, 1978, p. 51)

Such an approach does not seek to eliminate biology from human life, but to absorb it into a unity with social reality. Biology as a set of potentialities and insuperable necessities (see Timpanaro, 1978) provides the material of social interpretations and extensions; it does not cause human behaviour, but conditions and limits it. Biology is not a narrow set of absolute imperatives. That it is malleable and broad is as obvious for animals, whose nature is altered with changing environment, as for human beings (Lambert, 1978). The uniqueness of human beings lies in their ability to create the environment that alters their own – and indeed other animals' – biological nature.

Human biology and culture are both necessary for the creation of human society. It is as important to avoid a rigid separation of 'Nature' and 'Culture' as it is to avoid reducing one to the other, or simply uniting them as an undifferentiated reality. Human beings are doubly determined by a permanent (but not immutable) natural base and by a permanent social mediation and transformation of it. An attempt to eliminate the biological aspect is misleading because it denies that social behaviour takes place within nature and by extension of natural processes. Marx's insistence that 'men make their own history but they do not make it just as they please' applies as well to biological as to inherited social realities (see Timpanaro, 1978; see also Williams, 1978). An attempt – as in such disparate movements as Reichian analysis or the currently fashionable 'sociobiology' – to absorb culture into biology is equally misleading, because, as Sahlins puts it,

> Biology, while it is an absolutely necessary condition for culture, is equally and absolutely insufficient; it is completely unable to specify the cultural properties of human behaviour or their variations from one human group to another.
>
> (Sahlins, 1976, p. xi)

It is clear that, within certain limits, human beings have no fixed, inherited nature. We become human only in human society. Lucien Malson may overstate his case when he writes, 'The idea that man has no nature is now beyond dispute. He has or rather is a history' (Malson, 1972, p. 9), but he is correct to focus on history and change in the creation of human culture and personality. Social reality cannot simply be peeled off to reveal 'natural man' lurking beneath (Malson, 1972, p. 10).

This is true of sexuality in all its forms, from what seem to be the most purely 'natural' acts of intercourse (Malson, 1972, p. 48) or gender differentiation and hierarchy to the most elaborated forms of fantasy or kinship relations. Contrary to a common belief that sexuality is simply 'natural behaviour', nothing is more essentially transmitted by a social process of learning than sexual behaviour, as Mary Douglas notes (1973, p. 93).

Even an act that is apparently so purely physical, individual, and biological as masturbation illustrates this point. Doubtless we stroke our genitals because the act is pleasurable and the pleasure is physiologically rooted, but from that to masturbation, with its large element of fantasy, is a social leap, mediated by a vast set of definitions, meanings, connotations, learned behaviour, and shared and learned fantasies.

Sexual reality is variable, and it is so in several senses. It changes within individuals, within genders, and within societies, just as it differs from gender to gender, from class to class, and from society to society. Even the very meaning and content of sexual arousal varies according to these categories (Davenport, 1977). Above all, there is continuous development and transformation of its realities. What Marx suggests for hunger is equally true of the social forms of sexuality: 'Hunger is hunger, but the hunger gratified by cooked meat eaten with a knife and fork is a different hunger from that which bolts down raw meat with the aid of hand, nail and tooth' (Marx, 1973, p. 92).

There do exist certain sexual forms which, at least at a high level of generality, are common to all human societies: love, intercourse, kinship, can be understood universally on a very general level. But that both 'saint and sinner' have erotic impulses, as Georges Bataille rightly claims (Bataille, 1962), or that Greece, medieval Europe, and modern capitalist societies share general sexual forms, does not make the contents and meaning of these impulses and forms identical or undifferentiated. They must be carefully distinguished and separately understood, since their inner structures and social meanings and articulations are very different. The content and meaning of the eroticism of Christian mysticism is by no means reducible to that of Henry Miller, nor is the asceticism of the monk identical to that of the Irish peasants who delay their marriages to a relatively late age.[4]

The forms, content, and context of sexuality always differ. There is no abstract and universal category of 'the erotic' or 'the sexual' applicable without change to all societies. Any view which suggests otherwise is hopelessly mired in one or another form of biologism, and biologism is easily put forth as the basis of normative attitudes toward sexuality, which, if deviated from, may be seen as rendering the deviant behaviour 'unhealthy' and 'abnormal'.

Such views are as unenlightening when dealing with Christian celibacy as when discussing Greek homosexual behaviour.

Sexuality as praxis (I)

When we look more directly at the social world itself, it becomes apparent that the general distinguishing mark of human sexuality, as of all social reality, is the unique role played in its construction by language, consciousness, symbolism, and labour, which, taken together – as they must be – are praxis, the production and reproduction of material life. Through praxis human beings produce an everchanging human world within nature and give order and meaning to it, just as they come to know and give meaning to, and, to a degree, change, the realities of their own bodies, their physiology (Vazquez, 1977). The content of sexuality is ultimately provided by human social relations, human productive activities, and human consciousness. The history of sexuality is therefore the history of a subject whose meaning and contents are in a continual process of change. It is the history of social relations.

For sexuality, although part of material reality, is not itself an object or thing. It is rather a group of social relations, of human interactions. Marx writes in the *Grundrisse* that 'Society does not consist of individuals, but expresses the sum of interrelations, the relations within which these individuals stand' (Marx, 1973, p. 265). This seems to put the emphasis precisely where it should be: individuals do exist as the constituent elements of society, but society is not the simple multiplication of isolated individuals. It is constituted only by the relationships between those individuals. On the other hand, society does not stand outside of and beyond the individuals who exist within it, but is the expression of their complex activity. The emphasis is on activity and relationships, which individuals ultimately create and through which, in turn, they are themselves created and modified. Particular individuals are both subjects and objects within the process, although in class societies the subjective aspect tends to be lost to sight and the processes tend to become reified as objective conditions working from outside.

Sexuality is relational.[5] It consists of activity and interactions active social relations – and not simply 'acts', as if sexuality were the enumeration and typology of an individual's orgasms (as it sometimes appears to be conceived in, for example, the work of Kinsey and others), a position that puts the emphasis back within the individual alone. 'It' does not do anything, combine with anything, appear anywhere; only people, acting within specific relationships create what we call sexuality. This is a significant aspect of what Marx means when he claims, in the famous Sixth Thesis on Feuerbach, that 'the essence of man is no abstraction inherent in each single individual. In its reality it is the ensemble of the social relations' (Marx and Engels, 1976, p. 4). Social relations, like the biological inheritance, at once create, condition, and limit the possibilities of individual activity and personality.

Praxis is fully meaningful only at the level of socio-historical reality The particular interrelations and activities which exist at any moment in a specific society create sexual and other categories which, ultimately, determine the broad range of modes of behaviour available to individuals who are born within that society. In turn, the social categories and interrelations are themselves altered over time by the activities and changing relationships of individuals. Sexual categories do not make manifest essences implicit within individuals, but are the expression of the active relationships of the members of entire groups and collectivities.

We can understand this most clearly by examining particular categories. We speak, for example, of homosexuals and heterosexuals as distinct categories of people, each with its sexual essence and personal behavioural characteristics. That these are not 'natural' categories is evident. Freud, especially in the *Three Essays on the Theory of Sexuality*, and other psychologists have demonstrated that the boundaries between the two groups in our own society are fluid and difficult to define. And, as a result of everyday experience as well as the material collected in surveys such as the Kinsey reports, we know that the categories of heterosexuality and homosexuality are by no means coextensive with the activities and personalities of heterosexuals and homosexuals. Individuals belonging to either group are capable of performing and, on more or less numerous occasions, do perform acts, and have behavioural characteristics and display social relationships thought specific to the other group.

The categories in fact take what are no more than a group of more or less closely related acts ('homosexual'/'heterosexual' behaviour) and convert them into case studies of people ('homosexuals'/'heterosexuals'). This conversion of acts into roles/personalities, and ultimately into entire subcultures, cannot be said to have been accomplished before at least the seventeenth century, and, as a firm belief and more or less close approximation of reality, the late nineteenth century.[6] What we call 'homosexuality' (in the sense of the distinguishing traits of 'homosexuals'), for example, was not considered a unified set of acts, much less a set of qualities defining particular persons, in precapitalist societies. Jeffrey Weeks, in discussing the act of Henry VIII of 1533 which first brought sodomy within the purview of statute law, argues that

> ... the central point was that the law was directed against a series of sexual acts, not a particular type of person. There was no concept of the homosexual in law, and homosexuality was regarded not as a particular attribute of a certain type of person but as a potential in all sinful creatures.

> (Weeks, 1977, p. 12)

The Greeks of the classical period would have agreed with the general principle, if not with the moral attitude. Homosexuality and heterosexuality for them were indeed groups of not necessarily very closely related acts, each of which could be performed by any person, depending upon his or her gender, status, or class.[7] 'Homosexuals' and 'heterosexuals' in the modern sense did not exist in their world, and to speak, as is common, of the Greeks as 'bisexual' is illegitimate as well, since that merely adds a new, intermediate category, whereas it was precisely the categories themselves which had no meaning in antiquity.

Heterosexuals and homosexuals are involved in social 'roles' and attitudes which pertain to a particular society, modern capitalism. These roles do have something in common with very different roles known in other societies – modern homosexuality and ancient pederasty, for example, share at least one feature: that the participants were of the same sex and that sexual intercourse is often involved – but the significant features are those that are not shared, including the entire range of symbolic, social, economic, and political meanings and functions each group of roles possesses.

'Homosexual' and 'heterosexual' behaviour may be universal; homosexual and heterosexual identity and consciousness are modern realities. These identities are not inherent in the individual. In order to be gay, for example, more than individual inclinations (however we might conceive of those) or homosexual activity is required; entire ranges of social attitudes and the construction of particular cultures, subcultures, and social relations are first necessary. To 'commit' a homosexual act is one thing; to be a homosexual is something entirely different.

By the same token, of course, these are changeable and changing roles. The emergence of a gay movement (like that of the women's movement) has meant major alterations in homosexual and heterosexual realities and self-perceptions. Indeed, it is abundantly clear that there has always existed in the modern world a dialectical interplay between those social categories and activities that ascribe to certain people a homosexual identity and the activities of those who are so categorized. The result is the complex constitution of 'the homosexual' as a social being within bourgeois society. The same is, of course, true of 'the heterosexual', although the processes and details vary (see Foucault, 1978; Hocquenghem, 1978).

The example of homosexuality/heterosexuality is particularly striking, since it involves a categorization that appears limited to modern societies. But even categories with an apparently more general application demonstrate the same social construction.

For example, as feminists have made abundantly clear, while every society does divide its members into 'men' and 'women', what is meant by these divisions and the roles played by those defined by these terms varies significantly from society to society and even within each society by class, estate, or social position. The same is true of kinship relations. All societies have some conception of kinship, and use it for a variety of purposes, but the conceptions differ widely and the institutions based on them are not necessarily directly comparable. Above all, the modern nuclear family, with its particular social and economic roles, does not appear to exist in other societies, which have no institution truly analogous to our own, either in conception, membership, or in articulation with other institutions and activities. Even within any single society, family/kinship patterns, perceptions, and activity vary considerably by class and gender.[8]

The point is clear: the members of each society create all of the sexual categories and roles within which they act and define themselves. The categories and the significance of the activity involved will vary as widely as do the societies within whose general social relations they occur, and categories appropriate to each society must be discovered by historians.

Not only must the categories of any single society or period not be hypostatized as universal, but even the categories that are appropriate to each society must be treated with care. Ultimately, they are only parameters within which sexual activity occurs or, indeed, against which it may be brought to bear. They tend to be normative, and ideological, in nature – that is, they are presented as the categories within which members of particular societies ought to act. The realities of any society only approximate the normative categories, as our homosexual/heterosexual example most clearly showed. It is both as norms, which determine the status of all sexual activity, and as approximations to actual social reality that they must be defined and explored.

Sexuality as praxis (II)

Within this broad approach, the relationship between sexual activity and its categories and those that are non-sexual, especially those that are economic in nature, becomes of great importance.

Too many Marxists have tried to solve this problem by placing it within a simplified version of the 'base/superstructure' model of society, in which the base is considered simply as 'the economy', narrowly defined, while sexuality is relegated to the superstructure; that is, sexuality is seen as a 'reflex' of an economic base.[9] Aside from the problems inherent in the base/superstructure model itself (see Williams, 1977), this approach not only reproduces the classic bourgeois division of society into private and public spheres, enshrining capitalist ideology as universal reality, but loses the basic insights inherent in viewing sexuality as social relations and activity.

Recently, many theorists, mainly working within a feminist perspective, began to develop a more sophisticated point of view, aiming, as Gayle Rubin put it in an important article, 'to introduce a distinction between "economic" system and "sexual" system, and to indicate that sexual systems have a certain autonomy and cannot always be explained in terms of economic forces' (Rubin, 1975, p. 167).[10] This view, which represented a great advance, nonetheless still partially accepted the contemporary distinction between a sphere of work and a sphere of sexuality.

The latest developments of socialist-feminist theory and practice have brought us still further, by demonstrating clearly that both sexuality in all its aspects and work/production are equally involved in the production and reproduction of all aspects of social reality, and cannot easily be separated out from one another.[11] Above all, elements of class and sexuality do not contradict one another or exist on different planes, but produce and reproduce each other's realities in complex ways, and both often take the form of activity carried out by the same persons working within the same institutions.

This means, among other things, that what we consider 'sexuality' was, in the pre-bourgeois world, a group of acts and institutions not necessarily linked to one another, or, if they were linked, combined in ways very different from our own. Intercourse, kinship and the family, and gender, did not form anything like a 'field' of sexuality. Rather, each group of sexual acts was connected directly or indirectly – that is, formed a part of – institutions and thought patterns that we tend to view as political, economic, or social in nature, and the connections cut across our idea of sexuality as a thing, detachable from other things, and as a separate sphere of private existence.

The Greeks, for example, would not have known how, and would not have sought, to detach 'sexuality' from the household (*oikos*), with its economic, political, and religious functions; from the state (especially as the reproduction of citizenship); from religion (as fertility cults or ancestor worship, for example); or from class and estate (as the determiner of the propriety of sexual acts, and the like). Nor would they have been able to distinguish a private realm of 'sexuality'; the Greek *oikos* or household unit was as much or more a public institution as a private one.[12] This is even more true of so-called primitive societies, where sexuality (mediated through kinship, the dominant form of social relations) seems to permeate all aspects of life uniformly.

It was only with the development of capitalist societies that 'sexuality' and the 'economy' became separable from other spheres of society and could be counterposed to one another as realities of different sorts.[13] To be sure, the reality of that separation is, in the fullest sense of the word, ideological; that is, the spheres do have a certain reality as autonomous areas of activity and consciousness, but the links between them are innumerable, and both remain significant in the production and reproduction of social reality in the fullest sense. The actual connections between sexuality and the economy must be studied in greater detail, as must the specific relations between class, gender, family, and intercourse,[14] if the Marxist and sexual liberation movements are to work in a cooperative and fruitful, rather than antagonistic and harmful, manner.

A second major problem-area stands in the way of a fuller understanding of sexuality as praxis. The approach to sexuality we have outlined does overcome the apparently insurmountable opposition between society and the individual that marks the ideological views with which we began our discussion. But it overcomes it at a general level, leaving many specific problems unsolved. The most important of these is the large and thorny problem of the determination of the specific ways in which specific individuals react to existing sexual categories and act within or against them. To deal with this vast subject fully, Marxists need to develop a psychology – or a set of psychologies – compatible with their social and economic analyses.[15]

Much the most common approach among Western Marxists since the mid-twentieth century toward creating a Marxist psychology has been an attempt, in one manner or another, to combine

Marx and Freud. Whether in the sophisticated and dialectical versions of the Frankfurt School, Herbert Marcuse, or Wilhelm Reich, or in what Richard Lichtman has called 'the popular view that Freud analysed the individual while Marx uncovered the structure of social reality' (Lichtman, 1976, p. 5),[16] these attempts arose out of the felt need for a more fully developed Marxist psychology in light of the failure of socialist revolutions in the West.

None of these attempts has, ultimately, been a success, and their failure seems to lie in real contradictions between Marxist and Freudian theory. Both present theories of the relationship between individual and society, theories that contradict each other at fundamental levels. Freud does accept the importance of social relations for individual psychology. For him, sexuality has its roots in physiology, especially in the anatomical differences between the sexes, but these distinctions are not in themselves constitutive of our sexuality. Sexuality is indeed a process of development in which the unconscious takes account of biology as well as of society (mediated through the family) to produce an individual's sexuality.[17]

The problems begin here. Society, for Freud, is the medium in which the individual psyche grows and operates, but it is also in fundamental ways antipathetical to the individual, forcing him or her to repress instinctual desires. Freud's theory preserves the bourgeois division between society and the individual, and ultimately gives primacy to inborn drives within an essentially ahistorical individual over social reality. In a revealing passage, Freud argues:

> Human civilization rests upon two pillars, of which one is the control of natural forces and the other the restriction of our instincts. The ruler's throne rests upon fettered slaves. Among the instinctual components which are thus brought into service, the sexual instincts, in the narrow sense of the word, are conspicuous for their strength and savagery. Woe if they should be set loose! The throne would be overturned and the ruler trampled under foot.
>
> (Freud, 1953–74b, p. 218)

In spite of the fact that Freud does not view instincts as purely biological in nature (Freud, 1953–74a, pp. 105–40), he certainly sees sexuality as an internal, biologically based force, a thing inherent in the individual. This is a view that makes it difficult to use Freud alongside of Marx in the elucidation of the nature of sexuality. This is not to say we need necessarily discard all of Freud. The general theory of the unconscious remains a powerful one. Zillah Eisenstein pointed in a useful direction when she wrote, 'Whether there can be a meaningful synthesis of Marx and Freud depends on whether it is possible to understand how the unconscious is reproduced and maintained by the relations of the society' (Eisenstein, 1979, p. 3). But it is uncertain whether the Freudian theory of the unconscious can be stripped of so much of its specific content and remain useful for Marxist purposes. The work of Lacan, which attempts to de-biologize the Freudian unconscious by focusing on the role of language, and that of Deleuze and Guattari, in their *Anti-Oedipus*, which attempts to provide it with a more fully socio-historical content, are significant beginnings in this process (Deleuze and Guattari, 1977; see also Brown, 1959; Marcuse, 1955).

At the present time, however, Marxism still awaits a psychology fully adequate to its needs, although some recent developments are promising, such as the publication in English of the important non-Freudian work of the early Soviet psychologist L.S. Vygotsky (Vygotsky, 1977; see also Toulmin, 1978). But if psychology is to play a significant role in Marxist thought, as a science whose object is one of the dialectical poles of the individual/society unity, then it must have a finer grasp of the nature of that object. At this point, we can only agree with Lucien Seve that the object of psychology has not yet been adequately explored (Seve, 1975).

Acknowledgements

This essay represents a condensed and reworked version of the introduction to a much longer work on the nature of sexuality in history. The author would like to thank Betsy Blackmar, Edwin Burrows, Victoria de Grazia, Elizabeth Fee, Joseph Interrante, Michael Merrill, David Varas, and Michael Wallace for their invaluable comments on earlier drafts. He dedicates the essay to David Varas, without whose help and encouragement it would have been impossible to write it.

Notes

1 As reported in Athenaeus, Deipnosophistase 12.450 d–f (= F. Jacoby, *Fragmente der griech. Historiker* no. 539, fragment no. 2).

2 See for other examples, Lucian, 'The Ship' (Loeb Classical Library edition of Lucian, vol. VI, 481), or the 'Love Stories', attributed to Plutarch (*Moralia* 771E–775E), which provide pairs of similar love tales, each consisting of one involving heterosexual love and one involving homosexual love.

3 The footnote was added in the 1910 edition.

4 See the important analysis of this and similar points in Rougement, 1956.

5 See the work of the so-called 'symbolic interactionalists', best exemplified by Plummer, 1975. Their work, although not Marxist and too focused on individuals *per se*, does represent a major step forward in our understanding of sexuality as interpersonal.

6 Mary McIntosh, 'The homosexual role' (1968), the pioneer work in this field, suggests the seventeenth century for the emergence of the first homosexual subculture. Randolph Trumbach, 'London's sodomites: homosexual behavior and Western culture in the eighteenth century' (1977/78), argues for the eighteenth century. Jeffrey Weeks, in two important works, 'Sins and disease' (1976) and *Coming Out* (1977), argues – correctly, I believe – that the full emergence of homosexual role and subculture occurs only in the second half of the nineteenth century. See the articles by Weeks (1979) and Hansen (1979) in the *Radical History Review*. All of these works deal with England, but there is little reason to suspect that the general phenomenon, at least, varies very considerably in other bourgeois countries.

7 The best work available on Greek homosexual behaviour is Dover, 1978, which contains further bibliography.

8 On the conceptualization of family, kinship, and household, see the important collective work by Rapp, Ross, and Bridenthal, 'Examining family history' (1979), as well as Rapp, 'Family and class in contemporary America' (1978). See Poster (1978), and the critique of it by Ellen Ross (1979).

9 This appears to be true even of such relatively unorthodox thinkers as Althusser (1971); Balibar (1970, pt III); Hindess and Hirst (1975, esp. ch. 1); and Meillassoux, (1981, pt I).

10 For other views similar to those of Rubin, on this point at least, see Bridenthal (1976); Chodorow (1979); and Mitchell (1972).

11 Among recent works that come to this conclusion, and whose bibliographies and notes are useful for further study, see Forman (1977); Kelly (1979); Rapp, Ross, and Bridenthal (1979); Vogel (1979) and Zaretsky (1976).

12 On the Greek *oikos* and related institutions, see Lacey (1968).

13 See Foucault (1978) and Zaretsky (1976) for attempts to conceptualize the emergence of these categories. On the non-emergence of a separate sphere of the economy in non-capitalist societies, see Amin (1977) and Lukacs (1968).

14 For works that begin this process, see those cited in notes 10 and 11 above, plus the articles collected in Eisenstein (1979).

15 For a full discussion of this need and what it involves, see Seve, 1975. Seve is best on the social conditioning of individual psychology and weakest on individual psychic processes themselves.

16 This article along with its successors in *Socialist Review*, 33 (1977), pp. 59–84, and 36 (1977), pp. 37–78, form a good introduction to the study of the relationship between Marx and Freud, arguing for their incompatibility.

17 An important recent attempt to demonstrate the social underpinnings of Freud's thought is Mitchell (1974); Zaretsky (1975) demonstrates several defects in Freud's understanding of socio-historical reality, but suggests that they are remediable.

References

ALTHUSSER, L. (1971) *Lenin and Philosophy*, New York: Monthly Review Press.

AMIN, S. (1977) 'In praise of socialism', in *Imperialism and Unequal Development*, New York: Monthly Review Press.

BALIBAR, E. (1970) *Reading Capital*, London: NLB.

BATAILLE, G. (1962) *Death and Sensuality: A Study of Eroticism and Taboo*, New York: Arno Press.

BRIDENTHAL, R. (1976) 'The dialectics of production and reproduction in history', *Radical America*, 10(2), pp. 3–11.

BROWN, N.O. (1959) *Life Against Death*, Middletown, CT: Wesleyan University Press.

CHODOROW, N. (1979) 'Mothering, male dominance and capitalism', in EISENSTEIN, Z. (ed.), *Capitalist Patriarchy and the Case for Social Feminism*, New York: Monthly Review Press.

DAVENPORT, W.H. (1977) 'Sex in cross-cultural perspective', in BEACH, F. (ed.), *Human Sexuality in Four Perspectives*, Baltimore, MD: Wiley.

DELEUZE, G. and GUATTARI, F. (1977) *Anti-Oedipus: Capitalism and Schizophrenia*, New York: Viking Press.

DOUGLAS, M. (1973) *Natural Symbols: Explorations in Cosmology*, New York: Pantheon.

DOVER, K.J. (1978) *Greek Homosexuality*, Cambridge, MA: Harvard University Press.

EISENSTEIN, Z. (ed.) (1979) *Capitalist Patriarchy and the Case for Socialist Feminism*, New York: Monthly Review Press.

ENGELS, F. (1972 [1884]) *The Origins of the Family, Private Property, and the State*, New York: International Publishers.

FORMAN, A. (1977) *Femininity as Alienation: Women and the Family in Marxism and Psychoanalysis*, London: Pluto.

FOUCAULT, M. (1978) *The History of Sexuality, Volume I: An Introduction*, New York: Pantheon.

FREUD, S. (1953–74a) 'Instincts and their vicissitudes', in *The Standard Edition of the Complete Psychological Works of Sigmund Freud*, ed. J. Strachey, vol. 14, London: Hogarth Press.

—— (1953–74b) 'The resistance to psycho-analysis', in *The Standard Edition of the Complete Psychological Works of Sigmund Freud*, ed. J. Strachey, vol. 19, London: Hogarth Press.

—— (1964) *Three Essays on the Theory of Sexuality*, New York: Basic Books.

GORDON, L. and HUNTER, A. (1977/1978) 'Sex, family and the new right', *Radical America*, 11/12, November 1977/February 1978, pp. 9–26.

HANSEN, B. (1979) 'Historical construction of homosexuality', *Radical History Review*, 20, pp. 66–73.

HINDESS, P. and HIRST, B. (1975) *Pre-Capitalist Modes of Production*, London: Routledge and Kegan Paul.

HOCQUENGHEM, G. (1978) *Homosexual Desire*, New York: Schoken.

KELLY, J. (1979) 'The doubled vision of feminist theory', *Feminist Studies*, 5, pp. 216–27.

KRAFFT-EBING, R. VON (1965 [1886 orig.]) *Psychopathia Sexualis: A Medico-Forensic Study*, New York: G.P. Putnam's & Sons.

LACEY, W.K. (1968) *The Family in Classical Greece*, London: Thames and Hudson.

LAMBERT, H.H. (1978) 'Biology and equality', *Signs*, 4, pp. 97–117.

LICHTMAN, R. (1976) 'Marx and Freud', *Socialist Review*, 30, pp. 3–56.

LUCIAN (1959) 'The ship', in *Lucian, volume IV*, London: Heinemann (Loeb Classical Library edition).

LUKACS, G. (1968) *History and Class Consciousness*, Cambridge, MA: MIT Press.

MCINTOSH, M. (1968) 'The homosexual role', *Social Problems*, 16, pp. 182–91.

MALSON, L. (1972) *Wolf Children and the Problem of Human Nature*, New York: Monthly Review Press.

MARCUS, S. (1974) *The Other Victorians: A Study of Sexuality and Pornography in Mid-Nineteenth Century England*, second edition, New York: Basic Books.

MARCUSE, H. (1955) *Eros and Civilization*, Boston, MA: Beacon Press.

MARX, K. (1973) *Grundrisse*, New York: Random House.

—— and ENGELS, F. (1976) *Collected Works*, vol. 5, New York: International Publishers.

MEILLASSOUX, C. (1981) *Maidens, Meal, and Money: Capitalism and the Domestic Community*, New York: Cambridge University Press.

MITCHELL, J. (1972) *Women's Estate*, New York: Pantheon.

—— (1974) *Psychoanalysis and Feminism*, New York: Pantheon.

PLUMMER, K. (1975) *Sexual Stigma*, London: Routledge and Kegan Paul.

PLUTARCH (attributed to) (1936) 'The love stories', in *Plutarch: Moralia – vol. X*, London: Heinemann.

POSTER, M. (1978) *Critical Theory of the Family*, New York: Seabury Press.

RAPP, R. (1978) 'Family and class in contemporary America', *Science and Society*, 42, pp. 278–300.

——, ROSS, E. and BRIDENTHAL, R. (1979) 'Examining family history', *Feminist Studies*, 5, pp. 174–200.

ROSS, E. (1979) 'Rethinking the family', *Radical History Review*, 20, pp. 76–84.

ROUGEMENT, D. (1956) *Love in the Western World*, New York: Pantheon.

RUBIN, G. (1975) 'The traffic in women: notes on the "political economy" of sex', in REITER, R. (ed.), *Towards an Anthropology of Women*, New York: Monthly Review Press.

SAHLINS, M. (1976) *The Use and Abuse of Biology*, Ann Arbor: University of Michigan Press.

—— (1978) [n.t.], *The New York Review of Books*, 23 November, p. 51.

SENNETT, R. (1977) *The Fall of Public Man*, New York: Random House.

SEVE, L. (1975) *Marxism and the Theory of Human Personality*, London: Lawrence and Wishart.

SMITH-ROSENBERG, C. (1976) 'The new woman and the new history', *Feminist Studies*, 3, p. 185.

TIMPANARO, S. (1978) *On Materialism*, London: NLB.

TOULMIN, S. (1978) 'The Mozart of psychology', *New York Review of Books*, 23 September, pp. 51–7.

TRUMBACH, R. (1977/78) 'London's sodomites: homosexual behaviour and Western culture in the eighteenth century', *Journal of Social History*, 11, pp. 1–33.

VAZQUEZ, A.S. (1977) *The Philosophy of Praxis*, London: Merlin Press.

VOGEL, L. (1979) 'Questions on the woman question', *Monthly Review*, June, pp. 39–60.

VYGOTSKY, L.S. (1977) *Mind in Society: The Development of Higher Psychological Processes*, Cambridge, MA: Harvard University Press.

WEEKS, J. (1976) 'Sins and disease: some notes on homosexuality in the nineteenth century', *History Workshop*, 1, pp. 211–19.

—— (1977) *Coming Out: Homosexual Politics in Britain from the Nineteenth Century to the Present*, London: Quartet Books.

—— (1979) 'Movements of affirmation: sexual meaning and homosexual identities', *Radical History Review*, 20, pp. 164–80.

WILLIAMS, R. (1977) *Marxism and Literature*, New York: Oxford University Press.

—— (1978) 'Problems of materialism', *New Left Review*, 109, pp. 3–18.

ZARETSKY, E. (1975) 'Male supremacy and the unconscious', *Socialist Review*, 21/22, pp. 7–55.

—— (1976) *Capitalism and Personal Life*, New York: Harper and Row.

3   Sexual scripts

William Simon and John H. Gagnon [1984]

Profoundly enlarged attention has been paid to the issues of human sexuality since World War Two. Yet discussions of these issues remain almost as theoretically barren as before. We say 'almost' because some progress has been made. Among Freudian revisionists, Kohut (1978) and Stoller (1979) have moved us beyond the rigidities of traditional libido theory. These developments have largely remained indifferent to the dramatic changes in the patterns and structures of everyday social life over the past half-century and to the impact these must have upon the developmental process.

Recent work in social history and psychohistory makes it less easy to treat the sexual as an unchanging constant, providing the illusion of a unifying thread in the human record. For the most part, work in this tradition has persisted in traditional metapsychological conservatisms, largely attempting to sustain a static model of the human within a landscape of changing ecologies and cultures. The history of the psyche remains the unfinished business of psychohistory. We attempt to move this discussion further by proposing an approach that allows us to consider human sexuality in ways that are responsive to both the sociohistorical process and the necessary understandings that preserve a sense of individually experienced lives.

Scripts are a metaphor for conceptualizing the production of behaviour within social life. Most of social life most of the time must operate under the guidance of an operating syntax, much as language is a precondition for speech. For behaviour to occur, something resembling scripting must occur on three distinct levels: cultural scenarios, interpersonal scripts, and intrapsychic scripts.

Cultural scenarios are the instructional guides that exist at the level of collective life. All institutions and institutionalized arrangements can be seen as systems of signs and symbols through which the requirements and the practice of specific roles are given. The enactment of virtually all roles must either directly or indirectly reflect the contents of appropriate cultural scenarios. These scenarios are rarely entirely predictive of actual behaviour, and they are generally too abstract to be applied in all circumstances.

The possibility of a lack of congruence between the abstract scenario and the concrete situation must be resolved by the creation of interpersonal scripts. This is a process that transforms the social actor from being exclusively an actor to being a partial scriptwriter or adapter shaping the materials of relevant cultural scenarios into scripts for behaviour in particular contexts. Interpersonal scripting is the mechanism through which appropriate identities are made congruent with desired expectations.

Where complexities, conflicts, and/or ambiguities become endemic at the level of cultural scenarios, much greater demands are placed on the actor than can be met by interpersonal scripts alone. The need to script one's behaviour, as well as the implicit assumption of the scripted nature of the behaviour of others, is what engenders a meaningful 'internal rehearsal', which becomes significant when alternative outcomes are available. This intrapsychic scripting creates fantasy in a rich sense of that word: the symbolic reorganization of reality in ways to more fully realize the actor's many-layered and sometimes multivoiced wishes. Intrapsychic scripting becomes a historical necessity, as a private world of wishes and desires that are experienced as originating in the deepest recesses of the self must be bound to social life: individual desires are linked to social meanings. Desire is not reducible to an appetite, a drive, an instinct; it does not create the self, rather it is part of the process of the creation of the self.

The relevance of the three levels of scripting – cultural scenarios, interpersonal scripts, and intrapsychic scripts – is far from identical in all social settings and/or for all individuals in any given setting. In traditional societies, cultural scenarios and a limited repertoire of what appear to be 'ritualized improvisations' may be all that is required for understanding by either participants or observers. Such societies might be termed paradigmatic societies. They are paradigmatic in a double sense: in the sense of a high degree of shared meanings and in the sense of specific or concrete meanings being perceived as consistently derived from a small number of highly integrated master meanings. Specific shared meanings are experienced substantially as being consistent both within and across distinct spheres of life.

Postparadigmatic societies are those in which there are substantially fewer shared meanings and, possibly of greater significance, potentially profound disjunctures of meaning between distinct spheres of life. As a result, the enactment of the same role within different spheres of life or different roles within the same sphere routinely requires different appearances, if not different organizations, of the self.

The cultural scenario that loses its coercive powers also loses its predictability and frequently becomes merely a legitimating reference or explanation. The failure of the coercive powers of cultural scenarios occasions anomie, personal alienation and uncertainty. Much of the passionate intensity associated with anomic behaviour might best be interpreted as restorative efforts, often desperate efforts at effecting a restoration of a more cohesive self, reinforced by effective social ties. Anomie feeds on the ultimate dependence upon collective life that describes all human experience. The integration of personal metaphors and social meanings that make social conduct possible is complex. Scripting becomes a useful metaphor for understanding this process.

The scripting of sexual behaviour implies a rejection of the idea that the sexual represents a very special, if not unique, quality of motivation. From a scripting perspective, the sexual is not viewed as an intrinsically significant aspect of human behaviour; rather, the sexual is viewed as becoming significant either when it is defined as such by collective life – sociogenic significance; or when individual experiences or development assign it a special significance – ontogenic significance. The significance of some aspect of behaviour does not determine the frequency with which that behaviour occurs, but only the amount and intensity of attention paid to it.

Sociogenic and ontogenic factors are closely interrelated. These are societal settings in which the sexual takes on a strong meaning and successful performance or avoidance of what is defined as sexual plays a major role in the evaluation of individual competence and worth. These should also be settings in which sexual meanings play a correspondingly significant role in the intrapsychic lives of individuals. Even in settings with a high density of external sexual cues, not all individuals need experience an equivalent density of internal cues. It is also possible for some individuals in settings marked by relatively little concern for the sexual to create a set of sexual meanings and referents far more intense than those apparent in the setting.

The motivation to perceive and respond in sexual terms need not be exclusively determined by what is essential to a given setting. For the most part, ontogenic variations from prevailing cultural scenarios tend to be limited to a universe largely created by such cultural scenarios – in other words, by the application of conventional sexual meanings to unconventional sexual objects or by the expression of unconventional motives through conventional sexual activities.

The most basic sources of sociogenic influence are the cultural scenarios that explicitly deal with the sexual or those that can implicitly be put to sexual uses. Such cultural scenarios not only specify appropriate objects, aims, and desirable qualities of self/other relations, but also instruct in times, places, sequences of gesture and utterance, and, among the most important, what the actor and coparticipants (real or imagined) are assumed to be feeling. These instructions make most of us far more committed and rehearsed at the time of our initial sexual encounters than we realize.

When there is a fundamental congruence between the sexual as it is defined by prevailing cultural scenarios and experienced intrapsychically, consequent behaviour is symbolic. It is entirely dependent upon the shared significant meanings of collective life. The sexual takes a natural air obscuring that virtually all the cues initiating sexual behaviour are embedded in the external environment. This reliance upon external cues may have made what later eras would define as 'sexual deprivation' – long periods during which sexual activities are not accessible – more easily managed in most historical settings than contemporary observers might think.

A lack of congruence between levels of scripting transforms the sexual into more obscurely metaphoric behaviour, as it may become a vehicle for meaning above and beyond conventionally shared meanings: private sexual cultures grow within the heart of public sexual cultures. It may well have been the growing number of individuals in Western societies experiencing such a lack of congruence that made prevailing eighteenth- and nineteenth-century discourses on the nature of the sexual so highly effective in gaining widespread adherence to modern Western sexual values and idealized patterns of behaviour.

Interpersonal scripting, representing the actor's response to the external world, draws heavily upon cultural scenarios, invoking symbolic elements expressive of such scenarios. Among other functions, interpersonal scripting serves to lower uncertainty and heighten legitimacy for both the other or others as well as the actor. Interpersonal scripts might be defined as the representations of self and the implied mirroring of the other that facilitates the occurrence of a sexual exchange. While such scripts generally imply things about the internal feelings of the participants, only the representation of appropriate feelings need be manifested or confirmed. For virtually all, at one time or other, desire will follow rather than precede behaviour.

Interpersonal scripts represent our definition of the immediate social context. The motives, conscious and unconscious, that underlie what appears to be manifestly sexual behaviour, may vary widely. As might also be said for any significant area of behaviour, there are many more reasons for behaving sexually than there are ways of behaving sexually. Almost half a century after the death of Freud, the quest for the sexual motives informing nonsexual behaviour tends to provoke far less anxiety than a quest for the nonsexual motives that upon occasion organize and sustain sexual behaviour. To the degree that for our time and place the most current conceptions of sexual behaviour imply a potential for sexual response, we also require an understanding of the less directly observable dimension of intrapsychic scripting: that which elicits and sustains sexual arousal, at times making orgasm possible.

There are some collective situations in which almost all interpersonal scripts represent, at best, minor variations of dominant cultural scenarios and in which the practised interpersonal scripts satisfy the requirements of intrapsychic scripting. Most typically these come close on the sexual patterns that Freud viewed as characterizing the world of antiquity, when emphasis was placed upon the drive and little attention was paid to the object of the drive. Writing as he did in a world of pervasive sexism, Freud failed to observe that this multiple congruence of scripting elements most often occurs when the concerns for sexual arousal and orgasm are the exclusive or nearly exclusive interests of only one participant – the male.

Part of the historical record of sexism is that women rarely have been selected for sexual roles on the basis of their own interest in sexual pleasure. The idea of female interest in, or commitment to, sexual pleasure was, and possibly still is, threatening to many men and women. Even Freud casually commented upon the ease with which women, presumably more so than men, accommodate to varied sexual 'perversions' once they have been sufficiently exposed to the potential pleasures. This is not to say that women in such settings did not have commitments to effectively utilizing or responding to interpersonal sexual scripts, but that these commitments rarely tended to be erotically or orgasmically focused.

In the modern era, Freud also noted, the drive is 'despised'; the emphasis is placed upon the object and, we would add, the quality of relationship with the object. This shift in focus from the drive to the object must inevitably occasion a growth of emphatic concerns. The transformation of the object into a participating other often requires the recognition of the other as another self. The sexual actor must not only recognize the behaviour of the other, he or she must also recognize the feelings communicated, however uncertainly, by that behaviour. The eroticized sexual act often represents for both self and other an act of offering and possession of what can only rarely, if ever, be wholly offered or possessed: a recognition of the intrapsychic experience of another person: for example, Did you really want it? Did you really enjoy it?

A social world requiring that we bargain for our identities inevitably trains us to bargain with ourselves. Desire, including the desire for desire, becomes one of the most pervasive currencies for negotiating exchanges across domains. The self in becoming a scripted actor becomes its own producer, managing resources, investing in long-term payoffs and short-term cash flow while becoming its own playwright. While nonerotic motives frequently organize and lead us through our selection of interpersonal sexual scripts, an increasing emphasis upon erotic pleasure characterizes much of contemporary sexual life not merely in response to the changing contents of available cultural scenarios, but as an expression of the changing experience of the self.

The estrangement of the erotic from the domain of everyday life, so fundamental a part of the modern Western tradition, made it available to fulfil the beliefs of those who sought its expulsion in the first place. The erotic became the badlands of desire; a domain in which the abstractions of moral discipline could find a concrete and persistent test. Ironically, for that reason, the erotic also became a realm in which the laws and identities governing everyday life could be suspended and the self be organized in ways that include aspects and qualities otherwise exiled or expressed through muted disguises and/or contrary uses. The puritan tradition created a road map where the dimensions of self that were to be excluded from the everyday self or were denied full expression could rally, enriching and enriched by the erotic. The erotic is to be experienced as having a domain, a licence of its own.

Erotic licence applies to both interpersonal scripts, wherein we are licensed to eroticize our ideals, and intrapsychic scripts, wherein we are licensed to idealize the erotic. This licence for elaboration more often than not makes accommodation more difficult. An example would be the common experience of wanting to express a commitment to elements of interpersonal scripting that are inconsistent with one's feelings – to simultaneously take possession of the object of desire (the male role) and to be the object of desire (the female role); to seduce and to be seductive, to conquer and to surrender, to desire and to be desirable.

The separation of an erotic identity from an everyday identity is reflected in the highly disjunctive experience that commonly occurs upon the entry into explicitly sexual acts. An experience of disjuncture usually occurs even among individuals who have had an extensive shared sexual history. This is reflected in the traditional and persistent practice of putting out the lights before initiating sexual activity – not to be seen, not to see, not to be seen seeing. The problem of disjunctive identities is also reflected in the questions, Who am I when I have sex? With whom am I having sex?

In the most pragmatic sense, sexual scripts must solve two problems. The first of these is gaining permission from the self to engage in desired forms of sexual behaviour. The second is that of access to the experiences that the desired behaviour is expected to generate. Frequently this requires that an actor's experience becomes contingent not only upon what his or her partner appears to be doing, but also upon what the partner appears to be experiencing. This emphatic inference derives partly from available cultural scenarios and partly from what is perceived as the actual experience of the other. It also derives from what the actor requires the other to be in order to maintain sexual excitement. Sometimes the actor, in his or her presented guise, merely provides the plausible access to behaviour, while the desired experience is to be gained not from, but from within the other: the not uncommon experience of the other becoming a metaphor for the self. This response is typified by a transsexual who when asked how she could have fathered several children while she was a he, replied, 'There was always a penis there, but it never was mine'.

What Freud saw as fundamental to the 'psychological novel' also describes the scripting of the sexual:

> The psychological novel in general probably owes its peculiarities to the tendency of modern writers to split up their ego by self-observation into many component egos, and in this way personify the conflicting trends in their own mental life in many heroes.

The phrase 'self-observation' points to the process that must follow the fashioning of an interpersonal script out of sometimes incongruous material: self-observation, often very careful self-observation. Self-observation represents incipient self-control, and self-control becomes synonymous with the staging of the self. The actor ultimately must submit to the playwright, while both nervously anticipate the response of overlapping, but not always harmonious, internal and external critics.

The concept of scripting can take on a literal meaning: not the creation and performance of a role, but the creation and staging of a drama. Roles are meaningless in themselves and take on meaning only in relation to the enactment of related roles. What the actor/ego is (including what the actor/ego feels he or she should be feeling) is dependent upon the creation of a cast of others (including what they should be feeling), the others who complete the meaning of the actor; others may be required to experience what the actor sometimes cannot experience in his or her own name. To use the language of Laplanche and Pontalis (1974), the sexual script can be seen as 'the mise-en-scène of desire'.

This complex process of sexual scripting encourages the conservative, highly ritualized, or stereotyped character that sexual behaviour often takes. This conservative character is often cited as support for the view that the sexual is shaped early and possesses only a limited capacity for subsequent change. This conservative aspect may depend more on the stability of social and personal history than on an ironhanded legacy of the early developmental process.

Few individuals, like few novelists or dramatists, wander far from the formulas of their most predictable successes. Once they have found a formula that works – in other words, the realization of sexual pleasure, as well as the realization of sociosexual competence – there is an obvious tendency on some levels to pararitualize that formula. Variations can occur, but variations generally occur within the limits of a larger, stabilizing body of scripts both interpersonal and intrapsychic. The stabilizing of sexual scripts, often confused with the crystallization of a sexual identity, occurs partly because it works by insuring adequate sexual performance and providing adequate sexual pleasure. It also represents an effective accommodation with the larger self process, in which sexual practice and sexual identity do not disturb the many components of one's nonsexual identities.

Changes in status or context, expected or unexpected, as Kohut (1978) has observed, have the capacity to call into question the organization of the self. A potential crisis of the self-formation process and the production of scripts – sexual and nonsexual – is occasioned by change not merely because some aspect of the self is under pressure to change, but also because the ecology of the self has been disturbed. Such moments require renegotiation of aspects of the self involved in or related to change: all aspects of the self that previously required a negotiated outcome must be reestablished. In modern societies there are relatively few individuals for whom the self-formation process does not involve such negotiated outcomes or outcomes of either compromise or dominance and repression.

Much of the process of sexual scripting, while appearing in the obscurity of individual behaviour, remains in most critical aspects a derivative of the social process. What appears to be the freedom of the individual from the determination of the social process may be little (and yet a great deal) more than a reflection of the increased complexity of collective life.

Few cultural scenarios are without implications for age or life-cycle stage. While rarely complete in the sense of specifying the full range of expected behaviours and responses to behaviour, it is hard to designate a role that is without life-cycle requirements in the double sense of (1) having entry and exiting requirements that are specific to a life-cycle stage or (2) having expectations that systematically vary with attributions of the life-cycle stage.

Some roles are very specific with respect to age requirements – for example, 'you cannot until age X', 'at age Y you must'. For many roles and activities, particularly those that are universal or nearly universal, standards of evaluation can vary dramatically in terms of the presumed life-cycle stage of the actor. For example, only the very young and very old are allowed to be sloppy, self-preoccupied ingestors of food. The commonplace admonition, 'act your age', speaks directly to the pervasive relevance of conceptualizations of life-cycle stages to virtually all behaviour. There are few roles or dimensions of identity other than the sexual that are so troubled by the transformations accompanying life-cycle stage changes.

Conceptualizations of life-cycle stages are implicit in the multiple roles most people are expected to play. This makes them an effective instrument for assessing the degree to which a collectivity might legitimately be called 'paradigmatic'. The term paradigmatic can be applied when there is a high degree of consensus regarding the boundaries and the differential expectations associated with each life-cycle stage, when there is near universal respect for boundaries and expectations, and when the application of these causes little conflict in integrating the several roles an individual occupies.

Failing all else, highly differentiated or postparadigmatic societies, such as the industrial and post-industrial countries of the West, have great difficulty in effectively sustaining this kind of integration. While much that is involved in the association of age with status persists, particularly in sexual domains, confusions, uncertainties, and flexibilities abound. Not only do the contents of age-specific expectations become ambiguously complex, but even when there is consensus regarding such expectations, the applicability of them frequently remains vague. What do we expect of the young? What do we expect of the old? Who is young? Who is old? The order in which these questions must be asked differs radically between paradigmatic and postparadigmatic social orders.

The translation of cultural sexual scenarios into interpersonal sexual scripts has the effect of empowering the actor who often realizes considerable discretion in invoking specific symbolic aspects of the life cycle. This empowering is shared with others who also have considerable discretion in confirming or disconfirming the actor's representations. An aging 'playboy' whose partners, like the *Playboy* centrefold, never age may simultaneously be an object of ridicule and envy. What were once coercive obligations increasingly become bargaining chips in negotiations with others, as well as in negotiation with the self. This is least troublesome at the extreme ends of the life cycle, the extremes which might be termed the presexual (childhood) and the postsexual (old age). Not that sexually significant events do not occur during these periods, but they are not or only rarely anticipated in prevailing cultural scenarios dealing with the very young and the very old.

Infancy, childhood, and until recently old age, were periods in which the appearance of sex-seeking behaviour was viewed as pathological; an assumption of pathology was made because those either too young or too old were assumed to be incapable of comprehending or experiencing the full meaning of the behaviour. Community outrage at the rape of an elderly woman or a female child is often greater than an even more brutal rape of a 'mature' woman, because, the inappropriateness of the object bespeaks its greater pathological origins and often precludes even the suspicion of initial complicity on the part of the victim.

For some individuals the sequence of life-cycle-based cultural scenarios continues to organize interpersonal sexual scripts in ways that facilitate the harmonizing of sexual commitments with more public role commitments. For such individuals, cultural scenarios covering conventional family careers serve as the organizing principle of sexual careers; for them, family careers, sexual careers, and the definition of life-cycle stages tend to coincide. Suggestive of this is that for Kinsey, and virtually all others, conceptualizations of heterosexual behaviour have been organized in terms of marital status: sexual careers are subsumed under the heading of premarital, marital, extramarital, or postmarital experiences.

Such a congruence of scripts and identities were once mandated by the institutional order. For increasing numbers this coincidence fails to occur or, when it occurs, it does so with the kinds of strains that undermine stability. The dramatic recent changes in patterns of sexual behaviours reflect not only profound change in the requirements and meaning attached to the sexual, but equally profound changes in the ordering of family careers and in the definition of the life cycle itself. Life-cycle stages once appeared to specify behaviour; now commitment to behaviour increasingly specifies one's life-cycle stage.

We commonly hear reference to a 'blurring of life-cycle stage boundaries', often accompanied by an admiring appreciation of more traditional societies that appear to maintain clear and nearly universal life-cycle stage distinctions. Not untypically, such groups are admired for facilitating the journey across the conventional life course by utilization of 'rites of passage'. The implied comparison is with contemporary societies that often appear to do very little to instruct individuals in how to manage such transitions; failing not only to provide training in the behaviours associated with a new stage, but to provide a clear basis for recognition by others.

What appears as a blurring of boundaries on the group level is not necessarily fully descriptive of what occurs on the individual level; it is often not fully descriptive of what is happening on the collective level as well. A highly differentiated society is unlikely to formulate instructive life-cycle scenarios that can simultaneously realize a level of abstraction sufficient to override existing difference and become an occasion for evoking powerful feelings. For example, the question of what constitutes minimal sexual maturity varies considerably across time and cultures; it varies dramatically across even the contemporary social landscape. Where serious involvement in sociosexual activities once marked the boundaries between adolescence and adulthood, it increasingly comes to mark the boundaries between childhood and adolescence.

Sexual cultural scenarios endure, but no longer provide the exclusive interpretive context. The specifics of person and place effectively compete for legitimating the appropriateness of a specific scenario. Age or life-cycle stage suggest the possibility of sexual activity at the same time that sexual activity affirms our claim to a specific stage of the life-cycle. If I do 'it', I am either old enough or young enough, depending on 'where I am coming from'. We can observe the commitment to the sexual following the essentially nonerotic motive of gaining interpersonal and/or intrapsychic confirmation. Current adolescent sexual patterns speak to this eloquently. The dramatic sexualization of early adolescence provides an exemplification of the desire for meaning, that is, confirmation of status competence, preceding a commitment to the meaning of erotic desire.

We do not imply that the sexual is entirely organized directly by the pressure of external requirements. Operative cultural scenarios substantially condition overt behaviour, both in behaviour and in the anticipation of behaviour. Internal rehearsals represent the trials or experiments in which a multitude of accumulated desires are tested for compatibility with each other, allowing for an initial crystallization of sexual identity.

The early eroticiszation of such trials through masturbatory reinforcement may serve to additionally strengthen the claims of the emergent intrapsychic scripts in seeking expression – however muted – in operative interpersonal scripts. Occurring most typically in contemporary society during a period of heightened narcissism, such fantasized rehearsals often find their narrative plausibility far more dependent upon personal ideals than upon social ideals. Occurring in the realm of fantasy, such emergent intrapsychic scripts have a capacity to more effectively harness social ideals to personal passions than may be possible in the enactment of interpersonal scripts that must simultaneously serve the erotic and the conventional.

While emotionally charged, not all – possibly very few – erotic rehearsals or fantasies are acted out. Many in varied representations continue necessarily to be acted within: the sexual dialogue with the other often bears little resemblance to the sexual dialogue with the self. Unfortunately, almost all of our concern with the sexual activities of adolescents centres upon overt behaviours – which have important consequences – while virtually none of this concern focuses upon the imagery informing that behaviour. With the exception of Stoller's work, virtually none of it focuses upon the sexual acts within sexual acts. Most people will find a negotiated compromise between the requirements of both levels of scripting, although the stability of that negotiated compromise is rarely assured.

The imagery of the intrapsychic yields to change far more slowly than the more externally monitored production of interpersonal scripts. With shifts in life-cycle status – from adolescence to adulthood in its varied stages, from being children to being parents, from engaging in violative behaviour to engaging in mandated behaviours – the accommodations effective at one stage become problematic at subsequent stages. Aside from its own intrinsic requirements, the sexual also shares the burden of demonstrating social, gender, and moral competence and, as a result, the demands placed upon interpersonal scripting often are compelling. Rather than being reciprocally reinforcing, the requirements of interpersonal and intrapsychic scripting of the sexual frequently represent a continuing – and for some a costly – dialectic.

One consequence of this partially narcissistic sexual repertoire is that it is highly responsive to subsequent narcissistic wounds or threats. The mid-life crisis, for example, often manifests itself in terms of reactivated sexual experiments, thought it may represent more of a renewal of the sexual rather than a failure of previous strategies of sexual repression or containment. Renewal may have roots in aspects of the self initially remote to the sexual, aspects of the self that link the individual to social life and his or her past and future far more critically than any burden the sexual may carry. Typical of these might be the conflicts between the self as child and the self as parent, as well as the crises attending both success and failure in the world of work.

The sexualization of this kind of 'crisis' serves two distinct functions. First, while appearing initially as a threat to the traditional social order, it actually lessens the estrangement of the individual by mandating a transformation of the self within the social order, not a transformation of the social order. It moves the individual towards a quality of interpersonal scripting that personalizes discontent and its solutions. For example, much, if not most, of the increase in female participation in extramarital sex may not be an expression of a feminist revolution so much as it is a more comfortable alternative to a revolution.

Second, as a postadolescent phenomenon, it generally follows the eroticization of the sexual and utilizes the powers of the intrapsychic to create new metaphors of desire – metaphors that effectively link the 'archaeology' of desire with new and often unanticipated social destinies. Both the anomie of deprivation and, even more profoundly, that of affluence focus the individual's attention upon available repertoires of gratification in ways that commonly highlight the promise of the erotic. The enlargement of psychic functions attending the anomic condition are attracted to the promises of erotic experience – promises of intensity, of confirmation.

For all the confusions attending both adolescence and the vaguely bounded 'mid-life crisis' or postadolescent identity crisis, it is easier to consider the role of the sexual within such contexts than it is during other segments of life. These have become matters of sufficient public concern to enable speculation on the scripting of the sexual within these contexts. Other segments of the life course remain largely uncharted domains. We suspect that even when life appears untraumatic – as it may for many – the problems of adapting sexual scripts to changed circumstances is an important, if relatively unattended issue.

The power of sexual scripts is tied to the extrasexual significances of confirming identities and making them congruent with appropriate relationships. Where identity is for the moment confirmed and relationships are stabilized, the meanings and uses of the sexual must shift in basic ways. Almost inevitably, for many there is a shift from the sexuality feeding off the excitement of uncertainty to a sexuality of reassurance. The stabilizing of identities and relationships tends to stabilize the structuring of interpersonal scripts. Even variations and elaborations take on a predictable character, accounting for what for most becomes a declining frequency of sexual activity. Possibly, the sources of sexual interest, if not sexual passion, increasingly depend upon materials drawn from aspects of intrapsychic scripting that can be embedded within the stereotyped interpersonal script. A useful, but potentially alienating adaptation encourages what has always been a potential aspect of sexual exchanges: we become dumb actors in one another's charades.

The problematic qualities of managing the scripting of the sexual by adults may be seen in two general ways. The major cultural scenarios that shape the most common interpersonal scripts tend to be almost exclusively drawn from the requirements of adolescence and young adulthood. There are virtually none tied to the issues of subsequent segments of life. The interpersonal scripts of these early stages, along with the intrapsychic elements they facilitate, may become in part the fantasied components of the intrapsychic at later stages, particularly the confirmation of attractiveness and displays of passionate romantic interest. While this transfer sustains sexual commitment and performance, it also has the capacity to provide a disenchanting commentary on such performances.

Partly derived from the process of evolving intrapsychic scripts and partly derived from the isolation of erotic realities from everyday reality, the imagery and content of intrapsychic scripts change very slowly. The language of accumulation and reorganization might be more accurate. Drawn from what we once were, as well as from what we were not and still are not allowed to be or express in more explicit form, the intrapsychic in muted form feeds our continuing sexual experiences and, not uncommonly, opportunistically enlarges its claims during moments of crisis, disjuncture, or transition.

Explorations such as this almost inevitably begin with promise and conclude with apology. What we offer is not a theory of sexual behaviour, but a conceptual apparatus with which to examine development and experience of the sexual. An examination must inevitably take us beyond inarticulate permanence of the body to the changing and diverse meanings and uses of the sexual. In doing so, we see the sexual not in traditional terms of biological imperatives, but in terms of the natural imperatives of the human: our natural dependence upon social meanings – upon symbol and metaphor – to give life to 'the body without organs'.

References and suggestions for further reading

DELEUZE, G. and GUATTARI, F. (1977) *Anti-Oedipus: Capitalism and Schizophrenia*, New York: Viking Press.

FOUCAULT, M. (1978) *The History of Sexuality, Volume 1: An Introduction*, New York: Pantheon Books.

FREUD, S. (1962) *Three Essays on the Theory of Sexuality*, New York: Harper/Colophon Books.

—— (1963) 'On the relation of the poet to day-dreaming', in RIEFF, P. (ed.), *Character and Culture*, New York: Collier.

KOHUT, H. (1978) 'Thoughts on narcissism and narcissistic rag', in ORNSTEIN, P.H. (ed.) *The Search for the Self*, New York: International University Press.

LAPLANCHE, J. and PONTALIS, J.B. (1974) *The Language of Psycho-Analysis*, New York: W.W. Norton.

LICHTENSTEIN, H. (1977) *The Dilemma of Human Identity*, New York: Jason Aronson.

STOLLER, R.J. (1979) *Sexual Excitement: Dynamics of Erotic Life*, New York: Pantheon Books.

4 Anthropology rediscovers sexuality

A theoretical comment

Carole S. Vance [1991]

> In the beginning was sex and sex will be in the end ... I maintain – and this is my thesis – that sex as a feature of man and society was always central and remains such ...
>
> (Goldenweiser, 1929, p. 53)

This opening sentence from Alexander Goldenweiser's essay, 'Sex and Primitive Society', suggests that sexuality has been an important focus for anthropological investigation. Indeed, such is the reputation anthropologists have bestowed upon themselves: fearless investigators of sexual customs and mores throughout the world, breaking through the erotophobic intellectual taboos common in other, more timid disciplines.

In reality, anthropology's relationship to the study of sexuality is more complex and contradictory. Anthropology as a field has been far from courageous or even adequate in its investigation of sexuality (Fisher, 1980; Davis and Whitten, 1987). Rather, the discipline often appears to share the prevailing cultural view that sexuality is not an entirely legitimate area of study, and that such study necessarily casts doubt not only on the research but on the motives and character of the researcher. In this, we have been no worse but also no better than other social science disciplines.

Manifestations of this attitude abound in graduate training and in the reward structure of the profession. Few graduate departments provide training in the study of human sexuality. As a result, there are no structured channels to transmit anthropological knowledge concerning sexuality to the next generation of students. The absence of a scholarly community engaged with issues of sexuality effectively prevents the field from advancing; students interested in the topic perceive that they must rediscover past generations' work on their own. Most advisors actively discourage graduate students from fieldwork or dissertations on sexuality for fear that the topic will prove a career liability. At best, students are advised to complete their doctoral degrees, build up reputations and credentials, and even obtain tenure, all of which are said to put one in a better position to embark on the study of sexuality (Fisher, 1980; Davis and Whitten, 1987). Rather than the collective effort needed to remedy a serious structural limitation in our discipline, this advice conveys the clear message that sexuality is so dangerous an intellectual terrain it can ruin the careers of otherwise competent graduate students and academics.

Nor is there any career track after graduate school for professional anthropologists interested in sexuality. Never attaining the status of an appropriate specialization, sexuality remains marginal. Funding is difficult, as agencies continue to be fearful of the subject's potential for public controversy. Colleagues often remain suspicious and hypercritical, as discomfort with the very subject of sexuality is cast instead in terms of scholarly adequacy or legitimacy.[1] Field projects rarely, if ever, focus fully or directly on sexuality; rather, field workers collect data as they can, some of which are never published for fear of harm to one's professional reputation. Some anthropologists retreat into sexology, more hospitable perhaps, yet seriously limited itself as an intellectual ghetto of disciplinary refugees (Vance, 1983; Irvine, 1990).

In light of these disincentives, it is perhaps not surprising that the recent development of a more cultural and non-essentialist discourse about sexuality has sprung not from the centre of anthropology but from its periphery, from other disciplines (especially history), and from theorizing done by marginal groups. The explosion of exciting and challenging work in what has come to be called social-construction theory during the past 15 years has yet to be felt in mainstream anthropology.

The intellectual history of social-construction theory is complex, and the moments offered here are for purposes of illustration, not comprehensive review (for basic texts, see Katz, 1976; Weeks, 1977; Padgug, 1979; Weeks, 1981; Katz, 1983; Snitow, Stansell and Thompson, 1983; Vance, 1984; Weeks, 1986; Peiss and Simmons, 1989; D'Emilio and Freedman, 1988; Altman *et al.*, 1989; Duberman, Vicinus and Chauncey, 1989). Social-construction theory drew on developments in several disciplines: social interactionism, labelling theory, and deviance in sociology (Gagnon and Simon, 1973; Plummer, 1982); social history, labour studies, women's history, and Marxist history (Duggan, 1990); and symbolic anthropology, cross-cultural work on sexuality, and gender studies in anthropology, to name only the most significant streams. In addition, theorists in many disciplines responded to new questions raised by feminist and lesbian/gay scholarship concerning gender and identity.

Sexuality and gender

Feminist scholarship and activism undertook the project of rethinking gender, which had a revolutionary impact on notions of what is natural. Feminist efforts focused on a critical review of theories which used reproduction to link gender with sexuality, thereby explaining the inevitability and naturalness of women's subordination (for anthropology, see Rosaldo and Lamphere, 1974; Reiter, 1975; Lamphere, 1977; Rapp, 1979; Atkinson, 1982; Moore, 1988).

This theoretical re-examination led to a general critique of biological determinism, in particular of received knowledge about the biology of sex differences (Hubbard, Henifin and Fried, 1982; Sayers, 1982; Lowe and Hubbard, 1983; Bleier, 1984; Fausto-Sterling, 1985; Tobach and Rosoft, 1978). Historical and cross-cultural evidence undermined the notion that women's roles, which varied so widely, could be caused by a seemingly uniform human reproduction and sexuality. In light of the diversity of gender roles in human society, it seemed unlikely that they were inevitable or caused by sexuality. The ease with which such theories had become accepted suggested that science was conducted within and mediated by powerful beliefs about gender and in turn provided ideological support for current social relations. Moreover, this increased sensitivity to the ideological aspects of science led to a wide-ranging inquiry into the historical connection between male dominance, scientific ideology, and the development of Western science and biomedicine (Barker-Benfield, 1976; Ehrenreich and English, 1979; Harding and Hintikka, 1983; Keller, 1984; Harding, 1986; Haraway, 1989; Jordanova, 1989; Schiebinger, 1989).

Feminist practice in grass-roots activism also fostered analyses that separated sexuality and gender. Popular struggles to advance women's access to abortion and birth control represented an attempt to separate sexuality from reproduction and women's gendered role as wives and mothers. Discussions in consciousness-raising groups made clear that what seemed to be a naturally gendered body was in fact a highly socially mediated product: femininity and sexual attractiveness were achieved through persistent socialization regarding standards of beauty, make-up and body language. Finally, discussions between different generations of women made clear how variable their allegedly natural sexuality was, moving within our own century from marital duty to multiple orgasm, vaginal to clitoral erotism, and Victorian passionlessness to a fittingly feminine enthusiasm. Sexuality and gender went together, it seemed, but in ways that were subject to change.

In 1975, anthropologist Gayle Rubin's influential essay, 'The Traffic in Women', made a compelling argument against essentialist explanations that sexuality and reproduction caused gender difference in any simple or inevitable way (1975). Instead, she explored the shape of 'a systematic social apparatus which takes up females as raw materials and fashions domesticated women as products' (Rubin, 1975, p. 158). She proposed the term 'sex/gender system' to describe 'the set of arrangements by which society transforms biological sexuality into products of human activity, and in which these transformed sexual needs are satisfied' (1975, p. 159).

In 1984, Rubin suggested a further deconstruction of the sex/gender system into two separate domains in which sexuality and gender were recognized as distinct systems (Rubin, 1984, p. 267). Most prior feminist analyses considered sexuality a totally derivative category whose organization was determined by the structure of gender inequality. According to Rubin's formulation, sexuality and gender were analytically distinct phenomena that required separate explanatory frames, even though they were interrelated in specific historical circumstances. Theories of sexuality could not explain gender, and, taking the argument to a new level, theories of gender could not explain sexuality.

This perspective suggested a novel framework: sexuality and gender are separate systems which are interwoven at many points. Although members of a culture experience this interweaving as natural, seamless and organic, the points of connection vary historically and cross-culturally. For researchers in sexuality, the task is not only to study changes in the expression of sexual behaviour and attitudes, but to examine the relationship of these changes to more deeply based shifts in how gender and sexuality were organized and interrelated within larger social relations.

Sexuality and identity

A second impetus for the development of social-construction theory arose from issues that emerged in the examination of male homosexuality in nineteenth-century Europe and America (Katz, 1976, 1983; Weeks, 1977, 1981). It is interesting to note that a significant portion of this early research was conducted by independent scholars, non-academics, and maverick academics usually working without funding or university support, since at this time the history of sexuality (particularly that of marginal groups) was scarcely a legitimate topic. As this research has recently achieved the barest modicum of academic acceptance, it is commonplace for properly employed academics to gloss these developments by a reference to Foucault and *The History of Sexuality* (1978). Without denying his contributions, such a singular genealogy obscures an important origin of social-construction theory, and inadvertently credits the university and scholarly disciplines with a development they never supported.

The first attempt to grapple with questions of sexual identity in a way now recognizable as social construction appears in Mary McIntosh's 1968 essay on the homosexual role in England (McIntosh, 1968). A landmark article offering many suggestive insights about the historical construction of sexuality in England, her observations initially vanished like pebbles in a pond until the mid-1970s, when they were again taken up by writers involved in the questions of feminism and gay liberation. It is at this time that an identifiably constructionist approach first appears.

The earliest scholarship in lesbian and gay history attempted to retrieve and revive documents, narratives and biographies that had been lost or made invisible due to historical neglect as well as active efforts to suppress the material by archivists, historians and estates. These documents and the lives represented therein were first conceived of as 'lesbian' or 'gay', and the enterprise as a search for historical roots. To their credit, researchers who started this enterprise sharing the implicit cultural ideology of fixed sexual categories then began to consider other ways of looking at their material and to ask more expansive questions.

Jeffrey Weeks, English historian of sexuality, first articulated this theoretical transition (Weeks, 1977). Drawing on McIntosh's concept of the homosexual role, he distinguished between homosexual behaviour, which he considered universal, and homosexual identity, which he viewed as historically and culturally specific and, in Britain, a comparatively recent development. His rich and provocative analysis of changing attitudes and identities also contextualized sexuality, examining its relationship to the reorganization of family, gender and household in nineteenth-century Britain.

Jonathan Katz's work also demonstrates this process. His first book, *Gay American History*, is in the tradition of a search for gay ancestors (Katz, 1976). In the course of researching his second book, however, he began to consider that the acts of sodomy reported in American colonial documents from the seventeenth century might not be equivalent to contemporary homosexuality (Katz, 1983). Colonial society did not seem to conceive of a unique type of person – a homosexual – who engaged in these acts. Nor was there any evidence of a homosexual subculture or individuals whose subjective sense of identity was organized around what we understand as sexual preference or identity. Katz's second book marks a sharp departure from the first, in that records or accounts that document same-sex emotional or sexual relations are not taken as evidence of 'gay' or 'lesbian' identity, but are treated as jumping-off points for a whole series of questions about the meanings of these acts to the people who engaged in them and to the culture and time in which they lived.

These intellectual developments are also evident in early work on the formation of lesbian identity (Rubin, 1979; Sahli, 1979; Rupp, 1980; Faderman, 1981) and work considering the question of sexual behaviour and identity in non-Western cultures, for example, Gilbert Herdt's work in New Guinea (1981, 1984, 1987). From this expanding body of work (Plummer, 1981; Bray, 1982; D'Emilio, 1983; Newton, 1984; Davis and Kennedy, 1986; Gerard and Hekma, 1988; Duberman, Vicinus and Chauncey, 1989; Vicinus, 1989, p. 171) came an impressive willingness to imagine: had the categories 'homosexual' and 'lesbian' always existed? And if not, what were their points of origin and conditions for development? If identical physical acts had different subjective meanings, how was sexual meaning constructed? If sexual subcultures come into being, what leads to their formation?

And although these questions were initially phrased in terms of homosexual identity and history, it is clear that they are equally applicable to heterosexual identity and history, implications just now being explored (Trimberger, 1983; Peiss, 1986, 1989; Stansell, 1986; Katz, 1990).

Sexuality as a contested domain

Continuing work on the history of the construction of sexuality in modern, state-level society shows that sexuality is an actively contested political and symbolic terrain in which groups struggle to implement sexual programmes and alter sexual arrangements and ideologies. The growth of state interest in regulating sexuality (and the related decline of religious control) made legislative and public policy domains particularly attractive fields for political and intellectual struggles around sexuality in the nineteenth and twentieth centuries. Mass movements mobilized around venereal disease, prostitution, masturbation, social purity and the double standard, employing grass-roots political organizing, legislative lobbying, mass demonstrations and cultural interventions utilizing complex symbols, rhetoric and representations (Pivar, 1972; Gordon, 1974; Bristow, 1977; Walkowitz, 1980; Weeks, 1981; Brandt, 1985; Kendrick, 1987; Peiss and Simmons, 1989). Because state intervention was increasingly formulated in a language of health, physicians and scientists became important participants in the newly developing regulatory discourses. They also actively participated in elaborating these discourses as a way to legitimize their newly professionalizing specialities.

Although socially powerful groups exercised more discursive power, they were not the only participants in sexual struggles. Minority reformers, progressives, suffragists and sex radicals also put forward programmes for change and introduced new ways of thinking about and organizing sexuality. The sexual subcultures that had grown up in urban areas were an especially fertile field for these experiments. Constructionist work shows how their attempt to carve out partially protected public spaces in which to elaborate and express new sexual forms, behaviours and sensibilities is also part of a larger political struggle to define sexuality. Subcultures give rise not only to new ways of organizing behaviour and identity but to new ways of symbolically resisting and engaging with the dominant order, some of which grow to have a profound impact beyond the small groups in which they are pioneered. In this respect, social-construction work has been valuable in exploring human agency and creativity in sexuality, moving away from uni-directional models of social change to describe complex and dynamic relationships among the state, professional experts, and sexual subcultures. This attempt to historicize sexuality has produced an innovative body of work to which historians, anthropologists, sociologists and others have contributed in an unusual interdisciplinary conversation

The development of social-construction models, 1975–90

The increasing popularity of the term 'social construction' obscures the fact that constructionist writers have used this term in diverse ways. It is true that all reject transhistorical and transcultural definitions of sexuality and suggest instead that sexuality is mediated by historical and cultural factors. But a close reading of constructionist texts shows that social constructionists differ in their views of what might be constructed, variously including sexual acts, sexual identities, sexual communities, the direction of erotic interest (object choice), and sexual desire itself. Despite these differences, all share the urge to problematize the terms and field of study.

At minimum, all social-construction approaches adopt the view that physically identical sexual acts may have varying social significance and subjective meaning depending on how they are defined and understood in different cultures and historical periods. Because a sexual act does not carry with it a universal social meaning, it follows that the relationship between sexual acts and sexual meanings is not fixed, and it is projected from the observer's time and place at great peril. Cultures provide widely different categories, schema and labels for framing sexual and affective experiences. These constructions not only influence individual subjectivity and behaviour, but they also organize and give meaning to collective sexual experience through, for example, the impact of sexual identities, definitions, ideologies and regulations. The relationship of sexual acts and identities to organized sexual communities is equally variable and complex. These distinctions, then, between sexual acts, identities and communities are widely employed by constructionist writers.

A further step in social-construction theory posits that even the direction of erotic interest itself, for example object choice (heterosexuality, homosexuality and bisexuality, as contemporary sexology would conceptualize it), is not intrinsic or inherent in the individual, but is constructed from more polymorphous possibilities. Not all constructionists take this step; and for those who do not, the direction of desire and erotic interest may be thought of as fixed, although the behavioural form this interest takes will be constructed by prevailing cultural frames, as will the subjective experience of individuals and the social significance attached to it by others.

The most radical form of constructionist theory[2] is willing to entertain the idea that there is no essential, undifferentiated sexual 'impulse', 'sex drive' or 'lust' that resides in the body due to physiological functioning and sensation. Sexual desire, then, is itself constructed by culture and history from the energies and capacities of the body. In this case, an important constructionist question concerns the origin of these impulses, since they are no longer assumed to be intrinsic or perhaps even necessary. This position, of course, contrasts sharply with more middle-ground constructionist theory, which implicitly accepts an inherent desire that is then constructed in terms of acts, identity, community and object choice. The contrast between middle-ground and radical positions makes it evident that constructionists may well have arguments with each other, as well as with those working in essentialist and cultural-influence traditions. Nevertheless, social-construction literature, making its first appearance in the mid-1970s, demonstrates gradual development of the ability to imagine that sexuality is constructed.

Cultural-influence models of sexuality, 1920–90

By contrast, conventional anthropological approaches to sexuality from 1920 to 1990 remained remarkably consistent. Just as sexuality itself remained an unexamined construct, the theoretical foundations remained unexamined, unnamed and implicit, as if they were so inevitable and natural that there could be little dispute or choice about this standard, almost generic, approach. For that reason I want to suggest the name 'cultural-influence model', to call attention to its distinctive features and promote greater recognition of this paradigm. In this model, sexuality is seen as the basic material – a kind of universal Play Doh – on which culture works, a naturalized category that remains closed to investigation and analysis.

On the one hand, the cultural-influence model emphasizes the role of culture and learning in shaping sexual behaviour and attitudes. In this respect, it rejects obvious forms of essentialism and universalizing. Variation was a key finding in many studies, in cross-cultural surveys (Ford and Beach, 1951; Minturn, Grosse and Haider, 1969; Broude and Greene, 1976; Gray, 1980; Frayser, 1985), in ethnographic accounts of single societies whose sexual customs stood in sharp contrast to those of the Euro-American reader (Mead, 1923; Malinowski, 1941 [1929 orig.]; Schapera, 1941; Goodenough, 1949; Berndt and Berndt, 1951; Levine, 1959; Howard and Howard, 1964; Davenport, 1965; Lessa, 1966; Suggs, 1966; Marshall and Suggs, 1972; Heider, 1976; Marshall, 1976), and in theoretical overviews (Goldenweiser, 1929; Bateson, 1947; Murdock, 1949; Honigman, 1954; Gebhard, 1976). Culture is viewed as encouraging or discouraging the expression of generic sexual acts, attitudes and relationships. Oral–genital contact, for example, might be a part of normal heterosexual expression in one group but taboo in another; male homosexuality might be severely punished in one tribe yet tolerated in another. Anthropological work from this period was characterized by a persistent emphasis on variability.

On the other hand, although culture is thought to shape sexual expression and customs, the bedrock of sexuality is assumed – and often quite explicitly stated – to be universal and biologically determined; in the literature, it appears as 'sex drive' or 'impulse'.[3] Although capable of being shaped, the drive is conceived of as powerful, moving toward expression after its awakening in puberty, sometimes exceeding social regulation, and taking a distinctively different form in men and women.

The core of sexuality is reproduction. Although most anthropological accounts by no means restrict themselves to analysing reproductive behaviour alone, reproductive sexuality (glossed as heterosexual intercourse) appears as the meat and potatoes in the sexual menu, with other forms, both heterosexual and homosexual, arranged as appetizers, vegetables and desserts. (These metaphors are not unknown in anthropological narratives.) Ethnographic and survey accounts almost always follow a reporting format that deals first with 'real sex' and then moves on to the 'variations'. Some accounts supposedly about sexuality are noticeably short on details about non-reproductive behaviour; Margaret Mead's (1961) article about the cultural determinants of sexual behaviours (in a wonderfully titled volume called *Sex and Internal Secretions*), travels a dizzying trail that includes pregnancy, menstruation, menopause and lactation but very little about non-reproductive sexuality or eroticism. Similarly, a more recent book, expansively titled *Varieties of Sexual Experience*, devotes virtually all but a few pages to reproduction, marriage and family organization (Frayser, 1985).

Within the cultural-influence model, the term 'sexuality' covers a broad range of topics. Its meaning is often taken for granted, left implicit as a shared understanding between the reader and author. Tracking its use through various articles and books shows that sexuality includes many wildly different things: intercourse, orgasm, foreplay; erotic fantasies, stories, humour; sex differences and the organization of masculinity and femininity, and gender relations (often called sex roles in the earlier literature).

In this model, sexuality is not only related to gender but blends easily, and is often conflated, with it. Sexuality, gender arrangements, masculinity and femininity are assumed to be connected, even interchangeable. This assumption, however, never illuminates their culturally and historically specific connections; it obscures them. The confusion springs from our own folk beliefs that (1) sex causes gender, that is, male–female reproductive differences and the process of reproduction (framed as and equated with 'sexuality') give rise to gender differentiation, and (2) gender causes sex, that is, women as a marked gender group constitute the locus of sexuality, sexual desire and motivation. Reproduction and its organization become the prime movers in all other male/female differentiation and in the flowering of the gender system. Gender and sexuality are seamlessly knit together.

Finally, the cultural-influence model assumes that sexual acts carry stable and universal significance in terms of identity and subjective meaning. The literature routinely regards opposite-gender sexual contact as 'heterosexuality' and same-gender contact as 'homosexuality', as if the same phenomena were being observed in all societies in which these acts occurred. With hindsight, these assumptions are curiously ethnocentric, since the meanings attached to these sexual behaviours are those of the observers and twentieth-century complex, industrial society. Cross-cultural surveys could fairly chart the distribution of same- or opposite-gender sexual contact or the frequency of sexual contact before marriage. But when investigators report instead on the presence or absence of 'homosexuality' or 'sexual permissiveness', they engage in a spurious translation from sexual act or behaviour to sexual meaning and identity, something later theoretical developments would come to reject.

To summarize, the cultural-influence model recognizes variations in the occurrence of sexual behaviour and in cultural attitudes that encourage or restrict behaviour, but not in the meaning of the behaviour itself. In addition, anthropologists working within this framework accept without question the existence of universal categories such as heterosexual and homo-sexual, male and female sexuality, and sex drive.

Despite these many deficiencies, it is important to recognize the strengths of this approach, particularly in its intellectual, historical and political context. Anthropology's commitment to cross-cultural comparison made it the most relativistic of social science disciplines in regard to the study of sexuality. Its finding of variation called into question prevailing notions about the inevitability or naturalness of sexual norms and behaviour common in America and Europe, and the connection between sexual regulation and social or familial stability. The variability it reported suggested that human sexuality was malleable and capable of assuming different forms. Work in the cultural-influence tradition undercut more mechanistic theories of sexual behaviour, still common in medicine and psychiatry, that suggested sexuality was largely a function of physiological functioning or instinctual drives. It began to develop social and intellectual space in which it was possible to regard sexuality as something other than a simple function of biology.

Although work in the cultural-influence model contributed to the development of social-construction theory, there is a sharp break between them in many respects. This difference has not been recognized by many anthropologists still working within the cultural-influence tradition. Indeed, many mistakenly seem to regard these new developments as theoretically compatible, even continuous with earlier work. Some have assimilated terms or phrases (such as 'social construction' or 'cultural construction') in their work, yet their analytic frames still contain many unexamined essentialist elements.[4] It is not the case that the cultural-influence model, because it recognizes cultural variation, is the same as social-construction theory. The cultural-influence model, then, no longer remains the only anthropological paradigm, although it still dominates contemporary work (Frayser, 1985; Mascia-Lees, 1989).

It would seem that the development of anthropology in this century – a general movement away from biologized frameworks toward perspectives that are denaturalizing and anti-essentialist – would foster the application of social-construction theory to the study of sexu-ality. Despite its challenge to the natural and universalized status of many domains, however, anthropology has largely excluded sexuality from this endeavour of suggesting that human actions have been and continue to be subject to historical and cultural forces and, thus, to change.

A social-construction approach to sexuality would examine the range of behaviour, ideology and subjective meaning among and within human groups, and would view the body, its functions and sensations as potentials (and limits) that are incorporated and mediated by culture. The physiology of orgasm and penile erection no more explains a culture's sexual schema than the auditory range of the human ear explains its music. Biology and physio-logical functioning are determinative only at the most extreme limits, and there to set the boundary of what is physically possible. The more interesting question for anthropological research on sexuality is to chart what is culturally possible – a far more expansive domain. Ecological adaptation and reproductive demands similarly explain only a small portion of sexual organization, since fertility adequate for replacement and even growth is relatively easy for most groups to achieve. More important, sexuality is not coterminous with or equiva-lent to reproduction: reproductive sexuality constitutes a small portion of the larger sexual universe.

In addition, a social-construction approach to sexuality must also problematize and ques-tion Euro-American folk and scientific beliefs about sexuality, rather than project them onto other groups in a manner that would be most unacceptably ethnocentric in any other subject area. Thus, statements about the universally compelling force of sexual impulse, the importance of sexuality in human life, the universally private status of sexual behaviour, or its quintessentially reproductive nature need to be presented as hypotheses, not *a priori* assumptions. Anthropology seems especially well suited to problematize these most naturalized categories, yet sexuality has been the last domain (trailing even gender) to have its natural, biologized status called into question. For many of us, essentialism was our first way of thinking about sexuality and still remains hegemonic.

Social-construction theory offers a radically different perspective in the study of sexuality, encouraging novel and fruitful research questions. Its influence has been increasing in anthropology (see Newton, 1979; Whitehead, 1981; Carrier, 1985; Fry, 1985; Blackwood, 1986; Caplan, 1987; Davis and Kennedy, 1989; Vance, 1990; Parker, 1991), although cultural-influence models still dominate (see Frayser, 1985; Gregor, 1985; Cohen and Mascia-Lees, 1989; Frayser, 1989; Mascia-Lees, Tierson and Relethford, 1989; Perper, 1989). One might have predicted a gradually intensifying competition between paradigms, possibly even a paradigm shift. The appearance of AIDS, however, has altered this dynamic.

AIDS and research on sexuality

The great concern about AIDS has dramatically increased the interest in conducting and funding sex research. Early in the epidemic, epidemiologists routinely began to include batteries of questions concerning the frequency and nature of their subjects' sexual behaviour. Their problems in measurement and conceptualization, as well as their futile search for baseline data, highlighted the scientific neglect of sex research. Indeed, the fact no large-scale study on American sexual habits has been conducted since the Kinsey volumes (Kinsey, Pomeroy and Martin, 1948; Kinsey, Pomeroy, Martin and Gebhard, 1953) now stands as a major embarrassment, resulting in our inability to answer even the most basic questions. As scientific groups and policy-makers recognized the need for this information, they strongly recommended drastic increases in funding and research efforts in affected countries (Booth, 1989a, 1989b; Turner, Miller and Moses, 1989). Although in many ways a positive and necessary step, the rush to funding nevertheless raises the possibility that the inadequate essentialist and cultural-influence models of sexuality will be revived and strengthened.

AIDS encourages the resurgence of biomedical approaches to sexuality through the repeated association of sexuality with disease. The medicalization of sexuality is intensifying, as the public turns to medical authorities for sexual information and advice. In addition, biomedical investigators in medical schools and schools of public health are conducting a significant portion of AIDS-related research in sexuality.[5] This signals a shift from a general trend developing after World War Two, when research on sexuality increasingly moved out of medical arenas. Thus, medicine's interest in sexuality is expanding to new areas beyond the specialties to which it was traditionally confined: sexually transmitted diseases, obstetrics and gynaecology, and psychiatry.

This development poses several dangers. Biomedical approaches to sexuality often regard sexuality as derivative from physiology and supposedly universal functioning of the body. Biomedical models tend to be the most unreflective about the influence of science and medical practice in constructing categories such as 'the body' and 'health'. Social-construction approaches are virtually unknown, and the concept that sexuality varies with culture and history is expressed at best via primitive cultural-influence models. There is limited recognition that sexuality has a history and that its definitions and meanings change over time and within populations. The reliance on survey instruments and easily quantified data in biomedically based research increases the tendency to count acts rather than explore meaning.

Such surveys have frequently equated sexual identities with sexual acts, for example, and treated 'gay men' and 'heterosexuals' as unproblematic categories. In addition, the high status of medical practitioners in the twentieth century and their recruitment from privileged class, gender and racial groups has resulted historically in their close alliances with dominant ideologies, including the sexual. Should this pattern persist, they are as unlikely to be aware of marginal sexual subcultures and sensibilities as they are to be sensitive to them.

Framing sexual research within a biomedical model and the perspective of disease also threatens to re-pathologize sexuality. This promises to return sexuality to the position it occupied in the late nineteenth and early twentieth centuries, where its public discussion was largely motivated and circumscribed by the discourses of venereal disease, prostitution and masturbation. These public discussions framed by medical experts, ostensibly about health and disease, were implicitly discussions about morality, gender and social order. This danger is heightened by the respect accorded medicine and science and the widespread public belief that science contains no values. The expansion of a supposedly objective and value-free discourse about sexuality organized under the guise of health opens the door to vastly increased governmental and professional intervention.

The emphasis placed on gay men and their sexual behaviour in the early stages of the epidemic constitutes a sharp departure from previous inattention to subordinate sexual groups. This attention, however, highlights their otherness in a manner reminiscent of nineteenth-century pathology models of homosexuality (Gever, 1989), emphasizing the naturalness of identity and reinforcing the sharp dichotomy between heterosexuality and homosexuality. This otherness is expanding to involve additional stigmatized groups at risk for AIDS, such as IV drug users, their partners, and inner-city minority women, drawing on historically and culturally resonant stereotypes (Gilman, 1988).

The danger posed by increased funding for research on sexuality connected with AIDS is not restricted to biomedicine. Within anthropology, it is unlikely that essentialist models will make a comeback; however, the field may well experience the impact of increasingly biomedical approaches to sexuality in interdisciplinary work conducted in medical settings. More important, increased funding and urgent calls for research are likely to strengthen cultural-influence models of sexuality, as more and more anthropologists will be drawn into work on AIDS (Feldman and Johnson, 1986; Gorman, 1986; Bateson and Goldsby, 1988; Bolton, 1989; Marshall and Bennett, 1990).

Most of these are likely to be medical anthropologists or specialists in affected geographic areas without specialized training in sexuality. As anthropologists, they can be relied on to bring with them an expectation of human diversity, sensitivity to ethnocentrism, and a respect for the role of culture in shaping behaviour, sexuality included. But this is precisely the problem, as these perspectives will reinvent the cultural-influence model as the common-sense, anthropological approach to sexuality. Anthropologists new to sex research may easily think that, because it allows for cultural variation, their own cultural-influence approach is identical to social-construction theory. Their own comparisons with work done from more biologized, biomedical approaches, particularly in non-Western cultures, will make cultural-influence models seem advanced, even cause for self-congratulation.

In all fields, the belated recognition of serious gaps in knowledge about sexual behaviour may emphasize the importance of behavioural data, which appear more easily measured than fantasy, identity and subjective meaning. Behavioural data lend themselves to easy quantification, fitting into the methodological biases of positivist social science. Amid an epidemic, researchers press for rapid results and reject the time, patience and tolerance for uncertainty that ethnographic and deconstructive techniques seem to require.

Despite these tendencies that reinforce cultural-influence and biologized approaches, the picture remains complex and contradictory. AIDS-inspired investigations into the realities of people's sexual worlds have already disclosed discrepancies between ideologies about sexuality and lived experience. Contradictions increase exponentially in other cultural contexts. These gaps exist in many areas, but are particularly insistent in regard to classificatory systems, identity, congruence between behaviour and self-definition, the meaning of sexual acts, and the stability of sexual preference. These inconsistencies point to the usefulness of social-construction theory and have spurred new work in anthropology (see Parker, 1987; Carrier, 1989; Murray and Payne, 1989; Asencio, 1990; Hawkeswood, 1990; Kane, 1990; Singer *et al.*, 1990). Much as was the case with early gay history, researchers in sexuality and AIDS may confront the limitations of their models, generating provocative and imaginative work.

Moreover, the entire phenomenon of 'safer sex' has emphasized the culturally malleable aspects of sexual behaviour. The safer sex campaign mounted by the gay community, surely one of the most dramatic and effective public health campaigns on record, made clear that sexual acts can only be understood within a cultural and subcultural context and that careful attention to meaning and symbolism allows the possibility of change even for adults (Patton, 1985; Altman, 1986; Watney, 1987; Crimp, 1989). The self-conscious leadership and participation of gay men, as opposed to biomedical experts, in this endeavour suggests that individuals actively participate in creating and changing cultural and erotic meanings, particularly when they have a stake in doing so. Safer sex campaigns reveal active sexual agents with an awareness of their symbolic universe and an ability to manipulate and re-create it, rather than passively receive a static sexual enculturation.

The political and symbolic mobilizations around the sexual dimensions and meanings of AIDS on the part of many different constituencies also belie the notion that sexuality and its meaning are derived simply from the body, unchanging or easily read. Yet various groups proffer their interpretations of AIDS and its sexual significance as lessons to be read from nature and the body (Patton, 1985; Altman, 1986; Treichler, 1987; Watney, 1987; Treichler, 1988; Gilman, 1989; Grover, 1989; Watney, 1989; Williamson, 1989; Juhasz, 1990). The multiplicity of competing lessons and the ferocious struggle for whose interpretation will prevail suggest that sexual meaning is a hotly contested, even political terrain. That dominant sectors, particularly the state, religion and the professional groups, exercise a disproportionate influence on the sexual discourse does not mean that their views are hegemonic or unchallenged by other groups. Nor does it mean that marginal groups only respond reactively and do not create their own subcultures and worlds of meaning.

In the midst of the creation of new discourses about sexuality, it is crucial that we become conscious of how these discourses are created and our own role in creating them. Anthropologists have a great deal to contribute to research in sexuality. The new situation brought about by AIDS in regard to sex research is filled with possibilities: to build on the challenging questions social-construction theory has raised, or to fall back onto cultural-influence and essentialist models. The stakes are not low – for research in sexuality, for applied work in AIDS education and prevention, for sexual politics, for human lives. If this is a moment in which anthropology 'rediscovers' sex, we need to consider two questions: who will do the looking? And more to the point, what will we be able to see? We need to be explicit about our theoretical models, mindful of their history, and self-conscious about our practice.

Acknowledgements

I would like to thank Frances M. Doughty for helpful conversations, invaluable editorial suggestions, and generous encouragement. I am appreciative of Shirley Lindenbaum's comments, patience and enthusiasm. Thanks also to Lisa Duggan, Gayle Rubin, David Schwartz, Gilbert Zicklin, Jonathan Katz, Janice Irvine, Ann Snitow, Nan Hunter, Jennifer Terry, Jacqueline Urla, Libbett Crandon, William Hawkeswood, Jeanne Bergman, Faye Ginsburg, and the anonymous reviewers from *Social Science and Medicine* for their comments. Thanks to Pamela Brown-Peterside for research assistance.

This paper was presented at the panel 'Anthropology Rediscovers Sex' at the 1988 annual meeting of the American Anthropological Association. Thanks to the convener, Shirley Lindenbaum, and participants for a lively dialogue. I also benefited from comments made by the members of the Medical Anthropology Colloquium at Columbia University. The responsibility for views expressed in this paper remains mine.

Notes

1 This resistance can have paradoxical effects, to judge from personal experience. My own grant application in 1977 to complete a conventional annotated anthropological bibliography on biocultural influences on sexuality was rejected on the grounds that the investigator 'was too young to engage in research on this topic' and, being unable to read Japanese, 'could not read the important new literature on Japanese macaques in the original'. Far from being discouraging, these comments piqued my interest all the more, since it appeared that anthropologists' volatile reactions deserved scrutiny at least as much as the cross-cultural material.

2 There is no suggestion here that the most radical forms of social-construction theory are necessarily the best, although the exercise of totally deconstructing one of the most essential categories, sexuality, often has an electrifying and energizing effect on one's thinking. Whether this degree of deconstruction can be plausibly maintained is another question.

3 Heider's work on the Dani is an exception in regard to conceptualizing variable levels of sexual energy.

4 A different attempt at assimilation is found in the assertion that the debate between essentialists and social constructionists in regard to sexuality is a replay of the nature–nurture controversy. This is a profound misunderstanding of social construction theory. In nature–nurture debates, researchers are proposing alternative biological or cultural mechanisms to explain phenomena they observe. At present, most observers agree that human behaviour is produced by a complex interaction of biological and cultural factors; they differ on the relative weight they assign to each. Although it might be appropriate to find some similarity between essentialists and the nature camp, to equate social construction to the nurture camp is mistaken. Social construction theory is not simply arguing for cultural causation. In addition, and more important, it encourages us to deconstruct and examine the behaviour or processes that both nature and nurture camps have reified and want to 'explain'. Social construction suggests that the object of study deserves at least as much analytic attention as the suspected causal mechanism.

5 This is not to say that research is not also being conducted by social scientists outside of medical institutions or that social scientists do not also contribute to studies based in medical schools, albeit usually in a lesser role. However, the sheer number of biomedically oriented population surveys coupled with their large sample sizes and budgets threatens to overshadow and displace sexuality research conducted by less biomedically oriented investigators. In addition, medical doctors are perceived to speak more authoritatively than social scientists about the body. Given this, increasingly essentialist perspectives that frame sexuality in relation to AIDS as a bodily matter will automatically increase the legitimacy of medical speakers and texts.

References

ALTMAN, D. (1986) *AIDS in the Mind of America: The Social, Political, and Psychological Impact of a New Epidemic*, New York: Anchor Press/Doubleday.

—— *et al.* (eds) (1989) *Homosexuality, Which Homosexuality?*, Amsterdam: An Dekker/Schorer.

ASENCIO, M. (1990) 'Puerto Rican adolescents playing by the rules', unpublished paper presented at the Annual Meeting of the American Anthropological Association.

ATKINSON, J.M. (1982) 'Anthropology: a review essay', *Signs*, 8, pp. 236–58.

BARKER-BENFIELD, G.J. (1976) *The Horrors of the Half-Known Life*, New York: Harper and Row.

BATESON, G. (1947) 'Sex and culture', *Annual New York Academy of Sciences*, XLVII, p. 647.

BATESON, M.C. and GOLDSBY, R. (1988) *Thinking AIDS: The Social Response to Biological Threat*, Reading, MA: Addison-Wesley.

BERNDT, R.M. and BERNDT, C. (1951) *Sexual Behaviour in Western Arnhem Land*, New York: Viking Fund.

BLACKWOOD, E. (ed.) (1986) *Anthropology and Homosexuality*, New York: Haworth Press.

BLEIER, R. (1984) *Science and Gender: A Critique of Biology and its Theories on Women*, New York: Pergamon Press.

BOLTON, R. (1989) 'The AIDS pandemic: a global emergency', *Medical Anthropology*, 10 (special issue), pp. 1–12.

BOOTH, W. (1989a) 'Asking America about its sex life', *Science*, 242, 20 January, p. 304.

—— (1989b) 'WHO seeks global data on sexual practices', *Science*, 244, 28 April, p. 418.

BRANDT, A.M. (1985) *No Magic Bullet: A Social History of Venereal Disease in the United States since 1880*, New York: Oxford University Press.

BRAY, A. (1982) *Homosexuality in Renaissance England*, London: Gay Men's Press.

BRISTOW, E.J. (1977) *Vice and Vigilance: Purity Movements in Britain since 1700*, New Jersey: Rowman and Littlefield.

BROUDE, G.J. and GREENE, S.J. (1976) 'Cross-cultural codes on twenty sexual attitudes and practices', *Ethnology*, 15, pp. 409–29.

CAPLAN, P. (ed.) (1987) *The Cultural Construction of Sexuality*, London: Tavistock.

CARRIER, J.M. (1985) 'Mexican male bisexuality', *Journal of Homosexuality*, 11, pp. 75–85.

—— (1989) 'Sexual behaviour and the spread of AIDS in Mexico', *Medical Anthropology*, 10, pp. 129–42.

COHEN, C.B. and MASCIA-LEES, F.E. (1989) 'Lasers in the jungle: reconfiguring questions of human and non-human primate sexuality', *Medical Anthropology*, 11, p. 351.

CRIMP, D. (ed.) (1989) *AIDS: Cultural Analysis, Cultural Activism*, Cambridge, MA: MIT Press.

DAVENPORT, W. (1965) 'Sexual patterns and their regulation in a society of the south west Pacific', in BEACH, F. (ed.) *Sex and Behaviour*, New York: Wiley.

DAVIS, D.L. and WHITTEN, R.G. (1987) 'The cross-cultural study of human sexuality', *Annual Review of Anthropology*, 16, pp. 69–98.

DAVIS, M. and KENNEDY, E. (1986) 'Oral history and the study of sexuality in the lesbian community: Buffalo, New York, 1940–60', *Feminist Studies*, 12, pp. 7–26.

—— (1989) 'The reproduction of butch-femme roles: a social constructionist approach', in PEISS, C. and SIMMONS, C. (eds) *Passion and Power: Sexuality in History*, Philadelphia: Temple University Press.

D'EMILIO, J. (1983) *Sexual Politics, Sexual Communities*, Chicago: University of Chicago Press.

—— and FREEDMAN, E.B. (1988) *Intimate Matters: A Social History of Sexuality in America*, New York: Harper and Row.

DUBERMAN, M.B., VICINUS, M. and CHAUNCEY, G. (eds) (1989) *Hidden from History: Reclaiming the Gay and Lesbian Past*, New York: New American Library.

DUGGAN, L. (1990) 'From instincts to politics: writing the history of sexuality in the US', *Journal of Sex Research*, 27, pp. 95–110.

EHRENREICH, B. and ENGLISH, D. (1979) *For Her Own Good: 150 Years of Experts' Advice to Women*, New York: Doubleday.

FADERMAN, L. (1981) *Surpassing the Love of Men*, New York: Morrow.

FAUSTO-STERLING, A. (1985) *Myths of Gender: Biological Theories about Women and Men*, New York: Basic Books.

FELDMAN, D.A. and JOHNSON, T.M. (eds) (1986) *The Social Dimension of AIDS: Method and Theory*, New York: Praeger.

FISHER, L. (1980) 'Relationships and sexuality in contexts and culture', in WOLMAN, B.B. and MONEY, J. (eds) *Handbook of Sexuality*, Englewood Cliffs, NJ: Prentice Hall.

FORD, C.S. and BEACH, F.A. (1951) *Patterns of Sexual Behaviour*, New York: Harper and Row.

FOUCAULT, M. (1978) *The History of Sexuality, volume I: An Introduction*, New York: Pantheon.

FRAYSER, S.G. (1985) *Varieties of Sexual Experience: An Anthropological Perspective on Human Sexuality*, New Haven, CT: HRAF Press.

—— (1989) 'Sexual and reproductive relationships: cross-cultural evidence and biosocial implications', *Medical Anthropology*, 11, pp. 385–408.

FRY, P. (1985) 'Male homosexuality and spirit possession in Brazil', *Journal of Homosexuality*, 11, pp. 137–53.

GAGNON, J.H. and SIMON, W. (1973) *Sexual Conduct: The Social Sources of Human Sexuality*, Chicago: Aldine.

GEBHARD, P.H. (1976) 'Human sexual behaviour: a summary statement', in GORDON, C. and JOHNSON, G. (eds) *Readings in Human Sexuality: Contemporary Perspectives*, New York: Harper and Row.

GERARD, K. and HEKMA, G. (eds) (1988) 'The pursuit of sodomy: male homosexuality in renaissance and enlightenment Europe', *Journal of Homosexuality*, 16 [special issue].

GEVER, M. (1989) 'Pictures of sickness: Stuart Marshall's bright eyes', in CRIMP, D. (ed.) *AIDS: Cultural Analysis, Cultural Activism*, Cambridge, MA: MIT Press.

GILMAN, S. (1988) *Disease and Representation: Images of Illness from Madness to AIDS*, Ithaca, NY: Cornell University Press.

—— (1989) 'AIDS and syphilis: the iconography of disease', in CRIMP, D. (ed.) *AIDS: Cultural Analysis, Cultural Activism*, Cambridge, MA: MIT Press.

GOLDENWEISER, A. (1929) 'Sex and primitive society', in CALVERTON, V.F. and SCHMALHAUNSEN, S.D. (eds) *Sex in Civilization*, New York: Macaulay Company.

GOODENOUGH, W.H. (1949) 'Premarital freedom on Truk: theory and practice', *American Anthropologist*, 51, pp. 615–20.

GORDON, L. (1974) *Woman's Body, Woman's Right: A Social History of Birth Control in America*, New York: Penguin.

GORMAN, E.M. (1986) 'The AIDS epidemic in San Francisco: epidemiological and anthropological perspectives', in JANES, C., STALL, R. and GIFFORD, S. (eds) *Anthropology and Epidemiology*, Dordrecht: Reidel.

GRAY, J.P. (1980) 'Cross-cultural factors associated with sexual foreplay', *Social Psychology*, 111, 3.

GREGOR, T. (1985) *Anxious Pleasures: The Sexual Lives of an Amazonian People*, Chicago: University of Chicago Press.

GROVER, J.Z. (1989) 'AIDS: keywords', in CRIMP, D. (ed.) *AIDS: Cultural Analysis, Cultural Activism*, Cambridge, MA: MIT Press.

HARAWAY, D. (1989) *Primate Visions: Gender, Race and Nature in the World of Modern Science*, New York: Routledge.

HARDING, S. (1986) *The Science Question in Feminism*, Ithaca, NY: Cornell University Press.

—— and HINTIKKA, M. (eds) (1983) *Discovering Reality: Feminist Perspectives on Epistemology, Metaphysics, Methodology and Philosophy of Science*, Dordrecht: Reidel.

HAWKESWOOD, W.G. (1990) 'I'm a black gay man who just happens to be gay: the sexuality of black gay men', unpublished paper presented at the Annual Meeting of the American Anthropological Association.

HEIDER, K.G. (1976) 'Dani sexuality: a low-energy system', *Man*, 11, pp. 188–201.

HERDT, G. (1981) *Guardians of the Flutes*, New York: McGraw Hill.

—— (1984) 'Semen transaction in Sambia culture', in HERDT, G. (ed.) *Ritualized Homosexuality in Melanesia*, Berkeley: University of California Press.

—— (1987) *The Sambia: Ritual and Gender in New Guinea*, New York: Holt, Rinehart, Winston.

HONIGMAN, J.J. (1954) 'An anthropological approach to sex', *Social Problems*, 2, pp. 7–16.

HOWARD, A. and HOWARD, I. (1964) 'Premarital sex and social control among the Rotumans', *American Anthropologist*, 66, p. 266.

HUBBARD, R., HENIFIN, M.S. and FRIED, B. (eds) (1982) *Biological Woman: The Convenient Myth*, Cambridge, MA: Schenkman.

IRVINE, J. (1990) *Disorders of Desire*, Philadelphia: Temple University Press.

JORDANOVA, L.J. (1989) *Sexual Visions: Images of Gender in Science and Medicine between the Eighteenth and Twentieth Centuries*, Madison: University of Wisconsin Press.

JUHASZ, A. (1990) 'The contained threat: women in mainstream AIDS documentary', *Journal of Sex Research*, 27, pp. 25–46.

KANE, S. (1990) 'AIDS, addiction and condom use: sources of sexual risk for heterosexual women', *Journal of Sex Research*, 27, pp. 427–44.

KATZ, J. (1976) *Gay American History*, New York: Crowell.

—— (1983) *Gay/Lesbian Almanac*, New York: Harper and Row.

—— (1990) 'The invention of heterosexuality', *Socialist Review*, 20, pp. 7–34.

KELLER, E.F. (1984) *Reflections on Gender and Science*, New Haven, CT: Yale University Press.

KENDRICK, W. (1987) *The Secret Museum*, New York: Viking.

KINSEY, A., POMEROY, W. and MARTIN, C.E. (1948) *Sexual Behavior in the Human Male*, Philadelphia, PA: Saunders.

——, POMEROY, W., MARTIN, C.E. and GEBHARD, R.H. (1953) *Sexual Behavior in the Human Female*, Philadelphia, PA: Saunders.

LAMPHERE, L. (1977) 'Anthropology: a review essay', *Signs*, 2(3), pp. 612–27.

LESSA, W.A. (1966) 'Sexual behaviour', in *Ulithi: A Design for Living*, New York: Holt, Rinehart, Winston.

LEVINE, R.A. (1959) 'Gusii sex offenses: a study in social control', *American Anthropologist*, 61, pp. 965–90.

LOWE, M. and HUBBARD, R. (1983) *Women's Nature: Rationalizations of Inequality*, New York: Pergamon Press.

MCINTOSH, M. (1968) 'The homosexual role', *Social Problems*, 16, pp. 182–92.

MALINOWSKI, B. (1941 [1929 orig.]) *The Sexual Life of Savages in North-Western Melanesia*, New York: Halcyon House.

MARSHALL, D.S. (1976) 'Too much in Mangaia', in GORDON, C. and JOHNSON, G. (eds) *Readings in Human Sexuality: Contemporary Perspectives*, New York: Holt, Rinehart, Winston.

—— and SUGGS, R.C. (eds) (1972) *Human Sexual Behaviour*, Englewood Cliffs, NJ: Prentice Hall.

MARSHALL, P.A. and BENNETT, L.A. (eds) (1990) 'Culture and behaviour in the AIDS epidemic', *Medical Anthropology Quarterly*, 4 [special issue], pp. 1–3.

MASCIA-LEES, F.E. (ed.) (1989) 'Human sexuality in biocultural perspective', *Medical Anthropology*, 11 [special issue].

——, TIERSON, F.D. and RELETHFORD, J.H. (1989) 'Investigating the biocultural dimensions of human sexual behaviour', *Medical Anthropology*, 11, pp. 367–80.

MEAD, M. (1923) *Coming of Age in Samoa*, New York: Morrow.

—— (1961) 'Cultural determinants of sexual behaviours', in YOUNG, W.C. (ed.) *Sex and Internal Secretions*, Philadelphia, PA: Williams and Wilkins.

MINTURN, L., GROSSE, M. and HAIDER, S. (1969) 'Culture patterning of sexual beliefs and behaviour', *Ethnology*, 8, pp. 301–18.

MOORE, H.L. (1988) *Feminism and Anthropology*, Minneapolis: University of Minnesota Press.

MURDOCK, G.P. (1949) 'The social regulation of sexual behaviour', in HOCH, P.H. and ZUBIN, J. (eds) *Psychosexual Development in Health and Disease*, New York: Grune and Straton.

MURRAY, S.O. and PAYNE, K. (1989) 'The social classification of AIDS in American epidemiology', *Medical Anthropology*, 10, pp. 115–28.

NEWTON, E. (1979) *Mother Camp: Female Impersonators in America*, Chicago: University of Chicago Press.

—— (1984) 'The mythic mannish lesbian: Radclyffe Hall and the new woman', *Signs*, 9, pp. 557–75.

PADGUG, R.A. (1979) 'Sexual matters: on conceptualizing sexuality in history', *Radical History Review*, 20, pp. 3–23.

PARKER, R. (1987) 'Acquired immunodeficiency syndrome in urban Brazil', *Medical Anthropology Quarterly*, 1, pp. 155–75.

—— (1991) *Bodies, Pleasures, and Passions: Sexual Culture in Contemporary Brazil*, Boston, MA: Beacon Press.

PATTON, C. (1985) *Sex and Germs*, Boston, MA: South End Press.

PEISS, C. (1986) *Cheap Amusements: Working Women and Leisure in Turn-of-the-Century New York*, Philadelphia: Temple University Press.

—— (1989) 'Charity girls and city pleasures: historical notes on working class sexuality, 1880–1920', in PEISS, C. and SIMMONS, C. (eds) *Passion and Power: Sexuality in History*, Philadelphia: Temple University Press.

—— and SIMMONS, C. (eds) (1989) *Passion and Power: Sexuality in History*, Philadelphia: Temple University Press.

PERPER, T. (1989) 'Theories and observations: sexual selection and female choice in human beings', *Medical Anthropology*, 11, pp. 409–54.

PIVAR, D. (1972) *1868–1900, Purity Crusade: Sexual Morality and Social Control*, Westport, CT: Greenwood Press.

PLUMMER, K. (ed.) (1981) *The Making of the Modern Homosexual*, London: Hutchinson.

—— (1982) 'Symbolic interactionism and sexual conduct: an emergent perspective', in BRAKE, M. (ed.) *Human Sexual Relations*, New York: Pantheon.

RAPP, R. (1979) 'Anthropology: a review essay', *Signs*, 4, pp. 497–513.

REITER, R. (ed.) (1975) *Toward an Anthropology of Women*, New York: Monthly Review Press.

ROSALDO, M.Z. and LAMPHERE, L. (eds) (1974) *Women, Culture and Society*, Stanford, CA: Stanford University Press.

RUBIN, G. (1975) 'The traffic in women: notes on the "political economy" of sex', in REITER, R. (ed.) *Toward an Anthropology of Women*, New York: Monthly Review Press.

—— (1979) 'Introduction', in VIVIER, R., *A Woman Appeared to Me*, Weatherby Lake: Naiad Press.

—— (1984) 'Thinking sex: notes for a radical theory in the politics of sexuality', in VANCE, C.S. (ed.) *Pleasure and Danger Exploring Female Sexuality*, New York: Routledge and Kegan Paul.

RUPP, L. (1980) '"Imagine my surprise": women's relationships in mid-twentieth century America', *Frontiers*, 5,

SAHLI, N. (1979) 'Smashing: women's relationships before the fall', *Chrysalis*, 8(17), [n.p.n.].

SAYERS, J. (1982) *Biological Politics: Feminist and Anti-Feminist Perspectives*, New York: Tavistock.

SCHAPERA, I. (1941) *Married Life in an African Tribe*, New York: Sheridan House.

SCHIEBINGER, L. (1989) *The Mind Has No Sex: Women in the Origin of Modern Science*, Cambridge, MA: Harvard University Press.

SINGER, M., FLORES, C., DAVISON, L., BURKE, G., CASTILLO, Z., SCANLON, K. and RIVERA, M. (1990) 'SIDA: the economic, social and cultural context of AIDS among Latinos', *Medical Anthropology Quarterly*, 4, pp. 72–114.

SNITOW, A., STANSELL, C. and THOMPSON, S. (eds) (1983) *Powers of Desire*, New York: Monthly Review Press.

STANSELL, C. (1986) *City of Women: Sex and Class in New York, 1789–1860*, New York: Knopf.

SUGGS, R.C. (1966) *Marquesan Sexual Behaviour*, New York: Harcourt, Brace and World.

TOBACH, E. and ROSOFT, B. (eds) (1978) *Genes and Gender*, Vols 1–4, New York: Gordian Press.

TREICHLER, P.A. (1987) 'AIDS, homophobia and biomedical discourse: an epidemic of signification', in CRIMP, D. (ed.) *AIDS: Cultural Analysis, Cultural Activism*, Cambridge, MA: MIT Press.

—— (1988) 'AIDS, gender, and biomedical discourse: current contests for meaning', in FEE, E. and FOX, D.M. (eds) *AIDS: The Burden of History*, Berkeley: University of California Press.

TRIMBERGER, E.K. (1983) 'Feminism, men and modern love: Greenwich Village, 1900–1925', in SNITOW, A., STANSELL, C. and THOMPSON, S. (eds) *Powers of Desire*, New York: Monthly Review Press.

TURNER, C.E., MILLER, H.G. and MOSES, L.E. (eds) (1989) *AIDS: Sexual Behaviour and Intravenous Drug Use*, Washington, DC: National Academy Press.

VANCE, C.S. (1983) 'Gender systems, ideology and sex research', in SNITOW, A., STANSELL, C. and THOMPSON, S. (eds) *Powers of Desire*, New York: Monthly Review Press.

—— (ed.) (1984) *Pleasure and Danger: Exploring Female Sexuality*, New York: Routledge and Kegan Paul.

—— (1990) 'Negotiating sex and gender in the Attorney General's commission on pornography', in GINSBURG, F. and TSING, A.L. (eds) *Uncertain Terms: Negotiating Gender in American Culture*, Boston, MA: Beacon Press.

VICINUS, M. (1989) '"They wonder to which sex I belong": the historical roots of the modern lesbian identity', in ALTMAN, D. *et al.* (eds) *Homosexuality, Which Homosexuality?*, Amsterdam: An Dekker/Schorer.

WALKOWITZ, J.R. (1980) *Prostitution and Victorian Society: Women, Class, and the State*, Cambridge: Cambridge University Press.

WATNEY, S. (1987) *Policing Desire: Pornography, AIDS and the Media*, Minneapolis: University of Minnesota Press.

—— (1989) 'The spectacle of AIDS', in CRIMP, D. (ed.) *AIDS: Cultural Analysis, Cultural Activism*, Cambridge, MA: MIT Press.

WEEKS, J. (1977) *Coming Out: Homosexual Politics in Britain from the 19th Century to the Present*, London: Quartet Books.

—— (1981) *Sex, Politics and Society: The Regulation of Sexuality Since 1800*, New York: Longman.

—— (1986) *Sexuality*, London: Tavistock.

WHITEHEAD, H. (1981) 'The bow and the burden strap: a new look at institutionalized homosexuality in native North America', in ORTNER, S.B. and WHITEHEAD, H. (eds) *Sexual Meanings*, Cambridge: Cambridge University Press.

WILLIAMSON, J. (1989) 'Every virus tells a story: the meanings of HIV and AIDS', in CARTER, E. and WATNEY, S. (eds) *Taking Liberties: AIDS and Cultural Politics*, London: Serpent's Tail.

Part 2

Gender and power

5 Gender as a useful category of historical analysis

Joan Wallach Scott [1986]

Gender, n. a grammatical term only. To talk of persons or creatures of the masculine or feminine gender, meaning of the male or female sex, is either a jocularity (permissible or not
according to context) or a blunder.

(Fowler's *Dictionary of Modern English Usage*)

Those who would codify the meanings of words fight a losing battle, for words, like the ideas
and things they are meant to signify, have a history. Neither Oxford dons nor the Académie
Française has been entirely able to stem the tide, to capture and fix meanings free of the play
of human invention and imagination. Mary Wortley Montagu added bite to her witty denunciation 'of the fair sex' ('my only consolation for being of that gender has been the assurance of
never being married to any one among them') by deliberately misusing the grammatical reference.[1] Through the ages, people have made figurative allusions by employing grammatical
terms to evoke traits of character or sexuality. For example, the usage offered by the
Dictionnaire de la Langue Française in 1876 was: 'On ne sait de quel genre il est, s'il est
mâle ou femelle, se dit d'un homme très-caché, dont on ne connait pas les sentiments' (Littré,
1876). And Gladstone made this distinction in 1878: 'Athene has nothing of sex except the
gender, nothing of the woman except the form' (Williams, 1983, p. 285). Most recently – too
recently to find its way into dictionaries or the *Encyclopedia of the Social Sciences* – feminists
have in a more literal and serious vein begun to use 'gender' as a way of referring to the social
organization of the relationship between the sexes. The connection to grammar is both
explicit and full of unexamined possibilities. Explicit because the grammatical usage
involves formal rules that follow from the masculine or feminine designation; full of unexamined possibilities because in many Indo-European languages there is a third category –
unsexed or neuter. In grammar, gender is understood to be a way of classifying phenomena, a
socially agreed upon system of distinctions rather than an objective description of inherent
traits. In addition, classifications suggest a relationship among categories that makes distinctions or separate groupings possible.

In its most recent usage, 'gender' seems to have first appeared among American feminists
who wanted to insist on the fundamentally social quality of distinctions based on sex. The
word denoted a rejection of the biological determinism implicit in the use of such terms as
'sex' or 'sexual difference'. 'Gender' also stressed the relational aspect of normative definitions of femininity. Those who worried that women's studies scholarships focused too
narrowly and separately on women used the term 'gender' to introduce a relational notion
into our analytic vocabulary. According to this view, women and men were defined in terms
of one another, and no understanding of either could be achieved by entirely separate study.

Thus Natalie Davis suggested in 1975, 'It seems to me that we should be interested in the history of both women and men, that we should not be working only on the subjected sex any more than a historian of class can focus entirely on peasants. Our goal is to understand the significance of the sexes, of gender groups in the historical past. Our goal is to discover the range in sex roles and in sexual symbolism in different societies and periods, to find out what meaning they had and how they functioned to maintain the social order or to promote its change' (Davis, 1975–76).

In addition, and perhaps most important, 'gender' was a term offered by those who claimed that women's scholarship would fundamentally transform disciplinary paradigms. Feminist scholars pointed out early on that the study of women would not only add new subject matter but would also force a critical reexamination of the premises and standards of existing scholarly work. 'We are learning', wrote three feminist historians, 'that the writing of women into history necessarily involves redefining and enlarging traditional notions of historical significance, to encompass personal, subjective experience as well as public and political activities. It is not too much to suggest that however hesitant the actual beginnings, such a methodology implies not only a new history of women, but also a new history' (Gordon, Buhle and Dye, 1976, p. 89). The way in which this new history would both include and account for women's experience rested on the extent to which gender could be developed as a category of analysis. Here the analogies to class and race were explicit; indeed, the most politically inclusive of scholars of women's studies regularly invoked all three categories as crucial to the writing of a new history.[2] An interest in class, race, and gender signalled, first, a scholar's commitment to a history that included stories of the oppressed and an analysis of the meaning and nature of their oppression and, second, scholarly understanding that inequalities of power are organized along at least three axes.

The litany of class, race, and gender suggests a parity for each term, but, in fact, that is not at all the case. While 'class' most often rests on Marx's elaborate (and since elaborated) theory of economic determination and historical change, 'race' and 'gender' carry no such associations. No unanimity exists among those who employ concepts of class. Some scholars employ Weberian notions, others use class as a temporary heuristic device. Still, when we invoke class, we are working with or against a set of definitions that, in the case of Marxism, involve an idea of economic causality and a vision of the path along which history has moved dialectically. There is no such clarity or coherence for either race or gender. In the case of gender, the usage has involved a range of theoretical positions as well as simple descriptive references to the relationships between the sexes.

Feminist historians, trained as most historians are to be more comfortable with description than theory, have nonetheless increasingly looked for usable theoretical formulations. They have done so for at least two reasons. First, the proliferation of case studies in women's history seems to call for some synthesizing perspective that can explain continuities and discontinuities and account for persisting inequalities as well as radically different social experiences. Second, the discrepancy between the high quality of recent work in women's history and its continuing marginal status in the field as a whole (as measured by textbooks, syllabi, and monographic work) points up the limits of descriptive approaches that do not address dominant disciplinary concepts, or at least that do not address these concepts in terms that can shake their power and perhaps transform them. It has not been enough for historians of women to prove either that women had a history or that women participated in the major political upheavals of Western civilization. In the case of women's history, the response of most nonfeminist historians has been acknowledgement and then separation or dismissal ('women had a history separate from men's, therefore let feminists do women's history, which need not concern us'; or 'women's history is about sex and the family and should be done separately from political and economic history'). In the case of women's participation, the response has been minimal interest at best ('my understanding of the French Revolution is not changed by knowing that women participated in it'). The challenge posed by these responses is, in the end, a theoretical one. It requires analysis not only of the relationship between male and female experience in the past, but also of the connection between past history and current historical practice. How does gender work in human social relationships? How does gender give meaning to the organization and perception of historical knowledge? The answers depend on gender as an analytic category.

For the most part, the attempts of historians to theorize about gender have remained within traditional social scientific frameworks, using long-standing formulations that provide universal causal explanations. These theories have been limited at best because they tend to contain reductive or overly simple generalizations that undercut not only history's disciplinary sense of the complexity of social causation but also feminist commitments to analyses that will lead to change. A review of these theories will expose their limits and make it possible to propose an alternative approach.

The approaches used by most historians fall into two distinct categories. The first is essentially descriptive; that is, it refers to the existence of phenomena or realities without interpreting, explaining, or attributing causality. The second usage is causal; it theorizes about the nature of phenomena or realities, seeking an understanding of how and why these take the form they do.

In its simplest recent usage, 'gender' is a synonym for 'women'. Any number of books and articles whose subject is women's history have, in the past few years, substituted 'gender' for 'women' in their titles. In some cases, this usage, though vaguely referring to certain analytic concepts, is actually about the political acceptability of the field. In these instances, the use of 'gender' is meant to denote the scholarly seriousness of a work, for 'gender' has a more neutral and objective sound than does 'women'. 'Gender' seems to fit within the scientific terminology of social science and thus dissociates itself from the (supposedly strident) politics of feminism. In this usage, 'gender' does not carry with it a necessary statement about inequality or power nor does it name the aggrieved (and hitherto invisible) party. Whereas the term 'women's history' proclaims its politics by asserting (contrary to customary practice) that women are valid historical subjects, 'gender' includes, but does not name women, and so seems to pose no critical threat. This use of 'gender' is one facet of what might be called the quest of feminist scholarship for academic legitimacy in the 1980s.

But only one facet. 'Gender' as a substitute for 'women' is also used to suggest that information about women is necessarily information about men, that one implies the study of the other. This usage insists that the world of women is part of the world of men, created in and by it. This usage rejects the interpretive utility of the idea of separate spheres, maintaining that to study women in isolation perpetuates the fiction that one sphere, the experience of one sex, has little or nothing to do with the other. In addition, gender is also used to designate social relations between the sexes. Its use explicitly rejects biological explanations, such as those that find a common denominator for diverse forms of female subordination in the facts that women have the capacity to give birth and men have greater muscular strength. Instead, gender becomes a way of denoting 'cultural constructions' – the entirely social creation of ideas about appropriate roles for women and men. It is a way of referring to the exclusively social origins of the subjective identities of men and women. Gender is, in this definition, a social category imposed on a sexed body.[3] Gender seems to have become a particularly useful word as studies of sex and sexuality have proliferated, for it offers a way of differentiating sexual practice from the social roles assigned to women and men. Although scholars acknowledge the connection between sex and (what the sociologists of the family called) 'sex roles', these scholars do not assume a simple or direct linkage. The use of gender emphasizes an entire system of relationships that may include sex, but is not directly determined by sex nor directly determining of sexuality.

These descriptive usages of gender have been employed by historians most often to map out a new terrain. As social historians turned to new objects of study, gender was relevant for such topics as women, children, families, and gender ideologies. This usage of gender, in other words, refers only to those areas – both structural and ideological – involving relations between the sexes. Because, on the face of it, war, diplomacy, and high politics have not been explicitly about those relationships, gender seems not to apply and so continues to be irrelevant to the thinking of historians concerned with issues of politics and power. The effect is to endorse a certain functionalist view ultimately rooted in biology and to perpetuate the idea of separate spheres (sex or politics, family or nation, women or men) in the writing of history. Although gender in this usage asserts that relationships between the sexes are social, it says nothing about why these relationships are constructed as they are, how they work, or how they change. In its descriptive usage, then, gender is a concept associated with the study of things related to women. Gender is a new topic, a new department of historical investigation, but it does not have the analytic power to address (and change) existing historical paradigms.

Some historians were, of course, aware of this problem, hence the efforts to employ theories that might explain the concept of gender and account for historical change. Indeed, the challenge was to reconcile theory, which was framed in general or universal terms, and history, which was committed to the study of contextual specificity and fundamental change. The result has been extremely eclectic: partial borrowings that vitiate the analytic power of a particular theory or worse, employ its precepts without awareness of their implications; or accounts of change that, because they embed universal theories, only illustrate unchanging themes; or wonderfully imaginative studies in which theory is nonetheless so hidden that these studies cannot serve as models for other investigations. Because the theories on which historians have drawn are often not spelled out in all their implications, it seems worthwhile to spend some time doing that. Only through such an exercise can we evaluate the usefulness of these theories and begin to articulate a more powerful theoretical approach.

Feminist historians have employed a variety of approaches to the analysis of gender, but the approaches come down to a choice among three theoretical positions.[4] The first, an entirely feminist effort, attempts to explain the origins of patriarchy. The second locates itself within a Marxian tradition and seeks there an accommodation with feminist critiques. The third, fundamentally divided between French post-structuralist and Anglo-American object-relations theorists, draws on these different schools of psychoanalysis to explain the production and reproduction of the subject's gendered identity.

Theorists of patriarchy have directed their attention to the subordination of women and found their explanation for it in the male 'need' to dominate the female. In Mary O'Brien's ingenious adaptation of Hegel, she defined male domination as the effect of men's desire to transcend their alienation from the means of the reproduction of the species. The principle of generational continuity restores the primacy of paternity and obscures the real labour and the social reality of women's work in childbirth. The source of women's liberation lies in 'an adequate understanding of the process of reproduction', an appreciation of the contradiction between the nature of women's reproductive labour and (male) ideological mystifications of it (O'Brien, 1981, pp. 8–15, 46). For Shulamith Firestone (1970), reproduction was also the 'bitter trap' (O'Brien, 1981, p. 8) for women. In her more materialist analysis, however, liberation would come with transformations in reproductive technology, which might in some not too distant future eliminate the need for women's bodies as the agents of species reproduction.

If reproduction was the key to patriarchy for some, sexuality itself was the answer for others. Catherine MacKinnon's bold formulations were at once her own and characteristic of a certain approach: 'Sexuality is to feminism what work is to Marxism: that which is most one's own, yet most taken away' (MacKinnon, 1982, p. 515). 'Sexual objectification is the primary process of the subjection of women. It unites act with word, construction with expression, perception with enforcement, myth with reality. Man fucks woman; subject verb object' (1982, p. 541). Continuing her analogy to Marx, MacKinnon offered, in the place of dialectical materialism, consciousness-raising as feminism's method of analysis. By expressing the shared experience of objectification, she argued, women come to understand their common identity and so are moved to political action. Although sexual relations are defined in MacKinnon's analysis as social, there is nothing except the inherent inequality of the sexual relation itself to explain why the system of power operates as it does. The source of unequal relations between the sexes is, in the end, unequal relations between the sexes. Although the inequality of which sexuality is the source is said to be embodied in a 'whole system of social relationships', how this system works is not explained (1982, p. 543).

Theorists of patriarchy have addressed the inequality of males and females in important ways, but, for historians, their theories pose problems. First, while they offer an analysis internal to the gender system itself, they also assert the primacy of that system in all social organization. But theories of patriarchy do not show what gender inequality has to do with other inequalities. Second, whether domination comes in the form of the male appropriation of the female's reproductive labour or in the sexual objectification of women by men, the analysis rests on physical difference. Any physical difference takes on a universal and unchanging aspect, even if theorists of patriarchy take into account the existence of changing forms and systems of gender inequality.[5] A theory that rests on the single variable of physical difference poses problems for historians: it assumes a consistent or inherent meaning for the human body – outside social or cultural construction – and thus the ahistoricity of gender itself. History becomes, in a sense, epiphenomenal, providing endless variations on the unchanging theme of a fixed gender inequality.

Marxist feminists have a more historical approach, guided as they are by a theory of history. But, whatever the variations and adaptations have been, the self-imposed require-ment that there be a 'material' explanation for gender has limited or at least slowed the devel-opment of new lines of analysis. Whether a so-called dual-systems solution is proffered (one that posits the separate but interacting realms of capitalism and patriarchy) or an analysis based more firmly in orthodox Marxist discussions of modes of production is developed, the explanation for the origins of and changes in gender systems is found outside the sexual divi-sion of labour. Families, households, and sexuality are all, finally, products of changing modes of production. That is how Engels concluded his explorations of the *Origins of the Family* (1972 [1884 orig.]); that is where economist Heidi Hartmann's analysis ultimately rests. Hartmann insists on the importance of taking into account patriarchy and capitalism as separate but interacting systems. Yet, as her argument unfolds, economic causality takes precedence, and patriarchy always develops and changes as a function of relations of produc-tion (Hartmann, 1976, 1979, 1981).

Early discussions among Marxist feminists circled around the same set of problems: a rejection of the essentialism of those who would argue that the 'exigencies of biological reproduction' determine the sexual division of labour under capitalism; the futility of inserting 'modes of reproduction' into discussions of modes of production (it remains an oppositional category and does not assume equal status with modes of production); the recognition that economic systems do not directly determine gender relationships, indeed, that the subordination of women pre-dates capitalism and continues under socialism; the search nonetheless for a materialist explanation that excludes natural physical differences.[6] An important attempt to break out of this circle of problems came from Joan Kelly in her essay 'The Doubled Vision of Feminist Theory', where she argued that economic and gender systems interact to produce social and historical experiences; that neither system was causal, but both 'operate simultaneously to reproduce the socioeconomic and male-dominant structures of … [a] particular social order' (Kelly, 1984, p. 61). Kelly's suggestion that gender systems have an independent existence provided a crucial conceptual opening, but her commitment to remain within a Marxist framework led her to emphasize the causal role of economic factors even in the determination of the gender system. 'The relation of the sexes operates in accordance with, and through, socioeconomic structures, as well as sex/gender ones' (1984, p. 61). Kelly introduced the idea of a 'sexually based social reality', but she tended to emphasize the social rather than the sexual nature of that reality, and, most often, 'social', in her usage, was conceived in terms of economic relations of production.

The most far-reaching exploration of sexuality by American Marxist feminists is in *Powers of Desire*, a volume of essays published in 1983 (Snitow, Stansell and Thompson, 1983). Influenced by increasing attention to sexuality among political activists and scholars, by French philosopher Michel Foucault's insistence that sexuality is produced in historical contexts, and by the conviction that the current 'sexual revolution' requires serious analysis, the authors make 'sexual politics' the focus of their inquiry. In so doing, they open the question of causality and offer a variety of solutions to it; indeed, the real excitement of this volume is its lack of analytic unanimity, its sense of analytic tension. If individual authors tend to stress the causality of social (by which is often meant 'economic') contexts, they nonetheless include suggestions about the importance of studying 'the psychic structuring of gender identity'. If 'gender ideology' is sometimes said to 'reflect' economic and social structures, there is also a crucial recognition of the need to understand the complex 'link between society and enduring psychic structure' (Ross and Rapp, 1983, p. 53). On the one hand, the editors endorse Jessica Benjamin's point that politics must include attention to 'the erotic, fantastic components of human life', but, on the other hand, no essays besides Benjamin's deal fully or seriously with the theoretical issues she raises (Snitow, Stansell and Thompson, 1983, p. 12; Benjamin, 1983, p. 297). Instead, a tacit assumption runs through the volume that Marxism can be expanded to include discussions of ideology, culture, and psychology and that this expansion will happen through the kind of concrete examination of evidence undertaken in most of the articles. The advantage of such an approach lies in its avoidance of sharp differences of position, the disadvantage in its leaving in place an already fully articulated theory that leads back from relations of the sexes to relations of production.

A comparison of American Marxist-feminist efforts, exploratory and relatively wide-ranging, to those of their English counterparts, tied more closely to the politics of a strong and viable Marxist tradition, reveals that the English have had greater difficulty in challenging the constraints of strictly determinist explanations. This difficulty can be seen most dramatically in the debates in the *New Left Review* between Michèle Barrett and her critics, who charge her with abandoning a materialist analysis of the sexual division of labour under capitalism (Brenner and Ramas, 1984; Barrett, 1984, 1985; Weir and Wilson, 1984; Lewis, 1985).[7] It can be seen as well in the replacement of an initial feminist attempt to reconcile psychoanalysis and Marxism with a choice of one or another of these theoretical positions by scholars who earlier insisted that some fusion of the two was possible.[8] The difficulty for both English and American feminists working within Marxism is apparent in the work I have mentioned here. The problem they face is the opposite of the one posed by patriarchal theory. For within Marxism, the concept of gender has long been treated as the by-product of changing economic structures; gender has had no independent analytic status of its own.

A review of psychoanalytic theory requires a specification of schools, since the various approaches have tended to be classified by the national origins of the founders and the majority of the practitioners. There is the Anglo-American school, working within the terms of theories of object-relations. In the United States, Nancy Chodorow is the name most readily associated with this approach. In addition, the work of Carol Gilligan has had a far-reaching impact on American scholarship, including history. Gilligan's work draws on Chodorow's, although it is concerned less with the construction of the subject than with moral development and behaviour. In contrast to the Anglo-American school, the French school is based on structuralist and post-structuralist readings of Freud in terms of theories of language (for feminists, the key figure is Jacques Lacan).

Both schools are concerned with the processes by which the subject's identity is created; both focus on the early stages of child development for clues to the formation of gender identity. Object-relations theorists stress the influence of actual experience (the child sees, hears, relates to those who care for it, particularly, of course, to its parents), while the post-structuralists emphasize the centrality of language in communicating, interpreting, and representing gender. (By 'language', post-structuralists do not mean words but systems of meaning – symbolic orders – that precede the actual mastery of speech, reading, and writing.) Another difference between the two schools of thought focuses on the unconscious, which for Chodorow is ultimately subject to conscious understanding and for Lacan is not. For Lacanians, the unconscious is a critical factor in the construction of the subject; it is the location, moreover, of sexual division and, for that reason, of continuing instability for the gendered subject.

In recent years, feminist historians have been drawn to these theories either because they serve to endorse specific findings with general observations or because they seem to offer an important theoretical formulation about gender. Increasingly, those historians working with a concept of 'women's culture' cite Chodorow's or Gilligan's work as both proof of and explanation for their interpretations; those wrestling with feminist theory look to Lacan. In the end, neither of these theories seems to me entirely workable for historians; a closer look at each may help explain why.

My reservation about object-relations theory concerns its literalism, its reliance on relatively small structures of interaction to produce gender identity and to generate change. Both the family division of labour and the actual assignment of tasks to each parent play a crucial role in Chodorow's theory. The outcome of prevailing Western systems is a clear division between male and female: 'The basic feminine sense of self is connected to the world, the basic masculine sense of self is separate' (Chodorow, 1978, p. 169). According to Chodorow, if fathers were more involved in parenting and present more often in domestic situations, the outcome of the oedipal drama might be different.[9]

This interpretation limits the concept of gender to family and household experience and, for the historian, leaves no way to connect the concept (or the individual) to other social systems of economy, politics, or power. Of course, it is implicit that social arrangements requiring fathers to work and mothers to perform most child-rearing tasks structure family organization. Where such arrangements come from and why they are articulated in terms of a sexual division of labour is not clear. Neither is the issue of inequality, as opposed to that of asymmetry, addressed. How can we account within this theory for persistent associations of masculinity with power, for the higher value placed on manhood than on womanhood, for the way children seem to learn these associations and evaluations even when they live outside nuclear households or in households where parenting is equally divided between husband and wife? I do not think we can without some attention to signifying systems, that is, to the ways societies represent gender, use it to articulate the rules of social relationships, or construct the meaning of experience. Without meaning, there is no experience; without processes of signification, there is no meaning.

Language is the centre of Lacanian theory; it is the key to the child's induction into the symbolic order. Through language, gendered identity is constructed. According to Lacan, the phallus is the central signifier of sexual difference. But the meaning of the phallus must be read metaphorically. For the child, the oedipal drama sets forth the terms of cultural interaction, since the threat of castration embodies the power, the rules of (the Father's) law. The child's relationship to the law depends on sexual difference, on its imaginative (or fantastic) identification with masculinity or femininity. The imposition, in other words, of the rules of social interaction is inherently and specifically gendered, for the female necessarily has a different relationship to the phallus than the male does. But gender identification, although it always appears coherent and fixed, is, in fact, highly unstable. As meaning systems, subjective identities are processes of differentiation and distinction, requiring the suppression of ambiguities and opposite elements in order to ensure (create the illusion of) coherence and common understanding. The principle of masculinity rests on the necessary repression of feminine aspects – of the subject's potential for bisexuality – and introduces conflict into the opposition of masculine and feminine. Repressed desires are present in the unconscious and are constantly a threat to the stability of gender identification, denying its unity, subverting its need for security. In addition, conscious ideas of masculine or feminine are not fixed, since they vary according to contextual usage. Conflict always exists, then, between the subject's need for the appearance of wholeness and the imprecision of terminology, its relative meaning, its dependence on repression (Mitchell and Rose, 1983; Alexander, 1984). This kind of interpretation makes the categories of 'man' and 'woman' problematic by suggesting that masculine and feminine are not inherent characteristics but subjective (or fictional) constructs. This interpretation also implies that the subject is in a constant process of construction, and it offers a systematic way of interpreting conscious and unconscious desire by pointing to language as the appropriate place for analysis. As such, I find it instructive.

I am troubled, nonetheless, by the exclusive fixation on questions of the individual subject and by the tendency to reify subjectively originating antagonism between males and females as the central fact of gender. In addition, although there is openness in the concept of how 'the subject' is constructed, the theory tends to universalize the categories and relationship of male and female. The outcome for historians is a reductive reading of evidence from the past. Even though this theory takes social relationships into account by linking castration to prohibition and law, it does not permit the introduction of a notion of historical specificity and variability. The phallus is the only signifier; the process of constructing the gendered subject is, in the end, predictable because it is always the same. If, as film theorist Teresa de Lauretis suggests, we need to think in terms of the construction of subjectivity in social and historical contexts, there is no way to specify those contexts within the terms offered by Lacan. Indeed, even in de Lauretis's attempt, social reality (that is, 'material, economic and interpersonal [relations] which are in fact social, and in a larger perspective historical') seems to lie outside, apart from the subject (de Lauretis, 1984, p. 159). A way to conceive of 'social reality' in terms of gender is lacking.

The problem of sexual antagonism in this theory has two aspects. First, it projects a certain timeless quality, even when it is historicized as well as it has been by Sally Alexander. Alexander's reading of Lacan led her to conclude that 'antagonism between the sexes is an unavoidable aspect of the acquisition of sexual identity ... If antagonism is always latent, it is possible that history offers no final resolution, only the constant reshaping, reorganizing of the symbolization of difference, and the sexual division of labour' (Alexander, 1984, p. 135). It may be my hopeless utopianism that gives me pause before this formulation, or it may be that I have not yet shed the episteme of what Foucault called the Classical Age. Whatever the explanation, Alexander's formulation contributes to the fixing of the binary opposition of male and female as the only possible relationship and as a permanent aspect of the human condition. It perpetuates rather than questions what Denise Riley refers to as 'the dreadful air of constancy of sexual polarity'. She writes: 'The historically constructed nature of the opposition [between male and female] produces as one of its effects just that air of an invariant and monotonous men/women opposition' (Riley, 1985, p. 11).[10]

It is precisely that opposition, in all its tedium and monotony, that (to return to the Anglo-American side) Carol Gilligan's work has promoted. Gilligan explains the divergent paths of moral development followed by boys and girls in terms of differences of 'experience' (lived reality). It is not surprising that historians of women have picked up her ideas and used them to explain the 'different voices' their work has enabled them to hear. The problems with these borrowings are manifold, and they are logically connected (Gilligan, 1982). The first is a slippage that often happens in the attribution of causality. the argument moves from a statement such as 'women's experience leads them to make moral choices contingent on contexts and relationships' to 'women think and choose this way because they are women'. Implied in this line of reasoning is the ahistorical, if not essentialist, notion of woman. Gilligan and others have extrapolated her description, based on a small sample of late twentieth-century American schoolchildren, into a statement about all women. This extrapolation is evident especially, but not exclusively, in the discussions by some historians of 'women's culture' that take evidence from early saints to modern militant labour activists and reduce it to proof of Gilligan's hypothesis about a universal female preference for relatedness.[11] This use of Gilligan's ideas provides sharp contrast to the more complicated and historicized conceptions of 'women's culture' evident in the *Feminist Studies* 1980 symposium (*Feminist Studies*, 1980). Indeed, a comparison of that set of articles with Gilligan's formulations reveals the extent to which her notion is ahistorical, defining woman/man as a universal, self-reproducing binary opposition – fixed always in the same way. By insisting on fixed differences (in Gilligan's case, by simplifying data with more mixed results about sex and moral reasoning to underscore sexual difference), feminists contribute to the kind of thinking they want to oppose. Although they insist on the revaluation of the category 'female' (Gilligan suggests that women's moral choices may be more humane than men's), they do not examine the binary opposition itself.

We need a refusal of the fixed and permanent quality of the binary opposition, a genuine historicization and deconstruction of the terms of sexual difference. We must become more self-conscious about distinguishing between our analytic vocabulary and the material we want to analyse. We must find ways (however imperfect) continually to subject our categories to criticism, our analyses to self-criticism. If we employ Jacques Derrida's definition of deconstruction, this criticism means analysing in context the way any binary opposition operates, reversing and displacing its hierarchical construction, rather than accepting it as real or self-evident or in the nature of things.[12] In a sense, of course, feminists have been doing this for years. The history of feminist thought is a history of the refusal of the hierarchical construction of the relationship between male and female in its specific contexts and an attempt to reverse or displace its operations. Feminist historians are now in a position to theorize their practice and to develop gender as an analytic category.

Concern with gender as an analytic category has emerged only in the late twentieth century. It is absent from the major bodies of social theory articulated from the eighteenth to the early twentieth century. To be sure, some of those theories built their logic on analogies to the opposition of male and female, others acknowledged a 'woman question', still others addressed the formation of subjective sexual identity, but gender as a way of talking about systems of social or sexual relations did not appear. This neglect may in part explain the difficulty that contemporary feminists have had incorporating the term 'gender' into existing bodies of theory and convincing adherents of one or another theoretical school that gender belongs in their vocabulary. The term 'gender' is part of the attempt by contemporary feminists to stake claim to a certain definitional ground, to insist on the inadequacy of existing bodies of theory for explaining persistent inequalities between women and men. It seems to me significant that the use of the word 'gender' has emerged at a moment of great epistemological turmoil that takes the form, in some cases, of a shift from scientific to literary paradigms among social scientists (from an emphasis on cause to one on meaning, blurring genres of inquiry, in anthropologist Clifford Geertz's phrase [1980]) and, in other cases, the form of debates about theory between those who assert the transparency of facts and those who insist that all reality is construed or constructed, between those who defend and those who question the idea that 'man' is the rational master of his own destiny. In the space opened by this debate and on the side of the critique of science developed by the humanities, and of empiricism and humanism by post-structuralists, feminists have begun to find not only a theoretical voice of their own but scholarly and political allies as well. It is within this space that we must articulate gender as an analytic category.

What should be done by historians who, after all, have seen their discipline dismissed by some recent theorists as a relic of humanist thought? I do not think we should quit the archives or abandon the study of the past, but we do have to change some of the ways we've gone about working, some of the questions we have asked. We need to scrutinize our methods of analysis, clarify our operative assumptions, and explain how we think change occurs. Instead of a search for single origins, we have to conceive of processes so interconnected that they cannot be disentangled. Of course, we identify problems to study, and these constitute beginnings or points of entry into complex processes. But it is the processes we must continually keep in mind. We must ask more often how things happened in order to find out why they happened; in anthropologist Michelle Rosaldo's formulation, we must pursue not universal, general causality but meaningful explanation: 'It now appears to me that women's place in human social life is not in any direct sense a product of the things she does, but of the meaning her activities acquire through concrete social interaction' (Rosaldo, 1980). To pursue meaning, we need to deal with the individual subject as well as social organization and to articulate the nature of their interrelationships, for both are crucial to understanding how gender works, how change occurs. Finally, we need to replace the notion that social power is unified, coherent, and centralized with something like Michel Foucault's concept of power as dispersed constellations of unequal relationships, discursively constituted in social 'fields of force' (Foucault, 1980a, 1980b). Within these processes and structures, there is room for a concept of human agency as the attempt (at least partially rational) to construct an identity, a life, a set of relationships, a society within certain limits and with language – conceptual language that at once sets boundaries and contains the possibility for negation, resistance, reinterpretation, the play of metaphoric invention and imagination.

My definition of gender has two parts and several subsets. They are interrelated but must be analytically distinct. The core of the definition rests on an integral connection between two propositions: gender is a constitutive element of social relationships based on perceived differences between the sexes, and gender is a primary way of signifying relationships of power. Changes in the organization of social relationships always correspond to changes in representations of power, but the direction of change is not necessarily one way. As a constitutive element of social relationships based on perceived differences between the sexes, gender involves four interrelated elements: first, culturally available symbols that evoke multiple (and often contradictory) representations – Eve and Mary as symbols of woman, for example, in the Western Christian tradition – but also, myths of light and dark, purification and pollution, innocence and corruption. For historians, the interesting questions are, which symbolic representations are invoked, how, and in what contexts? Second are the normative concepts that set forth interpretations of the meanings of the symbols, that attempt to limit and contain their metaphoric possibilities. These concepts are expressed in religious, educational, scientific, legal, and political doctrines and typically take the form of a fixed binary opposition, categorically and unequivocally asserting the meaning of male and female, masculine and feminine. In fact, these normative statements depend on the refusal or repression of alternative possibilities, and sometimes overt contests about them take place (at what moments and under what circumstances ought to be a concern of historians). The position that emerges as dominant, however, is stated as the only possible one. Subsequent history is written as if these normative positions were the product of social consensus rather than of conflict. An example of this kind of history is the treatment of the Victorian ideology of domesticity as if it were created whole and only afterwards reacted to instead of being the constant subject of great differences of opinion. Another kind of example comes from contemporary fundamentalist religious groups that have forcibly linked their practice to a restoration of women's supposedly more authentic 'traditional' role, when, in fact, there is little historical precedent for the unquestioned performance of such a role. The point of new historical investigation is to disrupt the notion of fixity, to discover the nature of the debate or repression that leads to the appearance of timeless permanence in binary gender representation. This kind of analysis must include a notion of politics and reference to social institutions and organizations – the third aspect of gender relationships.

Some scholars, notably anthropologists, have restricted the use of gender to the kinship system (focusing on household and family as the basis for social organization). We need a broader view that includes not only kinship but also (especially for complex modern societies) the labour market (a sex-segregated labour market is a part of the process of gender construction), education (all-male, single-sex, or coeducational institutions are part of the same process), and the polity (universal male suffrage is part of the process of gender construction). It makes little sense to force these institutions back to functional utility in the kinship system, or to argue that contemporary relationships between men and women are artifacts of older kinship systems based on the exchange of women.[13] Gender is constructed through kinship, but not exclusively; it is constructed as well in the economy and the polity, which, in our society at least, now operate largely independently of kinship.

The fourth aspect of gender is subjective identity. I agree with anthropologist Gayle Rubin's formulation that psychoanalysis offers an important theory about the reproduction of gender, a description of the 'transformation of the biological sexuality of individuals as they are enculturated' (Rubin, 1975, p. 189). But the universal claim of psychoanalysis gives me pause. Even though Lacanian theory may be helpful for thinking about the construction of gendered identity, historians need to work in a more historical way. If gender identity is based only and universally on fear of castration, the point of historical inquiry is denied. Moreover, real men and women do not always or literally fulfil the terms either of their society's prescriptions or of our analytic categories. Historians need instead to examine the ways in which gendered identities are substantively constructed and relate their findings to a range of activities, social organizations, and historically specific cultural representations. The best efforts in this area so far have been, not surprisingly, biographies: Biddy Martin's interpretation of Lou Andreas Salomé (1980), Kathryn Sklar's depiction of Catharine Beecher (1973), Jacqueline Hall's life of Jessie Daniel Ames (1974), and Mary Hill's discussion of Charlotte Perkins Gilman (1980). But collective treatments are also possible, as Mrinalina Sinha (1984, 1986) and Lou Ratté (1983) have shown in their respective studies of the terms of construction of gender identity for British colonial administrators in India and for British-educated Indians who emerged as anti-imperialist, nationalist leaders.

The first part of my definition of gender consists, then, of all four of these elements, and no one of them operates without the others. Yet they do not operate simultaneously, with one simply reflecting the others. A question for historical research is, in fact, what the relationships among the four aspects are. The sketch I have offered of the process of constructing gender relationships could be used to discuss class, race, ethnicity, or, for that matter, any social process. My point was to clarify and specify how one needs to think about the effect of gender in social and institutional relationships, because this thinking is often not done precisely or systematically. The theorizing of gender, however, is developed in my second proposition: gender is a primary way of signifying relationships of power. It might be better to say, gender is a primary field within which or by means of which power is articulated. Gender is not the only field, but it seems to have been a persistent and recurrent way of enabling the signification of power in the West, in the Judeo-Christian as well as the Islamic tradition. As such, this part of the definition might seem to belong in the normative section of the argument, yet it does not, for concepts of power, though they may build on gender, are not always literally about gender itself. French sociologist Pierre Bourdieu has written about how the 'di-vision du monde', based on references to 'biological differences and notably those that refer to the division of the labour of procreation and reproduction', operates as 'the best founded of collective illusions'. Established as an objective set of references, concepts of gender structure perception and the concrete and symbolic organization of all social life (Bourdieu, 1980, pp. 246–47, 333–461, esp. p. 366). To the extent that these references establish distributions of power (differential control over or access to material and symbolic resources), gender becomes implicated in the conception and construction of power itself. The French anthropologist Maurice Godelier has put it this way: 'It is not sexuality which haunts society, but society which haunts the body's sexuality. Sex-related differences between bodies are continually summoned as testimony to social relations and phenomena that have nothing to do with sexuality. Not only as testimony to, but also testimony for – in other words, as legitimation' (Godelier, 1981, p. 17).

The legitimizing function of gender works in many ways. Bourdieu, for example, showed how, in certain cultures, agricultural exploitation was organized according to concepts of time and season that rested on specific definitions of the opposition between masculine and feminine. Gayatri Spivak has done a pointed analysis of the uses of gender and colonialism in certain texts of British and American women writers.[14] Natalie Davis (1975) has shown how concepts of masculine and feminine related to understandings and criticisms of the rules of social order in early modern France. Historian Caroline Bynum has thrown new light on medieval spirituality through her attention to the relationships between concepts of masculine and religious behaviour. Her work gives us important insight into the ways in which these concepts informed the politics of monastic institutions as well as of individual believers (Bynum, 1982, 1985, 1987). Art historians have opened a new territory by reading social implications from literal depictions of women and men (see, for example, Clark, 1985). These interpretations are based on the idea that conceptual languages employ differentiation to establish meaning and that sexual difference is a primary way of signifying differentiation.[15] Gender, then, provides a way to decode meaning and to understand the complex connections among various forms of human interaction. When historians look for the ways in which the concept of gender legitimizes and constructs social relationships, they develop insight into the reciprocal nature of gender and society and into the particular and contextually specific ways in which politics constructs gender and gender constructs politics.

Politics is only one of the areas in which gender can be used for historical analysis. I have chosen the following examples relating to politics and power in their most traditionally construed sense, that is, as they pertain to government and the nation-state, for two reasons. First, the territory is virtually uncharted, since gender has been seen as antithetical to the real business of politics. Second, political history – still the dominant mode of historical inquiry – has been the stronghold of resistance to the inclusion of material or even questions about women and gender.

Gender has been employed literally or analogically in political theory to justify or criticize the reign of monarchs and to express the relationship between ruler and ruled. One might have expected that the debates of contemporaries over the reigns of Elizabeth I in England and Catherine de' Medici in France would dwell on the issue of women's suitability for political rule, but, in the period when kinship and kingship were integrally related, discussions about male kings were equally preoccupied with masculinity and femininity (Weil, 1985; see also Montrose, 1983; Hunt, 1983). Analogies to the marital relationship provide structure for the arguments of Jean Bodin, Robert Filmer, and John Locke. Edmund Burke's attack on the French Revolution is built around a contrast between ugly, murderous *sansculotte* hags ('the furies of hell, in the abused shape of the vilest of women') and the soft femininity of Marie Antoinette, who escaped the crowd to 'seek refuge at the feet of a king and husband' and whose beauty once inspired national pride (1909 [orig. 1790], pp. 208–9). (It was in reference to the appropriate role for the feminine in the political order that Burke wrote, 'To make us love our country, our country ought to be lovely' (1909 [orig. 1790], p. 214).)[16] But the analogy is not always to marriage or even to heterosexuality. In medieval Islamic political theory, the symbols of political power alluded most often to sex between man and boy, suggesting not only forms of acceptable sexuality akin to those that Foucault's last work described in classical Greece but also the irrelevance of women to any notion of politics and public life.[17]

Lest this last comment suggest that political theory simply reflects social organization, it seems important to note that changes in gender relationships can be set off by views of the needs of state. A striking example is Louis de Bonald's argument in 1816 about why the divorce legislation of the French Revolution had to be repealed:

> Just as political democracy, 'allows the people, the weak part of political society, to rise against the established power', so divorce, 'veritable domestic democracy', allows the wife, 'the weak part, to rebel against marital authority … in order to keep the state out of the hands of the people, it is necessary to keep the family out of the hands of wives and children'.

(Phillips, 1976, p. 217)

Bonald begins with an analogy and then establishes a direct correspondence between divorce and democracy. Harking back to much earlier arguments about the well-ordered family as the foundation of the well-ordered state, the legislation that implemented this view redefined the limits of the marital relationship. Similarly, in our own time, conservative political ideologues would like to pass a series of laws about the organization and behaviour of the family that would alter current practices. The connection between authoritarian regimes and the control of women has been noted but not thoroughly studied. Whether at a crucial moment for Jacobin hegemony in the French Revolution, at the point of Stalin's bid for controlling authority, the implementation of Nazi policy in Germany, or with the triumph in Iran of the Ayatollah Khomeini, emergent rulers have legitimized domination, strength, central authority, and ruling power as masculine (enemies, outsiders, subversives, weakness as feminine) and made that code literal in laws (forbidding women's political participation, outlawing abortion, prohibiting wage-earning by mothers, imposing female dress codes) that put women in their place.[18] These actions and their timing make little sense in themselves; in most instances, the state had nothing immediate or material to gain from the control of women. The actions can only be made sense of as part of an analysis of the construction and consolidation of power. An assertion of control or strength was given form as a policy about women. In these examples, sexual difference was conceived in terms of the domination or control of women. These examples provide some insight into the kinds of power relationships being constructed in modern history, but this particular type of relationship is not a universal political theme. In different ways, for example, the democratic regimes of the twentieth century have also constructed their political ideologies with gendered concepts and translated them into policy; the welfare state, for example, demonstrated its protective paternalism in laws directed at women and children (Wilson, 1977; Lewis, 1980; McDougall, 1983; Jenson, 1985). Historically, some socialist and anarchist movements have refused metaphors of domination entirely, imaginatively presenting their critiques of particular regimes or social organizations in terms of transformations of gender identities. Utopian socialists in France and England in the 1830s and 1840s conceived their dreams for a harmonious future in terms of the complementary natures of individuals as exemplified in the union of man and woman, 'the social individual' (see Taylor, 1983). European anarchists were long known not only for refusing the conventions of bourgeois marriage but for their visions of a world in which sexual difference did not imply hierarchy.

These examples are of explicit connections between gender and power, but they are only a part of my definition of gender as a primary way of signifying relationships of power. Attention to gender is often not explicit, but it is nonetheless a crucial part of the organization of equality or inequality. Hierarchical structures rely on generalized understandings of the so-called natural relationships between male and female. The concept of class in the nineteenth century relied on gender for its articulation. While middle-class reformers in France, for example, depicted workers in terms coded as feminine (subordinated, weak, sexually exploited like prostitutes), labour and socialist leaders replied by insisting on the masculine position of the working class (producers, strong, protectors of their women and children). The terms of this discourse were not explicitly about gender, but they were strengthened by references to it. The gendered 'coding' of certain terms established and 'naturalized' their meanings. In the process, historically specific, normative definitions of gender (which were taken as givens) were reproduced and embedded in the culture of the French working class (Rancière and Vaudray, 1975; Devance, 1977).

The subject of war, diplomacy, and high politics frequently comes up when traditional political historians question the utility of gender in their work. But here, too, we need to look beyond the actors and the literal import of their words. Power relations among nations and the status of colonial subjects have been made comprehensible (and thus legitimate) in terms of relations between male and female. The legitimizing of war – of expending young lives to protect the state – has variously taken the forms of explicit appeals to manhood (to the need to defend otherwise vulnerable women and children), of implicit reliance on belief in the duty of sons to serve their leaders or their (father the) king, and of associations between masculinity and national strength (Spivak, 1981; Bhabha, 1984; Hausen, 1987; see also Inglis, 1987). High politics itself is a gendered concept, the reasons for and the fact of its highest authority, precisely in its exclusion of women from its work. Gender is one of the recurrent references by which political power has been conceived, legitimated, and criticized. It refers to but also establishes the meaning of the male/female opposition. To vindicate political power, the reference must seem sure and fixed, outside human construction, part of the natural or divine order. In that way, the binary opposition and the social process of gender relationships both become part of the meaning of power itself; to question or alter any aspect threatens the entire system.

If significations of gender and power construct one another, how do things change? The answer in a general sense is that change may be initiated in many places. Massive political upheavals that throw old orders into chaos and bring new ones into being may revise the terms (and so the organization) of gender in the search for new forms of legitimation. But they may not; old notions of gender have also served to validate new regimes.[19] Demographic crises, occasioned by food shortages, plagues, or wars, may have called into question normative visions of heterosexual marriage (as happened in some circles, in some countries in the 1920s), but they have also spawned pronatalist policies that insist on the exclusive importance of women's maternal and reproductive functions.[20] Shifting patterns of employment may lead to altered marital strategies and to different possibilities for the construction of subjectivity, but they can also be experienced as new arenas of activity for dutiful daughters and wives.[21] The emergence of new kinds of cultural symbols may make possible the reinterpreting or, indeed, rewriting of the oedipal story, but it can also serve to reinscribe that terrible drama in even more telling terms. Political processes will determine which outcome prevails – political in the sense that different actors and different meanings are contending with one another for control. The nature of that process, of the actors and their actions, can only be determined specifically, in the context of time and place. We can write the history of that process only if we recognize that 'man' and 'woman' are at once empty and overflowing categories. Empty because they have no ultimate, transcendent meaning. Overflowing because even when they appear to be fixed, they still contain within them alternative, denied, or suppressed definitions.

Political history has, in a sense, been enacted on the field of gender. It is a field that seems fixed yet whose meaning is contested and in flux. If we treat the opposition between male and female as problematic rather than known, as something contextually defined, repeatedly constructed, then we must constantly ask not only what is at stake in proclamations or debates that invoke gender to explain or justify their positions but also how implicit understandings of gender are being invoked and reinscribed. What is the relationship between laws about women and the power of the state? Why (and since when) have women been invisible as historical subjects, when we know they participated in the great and small events of human history? Has gender legitimized the emergence of professional careers (see, for example, Rossiter, 1982)? Is (to quote the tide of a recent article by French feminist Luce Irigaray) the subject of science sexed (Irigaray, 1985a)? What is the relationship between state politics and the discovery of the crime of homosexuality?[22] How have social institutions incorporated gender into their assumptions and organizations? Have there ever been genuinely egalitarian concepts of gender in terms of which political systems were projected, if not built?

Investigation of these issues will yield a history that will provide new perspectives on old questions (about how, for example, political rule is imposed, or what the impact of war on society is), redefine the old questions in new terms (introducing considerations of family and sexuality, for example, in the study of economics or war), make women visible as active participants, and create analytic distance between the seemingly fixed language of the past and our own terminology. In addition, this new history will leave open possibilities for thinking about current feminist political strategies and the (utopian) future, for it suggests that gender must be redefined and restructured in conjunction with a vision of political and social equality that includes not only sex but class and race.

Acknowledgements

This essay was first prepared for delivery at the meetings of the American Historical Association in December 1985. It was subsequently published in its current form in Volume 91, Issue 5 of the *American Historical Review* (December 1986). Discussions with Denise Riley, Janice Doane, Yasmine Ergas, Anne Norton, and Harriet Whitehead helped formulate my ideas on the various subjects touched in the course of this paper. The final version profited from comments by Ira Karznelson, Charles Tilly, Louise Tilly, Elisabetta Galeotti, Rayna Rapp, Christine Stansell, and Joan Vincent. I am also grateful for the unusually careful editing done at the AHR by Allyn Roberts and David Ransell.

Notes

1 *Oxford English Dictionary*, 1961.
2 The best and most subtle example is from Kelly, 1984, especially p. 61.
3 For an argument against the use of gender to emphasize the social aspect of sexual difference, see Gatens, 1985. I agree with her argument that the sex/gender distinction grants autonomous or transparent determination to the body, ignoring the fact that what we know about the body is culturally produced knowledge.
4 For a different characterization of feminist analysis, see Nicholson, 1986.
5 For an interesting discussion of the strengths and limits of the term 'patriarchy', see the exchange among historians Sheila Rowbotham, Sally Alexander, and Barbara Taylor in Samuel, 1981.
6 Discussions of Marxist feminism include Eisenstein, 1981; Kuhn, 1978; Coward, 1983; Scott, 1974; Humphries, 1971, 1977; and see the debate on Humphries's work in *Review of Radical Political Economics*, 1980.
7 See also Armstrong and Armstrong, 1984; Jenson, 1985.
8 For early theoretical formulations, see *Papers on Patriarchy: Conference, London 76*. I am grateful to Jane Caplan for telling me of the existence of this publication and for her willingness to share with me her copy and her ideas about it. For the psychoanalytic position, see Alexander, 1984. In seminars at Princeton University in early 1986, Juliet Mitchell seemed to be returning to an emphasis on the priority of materialist analyses of gender. For an attempt to get beyond the theoretical impasse of Marxist feminism, see Coward, 1983. See also the brilliant American effort in this direction by anthropologist Gayle Rubin, 1975.

9 'My account suggests that these gender-related issues may be influenced during the period of the Oedipus complex, but they are not its only focus or outcome. The negotiation of these issues occurs in the context of broader object-relational and ego processes. These broader processes have equal influence on psychic structure formation, and psychic life and relational modes in men and women. They account for differing modes of identification and orientation to heterosexual objects, for the more asymmetrical oedipal issues psychoanalysts describe. These outcomes, like more traditional oedipal outcomes, arise from the asymmetrical organization of parenting, with the mother's role as primary parent and the father's typically greater remoteness and his investment in socialization especially in areas concerned with gender-typing' (Chodorow, 1978, p. 166). It is important to note that there are differences in interpretation and approach between Chodorow and British object-relations theorists who follow the work of D.W. Winnicott and Melanie Klein. Chodorow's approach is best characterized as a more sociological or sociologized theory, but it is the dominant lens through which object-relations theory has been viewed by American feminists. On the history of British object-relations theory in social policy, see Riley, 1984.

10 The argument is fully elaborated in Riley's brilliant book, *'Am I That Name?': Feminism and the Category of 'Women' in History* (Riley, 1988).

11 Useful critiques of Gilligan's book are: Auerbach *et al.*, 1985, and 'Women and Morality', a special issue of *Social Research*, 1983. My comments on the tendency of historians to cite Gilligan come from reading unpublished manuscripts and grant proposals, and it seems unfair to cite those here. I have kept track of the references for over five years, and they are many and increasing.

12 For a succinct and accessible discussion of Derrida, see Culler, 1982, especially pp. 156–79. See also Derrida, 1974, 1979, and a transcription of Pembroke Centre Seminar, 1983, in *Subjects/ Objects* (fall, 1984).

13 For this argument, see Rubin, 1975, p. 199.

14 Spivak, 1985. See also Millett, 1971. An examination of how feminine references work in major texts of Western philosophy is carried out by Irigaray, 1985b.

15 The difference between structuralist and post-structuralist theorists on this question rests on how open or closed they viewed the categories of difference. To the extent that post-structuralists do not fix a universal meaning for the categories or the relationship between them, their approach seems conducive to the kind of historical analysis I am advocating.

16 See Bodin, 1967 [1606 orig.]; Filmer, 1949 and Locke, 1970 [1690 orig.]. See also Fox-Genovese, 1977 and Shanley, 1979.

17 I am grateful to Bernard Lewis for the reference to Islam (Foucault, 1984). On women in classical Athens, see Arthur, 1977.

18 On the French Revolution, see Levy, Applewhite and Johnson, 1979, pp. 209–20; on Soviet legislation, see the documents in Schlesinger, 1949, pp. 62–71, 251–54; on Nazi policy, Mason, 1976a, 1976b.

19 On the French Revolution, see Levy, Applewhite and Johnson, 1979. On the American Revolution, see Hoff-Wilson, 1976; Kerber, 1980; Norton, 1980. On the French Third Republic, see Hause, 1984. An extremely interesting treatment of a recent case is Molyneux, 1985.

20 On pronatalism, see Riley, 1984 and Jenson, 1985. On the 1920s, see the essays in *Stratégies des Femmes*, 1984.

21 For various interpretations of the impact of new work on women, see Shorter, 1975; Tilly and Scott, 1978; and Dublin, 1979.

22 Crompton, 1985. This question is touched on also in Weeks, 1981.

References

ALEXANDER, S. (1984) 'Women, class and sexual difference', *History Workshop*, 17, pp. 125–35.

ARMSTRONG, H. and ARMSTRONG, P. (1984) 'Comments: more on marxist feminism', *Studies in Political Economy*, 15, pp. 179–84.

ARTHUR, M. (1977) '"Liberated woman": the classical era', in BRIDENTHAL, R. and KOONZ, C. (eds) *Becoming Visible: Women in European History*, Boston, MA: Houghton Mifflin.

AUERBACH, J. *et al.* (1985) 'Commentary on Gilligan's *In a Different Voice*', *Feminist Studies*, 11, pp. 149–62.

BARRETT, M. (1984) 'Rethinking women's oppression: a reply to Brenner and Ramas', *New Left Review*, 146, pp. 123–8.

—— (1985) 'A response to Weir and Wilson', *New Left Review*, 150, pp. 143–7.

BENJAMIN, J. (1983) 'Master and slave: the fantasy of erotic domination', in SNITOW, A., STANSELL, C. and THOMPSON, S. (eds) (1983) *Powers of Desire: The Politics of Sexuality*, New York: Monthly Review Press.

BHABHA, H. (1984) 'Of mimicry and man: the ambivalence of colonial discourse', *October*, 28, pp. 125–33.

BODIN, J. (1967 [1606 orig.]) *Six Books of the Commonwealth*, New York: Barnes and Noble.

BOURDIEU, P. (1980) *Le Sens pratique*, Paris: Les Editions de Minuit.

BRENNER, J. and RAMAS, M. (1984) 'Rethinking women's oppression', *New Left Review*, 144, pp. 33–71.

BURKE, E. (1909 [1790 orig.]) *Reflections on the Revolution in France*, New York: P.F. Collier.

BYNUM, C.W. (1982) *Jesus as Mother: Studies in the Spirituality of the High Middle Ages*, Berkeley: University of California Press.

—— (1985) 'Fast, feast, and flesh: the religious significance of food to Medieval women', *Representations*, 11, pp. 1–25.

—— (1987) 'Introduction', *Religion and Gender: Essays on the Complexity of Symbols*, Boston, MA: Beacon Press.

CHODOROW, N. (1978) *The Reproduction of Mothering: Psychoanalysis and the Sociology of Gender*, Berkeley: University of California Press.

CLARK, T.J. (1985) *The Painting of Modern Life*, New York: Knopf.

COWARD, R. (1983) *Patriarchal Precedents*, London: Routledge and Kegan Paul.

CROMPTON, L. (1985) *Byron and Greek Love: Homophobia in Nineteenth-Century England*, Berkeley: University of California Press.

CULLER, J. (1982) *On Deconstruction: Theory and Criticism after Structuralism*, Ithaca, NY: Cornell University Press.

DAVIS, N.Z. (1975) 'Women on top', in *Society and Culture in Early Modern France*, Stanford, CA: Stanford University Press.

—— (1975–76) 'Women's history in transition: the European case', *Feminist Studies*, 3, p. 90.

DE LAURETIS, T. (1984) *Alice Doesn't: Feminism, Semiotics, Cinema*, Bloomington: Indiana University Press.

DERRIDA, J. (1974) *Of Grammatology*, Baltimore, MD: Johns Hopkins University Press.

—— (1979) *Spurs*, Chicago: University of Chicago Press.

DEVANCE, L. (1977) 'Femme, famille, travail et morale sexuelle dans l'idéologie de 1848', in *Mythes et représentations de la femme au XIXe siècle*, Paris: Champion.

DUBLIN, T. (1979) *Women and Work: The Transformation of Work and Community in Lowell, Massachusetts, 1826–1860*, New York: Columbia University Press.

EISENSTEIN, Z. (1981) *Capitalist Patriarchy and the Case for Socialist Feminism*, New York: Longman.

ENGELS, F. (1972 [1884 orig.]) *The Origins of the Family, Private Property, and the State*, New York: International Publishers.

FEMINIST STUDIES (1980) 6, pp. 26–64.

FILMER, R. (1949) *Patriarchia and Other Political Works*, Oxford: Basil Blackwell.

FIRESTONE, S. (1970) *The Dialectic of Sex*, New York: Bantam Books.

FOUCAULT, M. (1980a) *The History of Sexuality, Volume I, An Introduction*, New York: Vintage.

—— (1980b) *Power/Knowledge: Selected Interviews and Other Writings, 1972–1977*, New York: Pantheon.

—— (1984) *Histoire de la sexualité, Vol. 2, L'Usage des plaisirs*, Paris: Gallimard.

FOX-GENOVESE, E. (1977) 'Property and patriarchy in classical bourgeois political theory', *Radical History Review*, 4, pp. 36–59.

GATENS, M. (1985) 'A critique of the sex/gender distinction', in ALLEN, J. and PATTON, P. (eds) *Beyond Marxism?*, Liechhardt, NSW: Intervention Publications.

GEERTZ, C. (1980) 'Blurred genres', *American Scholar*, 49, pp. 165–79.

GILLIGAN, C. (1982) *In a Different Voice: Psychological Theory and the Women's Development*, Cambridge, MA: Harvard University Press.

GODELIER, M. (1981) 'The origins of male domination', *New Left Review*, 127, 17.

GORDON, A.D., BUHLE, M.J. and DYE, N.S. (1976) 'The problem of women's history', in CARROLL, B. (ed.) *Liberating Women's History*, Urbana: University of Illinois Press.

HALL, J.D. (1974) *Revolt Against Chivalry: Jessie Daniel Ames and the Women's Campaign Against Lynching*, New York: Columbia University Press.

HARTMANN, H. (1976) 'Capitalism, patriarchy, and job segregation by sex', *Signs*, 1, p. 168.

—— (1979) 'The unhappy marriage of Marxism and feminism: towards a more progressive union', *Capital and Class*, 8, pp. 1–33.

—— (1981) 'The family as the locus of gender, class, and political struggle: the example of housework', *Signs*, 6, pp. 366–94.

HAUSE, S. (1984) *Women's Suffrage and Social Politics in the Third Republic*, Princeton: Princeton University Press.

HAUSEN, K. (1987) 'The German nation's obligations to the heroes' widows of World War I,' in HIGONNET, M.R. *et al.* (eds) *Behind the Lines: Gender and the Two World Wars*, New Haven, CT: Yale University Press.

HILL, M.A. (1980) *Charlotte Perkins Gilman: The Making of a Radical Feminist, 1860–1896*, Philadelphia, PA: Temple University Press.

HOFF-WILSON, J. (1976) 'The illusion of change: women and the American revolution', in YOUNG, A. (ed.) *The American Revolution: Explorations in the History of American Radicalism*, DeKalb: Northern Illinois University Press.

HUMPHRIES, J. (1971) 'Class struggle and the persistence of the working class family', *Cambridge Journal of Economics*, 1, pp. 241–58.

—— (1977) 'Working class family women's liberation and class struggle: the case of nineteenth-century British history', *Review of Radical Political Economics*, 9, pp. 25–41.

HUNT, L. (1983) 'Hercules and the radical image in the French Revolution', *Representations*, 1, pp. 95–117.

INGLIS, K. (1987) 'The representation of gender on Australian war memorials', *Daedalus*, 116, pp. 35–59

IRIGARAY, L. (1985a) 'Is the subject of science sexed?', *Cultural Critique*, 1, pp. 73–88.

—— (1985b) *Speculum of the Other Woman*, Ithaca, NY: Cornell University Press.

JENSON, J. (1985) 'Gender and reproduction: or, babies and the state', unpublished paper, pp. 1–7.

KELLY, J. (1984) 'The doubled vision of feminist theory', in *Women, History and Theory*, Chicago: University of Chicago Press.

KERBER, L. (1980) *Women of the Republic*, Chapel Hill: University of North Carolina Press.

KUHN, A. (1978) 'Structures of patriarchy and capital in the family', in KUHN, A. and WOLPE, A. (eds) *Feminism and Materialism: Women and Modes of Production*, London: Routledge and Kegan Paul.

LEVY, D.G., APPLEWHITE, H. and JOHNSON, M.D. (eds) (1979) *Women in Revolutionary Paris, 1789–1795*, Urbana: University of Illinois Press.

LEWIS, J. (1980) *The Politics of Motherhood: Child and Maternal Welfare in England, 1900–1939*, London. Croom Helm.

—— (1985) 'The debate on sex and class', *New Left Review*, 149, pp. 108–20.

LITTRE, E. (1876) *Dictionnaire de la langue française*, Paris.

LOCKE, J. (1970 [1690 orig.]) *Two Treatises of Government*, Cambridge: Cambridge University Press.

MCDOUGALL, M.L. (1983) 'Protecting infants: the French campaign for maternity leaves, 1890s–1913', *French Historical Studies*, 13, pp. 79–105.

MACKINNON, C. (1982) 'Feminism, Marxism, method, and state: an agenda for theory', *Signs*, 7, pp. 515–44.

MARTIN, B. (1980) 'Feminism, criticism and Foucault', *New German Critique*, 27, pp. 3–30.

MASON, T. (1976a) 'Women in Nazi Germany', *History Workshop*, 1, pp. 74–113.

—— (1976b) 'Women in Germany, 1925–40: family, welfare and work', *History Workshop*, 2, pp. 5–32.

MILLETT, K. (1971) *Sexual Politics*, London: Hart Davis.

MITCHELL, J. and ROSE, J. (eds) (1983) *Jacques Lacan and the Ecole Freudienne*, New York: Norton.

MOLYNEUX, M. (1985) 'Mobilization without emancipation?: women's interests, the state and revolution in Nicaragua', *Feminist Studies*, 11, pp. 227–54.

MONTROSE, L. (1983) 'Shaping fantasies: figurations of gender and power in Elizabethan culture', *Representations*, 1, pp. 61–94.

NICHOLSON, L.J. (1986) *Gender and History: The Limits of Social Theory in the Age of the Family*, New York: Columbia University Press.

NORTON, M.B. (1980) *Liberty's Daughters: The Revolutionary Experience of American Women*, Boston, MA: Little, Brown.

O'BRIEN, M. (1981) *The Politics of Reproduction*, London: Routledge and Kegan Paul.

PAPERS ON PATRIARCHY CONFERENCE, LONDON 76, (1976) London: [n.p.n.].

PHILLIPS, R. (1976) 'Women and family breakdown in eighteenth century France: Rouen, 1780–1800', *Social History*, 2, p. 217.

RANCIERE, J. and VAUDRAY, P. (1975) 'En allant a l'expo: l'ouvrier, sa femme et les machines', *Les Révokes logiques*, 1, pp. 5–22.

RATTE, L. (1983) 'Gender ambivalence in the Indian nationalist movement', unpublished paper, Pembroke Centre Seminar, spring.

RILEY, D. (1984) *War in the Nursery*, London: Virago.

—— (1985) 'Summary of preamble to interwar feminist history work', unpublished paper, presented to the Preamble Seminar, May.

—— (1988) *'Am I That Name?': Feminism and the Category of 'Women' in History*, Basingstoke: Macmillan.

ROSALDO, M.Z. (1980) 'The use and abuse of anthropology: reflections on feminism and cross-cultural understanding', *Signs*, 5, pp. 389–417.

ROSS, E. and RAPP, R. (1983) 'Sex and society: a research note from social history and anthropology', in SNITOW, A., STANSELL, C. and THOMPSON, S. (eds) *Powers of Desire: The Politics of Sexuality*, New York: Monthly Review Press.

ROSSITER, M. (1982) *Women Scientists in America: Struggles and Strategies to 1914*, Baltimore, MD: Johns Hopkins University Press.

RUBIN, G. (1975) 'The traffic in women: notes on the political economy of sex,' in REITER, R.R. (ed.) *Towards an Anthropology of Women*, New York: Monthly Review Press.

SAMUEL, R. (ed.) (1981) *People's History and Socialist Theory*, London: Routledge and Kegan Paul.

SCHLESINGER, R. (1949) *Changing Attitudes in Soviet Russia: Documents and Readings, vol. 1, The Family in USSR*, London: Routledge and Kegan Paul.

SCOTT, H. (1974) *Does Socialism Liberate Women?: Experiences from Eastern Europe*, Boston, MA: Beacon Press.

SHANLEY, M.L. (1979) 'Marriage contract and social contract in seventeenth century English political thought', *Western Political Quarterly*, 3, pp. 79–91.

SHORTER, E. (1975) *The Making of the Modern Family*, New York: Basic Books.

SINHA, M. (1984) 'Manliness: a Victorian ideal and the British imperial elite in India', unpublished paper, Department of History, State University of New York, Stony Brook.

—— (1986) 'The age of consent Act: the ideal of masculinity and colonial ideology in late 19th century Bengal', *Proceedings, Eighth International Symposium on Asian Studies*, pp. 1199–1214.

SKLAR, K.K. (1973) *Catharine Beecher: A Study in American Domesticity*, New Haven, CT: Yale University Press.

SNITOW, A., STANSELL, C. and THOMPSON, S. (eds) (1983) *Powers of Desire: The Politics of Sexuality*, New York: Monthly Review Press.

SOCIAL RESEARCH (1983) 'Women and morality' (special issue), 50.

SPIVAK, G.C. (1981) '"Draupadi" by Mahasveta Devi', *Critical Inquiry*, 8, pp. 381–401.

—— (1985) 'Three women's texts and a critique of imperialism', *Critical Inquiry*, 12, pp. 243–6.

STRATEGIES DES FEMMES (1984) Paris: Editions Tierce.

SUBJECTS/OBJECTS (1984) fall issue.

TAYLOR, B. (1983) *Eve and the New Jerusalem*, New York: Pantheon.

TILLY, L.A. and SCOTT, J. (1978) *Women, Work and Family*, New York: Holt, Rinehart and Winston.

WEEKS, J. (1981) *Sex, Politics and Society: The Regulation of Sexuality since 1800*, London: Leyman.

WEIL, R. (1985) 'The crown has fallen to the distaff: gender and politics in the age of Catherine de Medici', *Critical Matrix* (Princeton Working Papers in Women's Studies).

WEIR, A. and WILSON, E. (1984) 'The British women's movement', *New Left Review*, 148, pp. 74–103.

WILLIAMS, R. (1983) *Keywords*, New York: Oxford University Press.

WILSON, E. (1977) *Women and the Welfare State*, London: Tavistock.

6 'Gender' for a Marxist dictionary

The sexual politics of a word

Donna J. Haraway [1991]

In 1993, Nora Räthzel from the autonomous women's collective of the West German independent Marxist journal *Das Argument*, wrote to ask me to write a 'keyword' entry for a new
Marxist dictionary. An editorial group from *Das Argument* had undertaken an ambitious
project to translate the multi-volume *Dictionnaire Critique du Marxisme* (Labica and
Benussen, 1985) into German and also to prepare a separate German supplement that brought
in especially the new social movements that were not treated in the French edition.[1] These
movements have produced a revolution in critical social theory internationally in the last
twenty years. They have also produced – and been partly produced by – revolutions in political language in the same period. As Räthzel expressed it, 'We, that is the women's editorial
group, are going to suggest some keywords which are missing, and we want some others
rewritten because the women do not appear where they should' (personal communication, 2
December 1993). This gentle understatement identified a major arena of feminist struggle –
the canonization of language, politics, and historical narratives in publishing practices,
including standard reference works.

'The women do not appear where they should.' The ambiguities of the statement were potent
and tempting. Here was an opportunity to participate in producing a reference text. I had up to
five typed pages for my assignment: sex/gender. Foolhardy, I wrote to accept the task.

There was an immediate problem: I am anglophone, with variously workable but troubled
German, French, and Spanish. This crippled language accomplishment reflects my political
location in a social world distorted by US hegemonic projects and the culpable ignorance of
white, especially, US citizens. English, especially American English, distinguishes between
sex and gender. That distinction has cost blood in struggle in many social arenas, as the reader
will see in the discussion that follows. German has a single word, *Geschlecht*, which is not
really the same as either the English sex or gender. Further, the dictionary project, translating
foreign contributors' entries into German, proposed to give each keyword in German,
Chinese (both ideogram and transcription), English, French, Russian (in transcription only),
and Spanish. The commingled histories of Marxism and of imperialism loomed large in that
list. Each keyword would inherit those histories.

At least I knew that what was happening to sex and gender in English was not the same as
what was going on with *género*, *genre*, and *Geschlecht*. The specific histories of women's
movements in the vast global areas where these languages were part of living politics were
principal reasons for the differences. The old hegemonic grammarians – including the sexologists – had lost control of gender and its proliferating siblings. Europe and North America
could not begin to discipline the twentieth-century fate of its imperializing languages.
However, I did not have a clue what to make of my sex/gender problem in Russian or
Chinese. Progressively, it became clear to me that I had rather few clues what to make of sex/

gender in *English*, even in the United States, much less in the anglophone world. There are so many Englishes in the United States alone, and all of them suddenly seemed germane to this promised five-page text for a German Marxist dictionary that was splitting off from its French parent in order to pay attention to new social movements. My English was marked by race, generation, gender (!), region, class, education, and political history. How could that English be my matrix for sex/gender in general? Was there any such thing, even as words, much less as anything else, as 'sex/gender in general'? Obviously not. These were not new problems for contributors to dictionaries, but I felt, well, chicken, *politically* chicken. But the presses roll on, and a due date was approaching. It was time to pluck out a feather and write. In the late twentieth century, after all, we are ourselves literally embodied writing technologies. That is part of the implosion of gender in sex and language, in biology and syntax, enabled by Western technoscience.

In 1985 I was moderately cheered to learn that the editorial group really wanted an entry on the sex/gender system. That helped; there was a specific textual locus for the first use of the term – Gayle Rubin's (1975) stunning essay, written when she was a graduate student at the University of Michigan, 'The traffic in women: notes on the political economy of sex'. I could just trace the fate of the 'sex/gender system' in the explosion of socialist and Marxist feminist writing indebted to Rubin. That thought provided very brief consolation. First, the editors directed that each keyword had to locate itself in relation to the corpus of Marx and Engels, whether or not they used the precise words. I think Marx would have been amused at the dead hand guiding the living cursor on the video display terminal. Second, those who adopted Rubin's formulation did so out of many histories, including academic and political interests. US white socialist feminists generated the most obvious body of writing for tracing the 'sex/gender system' narrowly considered. That fact itself was a complex problem, not a solution. Much of the most provocative feminist theory in the last twenty years has insisted on the ties of sex and race in ways that problematized the birth pangs of the sex/gender system in a discourse more focused on the interweaving of gender and class.[2] It has seemed very rare for feminist theory to hold race, sex/gender, and class analytically together – all the best intentions, hues of authors, and remarks in prefaces notwithstanding. In addition, there is as much reason for feminists to argue for a race/gender system as for a sex/gender system, and the two are not the same kind of analytical move. And, again, what happened to class? The evidence is building of a need for a theory of 'difference' whose geometries, paradigms, and logics break out of binaries, dialectics, and nature/culture models of any kind. Otherwise, threes will always reduce to twos, which quickly become lonely ones in the vanguard. And no one learns to count to four. These things matter politically.

Also, even though Marx and Engels – or Gayle Rubin, for that matter – had not ventured into sexology, medicine, or biology for their discussions of sex/gender or the woman question, I knew I would have to do so. At the same time, it was clear that other BIG currents of modern feminist writing on sex, sexuality, and gender interlaced constantly with even the most modest interpretation of my assignment. Most of those, perhaps especially the French and British feminist psychoanalytic and literary currents, do not appear in my entry on *Geschlecht*. In general, the entry below focuses on writing by US feminists. That is not a trivial scandal.[3]

So, what follows shows the odd jumps of continual reconstructions over six years. The gaps and rough edges, as well as the generic form of an encyclopedia entry, should all call attention to the political and conventional processes of standardization. Probably the smooth passages are the most revealing of all; they truly paper over a very contentious field. Perhaps only I needed a concrete lesson in how problematic an entry on any 'keyword' must be. But I suspect my sisters and other comrades also have at times tended simply to believe what they looked up in a reference work, instead of remembering that this form of writing is one more process for inhabiting possible worlds – tentatively, hopefully, polyvocally, and finitely. Finally, the keyword entry exceeded five typed pages, and the chicken was plucked bare. The body had become all text, and the instrument for the inscription was not a feather, but a mouse. The new genitalia of writing will supply the analyst with her metaphors, as the sex/gender system transmogrifies into other worlds of consequential, powercharged difference.

Keyword

Gender (English), Geschlecht (German), Genre (French), Género (Spanish)

[The root of the English, French, and Spanish words is the Latin verb *generare*, to beget, and the Latin stem *gener-*, race or kind. An obsolete English meaning of 'to gender' is 'to copulate' (*Oxford English Dictionary*). The substantives 'Geschlecht', 'gender', 'genre', and 'género' refer to the notion of sort, kind, and class. In English, 'gender' has been used in this 'generic' sense continuously since at least the fourteenth century. In French, German, Spanish, and English, words for 'gender' refer to grammatical and literary categories. The modern English and German words, 'gender' and 'Geschlecht', adhere closely to concepts of sex, sexuality, sexual difference, generation, engendering, and so on, while the French and Spanish seem not to carry those meanings as readily. Words close to 'gender' are implicated in concepts of kinship, race, biological taxonomy, language, and nationality. The substantive 'Geschlecht' carries the meanings of sex, stock, race, and family, while the adjectival form 'geschlechtlich' means in English translation both sexual and generic. 'Gender' is at the heart of constructions and classifications of systems of difference. Complex differentiation and merging of terms for 'sex' and 'gender' are part of the political history of the words. Medical meanings related to 'sex' accrue to 'gender' in English progressively through the twentieth century. Medical, zoological, grammatical, and literary meanings have all been contested in modern feminisms. The shared categorical racial and sexual meanings of gender point to the interwoven modern histories of colonial, racist, and sexual oppressions in systems of bodily production and inscription and their consequent liberatory and oppositional discourses. The difficulty of accommodating racial and sexual oppressions in Marxist theories of class is paralleled in the history of the words themselves. This background is essential to understanding the resonances of the theoretical concept of the 'sex-gender system' constructed by Western anglophone feminists in the 1970s.[4] In all their versions, feminist gender theories attempt to articulate the specificity of the oppressions of women in the context of cultures which make a distinction between sex and gender salient. That salience depends on a related system of meanings clustered around a family of binary pairs: nature/culture, nature/history, natural/human, resource/product. This interdependence on a key Western political-philosophical field of binary oppositions – whether understood functionally, dialectically, structurally, or psychoanalytically – problematizes claims to the universal applicability of the concepts around sex and gender; this issue is part of the current debate about the cross-cultural relevance of Euro-American versions of feminist theory (Strathern, 1988). The value of an analytical category is not necessarily annulled by critical consciousness of its historical specificity and cultural limits. But feminist concepts of gender raise sharply the problems of cultural comparison, linguistic translation, and political solidarity.]

History

Articulation of the problem area in the writings of Marx and Engels

In a critical, political sense, the concept of gender was articulated and progressively contested and theorized in the context of the post-Second-World-War, feminist women's movements. The modern feminist concept for gender is not found in the writings of Marx and Engels, although their writings and other practice, and those of others in the Marxist tradition, have provided crucial tools for, as well as barriers against, the later politicization and theorization of gender. Despite important differences, all the modern feminist meanings of gender have roots in Simone de Beauvoir's claim that 'one is not born a woman' (de Beauvoir, 1949; 1952, p. 249) and in post-Second-World-War social conditions that have enabled constructions of women as a collective historical subject-in-process. Gender is a concept developed to contest the naturalization of sexual difference in multiple arenas of struggle. Feminist theory and practice around gender seek to explain and change historical systems of sexual difference, whereby 'men' and 'women' are socially constituted and positioned in relations of hierarchy and antagonism. Since the concept of gender is so closely related to the Western distinction between nature and society or nature and history, via the distinction between sex and gender, the relation of feminist gender theories to Marxism is tied to the fate of the concepts of nature and labour in the Marxist canon and in Western philosophy more broadly.

Traditional Marxist approaches did not lead to a political concept of gender for two major reasons: first, women, as well as 'tribal' peoples, existed unstably at the boundary of the natural and social in the seminal writings of Marx and Engels, such that their efforts to account for the subordinate position of women were undercut by the category of the natural sexual division of labour, with its ground in an unexaminable natural heterosexuality; and second, Marx and Engels theorized the economic property relation as the ground of the oppression of women in marriage, such that women's subordination could be examined in terms of the capitalist relations of class, but not in terms of a specific sexual politics between men and women. The classical location of this argument is Engels' *The Origins of the Family, Private Property and the State* (1884). Engels' analytic priority of the family as a mediating formation between classes and the state subsumed any separate consideration of the division of the sexes as an antagonistic division (Coward, 1983, p. 160).[5] Despite their insistence on the historical variability of family forms and the importance of the question of the subordination of women, Marx and Engels could not historicize sex and gender from a base of natural heterosexuality.

The German Ideology (Marx and Engels, 1970; Part I, Theses on Feuerbach) is the major locus for Marx and Engels' naturalization of the sexual division of labour, in their assumption of a pre-social division of labour in the sex act (heterosexual intercourse), its supposed natural corollaries in the reproductive activities of men and women in the family, and the consequent inability to place women in their relations to men unambiguously on the side of history and of the fully social. In *The Economic and Philosophic Manuscripts of 1844*, Marx refers to the relation of man and woman as the 'most natural relation of human being to human being' (Marx, 1964b, p. 34). This assumption persists in volume one of *Capital* (Marx, 1964a, p. 351). This inability fully to historicize women's labour is paradoxical in view of the purpose of *The German Ideology* and subsequent work to place the family centrally in history as the place where social divisions arise. The root difficulty was an inability to historicize sex itself; like nature, sex functioned analytically as a prime matter or raw material for the work of history. Relying on Marx's research on ethnographic writings, Engels' *Origins* (1972 [orig. 1884]) systematized Marx's views about the linked transitions of family, forms of property,

of the division of labour, and the state. Engels almost laid a basis for theo-
oppressions of women in his brief assertion that a fully materialist analysis
d reproduction of immediate life reveals a twofold character: the produc-
of existence and 'the production of human beings themselves' ([orig. 1884];
. An exploration of this latter character has been the starting point for many Euro-
ican Marxist-feminists in their theories of the sex/gender division of labour (Chodorow,
1978; Harding, 1983, 1986; Hartmann, 1981; Hartsock, 1983a, 1983b; Jaggar, 1983;
O'Brien, 1981; Rubin, 1975; Young and Levidow, 1981).

The 'woman question' was widely debated in the many European Marxist parties in the late
nineteenth and early twentieth centuries. In the context of the German Social Democratic
Party the other of the two most influential Marxist treatments of the position of women was
written, August Bebel's *Woman under Socialism* (1883; orig. *Women in the Past, Present and
Future*, 1878). Alexandra Kollontai drew on Bebel in her struggles for women's emancipation in Russia and the Soviet Union; and within German social democracy, Clara Zetkin, a
leader of the International Socialist Women's Movement, developed Bebel's position in her
1889 'The Question of Women Workers and Women at the Present Time'.[6]

Current problematic

The gender identity paradigm

The story of the political reformulations of gender by post-1960s Western feminists must
pass through the construction of meanings and technologies of sex and gender in normal-
izing, liberal, interventionist-therapeutic, empiricist, and functionalist life sciences, principally in the United States, including psychology, psychoanalysis, medicine, biology, and
sociology. Gender was located firmly in an individualist problematic within the broad
'incitement to discourse' (Foucault, 1978) on sexuality characteristic of bourgeois, male-
dominant, and racist society. The concepts and technologies of 'gender identity' were
crafted from several components: an instinctualist reading of Freud; the focus on sexual
somatic and psychopathology by the great nineteenth-century sexologists (Krafft-Ebing,
Havelock Ellis) and their followers; the ongoing development of biochemical and physiological endocrinology from the 1920s; the psychobiology of sex differences growing out of
comparative psychology; proliferating hypotheses of hormonal, chromosomal, and neural
sexual dimorphism converging in the 1950s; and the first gender reassignment surgeries
around 1960 (Linden, 1981). 'Second-wave' feminist politics around 'biological determinism' vs. 'social constructionism' and the biopolitics of sex/gender differences occur within
discursive fields pre-structured by the gender identity paradigm crystallized in the 1950s and
1960s. The gender identity paradigm was a functionalist and essentializing version of Simone
de Beauvoir's 1940s insight that one is not born a woman. Significantly, the construction of
what could count as a woman (or a man) became a problem for bourgeois functionalists and
pre-feminist existentialists in the same historical post-war period in which the social foundations of women's lives in a world capitalist, male-dominant system were undergoing basic
reformulations.

In 1958, the Gender Identity Research Project was established at the University of California at Los Angeles (UCLA) medical centre for the study of intersexuals and transsexuals.
The psychoanalyst Robert Stoller's work (1968, 1976) discussed and generalized the findings
of the UCLA project. Stoller (1964) introduced the term 'gender identity' to the International
Psychoanalytic Congress at Stockholm in 1963. He formulated the concept of gender identity

within the framework of the biology/culture distinction, such that sex was related to biology (hormones, genes, nervous system, morphology) and gender was related to culture (psychology, sociology). The product of culture's working of biology was the core, achieved, gendered person – a man or a woman. Beginning in the 1950s, the psychoendocrinologist, John Money, ultimately from the institutional base of the Johns Hopkins Medical School's Gender Identity Clinic (established 1965), with his colleague, Anke Ehrhardt, developed and popularized the interactionist version of the gender identity paradigm, in which the functionalist mix of biological and social causations made room for a myriad of 'sex/gender differences' research and therapeutic programmes, including surgery, counselling, pedagogy, social services, and so on. Money and Ehrhardt's (1972) *Man and Woman, Boy and Girl* became a widely used college and university textbook.

The version of the nature/culture distinction in the gender identity paradigm was part of a broad liberal reformulation of life and social sciences in the post-Second-World-War, Western, professional and governing élites' divestment of pre-war renditions of biological racism. These reformulations failed to interrogate the political-social history of binary categories like nature/culture, and so sex/gender, in colonialist Western discourse. This discourse structured the world as an object of knowledge in terms of the appropriation by culture of the resources of nature. Many recent oppositional, liberatory literatures have criticized this ethnocentric epistemological and linguistic dimension of the domination of those inhabiting 'natural' categories or living at the mediating boundaries of the binarisms (women, people of colour, animals, the non-human environment) (Harding, 1986, pp. 163–96; Fee, 1986). Second-wave feminists soon criticized the binary logics of the nature/culture pair, including dialectical versions of the Marxist-humanist story of the domination, appropriation, or mediation of 'nature' by 'man' through 'labour'. But these efforts hesitated to extend their criticism fully to the derivative sex/gender distinction. That distinction was too useful in combating the pervasive biological determinisms constantly deployed against feminists in urgent 'sex differences' political struggles in schools, publishing houses, clinics, and so on. Fatally, in this constrained political climate, these early critiques did not focus on historicizing and culturally relativizing the 'passive' categories of sex or nature. Thus, formulations of an essential identity as a woman or a man were left analytically untouched and politically dangerous.

In the political and epistemological effort to remove women from the category of nature and to place them in culture as constructed and self-constructing social subjects in history, the concept of gender has tended to be quarantined from the infections of biological sex. Consequently, the ongoing constructions of what counts as sex or as female have been hard to theorize, except as 'bad science' where the female emerges as naturally subordinate. 'Biology' has tended to denote the body itself, rather than a social discourse open to intervention. Thus, feminists have argued against 'biological determinism' and for 'social constructionism' and in the process have been less powerful in deconstructing how bodies, including sexualized and racialized bodies, appear as objects of knowledge and sites of intervention in 'biology'. Alternatively, feminists have sometimes affirmed the categories of nature and the body as sites of resistance to the dominations of history, but the affirmations have tended to obscure the categorical and overdetermined aspect of 'nature' or the 'female body' as an oppositional ideological resource. Instead, nature has seemed simply there, a reserve to be preserved from the violations of civilization in general. Rather than marking a categorically determined pole, 'nature' or 'woman's body' too easily then means the saving core of reality distinguishable from the social impositions of patriarchy, imperialism, capitalism, racism, history, language. That repression of the construction of the category 'nature' can be and has been both used by and used against feminist efforts to theorize women's agency and status as social subjects.

Judith Butler (1989) argued that gender identity discourse is intrinsic to the fictions of heterosexual coherence, and that feminists need to learn to produce narrative legitimacy for a whole array of noncoherent genders. Gender identity discourse is also intrinsic to feminist racism, which insists on the non-reducibility and antagonistic relation of coherent women and men. The task is to 'disqualify' the analytic categories, like sex or nature, that lead to univocity. This move would expose the illusion of an interior organizing gender core and produce a field of race and gender difference open to resignification. Many feminists have resisted moves like those Butler recommends, for fear of losing a concept of agency for women as the concept of the subject withers under the attack on core identities and their constitutive fictions. Butler, however, argued that agency is an instituted practice in a field of enabling constraints. A concept of a coherent inner self, achieved (cultural) or innate (biological), is a regulatory fiction that is unnecessary – indeed, inhibitory – for feminist projects of producing and affirming complex agency and responsibility.

A related 'regulatory fiction' basic to Western concepts of gender insists that motherhood is natural and fatherhood is cultural: mothers make babies naturally, biologically. Motherhood is known on sight; fatherhood is inferred. Analysing gender concepts and practices among Melanesians, Strathern (1988, pp. 311–39) went to great pains to show both the ethnocentric quality of the self-evident Western assertion that 'women make babies' and the inferential character of all vision. She showed the productionist core of the belief that women make babies (and its pair, that man makes himself), which is intrinsic to Western formulations of sex and gender. Strathern argued that Hagen men and women do not exist in permanent states as subjects and objects within Aristotelian, Hegelian, Marxist, or Freudian frames. Hagen agency has a different dynamic and geometry. For Westerners, it is a central consequence of concepts of gender difference that a person may be turned by another person into an object and robbed of her or his status as subject. The proper state for a Western person is to have ownership of the self, to have and hold a core identity as if it were a possession. That possession may be made from various raw materials over time, that is, it may be a cultural production, or one may be born with it. Gender identity is such a possession. Not to have property in the self is not to be a subject, and so not to have agency. Agency follows different pathways for the Hagen, who as persons 'are composed of multiple gendered parts, or multiple gendered persons, who are interacting with one another as donors and recipients in maintaining the flow of elements through the body' (Douglas, 1989, p. 17). Sexist domination between persons can and does systematically occur, but it cannot be traced or addressed by the same analytical moves that would be appropriate for many Western social fields of meaning (Strathern, 1988, pp. 334–9). Butler could – cautiously – use Strathern's ethnographic arguments to illustrate one way to disperse the coherence of gender without losing the power of agency.

So, the ongoing tactical usefulness of the sex/gender distinction in life and social sciences has had dire consequences for much feminist theory, tying it to a liberal and functionalist paradigm despite repeated efforts to transcend those limits in a fully politicized and historicized concept of gender. The failure lay partly in not historicizing and relativizing sex and the historical-epistemological roots of the logic of analysis implied in the sex/gender distinction and in each member of the pair. At this level, the modern feminist limitation in theorizing and struggling for the empirical life and social sciences is similar to Marx and Engels' inability to extricate themselves from the natural sexual division of labour in heterosexuality despite their admirable project of historicizing the family.

Sex/gender differences discourse exploded in US sociological and psychological literature in the 1970s and 1980s. (This is shown, for example, in the occurrence of the word gender as a keyword in the abstracts for articles indexed in *Sociological Abstracts* [from 0 entries between

1966 and 1970, to 724 entries between 1981 and 1985], and in *Psychological Abstracts* [from 50 keyword abstract entries from 1966 to 1970, to 1326 such entries from 1981 to 1985].) The explosion is part of a vigorous political and scientific contestation over the construction of sex and gender, as categories and as emergent historical realities, in which feminist writing becomes prominent about the mid-1970s, primarily in criticisms of 'biological determinism' and of sexist science and technology, especially biology and medicine. Set up within the epistemological binary framework of nature/culture and sex/gender, many feminists (including socialist and Marxist feminists) appropriated the sex/gender distinction and the interactionist paradigm to argue for the primacy of culture-gender over biology-sex in a panoply of debates in Europe and the United States. These debates have ranged from genetic differences in mathematics ability of boys and girls, the presence and significance of sex differences in neural organization, the relevance of animal research to human behaviour, the causes of male dominance in the organization of scientific research, sexist structures and use patterns in language, sociobiology debates, struggles over the meanings of sex-chromosomal abnormalities, to the similarities of racism and sexism. By the mid-1980s, a growing suspicion of the category of gender and the binarism sex/gender entered the feminist literature in these debates. That scepticism was partly an outgrowth of challenges to racism in the Euro-American women's movements, such that some of the colonial and racist roots of the framework became clearer.[7]

The sex-gender system

Another stream of feminist sex-gender theory and politics came through appropriations of Marx and Freud read through Lacan and Lévi-Strauss in an influential formulation by Gayle Rubin (1975) of the 'sex-gender system'. Her paper appeared in the first anthology of socialist/Marxist feminist anthropology in the United States. Rubin and those indebted to her theorization adopted a version of the nature/culture distinction, but one flowing less out of US empiricist life and social science, and more from French psychoanalysis and structuralism. Rubin examined the 'domestication of women', in which human females were the raw materials for the social production of women, through the exchange systems of kinship controlled by men in the institution of human culture. She defined the sex-gender system as the system of social relations that transformed biological sexuality into products of human activity and in which the resulting historically specific sexual needs are met. She then called for a Marxian analysis of sex/gender systems as products of human activity which are changeable through political struggle. Rubin viewed the sexual division of labour and the psychological construction of desire (especially the oedipal formation) as the foundations of a system of production of human beings vesting men with rights in women which they do not have in themselves. To survive materially where men and women cannot perform the other's work and to satisfy deep structures of desire in the sex/gender system in which men exchange women, heterosexuality is obligatory. Obligatory heterosexuality is therefore central to the oppression of women.

> If the sexual property system were reorganized in such a way that men did not have overriding rights in women (if there was no exchange of women) and if there were no gender, the entire Oedipal drama would be a relic. In short, feminism must call for a revolution in kinship.
>
> (Rubin, 1975, p. 199)

Adrienne Rich (1980) also theorized compulsory heterosexuality to be at the root of the oppression of women. Rich figured 'the lesbian continuum' as a potent metaphor for grounding a new sisterhood. For Rich, marriage resistance in a cross-historical sweep was a defining practice constituting the lesbian continuum. Monique Wittig (1981) developed an independent argument that also foregrounded the centrality of obligatory heterosexuality in the oppression of women. In a formulation that its authors saw as the explanation for the decisive break with traditional Marxism of the Mouvement pour la Libération des Femmes (MLF) in France, the group associated with Wittig argued that all women belong to a class constituted by the hierarchical social relation of sexual difference that gives men ideological, political and economic power over women (Editors of *Questions féministes*, 1980).[8] What makes a woman is a specific relation of appropriation by a man. Like race, sex is an 'imaginary' formation of the kind that produces reality, including bodies then perceived as prior to all construction. 'Woman' only exists as this kind of imaginary being, while women are the product of a social relation of appropriation, naturalized as sex. A feminist is one who fights for women as a class and for the disappearance of that class. The key struggle is for the destruction of the social system of heterosexuality, because 'sex' is the naturalized political category that founds society as heterosexual. All the social sciences based on the category of 'sex' (most of them) must be overthrown. In this view, lesbians are not 'women' because they are outside the political economy of heterosexuality. Lesbian society destroys women as a natural group (Wittig, 1981).

Thus, theorized in three different frames, withdrawal from marriage was central to Rubin's, Rich's, and Wittig's political visions in the 1970s and early 1980s. Marriage encapsulated and reproduced the antagonistic relation of the two coherent social groups, men and women. In all three formulations both the binary of nature/culture and the dynamic of productionism enabled the further analysis. Withdrawal of women from the marriage economy was a potent figure and politics for withdrawal from men, and therefore for the self-constitution of women as personal and historical subjects outside the institution of culture by men in the exchange and appropriation of the products (including babies) of women. To be a subject in the Western sense meant reconstituting women outside the relations of objectification (as gift, commodity, object of desire) and appropriation (of babies, sex, services). The category-defining relation of men and women in objectification, exchange, and appropriation, which was the theoretical key to the category 'gender' in major bodies of feminist theory by white women in this period, was one of the moves that made an understanding of the race/gender or race/sex system and the barriers to cross-racial 'sisterhood' hard for white feminists analytically to grasp.

However, these formulations had the powerful virtue of foregrounding and legitimating lesbianism at the heart of feminism. The figure of the lesbian has been repeatedly at the contentious, generative centre of feminist debate (King, 1986). Audre Lorde put the black lesbian at the heart of her understanding of the 'house of difference':

> Being women together was not enough. We were different. Being gay-girls together was not enough. We were different. Being Black together was not enough. We were different. Being Black women together was not enough. We were different. Being Black dykes together was not enough. We were different … It was a while before we came to realize that our place was the very house of difference rather than the security of any one particular difference.
>
> (Lorde, 1982, p. 226)

This concept of difference grounded much US multi-cultural feminist theorizing on gender in the late 1980s.

There have been many uses and criticisms of Rubin's sex-gender system. In an article at the centre of much Euro-American Marxist and socialist-feminist debate, Hartmann (1981) insisted that patriarchy was not simply an ideology, as Juliet Mitchell seemed to argue in her seminal 'Women: the Longest Revolution' (1966) and its expansion in *Women's Estate* (1972), but a material system that could be defined 'as a set of social relations between men, which have a material base, and which, though hierarchical, establish or create interdependence and solidarity among men that enable them to dominate women' (Hartmann, 1981, p. 14). Within this frame, Hartmann attempted to explain the partnership of patriarchy and capital and the failure of male-dominated socialist labour movements to prioritize sexism. Hartmann used Rubin's concept of the sex-gender system to call for an understanding of the mode of production of human beings in patriarchal social relations through male control of women's labour power.

In the debate stimulated by Hartmann's thesis, Iris Young (1981) criticized the 'dual systems' approach to capital and patriarchy, which were then allied in the oppressions of class and gender. Note how race, including an interrogation of white racial positioning, remained an unexplored system in these formulations. Young argued that 'patriarchal relations are internally related to production relations as a whole' (1981, p. 49), such that a focus on the gender division of labour could reveal the dynamics of a single system of oppression. In addition to waged labour, the gender division of labour also included the excluded and unhistoricized labour categories in Marx and Engels, that is, bearing and rearing children, caring for the sick, cooking, housework, and sex-work like prostitution, in order to bring gender and women's specific situation to the centre of historical materialist analysis. In this theory, since the gender division of labour was also the first division of labour, one must give an account of the emergence of class society out of changes in the gender division of labour. Such an analysis does not posit that all women have a common, unified situation; but it makes the historically differentiated positions of women central. If capitalism and patriarchy are a single system, called capitalist patriarchy, then the struggle against class and gender oppressions must be unified. The struggle is the obligation of men and women, although autonomous women's organization would remain a practical necessity. This theory is a good example of strongly rationalist, modernist approaches, for which the 'postmodern' moves of the desegregation of metaphors of single systems in favour of complex open fields of criss-crossing plays of domination, privilege, and difference appeared very threatening. Young's 1981 work was also a good example of the power of modernist approaches in specific circumstances to provide political direction.

In exploring the epistemological consequences of a feminist historical materialism, Nancy Hartsock (1983a, 1983b) also concentrated on the categories that Marxism had been unable to historicize: (1) women's sensuous labour in the making of human beings through child-bearing and raising; and (2) women's nurturing and subsistence labour of all kinds. But Hartsock rejected the terminology of the gender division of labour in favour of the sexual division of labour, in order to emphasize the bodily dimensions of women's activity. Hartsock was also critical of Rubin's formulation of the sex-gender system because it emphasized the exchange system of kinship at the expense of a materialist analysis of the labour process that grounded women's potential construction of a revolutionary standpoint. Hartsock relied on versions of Marxist humanism embedded in the story of human self-formation in the sensuous mediations of nature and humanity through labour. In showing how women's lives differed systematically from men's, she aimed to establish the ground for a feminist materialist standpoint, which would be an engaged position and vision, from which the real relations of domination could be unmasked and a liberatory reality struggled for. She called for exploration of the relations between the exchange abstraction and abstract masculinity in the hostile systems of power characterizing phallocratic worlds. Several other Marxist feminists have contributed to intertwined and independent versions of feminist standpoint theory, where the debate on the sex/gender division of labour is a central issue. Fundamental to the debate is a progressive problematization of the category labour, or its extensions in Marxist-feminist meanings of reproduction, for efforts to theorize women's active agency and status as subjects in history.[9] Collins (1989a) adapted standpoint theory to characterize the foundations of black feminist thought in the self-defined perspective of black women on their own oppression.

Sandra Harding (1983) took account of the feminist theoretical flowering as a reflection of a heightening of lived contradictions in the sex-gender system, such that fundamental change can now be struggled for. In extending her approach to the sex-gender system to *The Science Question in Feminism* (1986), Harding stressed three variously interrelated elements of gender: (1) a fundamental category through which meaning is ascribed to everything, (2) a way of organizing social relations, and (3) a structure of personal identity. Desegregating these three elements has been part of coming to understand the complexity and problematic value of politics based on gender identities. Using the sex-gender system to explore post-Second-World-War politics of sexual identity in gay movements, Jeffrey Escoffier (1985) argued for a need to theorize the emergence and limitations of new forms of political subjectivity, in order to develop a committed, positioned politics without metaphysical identity closures. Haraway's (1985) 'Manifesto for Cyborgs' developed similar arguments in order to explore Marxist-feminist politics addressed to women's positionings in multi-national science and technology mediated social, cultural, and technical systems.

In another theoretical development indebted to Marxism, while critical both of it and of the language of gender, Catherine MacKinnon argued that

> Sexuality is to feminism what work is to marxism: that which is most one's own, yet most taken away ... Sexuality is that social process which creates, organizes, expresses, and directs desire, creating the social beings we know as women and men, as their relations create society ... As the organized expropriation of the work of some for the benefit of others defines a class – workers – the organized expropriation of the sexuality of some for the use of other defines the sex, woman.
>
> (MacKinnon, 1982, p. 515)

MacKinnon's position has been central to controversial approaches to political action in much of the US movement against pornography, defined as violence against women and/or as a violation of women's civil rights; that is, a refusal to women, via their construction as woman, of the status of citizen. MacKinnon saw the construction of woman as the material and ideological construction of the object of another's desire. Thus women are not simply alienated from the product of their labour; in so far as they exist as 'woman', that is to say, sex objects, they are not even potentially historical subjects. 'For women, there is no distinction between objectification and alienation because women have not authored objectifications, we have been them' (1982, pp. 253–4). The epistemological and political consequences of this position are far reaching and have been extremely controversial. For MacKinnon, the production of women is the production of a very material illusion, 'woman'. Unpacking this material illusion, which is women's lived reality, requires a politics of consciousness-raising, the specific form of feminist politics in MacKinnon's frame. 'Sexuality determines gender', and 'women's sexuality is its use, just as our femaleness is its alterity' (1982, p. 243). Like independent formulations in Lacanian feminisms, MacKinnon's position has been fruitful in theorizing processes of representation, in which 'power to create the world from one's point of view is power in its male form' (1982, p. 249).

In an analysis of the gendering of violence sympathetic to MacKinnon's, but drawing on different theoretical and political resources, Teresa de Lauretis's (1984, 1985) approaches to representation led her to view gender as the unexamined tragic flaw of modern and postmodern theories of culture, whose faultline is the heterosexual contract. De Lauretis defined gender as the social construction of 'woman' and 'man' and the semiotic production of subjectivity; gender has to do with 'the history, practices, and imbrication of meaning and experience'; that is, with the 'mutually constitutive effects in semiosis of the outer world of social reality with the inner world of subjectivity' (1984, pp. 158–86). De Lauretis drew on Charles Peirce's theories of semiosis to develop an approach to 'experience', one of the most problematic notions in modern feminism, that takes account both of experience's intimate embodiment and its mediation through signifying practices. Experience is never *im-mediately* accessible. Her efforts have been particularly helpful in understanding and contesting inscriptions of gender in cinema and other areas where the idea that gender is an embodied semiotic difference is crucial and empowering. Differentiating technologies of gender from Foucault's formulation of technologies of sex, de Lauretis identified a specific feminist gendered subject position within sex/gender systems. Her formulation echoed Lorde's understanding of the inhabitant of the house of difference: 'The female subject of feminism is one constructed across a multiplicity of discourses, positions, and meanings, which are often in conflict with one another and inherently (historically) contradictory' (de Lauretis, 1987, pp. ix–x).

Offering a very different theory of consciousness and the production of meanings from MacKinnon or de Lauretis, Hartsock's (1983a) exploration of the sexual division of labour drew on anglophone versions of psychoanalysis that were particularly important in US feminist theory, that is, object relations theory as developed especially by Nancy Chodorow (1978). Without adopting Rubin's Lacanian theories of always fragmentary sexed subjectivity, Chodorow adopted the concept of the sex-gender system in her study of the social organization of parenting, which produced women more capable of non-hostile relationality than men, but which also perpetuated the subordinate position of women through their production as people who are structured for mothering in patriarchy. Preferring an object relations psychoanalysis over a Lacanian version is related to neighbouring concepts like 'gender identity', with its empirical social science web of meanings, over 'acquisition of positions of sexed subjectivity', with this concept's immersion in Continental cultural/textual theory. Although criticized as an essentializing of woman-as-relational, Chodorow's feminist object relations theory has been immensely influential, having been adapted to explore a wide range of social phenomena. Drawing on and criticizing Lawrence Kohlberg's neo-Kantian theories, Gilligan (1982) also argued for women's greater contextual consciousness and resistance to universalizing abstractions, for example in moral reasoning.

Evelyn Keller developed a version of object relations theory to theorize systematic epistemological, psychic, and organizational masculine dominance of natural science (Keller, 1985). Keller foregrounded the logical mistake of equating *women* with *gender*.[10] Gender is a system of social, symbolic, and psychic relations, in which men and women are differentially positioned. Looking at the expression of gender as a cognitive experience, in which masculine psychic individuation produces an investment in impersonality, objectification, and domination, Keller described her project as an effort to understand the 'science-gender system' (1985, p. 8). Emphasizing social construction and concentrating on psychodynamic aspects of that construction, Keller took as her subject 'not women *per se*, or even women and science: it is the making of men, women, and science, or, more precisely, how the making of men and women has affected the making of science' (1985, p. 4). Her goal was to work for science as a human project, not a masculine one. She phrased her question as, 'Is sex to gender as nature is to science?' (Keller, 1987).

Chodorow's early work was developed in the context of a related series of sociological and anthropological papers theorizing a key role for the public/private division in the subordination of women (Rosaldo and Lamphere, 1974). In that collection, Rosaldo argued the universal salience of the limitation of women to the domestic realm, while power was vested in the space men inhabit, called public. Sherry Ortner (1974) connected that approach to her structuralist analysis of the proposition that women are to nature as men are to culture. Many Euro-American feminist efforts to articulate the social positioning of women that followed *Woman, Culture, and Society* and *Toward an Anthropology of Women* (Reiter, 1975), both strategically published in the mid-1970s, were deeply influenced by the universalizing and powerful theories of sex and gender of those early collections. In anthropology as a discipline, criticisms and other outgrowths of the early formulations were rich, leading both to extensive cross-cultural study of gender symbolisms and to fundamental rejection of the universal applicability of the nature/culture pair. Within the disciplines, there was growing criticism of universalizing explanations as an instance of mistaking the analytical tool for the reality (MacCormack and Strathern, 1980; Ortner and Whitehead, 1981; Rosaldo, 1980; Rubin, 1984). As feminist anthropology moved away from its early formulations, they none the less persisted in much feminist discourse outside anthropological disciplinary circles, as if the mid-1970s positions were permanently authoritative feminist anthropological theory, rather than a discursive node in a specific political-historical disciplinary moment.

The universalizing power of the sex-gender system and the analytical split between public and private were also sharply criticized politically, especially by women of colour, as part of the ethnocentric and imperializing tendencies of European and Euro-American feminisms. The category of gender obscured or subordinated all the other 'others'. Efforts to use Western or 'white' concepts of gender to characterize a 'Third World Woman' often resulted in reproducing orientalist, racist, and colonialist discourse (Amos *et al.*, 1984; Mohanty, 1984). Furthermore, US 'women of colour', itself a complex and contested political construction of sexed identities, produced critical theory about the production of systems of hierarchical differences, in which race, nationality, sex, and class were intertwined, both in the nineteenth and early twentieth centuries and from the earliest days of the women's movements that emerged from the 1960s civil rights and anti-war movements.[11] These theories of the social positioning of women ground and organize 'generic' feminist theory, in which concepts such as 'the house of difference' (Lorde), 'oppositional consciousness' (Sandoval), 'womanism' (Walker), 'shuttle from center to margin' (Spivak), 'Third World feminism' (Moraga and Smith), 'el mundo zurdo' (Anzaldúa and Moraga), 'la mestiza' (Anzaldúa), 'racially-structured patriarchal capitalism' (Bhavnani and Coulson, 1986), and 'inappropriate/d other' (Trinh, 1986–87, 1989) structure the field of feminist discourse, as it decodes what counts as a 'woman' within as well as outside 'feminism'. Complexly related figures have emerged also in feminist writing by 'white' women: 'sex-political classes' (Sofoulis, 1987); 'cyborg' (Haraway, 1985; 1991, pp. 149–81); the female subject of feminism (de Lauretis, 1987).

In the early 1980s, Kitchen Table: Women of Color Press was established in New York and began to publish the critical theoretical and other writings of radical women of colour. This development must be seen in the context of international publishing in many genres by women writing into consciousness the stories of their constructions, and thereby destabilizing the canons of Western feminism, as well as those of many other discourses. As the heterogeneous and critical subject positions of 'women of colour' were progressively elaborated in diverse publishing practices, the status of 'white' or 'Western' also was more readily seen as a contestable location and not as a given ethnicity, race, or inescapable destiny. Thus, 'white' women could be called to account for their active positioning.

Rubin's 1975 theory of the sex/gender system explained the complementarity of the sexes (obligatory heterosexuality) and the oppression of women by men through the central premise of the exchange of women in the founding of culture through kinship. But what happens to this approach when women are not positioned in similar ways in the institution of kinship? In particular, what happens to the idea of gender if whole groups of women and men are positioned outside the institution of kinship altogether, but in relation to the kinship systems of another, dominant group?

Carby (1987), Spillers (1987), and Hurtado (1989) interrogated the concept of gender through an exploration of the history and consequences of these matters. Carby clarified how in the New World, and specifically in the United States, black women were not constituted as 'woman', as white women were. Instead, black women were constituted simultaneously racially and sexually – as marked female (animal, sexualized and without rights), but not as woman (human, potential wife, conduit for the name of the father) – in a specific institution, slavery, that excluded them from 'culture' defined as the circulation of signs through the system of marriage. If kinship vested men with rights in women that they did not have in themselves, slavery abolished kinship for one group in a legal discourse that produced whole groups of people as alienable property (Spillers, 1987). MacKinnon (1982, 1987) defined woman as an imaginary figure, the object of another's desire, made real. The 'imaginary' figures made real in slave discourse were objects in another sense that made them different from either the Marxist figure of the alienated labourer or the 'unmodified' feminist figure of the object of desire. Free women in US white patriarchy were exchanged in a system that oppressed them, but white women inherited black women and men. As Hurtado (1989, p. 841) noted, in the nineteenth century prominent white feminists were married to white men, while black feminists were owned by white men. In a racist patriarchy, white men's 'need' for racially pure offspring positioned free and unfree women in incompatible, asymmetrical symbolic and social spaces.

The female slave was marked with these differences in a most literal fashion – the flesh was turned inside out, 'add[ing] a lexical dimension to the narratives of woman in culture and society' (Spillers, 1987, pp. 67–8). These differences did not end with formal emancipation; they have had definitive consequences into the late twentieth century and will continue to do so until racism as a founding institution of the New World is ended. Spillers called these founding relations of captivity and literal mutilation 'an American grammar' (1987, p. 68). Under conditions of the New World conquest, of slavery, and of their consequences up to the present, 'the lexis of reproduction, desire, naming, mothering, fathering, etc. [are] all thrown into extreme crisis' (1987, p. 76). 'Gendering, in its coeval reference to African-American women, *insinuates* an implicit and unresolved puzzle both within current feminist discourse *and* within those discursive communities that investigate the problematics of culture' (1987, p. 78).

Spillers foregrounded the point that free men and women inherited their name from the father, who in turn had rights in his minor children and wife that they did not have in themselves, but he did not own them in the full sense of alienable property. Unfree men and women inherited their condition from their mothers, who in turn specifically did not control their children. They had no name in the sense theorized by Lévi-Strauss or Lacan. Slave mothers could not transmit a name; they could not be wives; they were outside the system of marriage exchange. Slaves were unpositioned, unfixed, in a system of names; they were, specifically, unlocated and so disposable. In these discursive frames, white women were not legally or symbolically fully human; slaves were not legally or symbolically human at all. 'In this absence from a subject position, the captured sexualities provide a physical and biological expression of "otherness"' (Spillers, 1987, p. 67). To give birth (unfreely) to the heirs of property is not the same thing as to give birth (unfreely) to property (Carby, 1987, p. 53).

This little difference is part of the reason that 'reproductive rights' for women of colour in the US prominently hinge on comprehensive control of children – for example, their freedom from destruction through lynching, imprisonment, infant mortality, forced pregnancy, coercive sterilization, inadequate housing, racist education, or drug addiction (Hurtado, 1989, p. 853). For white women the concept of property in the self, the ownership of one's own body, in relation to reproductive freedom has more readily focused on the field of events around conception, pregnancy, abortion, and birth, because the system of white patriarchy turned on the control of legitimate children and the consequent constitution of white females as woman. To have or not have children then becomes literally a subject-defining choice for women. Black women specifically – and the women subjected to the conquest of the New World in general – faced a broader social field of reproductive unfreedom, in which their children did not inherit the status of human in the founding hegemonic discourses of US society. The problem of the black mother in this context is not simply her own status as subject, but also the status of her children and her sexual partners, male and female. Small wonder that the image of uplifting the race and the refusal of the categorical separation of men and women – without flinching from an analysis of coloured and white sexist oppression – have been prominent in New World black feminist discourse (Carby, 1987, pp. 6–7; hooks, 1981, 1984).

The positionings of African-American women are not the same as those of other women of colour; each condition of oppression requires specific analysis that refuses the separations but insists on the non-identities of race, sex, and class. These matters make starkly clear why an adequate feminist theory of gender must *simultaneously* be a theory of racial difference in specific historical conditions of production and reproduction. They also make clear why a theory and practice of sisterhood cannot be grounded in shared positionings in a system of sexual difference and the cross-cultural structural antagonism between coherent categories called women and men. Finally, they make clear why feminist theory produced by women of colour has constructed alternative discourses of womanhood that disrupt the humanisms of many Western discursive traditions.

> [I]t is our task to make a place for this different social subject. In so doing we are less interested in joining the ranks of gendered femaleness than gaining the insurgent ground as female social subject. Actually *claiming* the monstrosity of a female with the potential to 'name' ... 'Sapphire' might rewrite after all a radically different text of female empowerment.
>
> (Spillers, 1987, p. 80)

While contributing fundamentally to the breakup of any master subject location, the politics of 'difference' emerging from this and other complex reconstructings of concepts of social subjectivity and their associated writing practices is deeply opposed to levelling relativisms. Non-feminist theory in the human sciences has tended to identify the breakup of 'coherent' or masterful subjectivity as the 'death of the subject'. Like others in newly unstably subjugated positions, many feminists resist this formulation of the project and question its emergence at just the moment when raced/sexed/colonized speakers begin 'for the first time', that is, they claim an originary authority to represent themselves in institutionalized publishing practices and other kinds of self-constituting practice. Feminist deconstructions of the 'subject' have been fundamental, and they are not nostalgic for masterful coherence. Instead, necessarily political accounts of constructed embodiments, like feminist theories of gendered racial subjectivities, have to take affirmative and critical account of emergent, differentiating, self-representing, contradictory social subjectivities, with their claims on action, knowledge, and belief. The point involves the commitment to transformative social change, the moment of hope embedded in feminist theories of gender and other emergent discourses about the breakup of masterful subjectivity and the emergence of inappropriated others (Trinh, 1986–87, 1989).

The multiple academic and other institutional roots of the literal (written) category 'gender', feminist and otherwise, sketched in this entry have been part of the race-hierarchical system of relations that obscures the publications by women of colour because of their origin, language, genre – in short, 'marginality', 'alterity', and 'difference' as seen from the 'unmarked' positions of hegemonic and imperializing ('white') theory. But 'alterity' and 'difference' are precisely what 'gender' is 'grammatically' about, a fact that constitutes feminism as a politics defined by its fields of contestation and repeated refusals of master theories. 'Gender' was developed as a category to explore what counts as a 'woman', to problematize the previously taken-for-granted. If feminist theories of gender followed from Simone de Beauvoir's thesis that one is not born a woman, with all the consequences of that insight, in the light of Marxism and psychoanalysis, for understanding that any finally coherent subject is a fantasy, and that personal and collective identity is precariously and constantly socially reconstituted (Coward, 1983, p. 265), then the title of bell hooks's provocative book, echoing the great nineteenth-century black feminist and abolitionist, Sojourner Truth, *Ain't I a Woman* (1981), bristles with irony, as the identity of 'woman' is both claimed and deconstructed simultaneously. Struggle over the agents, memories, and terms of these reconstitutions is at the heart of feminist sex/gender politics.

The refusal to become or to remain a 'gendered' man or a woman, then, is an eminently political insistence on emerging from the nightmare of the all-too-real, imaginary narrative of sex and race. Finally and ironically, the political and explanatory power of the 'social' category of gender depends upon historicizing the categories of sex, flesh, body, biology, race, and nature in such a way that the binary, universalizing opposition that spawned the concept of the sex/gender system at a particular time and place in feminist theory implodes into articulated, differentiated, accountable, located, and consequential theories of embodiment, where nature is no longer imagined and enacted as resource to culture or sex to gender. Here is my location for a Utopian intersection of heterogeneous, multi-cultural, 'Western' (coloured, white, European, American, Asian, African, Pacific) feminist theories of gender hatched in odd siblingship with contradictory, hostile, fruitful, inherited binary dualisms. Phallogocentrism was the egg ovulated by the master subject, the brooding hen to the permanent chickens of history. But into the nest with that literal-minded egg has been placed the germ of a phoenix that will speak in all the tongues of a world turned upside down.

Notes

1 The project is so daunting that the 'supplement' split off from the translation project and is underway as a two-volume work of its own, the *Marxistisches Wörterbuch*, under the general editorship of Wolfgang F. Haug of the Institut für Philosophie, Freie Universität, Berlin. There are hundreds of contributors from Germany and many other countries. Taken from a list compiled in 1985, some of the planned keywords of particular interest to feminists include: *Diskurs, Dritte Welt, Familie, Feminismus, feministische Theologie, Frauen, Frauenbewegung, Geschlecht, Homosexualität, Kulturarbeit, Kybernetik, Luxemburgismus, Marxismus-Feminismus, Natur, Ökologie, Patriarchal,*

Post-modernismus, Rasse, Rassismus, Repräsentation, Sex/gender system, Sexismus, Sexpol, Sister-hood, technologische Rationalität, weibliche Ästhetik, and *weibliche Bildung.* This was, indeed, not the daily vocabulary of Marx and Engels. But they do, emphatically, belong in a late twentieth-century Marxist dictionary.

2 A curious linguistic point shows itself here: there is no marker to distinguish (biological) race and (cultural) race, as there is for (biological) sex and (cultural) gender, even though the nature/culture and biology/society binarisms pervade Western race discourse. The linguistic situation highlights the very recent and uneven entry of gender into the political, as opposed to the grammatical, lexicon. The non-naturalness of race – it is always and totally an arbitrary, cultural construction – can be empha-sized from the lack of a linguistic marker. But, as easily, the total collapse of the category of race into biologism is linguistically invited. All these matters continue to hinge on unexamined functioning of the productionist, Aristotelian logic fundamental to so much Western discourse. In the linguistic, political, and historical matrix, matter and form, act and potency, raw material and achieved product play out their escalating dramas of production and appropriation. Here is where subjects and objects get born and endlessly reincarnated.

3 Although not mutually exclusive, the language of 'gender' in Euro-American feminist discourse usually is the language of 'sexed subject position' and 'sexual difference' in European writing. For British Marxist feminism on the 'sexed subject in patriarchy', see Kuhn and Wolpe (1978), Marxist-Feminist Literature Collective (1978), Brown and Adams (1979), the journal *m/f*, Barrett (1980). German socialist-feminist positions on sexualization have stressed the dialectic of women's self-constructing agency, already structured social determination, and partial restructurings. This literature examines how women construct themselves into existing structures, in order to find the point where change might be possible. If women are theorized as passive victims of sex and gender as a system of domination, no theory of liberation will be possible. So social constructionism on the question of gender must not be allowed to become a theory of closed determinism (Haug, 1980, 1982; Haug *et al.*, 1983, 1987; Mouffe, 1983). Looking for a theory of experience, of how women actively embody themselves, the women in the collective writing the *Frauenformen* publications insisted on a descriptive/theoretical practice showing 'the ways we live ourselves in bodily terms' (Haug *et al.*, 1987, p. 30). They evolved a method called 'memory work' that emphasizes collectively criticized, written narratives about 'a stranger', a past 'remembered' self, while problematizing the self-deluding assumptions of autobiography and other causal accounts. The problem is how to account for emergence of 'the sexual itself as the process that produces the insertion of women into, and their subordination within, determinate social practices' (Haug *et al.*, 1987, p. 33). Ironically, self-consti-tuted as sexualized, as woman, women cannot be accountable for themselves or society (1987, p. 27). Like all the theories of sex, sexuality, and gender surveyed in this effort to write for a standard refer-ence work that inevitably functions to canonize some meanings over others, the *Frauenformen* versions insist on gender as a gerund or a verb, rather than a finished noun, a substantive. For femi-nists, gender means making and unmaking 'bodies' in a contestable world; an account of gender is a theory of experience as signifying and significant embodiment.

4 Joan Scott (1988, pp. 28–50 [also reprinted as Chapter 5 in this volume]) wrote an incisive treatment of the development of gender as a theoretical category in the discipline of history. She noted the long history of play on the grammatical gender difference for making figurative allusions to sex or character (1988, p. 28). Scott quoted as her epigram *Fowler's Dictionary of Modern English Usage*'s insistence that to use gender to mean the male or female sex was either a mistake or a joke. The ironies in this injunction abound. One benefit of the inheritance of feminist uses of gender from grammar is that, in that domain, 'gender is understood to be a way of classifying phenomena, a socially agreed-upon system of distinction, rather than an objective description of inherent traits' (Scott, 1988, p. 29).

5 See Coward (1983, Chapters 5 and 6) for a thorough discussion of the concepts of the family and the woman question in Marxist thought from 1848 to about 1930.

6 See *The Woman Question* (1951); Marx and Avelling (1885–86); Kollontai (1977).

7 To sample the uses and criticisms, see Bleier (1984, 1986), Brighton Women and Science Group (1980), Fausto-Sterling (1985), Henifin and Fried (1982), Hubbard, Kessler and McKenna (1978), Lewontin, Rose and Kamin (1984), Lowe and Hubbard (1983), Morawsky (1987), Sayers (1982), Thorne and Henley (1975), West and Zimmermann (1987).

8 Several streams of European feminisms (some disavowing the name) were born after the events of May '68. The stream drawing from Simone de Beauvoir's formulations, especially work by Monique

Wittig, Monique Plaza, Colette Guillaumin, and Christine Delphy, published in *Questions féministes*, *Nouvelles questions féministes*, and *Feminist Issues*, and the stream associated complexly with the group 'Psychanalyse et Politiques' and/or with Julia Kristeva, Luce Irigaray, Sarah Kofman, and Hélène Cixous have been particularly influential in international feminist development on issues of sexual difference. (For introductory summaries, see Duchen, 1986; Gallop, 1982; Marks and de Courtivron, 1980; Moi, 1985). These streams deserve large, separate treatments; but in the context of this entry two contributions to theories of 'gender' from these writers, who are deeply opposed among themselves on precisely these issues, must be signalled. First, there are Wittig's and Delphy's arguments for a materialist feminism, which insist that the issue is 'domination', not 'difference'. Second, there are Irigaray's, Kristeva's, and Cixous's various ways (intertextually positioned in relation to Derrida, Lacan and others) of insisting that the subject, which perhaps is best approached through writing and textuality, is always in process, always disrupted, that the idea of woman remains finally unclosed and multiple. Despite their important opposition between and within the francophone streams, all these theorists are possessed with flawed, contradictory, and critical projects of denaturalization of 'woman'.

9 Flax (1983), Harding (1983), O'Brien (1981), Rose (1983, 1986), Smith (1974).

10 Similarly, it is an error to equate 'race' with people of colour; whiteness is a racial construction as well, invisible as such because of its (like man's) occupation of the unmarked category (Carby, 1987, p. 18; Frankenberg, 1988; Haraway, 1989, pp. 152, 401–2).

11 See, for example, Anzaldúa (1987); Aptheker (1982); Bethel and Smith (1979); Bulkin, Pratt and Smith (1984); Carby (1987); Christian (1985); Collins (1989a, 1989b); Combahee River Collective (1979); Davis (1982); Giddings (1985); hooks (1981, 1984); Hull, Scott and Smith (1982); Hurtado (1989); Joseph and Lewis (1981); Lorde (1982, 1984); Moraga (1983); Moraga and Anzaldúa (1981); Sandoval (n.d.); Smith (1983); Spillers (1987); Walker (1983); Ware (1970).

References

AMOS, V., LEWIS, G., MAMA, A. and PARMAR, P. (eds) (1984) 'Many voices, one chant: black feminist perspectives', *Feminist Review*, 17, pp. 1–118.

ANZALDÚA, G. (1987) *Borderlands/La Frontera*, San Francisco: Spinters/Aunt Lute.

APTHEKER, B. (1982) *Woman's Legacy: Essays on Race, Sex and Class in American History*, Amherst: University of Massachusetts Press.

BARRETT, M. (1980) *Women's Oppression Today*, London: Verso.

DE BEAUVOIR, S. (1949) *Le Deuxième Sexe*, Paris: Gallimard.

—— (1952) *The Second Sex*, New York: Bantam.

BEBEL, A. (1883) *Woman under Socialism*, New York: Schoken, 1971 (orig. *Women in the Past, Present and Future*, 1878).

BETHEL, L. and SMITH, B. (eds) (1979) The Black Woman's Issue, *Conditions*, 5.

BHAVNANI, K.K. and COULSON, M. (1986) 'Transforming socialist-feminism: the challenge of racism', *Feminist Review*, 23, pp. 81–92.

BLEIER, R. (1984) *Science and Gender: A Critique of Biology and its Themes on Women*, New York: Pergamon.

—— (ed.) (1986) *Feminist Approaches to Science*, New York: Pergamon.

BRIGHTON WOMEN AND SCIENCE GROUP (1980) *Alice through the Microscope*, London: Virago.

BROWN, B., and ADAMS, P. (1979) 'The feminine body and feminist polities', *m/f*, 3, pp. 35–57.

BULKIN, E., PRATT, M.B. and SMITH, B. (1984) *Yours in Struggle: Three Feminist Perspectives on Racism and Anti Semitism*, New York: Long Haul.

BUTLER, J. (1989) *Gender Trouble: Feminism and the Subversion of Identity*, New York: Routledge.

CARBY, H. (1987) *Reconstructing Womanhood: The Emergence of the Afro-American Woman Novelist*, New York: Oxford University Press.

CHODOROW, N. (1978) *The Reproduction of Mothering: Psychoanalysis and the Sociology of Gender*, Los Angeles: University of California Press.

CHRISTIAN, B. (1985) *Black Feminist Criticism: Perspectives on Black Women Writers*, New York: Pergamon.

COLLINS, P.H. (1989a) 'The social construction of black feminist thought', *Signs*, 14, pp. 745–73.

—— (1989b) 'A comparison of two works on black family life', *Signs*, 14, pp. 875–84.

COMBAHEE RIVER COLLECTIVE (1979) 'A black feminist statement', in EISENSTEIN, Z. (ed.) *Capitalist Patriarchy and the Case for Socialist Feminism*, New York: Monthly Review.

COWARD, R. (1983) *Patriarchal Precedents: Sexuality and Social Relations*, London: Routledge and Kegan Paul.

DAVIS, A. (1982) *Women, Race and Class*, London: Women's Press.

DOUGLAS, M. (1989) 'A gentle deconstruction', *London Review of Books*, 4 May, pp. 17–18.

DUCHEN, C. (1986) *Feminism in France from May '68 to Mitterrand*, London: Routledge and Kegan Paul.

ENGELS, F. (1972 [orig. 1884]) *The Origins of the Family, Private Property and the State*, New York: International.

ESCOFFIER, J. (1985) 'Sexual revolution and the politics of gay identity', *Socialist Review*, 82/83, pp. 119–53.

FAUSTO-STERLING, A. (1985) *Myths of Gender: Biological Theories about Women and Men*, New York: Basic.

FEE, E. (1986) 'Critiques of modern science: the relationship of feminism to other radical epistemologies', in BLEIER, R. (ed.) *Feminist Approaches to Science*, New York: Pergamon.

FLAX, J. (1983) 'Political philosophy and the patriarchal unconscious: a psychoanalytic perspective on epistemology and metaphysics', in HARDING, S. and HINTIKKA, M. (eds) *Discovering Reality: Feminist Perspectives on Epistemology, Metaphysics, Methodology, and Philosophy of Science*, Dordrecht: Reidel.

FOUCAULT, M. (1978) *The History of Sexuality, Volume 1: An Introduction*, New York: Pantheon.

FRANKENBERG, R. (1988) 'The social construction of whiteness', PhD thesis, University of California at Santa Cruz.

GALLOP, J. (1982) *The Daughter's Seduction: Feminism and Psychoanalysis*, New York: Macmillan.

GIDDINGS, P. (1985) *When and Where I Enter: The Impact of Black Women on Race and Sex in America*, Toronto: Bantam.

GILLIGAN, C. (1982) *In a Different Voice*, Cambridge, MA: Harvard University Press.

HARAWAY, D.J. (1985) 'Manifesto for cyborgs: science, technology, and socialist feminism in the 1980s', *Socialist Review*, 80, pp. 65–108.

—— (1989) *Primate Visions: Gender, Race, and Nature in the World of Modern Science*, New York: Routledge.

—— (1991) 'A cyborg manifesto: science, technology, and socialist-feminism in the late twentieth century', in *Simians, Cyborgs, and Women: The Reinvention of Nature*, New York: Routledge.

HARDING, S. (1983) 'Why has the sex/gender system become visible only now?', in HARDING, S. and HINTIKKA, M. (eds) *Discovering Reality: Feminist Perspectives on Epistemology, Metaphysics, Methodology, and Philosophy of Science*, Dordrecht: Reidel.

—— (1986) *The Science Question in Feminism*, Ithaca, NY: Cornell University Press.

—— and HINTIKKA, M. (eds) (1983) *Discovering Reality: Feminist Perspectives on Epistemology, Metaphysics, Methodology, and Philosophy of Science*, Dordrecht: Reidel.

HARTMANN, H. (1981) 'The unhappy marriage of marxism and feminism', in SARGENT, L., *Women and Revolution*, Boston, MA: South End.

HARTSOCK, N. (1983a) 'The feminist standpoint: developing the ground for a specifically feminist historical materialism', in HARDING, S. and HINTIKKA, M. (eds) *Discovering Reality: Feminist Perspectives on Epistemology, Metaphysics, Methodology, and Philosophy of Science*, Dordrecht: Reidel.

—— (1983b) *Money, Sex, and Power*, New York: Longman.

HAUG, F. (ed.) (1980) *Frauenformen: Alltagsgeschichten und Entwurf einer Theorie weiblicher Sozialisation*, Berlin: Argument Sonderband 45.

—— (1982) 'Frauen und Theorie', *Das Argument*, 136, pp. 11–12.

HAUG, F. *et al.* (1983) *Sexualisierung: Frauenformen 2*, Berlin: Argument-Verlag.

—— *et al.* (1987) *Female Sexualization: A Collective Work of Memory*, London: Verso.

HOOKS, B. (1981) *Ain't I a Woman*, Boston, MA: South End.

—— (1984) *Feminist Theory: From Margin to Centre*, Boston, MA: South End.

HUBBARD, R., HENIFIN, M.S. and FRIED, B. (eds) (1982) *Biological Woman: The Convenient Myth*, Cambridge, MA: Schenkman.

HULL, G., SCOTT, P.B. and SMITH, B. (eds) (1982) *All the Women Are White, All the Men Are Black, but Some of Us Are Brave*, Old Westbury, NY: The Feminist Press.

HURTADO, A. (1989) 'Relating to privilege: seduction and rejection in the subordination of white women and women of colour', *Signs*, 14, pp. 833–55.

JAGGAR, A. (1983) *Feminist Politics and Human Nature*, Totowa, NJ: Roman & Allenheld.

JOSEPH, G. and LEWIS, J. (1981) *Common Differences*, New York: Anchor.

KELLER, E.F. (1985) *Reflections on Gender and Science*, New Haven, CT: Yale University Press.

—— (1987) 'The gender/science system: or, is sex to gender as nature is to science?', *Hypatia*, 2, pp. 37–49.

KESSLER, S. and MCKENNA, W. (1978) *Gender: An Ethnomethodological Approach*, Chicago: University of Chicago Press.

KING, K. (1986) 'The situation of lesbianism as feminism's magical sign: contests for meaning and the US women's movement, 1968–72', *Communication*, 9, pp. 65–92.

KOLLONTAI, A. (1977) *Selected Writings*, London: Allison & Busby.

KUHN, A. and WOLPE, A.M. (eds) (1978) *Feminism and Materialism*, London: Routledge and Kegan Paul.

LABICA, G. and BENUSSEN, G. (1985) *Dictionnaire critique du Marxisme*, 8 vols, Paris: Presses Universitaires de France.

DE LAURETIS, T. (1984) *Alice Doesn't: Feminism, Semiotics, Cinema*, Bloomington: Indiana University Press.

—— (1985) 'The violence of rhetoric: considerations on representation and gender', *Semiotica*, 54, pp. 11–31.

—— (1987) *Technologies of Gender: Essays on Theory, Film and Fiction*, Bloomington: Indiana University Press.

LEWONTIN, R.C., ROSE, S. and KAMIN, L.J. (1984) *Not in Our Genes: Biology, Ideology, and Human Nature*, New York: Pantheon.

LINDEN, R.R. (1981) 'The social construction of gender: a methodological analysis of the gender identity paradigm', University of California at Santa Cruz, unpublished essay.

LORDE, A. (1982) *Zami: A New Spelling of My Name*, Trumansberg, NY: Crossing.

—— (1984) *Sister Outsider*, Trumansberg, NY: Crossing.

LOWE, M. and HUBBARD, R. (eds) (1983) *Woman's Nature: Rationalization of Inequality*, New York: Pergamon.

MACCORMACK, C. and STRATHERN, M. (eds) (1980) *Nature, Culture, Gender*, Cambridge: Cambridge University Press.

MACKINNON, C. (1982) 'Feminism, marxism, method, and the state: an agenda for theory', *Signs*, 7, pp. 515–44.

—— (1987) *Feminism Unmodified: Discourses on Life and Law*, Cambridge, MA: Harvard University Press.

MARKS, E. and DE COURTIVRON, I. (eds) (1980) *New French Feminisms*, Amherst: University of Massachusetts Press.

MARX, E. and AVELING, E. (1885–86) *The Woman Question*, London: Swann & Sonnenschein.

MARX, K. (1964a) *Capital*, Vol. 1, New York: International.

—— (1964b) *The Economic and Philosophic Manuscripts of 1844*, New York: International.

—— and ENGELS, F. (1970) *The German Ideology*, London: Lawrence & Wishart.

MARXIST-FEMINIST LITERATURE COLLECTIVE (1978) 'Women's writing', *Ideology and Consciousness*, 1, pp. 27–48.

MITCHELL, J. (1966) 'Women: the longest revolution', *New Left Review*, 40, pp. 11–37.

—— (1972) *Women's Estate*, New York: Pantheon.

MOHANTY, C.T. (1984) 'Under Western eyes: feminist scholarship and colonial discourse', *Boundary*, 2, 3, pp. 333–58.

MOI, T. (1985) *Sexual/Textual Politics*, New York: Methuen.

MONEY, J. and EHRHARDT, A. (1972) *Man and Woman, Boy and Girl*, New York: New American Library.

MORAGA, C. (1983) *Loving in the War Years: Lo que nunca pasó por sus labios*, Boston, MA: South End.

—— and ANZALDÚA, G. (eds) (1981) *This Bridge Called My Back: Writings by Radical Women of Colour*, Watertown, MA: Persephone Press.

MORAWSKY, J.G. (1987) 'The troubled quest for masculinity, femininity and androgyny', *Review of Personality and Social Psychology*, 7, pp. 44–69.

MOUFFE, C. (1983) 'The sex-gender system and the discursive construction of women's subordination', *Rethinking Ideology*, Berlin: Argument Sonderband 84.

O'BRIEN, M. (1981) *The Politics of Reproduction*, New York: Routledge and Kegan Paul.

ORTNER, S.B. (1974) 'Is female to male as nature is to culture?', in ROSALDO, M. and LAMPHERE, L. (eds) *Woman, Culture, and Society*, Palo Alto, CA: Stanford University Press.

—— and WHITEHEAD, H. (eds) (1981) *Sexual Meanings: The Cultural Construction of Gender and Sexuality*, Cambridge: Cambridge University Press.

REITER, R.R. (ed.) (1975) *Toward an Anthropology of Women*, New York: Monthly Review.

RICH, A. (1980) 'Compulsory heterosexuality and lesbian existence', *Signs*, 5, pp. 631–60.

ROSALDO, M. (1980) 'The use and abuse of anthropology', *Signs*, 5, pp. 389–417.

—— and LAMPHERE, L. (eds) (1974) *Woman, Culture and Society*, Palo Alto, CA: Stanford University Press.

ROSE, H. (1983) 'Hand, brain, and heart: a feminist epistemology for the natural sciences', *Signs*, 9, pp. 73–90.

—— (1986) 'Women's work: women's knowledge', in MITCHELL, J. and OAKLEY, A. (eds) *What is Feminism?: A Re-Examination*, New York: Pantheon.

RUBIN, G. (1975) 'The traffic in women: notes on the political economy of sex', in REITER, R.R. (ed.) *Toward an Anthropology of Women*, New York: Monthly Review.

—— (1984) 'Thinking sex: notes for a radical theory of the politics of sexuality', in VANCE, C.S. (ed.) *Pleasure and Danger: Exploring Female Sexuality*, New York: Routledge and Kegan Paul.

SANDOVAL, C. (n.d.) *Yours in Struggle: Women Respond to Racism, a Report on the National Women's Studies Association*, Oakland, CA: Center for Third World Organization.

SARGENT, L. (ed.) (1981) *Women and Revolution*, Boston, MA: South End.

SAYERS, J. (1982) *Biological Politics: Feminist and Anti-Feminist Perspectives*, London: Tavistock.

SCOTT, J.W. (1988) *Gender and the Politics of History*, New York: Columbia University Press.

SMITH, B. (ed.) (1983) *Home Girls: A Black Feminist Anthology*, New York: Kitchen Table, Women of Colour Press.

SMITH, D. (1974) 'Women's perspective as a radical critique of sociology', *Sociological Inquiry*, 44, pp. 7–14.

SOFOULIS, Z. (1987) 'Lacklein', University of California at Santa Cruz, unpublished essay.

SPILLERS, H. (1987) 'Mama's baby, papa's maybe: an American grammar book', *Diacritics*, 17, pp. 65–81.

SPIVAK, G.C. (1985) 'Three women's texts and a critique of imperialism', *Critical Inquiry*, 12, pp. 243–61.

STOLLER, R. (1964) 'A contribution to the study of gender identity', *International Journal of Psycho-analysis*, 45, pp. 220–6.

—— (1968) *Sex and Gender*, vol. I, New York: Science House.

—— (1976) *Sex and Gender*, vol. II, New York: Janson Aronson.

STRATHERN, M. (1988) *The Gender of the Gift: Problems with Women and Problems with Society in Melanesia*, Berkeley: University of California Press.

THORNE, B. and HENLEY, N. (eds) (1975) *Language and Sex: Difference and Dominance*, Rowley, MA: Newbury.

TRINH, T.M. (1986–87) 'Introduction' and 'Difference: a special third world women issue', *Discourse: Journal for Theoretical Studies in Media and Culture*, 8, pp. 3–38.

—— (1989) *Woman, Native, Other: Writing Postcoloniality and Feminism*, Bloomington: Indiana University Press.

WALKER, A. (1983) *In Search of Our Mother's Gardens*, New York: Harcourt Brace Jovanovitch.

WARE, C. (1970) *Woman Power*, New York: Tower.

WEST, C. and ZIMMERMANN, D.H. (1987) 'Doing gender', *Gender and Society*, 1, pp. 125–51.

WITTIG, M. (1981) 'One is not born a woman', *Feminist Issue*, 2, pp. 47–54.

THE WOMAN QUESTION: SELECTED WRITINGS OF MARX, ENGELS, LENIN AND STALIN (1951) New York: International.

YOUNG, I. (1981) 'Beyond the unhappy marriage: a critique of the dual systems theory', in SARGENT, L. (ed.) *Women and Revolution*, Boston, MA: South End.

YOUNG, R.M. and LEVIDOW, L. (eds) (1981, 1985) *Science, Technology and the Labour Process*, 2 vols, London: CSE and Free Association Books.

7 'That we should all turn queer?'

Homosexual stigma in the making
of manhood and the breaking of a
revolution in Nicaragua

Roger N. Lancaster [1995]

In a broad sense, the Sandinista revolution was undermined by an all-round war of aggression. On the military front, the US-sponsored Contra war had left 30,000 people dead in a country of some three million. Contra attacks targeted schools, clinics, electrical facilities, bridges and farms, traumatizing the country's economic infrastructure and disrupting social services. On the economic front, the US economic embargo deprived Nicaragua of its historical market for agricultural products and, more importantly, of direct access to spare parts for its US-manufactured machinery. And on the international front, US vetoes deprived Nicaragua of any relief it might have received from lending agencies.

As a result of this three-pronged attack, Nicaragua's per capita gross domestic product fell to roughly half its pre-war level. By the late 1980s, defence was consuming over 60 per cent of government expenditures, and in 1988 the annual rate of inflation soared to 35,000 per cent. The cumulative effects of war and embargo totalled up to $17 billion in direct and indirect damages – in a country whose gross domestic product never much exceeded three billion, even in good years. The result was social, economic, and personal discombobulation.[1]

In a narrower sense, though, Nicaraguan families, structured by a 'culture of machismo' and rent by unresolved gender conflicts, proved the most effective medium of an intimate, low-intensity conflict that ate away at the revolution's base of popular support. Nicaraguan family life has long been characterized by widespread patterns of male abandonment. At the time of the revolution, some 34 per cent of Nicaraguan families were headed by women, and the figure was closer to 50 per cent in the cities. Brittle conjugal relations, in the context of a patriarchal economic structure, necessarily put women and children in a structurally disadvantageous social position.[2]

Such patterns of oppression had provided the context for the dramatic and unprecedented mobilization of women and youth in the Sandinista revolution. By the 1979 revolution, women constituted some 30 per cent of the FSLN guerrilla combatants (Molyneux, 1985, p. 227). Women and young people were active in the ensuing revolutionary process of the 1980s. In many civic projects – literacy campaigns, grass-roots health-care initiatives – women's participation far exceeded men's (Collinson, 1990, pp. 97, 124). And from the beginning, the Sandinista revolution included a strong current devoted to women's, even feminist, issues. The Nicaraguan women's organization AMNLAE (Asociación de Mujeres Nicaragüenses 'Luisa Amanda Espinoza') politicized a broad array of gender questions and family issues. Legal reforms and political mobilizations sponsored by AMNLAE attempted to change what AMNLAE and the Sandinistas called 'the culture of machismo'.

Under the Sandinistas, new legislation attempted to redress the obvious gender inequalities. A diverse package of laws, collectively known as the 'new family laws', aimed (1) to enhance the legal, social, and political position of women and children; (2) to secure the protection and well-being of children; and (3) to stabilize the Nicaraguan family, seen by many as being 'in crisis'. The reforms of this period have been criticized for not going far enough. But on paper, and by comparison with past precedent, they appear radical and far-reaching indeed. New laws outlawed sex discrimination, declared legal equality for women, treated domestic violence as a serious criminal offence, established equal social and economic rights for illegitimate children, and specified procedures for establishing paternity in cases of abandonment.[3] Family life was a site of multiple personal conflicts, vigorous political contestations, and frequently ambiguous power plays.

The results of these legal reforms were mixed. More women went to school, entered the labour force, and became involved in politics. However, women enjoyed increased educational and job opportunities in a context where real wages declined precipitously. Women and children benefited early on from consumer subsidies, but those subsidies largely disappeared as the war and crisis dragged on. Despite greater legal remedies at their disposal, women and children bore the brunt of the economic crisis. And despite legal reforms and good faith efforts, families were in no sense 'stabilized' – and it is difficult to see how they might have been. Traditional patterns of male abandonment were probably exacerbated under conditions of war and hardship. Only now, men left home, not to live in another Nicaraguan town or province, but to take up residency in Miami, or New York, or Los Angeles, where they were far from both traditional pressures to provide some assistance to abandoned families, and beyond the scope of new child-support laws.

In the context of the extended social, political, and personal crises of the 1980s, it would be difficult to overstate the effects of gender politics on the national-level politics of state. In a political strategy that duplicated the appeal of the New Right in the United States, conservative elites in Nicaragua attacked AMNLAE/Sandinista reform efforts as 'communistic attacks on the sanctity of the family'. Such diatribes targeted logical audiences: more traditional elements of society, whose values were being contested, and especially men, whose powers and prerogatives were being legally restricted. At the same time, however, in the popular classes, poor, middle-aged housewives and mothers emerged as a bulwark of opposition to Sandinismo (see IHCA, 1988). The reason for this development is not mysterious. As war and crisis dragged on, single mothers plainly bore the brunt of economic hardships. And mothers in general, in their role as care-providers, were most acutely confronted with soaring food prices, diminishing resources, and attendant difficulties in providing for families. Moreover, mothers became the main source of overt opposition to the unpopular military draft. What few anti-draft demonstrations occurred were organized by mothers, not by teenagers. The combination of open yet unresolved gender conflicts and a declining real standard of living encouraged some people – men and women, old and young – to entertain a nostalgic, conservative, Catholic traditionalism on gender issues.[4]

Such political openings were well understood by the internal opposition, and by the US State Department. Violeta Chamorro – mother, grandmother, widow – was an effective symbol from many angles. Her 1990 presidential campaign simultaneously rallied culturally conservative opposition to the Sandinistas, mobilized poor and working-class frustration with economic conditions, and articulated maternal opposition to the draft (Lancaster, 1992, pp. 290–3). In short, Chamorro's campaign actively trafficked in the traditional cult of motherhood: in its appeal to and through Nicaraguan women as domestic peacemakers, and in its promise to restore the 'true dignity of womanhood'.

My ethnography, *Life is Hard: Machismo, Danger, and the Intimacy of Power* (1992), traces the fissures and fault lines that existed within Nicaraguan families before the revolution and gradually widened in postrevolutionary society – the divides of gender, generation, and sexuality. My use of the term 'culture of machismo' not only quotes my informants, but deliberately echoes Oscar Lewis's phrase, 'culture of poverty'. Lewis (1966, p. 8) argued that what he called 'the culture of poverty' would not simply go away with a transformation of the economic conditions that create poverty. He argued that 'any movement – be it religious, pacifist, or revolutionary – that organizes and gives hope to the poor … must effectively destroy the psychological and social core of the culture of poverty'.

I would argue that many of the characteristics Lewis attributed to a 'culture of poverty' belong not to some special culture of poor people in Latin America, but to an overarching gendered world that might more accurately be called the 'culture of machismo'. Whether one even grants the existence of a culture of poverty, and despite the troubled and troubling legacy of this concept,[5] Lewis's basic argument provides a reasonable analogy with the case I make concerning Nicaragua. No one should slight the importance of certain structural factors (US aggression, Nicaragua's dependency on agroexports, a long-term agricultural recession in the international marketplace) in shaping the outcome of the revolution. But surely, the culture of machismo was itself one such factor. A pre-existing pattern of gender and sexuality did not simply 'wither away' after the revolution; it proved more resilient than the revolutionaries. Many of the conflicts and frustrations that eroded the revolutionary project belong most logically and most directly to the culture of machismo. And changing it would have required a revolution within the revolution.

Literal readings and everyday occurrences

What this paper addresses in detail is a dimension of gender studies that remains to be fully addressed in the ethnographic literature: not the role of male–female interaction in generating gender norms, but the role of male–male interaction; specifically, not the role of heterosexual norms in establishing homosexual stigma and a minority status, but the role of homosexual stigma in structuring male sexual and gender norms; and finally, not simply the role of homosexual stigma in thus producing and consolidating masculinity, but also its role as a crucial requirement in the reproduction of gender relations at large.

Nicaraguans themselves sometimes comment on such connections. I was interviewing Jaime, then a teenager, on the conception of masculinity within the culture of machismo. Jaime contrasted the current, changing situation with the past, and illustrated his argument as follows:

> A man helping his wife out around the house was unthinkable before the revolution. No man would be caught dead washing dishes or cooking or ironing. If his wife asked him to give her a hand, he would just say, 'Yo no soy cochón' (I'm not queer) and that would be the end of it …

What happens to our analysis of gender relations if we take this statement literally? Whence come the distinctions that, from men's perspective, define gender differences and reinforce appropriate masculinity? In an age of increasingly subtle reading strategies, it might be interesting to try the novel approach of listening straightforwardly to such remarks.

Or, consider an event I observed during a visit between neighbours. Guto, a teenage boy, was holding Esperanza's and Pedro's daughter, Auxiliadora. Guto's sister Aida was holding her son, Ervin. Guto decided to have the children, both of them two, 'fight' a mock battle. He manipulated the smaller girl's hands into lightly hitting Ervin. The boy began to cry. 'Veni, cochón!' ('Come on, *cochón* [queer]!'), Guto cajoled, mimicking the voice of a small girl, 'Come on, *cochón*!' The baby in his arms seemed confused by the goings-on around her. Embarrassed by such antics, but responding nonetheless, Aida pushed her son Ervin forward and began manipulating his hands in mock battle. The four of them played this way for a few seconds until Ervin began to cry again. 'Cochón, cochón!' Guto chastised, while Aida soothed her son.

Only a couple of days before, in the rowdy and drunken atmosphere of Santo Domingo, there had been what could only be described as a collective outbreak of domestic violence in the neighbourhood. Several couples fought; several women were beaten by their husbands. Indeed, Esperanza and her *compañero* (companion) had exchanged blows after Pedro had punched her in the face. With events of the other day still no doubt very much on her mind, Esperanza said to me: 'Now just look at that. They're teaching him how to beat women.' And so they were.

Again, what happens to our analysis of gender if we give such an event the literal reading it was given by Esperanza? Esperanza was commenting narrowly on the lesson Guto was teaching Aida's son; more generally and most tellingly, she might have been commenting on a whole structure of child socialization. The lesson for Ervin – an inescapable one, reinforced at every juncture of a boy's experience – is: show aggressiveness, dominate women, or be deprived of your masculinity. Despite the best intentions and reform efforts, even in politically conscious households (like the one described above: Esperanza and Pedro were labour unionists and activists; Aida was a member of AMNLAE), the overall regimen of child-rearing remains highly gendered, and is very much designed to instill the core values of machismo in successive generations:

1   Boys are typically teased, taunted and provoked by their older siblings until they display an appropriate rage; once solicited, these rages are tolerated, and are punished only when they exceed broadly defined limits. Girls receive no such training, and their signs of rage are neither indulged nor tolerated.
2   When young male children are learning to speak, and pick up profane language from the adults and older children around them, their outbursts are greeted with amused tolerance, even encouragement; punishment ensues only when they direct their invective against adults. Female children receive no such indulgence, and even mild vulgarities from them receive swift punishment.
3   Boys who are still toddling and scarcely able to talk might be sent on various short errands or allowed to play without adult supervision at some distance from the house. Girls are not pushed toward personal autonomy at such an early age; when they wander from the house, they are more quickly retrieved, and are frequently punished for doing so.
4   Past adolescence, teenage boys are allowed to roam the neighbourhood in the evening and to socialize with their friends in a relatively unsupervised manner; teenage girls absolutely are *not* allowed to do so.
5   Indeed, boys are given great leeway in ignoring or flouting their mothers' orders; girls are issued many fewer warnings before being whipped.
6   Corporal punishment diminishes and ceases for a boy at a much younger age than it does for a girl.
7   And when a teenage boy comes home in the evening smelling of alcohol, his mother is unlikely to make too many inquiries; if a teenage girl comes home smelling of alcohol, her mother is almost certain to beat her with a belt.

By many means over many years, a boy's training actively solicits the hallmark traits of machismo: an ideal of masculinity defined by assertiveness, aggression, and competition; relatively privileged access to space and mobility; disproportionate control over resources; and a willingness to take risks … But how is such a routine concretely maintained? Not simply a system of rewards – for most males at any age, the rewards are minimal, and the costs (in injury, humiliation, exertion, and fiscal expenses) can be quite high. What sanctions, then, are invoked? What disciplinary measures force compliance with machismo's gender norms for males? The answer is clear: boys are constantly disciplined by their elders – by parents and siblings alike – with the humiliating phrase, 'No sea cochón!' ('Don't be a queer!') when their demeanour falls short of the assertive, aggressive, masculine ideal. Any show of sensitivity, weakness, reticence – or whatever else is judged to be a feminine charac-teristic – is swiftly identified and ridiculed. By adolescence, boys enter a competitive arena, where the signs of masculinity are actively struggled for, and can only be won by wresting them away from other boys around them (see Lancaster, 1992, pp. 245–7).

Justifiably, the regimen of this socialization might be called 'brutal'; its whole purpose is to induce a certain insensitivity – and its effect is to produce an irresponsibility – in men. That conjugal pairings are so often volatile, violent, and brief is a logical consequence of this form of masculine socialization. That the fate of so many Nicaraguan men is alcoholism, broken health, loneliness and early death is also a direct consequence of this atomizing and isolating socialization.

This routine, its disciplinary forces, the values it incubates, all set in motion cultural devices from which even women find it difficult to extract themselves, despite their obvious victimization in the culture of machismo. For example, women do indeed speak ill of men – for excessive drinking, for womanizing, for beating women – but when men gather, it is usually the women who send for liquor and prepare the chasers, and they usually do so without being asked. By and large, men who are considered too mild-mannered or too passive in their personal interactions are not considered good prospects for husbands – even if they are demonstrably industrious and hard-working. Although women frequently mitigate the discipline of harsh fathers, it is nonetheless to some extent women – mothers – who solicit independent, aggressive, even violent behaviour in their sons, while keeping their daughters on a far shorter leash: they want their sons to be strong and independent, not soft, and they want their daughters to behave like acquiescent young ladies.

Yet a final literal reading of the situation: even while the Sandinistas devoted themselves to combatting machismo in some arenas, the logic of this sexual construct, and its disciplinary force in creating and consolidating a genre of masculinity, was ultimately reinforced by conditions of war. In 1986, I asked Charlie what he was going to do in another year or so, when he would reach the age of mandatory military service. What he said, and how he said it were both indicative. 'When it's my time, I'm not going to run. I'd rather stay in school and study, but when I have to, I'll go into the service, and do my time. Only the *cochones* run.' Charlie (reluctantly) struck the machista pose: only a queer would run. Charlie's sentiments were almost stereotypical of my conversations with young men. It is clear that most young men would have preferred not to serve. Most said as much. The Sandinistas were aware of this. So in addition to the usual appeals to patriotism and revolutionary ardour, the govern-ment and the Sandinista mass organizations occasionally manipulated prevailing conceptions of masculinity as an additional measure to discourage draft evasion. The following graffiti, splashed on a prominent wall in Granada, is typical of its genre and carries this force: 'Sólo las maricas son evasores' ('Only sissies are evaders').

Gender, sexuality and the body: theoretical approaches and impasses

Most previous theoretical approaches to the production of masculinity have generally failed to explore the dimension that I have been sketching.

The classical research on patterns of machismo in Central America (and similarly situated geographies) views it, effectively, as a cultural and ideological superstructure, resting atop an economic base.[6] The historical thrust of this paradigm can be readily summarized: the rise of large-scale, capital-intensive agriculture in the nineteenth century deprived peasants and small farmers of land, thus creating a popular class of landless, mobile, male labourers. Women and children became the 'fixed' pieces of family structure, men the detachable parts, and an ideology arose to justify the resulting flexible patterns of householding. This explanation has the advantage of a certain materiality, but the disadvantage of reducing gender relations to an ideological gloss on economic relations. It never makes inquiries into the materiality of the body in the production of gender, sexuality, and other cultural values. It also takes gender inequality almost as a given, and proposes only to understand the brittle nature of conjugal pairs and the prevalence of informal unions.

Beyond Latin American studies, most existing efforts at theorizing gender have viewed gender relations through the lens of relations between men and women. Moreover, since gender studies emerged first and primarily from feminism, the literature has tended to concentrate on the female side of the question. Women's studies has offered important theoretical contributions and practical correctives to androcentric bias. But gender is not simply feminine. Contemporary gender studies should seriously theorize masculinity, as well, and it needs to theorize both masculinity and femininity beyond the simple dyadic models that have repeatedly devolved into essentialist and biologically grounded arguments.

An exception to the usual pattern of research is Gilmore's (1990) cross-cultural study of masculinity. Yet whatever its merits might be in other settings, Gilmore's hypothetically typical construction of masculinity seems not at all applicable to machismo in Nicaragua. Gilmore's notion of manhood, like Chodorow's (1974, 1978), emphasizes its achieved and competitive orientation; but Gilmore also attributes to it a protective, nurturing effect: as women are to children, so men are to women and children. None of my female informants invokes such qualities when describing traditional patterns of masculinity in Nicaragua. Nor, for that matter, do men. Both speak of 'the macho' in terms of risktaking, gambling, self-assertion, and violence. The underlying theme is irresponsibility, not nurture.

Those approaches that have attempted to consider both gender and sexuality as part of a single cultural system have produced mixed results, owing in part to the simplicity of the models proposed. Especially in the work of Dworkin (1987, 1989) and MacKinnon (1987, 1989), crucial distinctions are lost, not simply between gender and sexuality, but also between innumerable oppositions: between the system as a whole and individual experience; between the existing system of sexuality and the sex act for any two people; between the hegemony of the sexual code and sexual reinscription and subversion ... In a paradoxical move that would seem to enhance the existential responsibility of theory, such analyses have actually unhinged theory altogether from the responsibility of human reciprocity. In this iron cage of analysis, every sex act becomes indistinguishable from rape and terrorism. So extreme have been the abuses of this model that even Gayle Rubin, who first popularized the gender/sexuality model (1975), has expressly urged their more rigorous separation into distinct analytical domains (Rubin, 1984). And there is a real danger here, if distinctions are not maintained – if every sex act without exception is taken as nothing other than the simple and direct expression of a pre-existing system. A theory incapable of differentiations is inadequate to any task of cultural criticism. Haraway (1990, pp. 200–1) has described such work as a virtual parody of feminism; others have remarked on its affinities with Puritanism. Its fundamental and recurring structure duplicates the logic of Stalinism, in the sense described by Sartre (1963): everything specific, individual, and particular, must be made to defer to the general, the systemic, the totality. And what will not readily defer to theory is dissolved 'in a bath of sulfuric acid'.

Gay theory has since its inception theorized sexuality, especially male–male sexuality. It has frequently done so in connection with the prevailing system of gender norms, and without the indulgences of an anti-sex Puritanism. Gay and lesbian theory provides a good starting point for the kind of analysis I have been pointing toward. But gay theory, especially its essentialist and universalist varieties, too often begins and ends with the experiences of a sexual minority. At its most sophisticated – that is, in social constructionism – it marks the historical limits and describes the social conditions of homosexual identity and resistance.[7] But in either case, as long as it is motivated primarily by the politics of identity, it retains both a minority and *minoritizing* perspective.

Poststructural theory and postmodern experimentation afford analytical mobility, a turn from the facile temptations of 'depth models', a romp of differentiations, and a rigorous challenge to the politics of identity. Foucault's *History of Sexuality* (1980) provides a rough draft of what a genuine political economy of the sexual body might be. I have drawn freely on his 'productive' view of sexuality – not sexuality as productive in the sense of producing something else (wealth, class, commodities), but as itself, in itself, directly, productive. Productive, indeed, of identities and statuses and values which are themselves arbitrary, contrived, relational, conventional, and ephemeral.

However, much of postmodern academic discourse duplicates the process of abstraction, reification, and fetishization inherent in the commodification process (Marx, 1967, pp. 71–83; Lukács, 1971). Fredric Jameson (1991) thus describes postmodernism as 'the cultural logic of late capitalism'. For cultural criticism, we need a theory of fetishes, not theoretical fetishism. Even Foucault's work, which properly treats power as a relational realm, also has the effect of virtually severing power relations from the real human beings who produce, maintain, and transform them. In such theory, human agency and social practice have been disengaged from our understanding of the world. Little wonder that the system appears all-powerful in the postmodern politics of disengagement.

To unfashionably invoke a return of the repressed, we might today consider the example a currently eclipsed approach. Critical Marxism, especially the work of Marcuse (1966) and Brown (1990), attempted to articulate Freud's 'economy of desire' with Marx's critique of political economy. Marcuse maintained a conception of 'really existing sexuality' as systematically distorted, but he never viewed pleasure – sexual or otherwise – as inherently exploitative. Rather, he tried to theorize the conditions under which pleasure was either repressed or made to serve the ends of exploitation. Unfortunately, the limitations of Marcuse's analysis are coterminous with Freud's view of human nature, based on a theory of innate drives. The ballast for Marcuse's critical mission was always a conception of Nature, against which was pitted the Un-Natural excrescences of capitalism: commodities, exploitation, sublimation. But at its broadest, and read at a novel angle, Marcuse's work wrestled with fundamental questions that need to be re-asked: not simply, What are the productive applications of repression? But also, and more enduringly: Can one distinguish, rigorously and *a priori*, between eros and economics, desire and consumption, love and political economy? And how might we integrate these elements into a comprehensive yet subtle critical theory?

These approaches, taken individually, are not 'wrong', but even taken collectively, they are not quite adequate, either. They are not quite adequate for understanding the gendered body as a locus of cultural meanings, historical practices, and physical sensations – as simultaneously ambiguous, yet concrete; as socially constructed, but at the same time constituent of social structures. Previous approaches have not provided the conceptual tools for diagramming the multiple links between everyday life and the system of gender/sexuality in various social formations. And up until very recently, existing approaches have scarcely attempted to theorize how male–male transactions structure masculinity, what homosexuality has to do with homosociality, or how these affect gender and (hetero)sexual relations. But increasingly, such topics define the horizon of research in many disciplines.

All theory arises from a context, addresses questions of immediate concern, and carries traces of its own birth, omens of its own death. The coming body of critical theory emerges against a political and cultural backdrop: the maturing and diversification of second-wave feminism; the simultaneous globalization and decentring of the gay and lesbian political movements; responses to the worldwide AIDS epidemic by those most affected; the new technologies of body discipline, and new tactics of body rebellion; the development of a 'late Marxism' amid these conditions of late capitalism; the fragmentation of modern, totalizing political projects, including Marxism, in a 'postcolonial' world that nonetheless remains colonial because it remains capitalist.

These decentred conditions pose new questions, whose answers might be sought by innovating recombinant, practical variations of pre-existing theory. We need a theoretical approach faithful to the humane spirit of critical Marxism, steeped in the lessons of gender studies and gay studies, observant of the real contributions of poststructural and postmodern theory – yet without all the latter's distracting bells and whistles. We need a model with the theoretical mobility and sophistication of modern cultural studies, but ethnographically attentive to the mundane conditions of everyday life – an epistemologically 'grounded' critical method (Scheper-Hughes, 1992, pp. 4, 24) that dares to engage in issues that are of real interest to real people while always remaining concretely connected to their fundamental life experiences. To follow the circuitries of power in culture, we need an approach that can demonstrate concrete links between gender and sexuality, where those links exist, but without collapsing distinctions between the two or naturalizing their interrelationships. That is, we need 'a political economy of the body' that neither confuses itself with the more standard political economy of an economic mode of production, nor attempts to duplicate its every move, and is unwilling to say – before the fact – where the one ends and the other begins, or even whether there is a logical demarcation at all between the two. There is indeed a growing literature that engages the body in the same spirit that Marx engaged political economy

which is to say, as a critique of existing political economy. Not all of this literature belongs to gay/lesbian studies, but it all entails a certain 'denaturalization' of the body, its care, meanings and habits. These works allow us to view the body itself as an ensemble of social practices. Jean Comaroff (1985) puts a modified conception of Bourdieu's (1977) habitus at the centre of anthropological concerns with the social process of embodiment (see also Comaroff and Comaroff, 1991, pp. 19–39). Much of Thomas Lacquer's (1990, 1992) emphasis is to historicize the body in a political-economic sense. M. Elaine Combs-Schilling (1989) diagrams a multi-levelled political economy of gender and sexuality in Morocco, and Richard Parker (1991) surveys the physical and social terrain of Brazilian sexual culture as enacted through carnival. The works of the Bakhtin school have provided a most productive site for recent attempts at theorizing the body, discourse, and culture (Bakhtin, 1981, 1984; Vološinov, 1993), while Donna Haraway's (1989, 1991) original work explores postmodernity's pliable borders, where nature and artifice, biology and technology, increasingly blur. Much of Nancy Scheper-Hughes' (1979, 1992; Scheper-Hughes and Lock, 1987) work collectively points toward a critical political economy of the body, its practices, and regimes of family life.

Closer to the topic at hand, Gilbert Herdt's (1981, 1982) research in Papua New Guinea clearly establishes links between sexuality and the production of appropriate gender, but the configuration is very different from that which obtains in either Nicaragua or in the countries of the North. Dennis Altman (1972, 1982) was an early practitioner of this radical political economy of the body, and Jeffrey Weeks (1977, 1981, 1985) has long laboured on this overall project. Judith Butler's *Gender Trouble* (1990) represents an attempt at theorizing the relationship between the system of asymmetrical gender relations and compulsory heterosexuality. Eve Sedgwick's *Between Men* (1985) and *Epistemology of the Closet* (1990) are direct attempts at theorizing the articulation of the homosocial, the homosexual, and the hetero-sexual in Western society, although these books' emphasis on elite literary texts leaves them with few points of access to forms of everyday life.[8]

It might be objected that this angle is an improbable one; that it stretches metaphors to speak of a 'political economy of the body'. Clearly, the literal mechanics of appropriation, exploitation, and production are different in the two domains connected by this metaphor.[9] What 'political economy' usually designates is material production and consumption, along with the attendant political regime that both supports and is supported by a given mode of production. The 'political economy of the body' alludes to that ensemble of representations and relations configured around the human body; to all the social, cultural, and economic values produced out of the raw material of the physical body; to the sum of gender transactions and sexual exchanges that collectively constitute the social body; and to all those power relations supported by and which support a given body regime. I would argue that the 'mechanics' are roughly comparable in either case. Any mode of production works over some raw material – whether it be physical material, or the matter of the physiology – to produce products of some value. Those products – whether they embody the value of commodities or the values of men and women – are circulated and exchanged according to certain implicit rules. All exploitative and inegalitarian modes of production and exchange produce certain conflicts over the allocation of goods, rewards, and powers. In any given political economy, these relations and conflicts give rise to an ensemble of political, repre-sentational, and juridical relationships. Acting as transactors and following the logic of the system they inhabit, humans are produced – or, rather, they produce themselves, and their consciousness, in the process of their overall activity.

To speak of a political economy of the body, or to conceive the body as a field of produc-tive relations, is not to draw rigorous, one-to-one analogies with material production but to re-iterate that what is produced in any case is not a 'good' but a 'value'. What 'economy' means in all cases is a system where value is assigned based not on any 'intrinsic' worth of an object but rather on the object's position in the system of production and exchange. Thus, the value of a commodity is calculated in relation to other commodities and by the comparative social labour that produced it. Classes, too, are defined relationally: by their relations to each other in the social production process. In the political economy of 'colorism' (Lancaster, 1991), one's value as a person is determined within a system of material and symbolic exchanges, in terms of relations between the lexical clusters around *blanco* (white) and *negro* (black).

All theory is metaphorical, but to keep closely to Marx's arguments, it is no less metaphor-ical, no less concrete, to speak of a 'political economics of the body' than to speak of a 'polit-ical economy of material production'. Such an emphasis returns Marxism to its original reflections on the production of the human condition (Marx and Engels, 1964): it is a given form of humanity that is ultimately produced by any given mode of production.[10]

The culmination of these theoretical developments and mediations should result not simply in some well-demarcated 'queer theory', but in the *queering of theory* as we all know and use it. Without forgetting the limits and conditions of homosexual identity, such an approach would consider the circulation of stigma in, through, and around sexuality – not simply how a minority identity is constructed, but how the stigmatization process affects everyone. Such theory begins but does not end with the simple affirmation of identities; it understands its subjects in the context of a general political economy of sexuality. It is capable of discovering concrete links beyond the realm of sexuality proper. As is implicit in the term 'political econ-omy', this model links sexuality to systems of gender, to modes of economic production and distribution, and to the corpus of bureaucratic and military coercions that constitute the state. A practical theory so conceived might allow us to develop a different kind of politics: a politics of solidarity, not identity, whose purpose is to change systems of practice and meaning rather than to simply carve out new minority rights within a preexisting system.

Toward a political economy of machismo

To return, then, to the line of questions that prompted this essay: What, concretely, is machismo? What does it mean to be a man in the culture of machismo? And why do Nicaraguan men behave as they so often do (and as Nicaraguan women so vigorously complain): beating their wives, simultaneously fathering multiple households of children, abandoning *compañeras* and children, gambling away hard-earned money, and drinking to excess? And why did a decade of efforts to roll back the culture of machismo achieve so few tangible results? An easy answer to the final question would be that the strain on Nicaragua's economic resources has made social restructuring impossible for the time being. That is indeed a partial answer. For those men already engaged in the culture of machismo, what AMNLAE and the Sandinistas call 'responsibility' would prove costly, even under the best of circumstances. Under the current economy of scarcity, it would perhaps be prohibitively costly. Perhaps under a recovered economy, men might be more likely to support the children they father, and perhaps under better circumstances, sex education and contraception might make alternatives to the status quo available. Amidst the dislocations of war and hyper-inflation, however, and among all the personal turmoils thus engendered, it is difficult to imagine any systematic restructuring of the personal life and of personal relations.

But there is more to the matter than that, for the arrangement of interpersonal relationships is dependent on far more than the immediate state of the economy. The question of machismo cannot be addressed adequately if it is viewed as an ideology in the classical sense of the term. Machismo is not merely a set of erroneous ideas that somehow got lodged in people's heads. Rather, it is an organization of social relations that generates ideas. Machismo, therefore, is more than an 'effect' produced by other material causes. It has its own materiality, its own power to produce effects. The resilience of machismo has nothing to do with the tendency of ideology to 'lag' behind changes in the system of economic production, for machismo itself is a real political economy of the body. In the political economy of machismo – that is, within the horizon of the masculinized, male body – one's standing as a man is gauged by the execution of certain transactions (drinking, gambling, womanizing) in relation to other men.

As a field of power relations, machismo entails every bit as much force as economic production, and no less influences economic production than it is influenced by it – otherwise, why would poverty have a feminine face in Nicaragua? Why would women and children be specially disadvantaged? Why else would weakness, failure, and fear be conceived within the logic of the *cochón*? And why would local understandings of wealth, success, and effective politics revolve around a blurred constellation of male dreams of omnipotence: *el hombre grande*, it goes without saying, is *un gran macho*, who is, naturally, also a *caudillo* … Although we might acknowledge the difficulty in domesticating masculinity under conditions of acute crisis, there is no particular reason to believe that men could be brought into the fold of the family more readily under conditions of surplus than under conditions of scarcity, for machismo produces its own surpluses and scarcities. And we cannot even begin to prejudge which activities characterize the political economy of the body and which ones characterize the economic relations of production; where machismo leaves off as a system, and where this distinct region of peripheral neocolonial capitalism begins.

Nor can the question of machismo be fully addressed as a matter of relations between men and women. It is that, but it is also more. Machismo (no less than North American concepts of masculinity and appropriate sexuality) is not exclusively or even primarily a means of structuring power relations between men and women. Indeed, men are never in a situation of direct competition with women for male honour. The rules of the game effectively exclude women from this male domain; by definition, it is only with other men that a man directly competes. Machismo, then – and the conception of masculinity it implies – is a means of structuring power between and among men. Like drinking, gambling, risk-taking, asserting one's opinion, and fighting, the conquest of women is a feat performed with two audiences in mind: first, other men, to whom one must constantly prove one's masculinity and virility; and second, to one's self, to whom one must also show all the signs of masculinity.[11]

Machismo, then, is a matter of constantly asserting one's masculinity by way of practices that show the self to be 'active', not 'passive' (as defined in a given milieu). Every gesture, every posture, every stance, every way of acting in the world, is immediately seen as 'masculine' or 'feminine', depending on whether it connotes activity or passivity. Every action is governed by a relational system – a code – which produces its meanings out of the subject matter of the body, its form, its engagement with other bodies. Every act is, effectively, part of an ongoing exchange-system between men (in which women very often figure as intermediaries, but never directly as transactors). To maintain one's masculinity, one must successfully come out on top of these exchanges. To lose in this ongoing exchange system entails a loss of face, which is to say, a loss of status, and a loss of masculinity. The threat, and the fear, is a total loss of status, whereby one descends to the zero point of the game, and either literally or effectively becomes a *cochón*.

The *cochón*, itself a product of machismo, thus grounds the system of machismo, holds it in its place, and vice versa.

Embodying power: homosexuality as medium of exchange

An earlier paper of mine diagrams the construction of homosexual stigma in Nicaragua (Lancaster, 1988). There, as in much of Latin America, the stigmatized identity is configured not simply around homosexual intercourse, but in terms of the receptive, especially anal-'passive' role in sexual intercourse.[12] Whatever else a *cochón* might or might not do, he is tacitly understood as one who assumes the receptive role in anal intercourse. His partner, defined as 'active' in the terms of their engagement, is not stigmatized, nor does he necessarily acquire a special identity of any sort.

This implies a very different demarcation for the *cochón* than that which circumscribes the North American homosexual. In the United States, outside of a few well-defined contexts, homosexual intercourse – indeed, homosexual desire – of any sort in any position marks one as a homosexual. But it is not simply a minority status which is differentially produced. What is also produced, in either case, is a majority, 'normative' status. It is heterosexual honour in the United States to never, under any circumstances, feel or express homosexual desire. Masculinity here is constructed atop the repression of homosexuality.

In Nicaragua, however, homosexual activity – both figuratively and literally – is the very medium of a masculinity defined most bluntly in terms of use-values (not the value of repression). This is not to say that there are not other media; there are. What is unique about the homosexual medium is that it signifies most directly and without intermediaries the male–male nature of machismo. Figuratively, the *cochón* is held to represent the degradation of a fallen man. At every turn, and in innumerable discourses, the honour of 'los machos' is measured against his shame. This gauging is never simply a passive comparison. Masculinity is relational: not simply as a 'vis-à-vis', but as a practice of imposition and domination; it must therefore be actively demonstrated, enacted, and maintained. Literally, in terms of male–male sexual relations, when one 'uses' a *cochón*, one acquires masculinity; when one is 'used' as a *cochón*, one expends it. The same act, then, makes one man an *hombre-hombre*, a manly man, and the other a *cochón*.

The machista's 'honour' and the *cochón*'s 'shame' are opposite sides of the same coin, alternate angles of the same transaction. A value is produced, circulated, and reproduced in sexual transactions between men, and so is a stigma. Indeed, this value can only be measured against stigma. (Put in political-economic terms: in systems of exploitation, every 'surplus' value is produced by an act of appropriation, and thus implies the creation of a 'deficit' somewhere else.) Each act of intercourse 'produces' moreover a system of masculinity – a system that explicitly regulates relations between men, but which no less conditions relations between men and women. Whatever the private sentiments of those involved – and relations between machistas and *cochones* are sometimes quite tender – these terms unambiguously denote winners and losers in the public game of masculinity: a game which structures male actions and interactions.

To open up the question of homosexual stigma to its farthest parameters: what is at stake is not simply a question of the construction of minority sexual identity through stigma, but moreover the elaboration of a majority status and a prevailing culture through the circulation of stigma. The definition of masculinity rides piggy-back, as it were, on the stigma of the *cochón*.[13]

The circulation of stigma

That being said, of course, sex is never so precise, and the real circulation of stigma is never so categorical. The stigma of the *cochón* applies, in its strictest and most limited sense, to a relatively small minority of men: those who are the 'passive' participants in anal intercourse. In its broadest sense, however, the stigma threatens, even taints, all men.

The circulation of stigma implies a complex economy, an ambiguous discourse, and incessant power-struggles. In the words of Erving Goffman, stigma requires of us a carefully staged 'presentation of self in everyday life' (1959); it entails multiple levels of public, private, and intermediate transactions. To extend the dramaturgic metaphor, it brings into play many stages, many backstages, and many choruses. Or, to employ a game analogy: everyone wishes to pass the stigma along; no one wishes to be left holding it. As cunning and artful as are those who dodge it, by that very token must the invocation of stigma be coarse, generalized, and to some degree non-discriminating. While the system of stigma produces certain distinct categories, then, its operation is never entirely categorical, for stigma is necessarily 'sticky'.

In the culture of machismo, the *cochón* is narrowly defined as anal-passive, but the concept of anal passivity serves more loosely as a sort of extreme case of 'passivity'. The term 'cochón' thus may be invoked in both a strict and a loose sense. Which aspect of the concept is emphasized – anality or passivity – will determine whether it encompasses a small minority or a potentially large majority of men. Therein lies the peculiar power of stigma to regulate conduct and generate effects: it ultimately threatens all men who fail to maintain a proper public face. In machismo, the ambiguity of discourse is a highly productive feature of the system.

Thus, the *hombre-hombre*'s exemption from stigma is never entirely secure. He might find his honour tainted under certain circumstances. If an *hombre-hombre*'s sexual engagement with a *cochón* comes to light, for example, and if the nature of that relationship is seen as compromising the former's strength and power – in other words, if he is seen as being emotionally vulnerable to another man – his own masculinity would be undermined, regardless of his physical role in intercourse, and he might well be enveloped within the *cochón*'s stigma. Or if the *activo*'s attraction to men is perceived as being so great as to define a clear preference for men, and if this preference is understood to mitigate his social and sexual dominion over women, he would be seen as eschewing his masculine prerogatives and would undoubtedly be stigmatized. However, the Nicaraguan *hombre-hombre* retains the tools and strategies to ward off such stigma, both within and even through his sexual relationships with other men, and his arsenal is not much less than that which is available to other men who are not sleeping with *cochones*.

This is a crucial point. These kinds of circumstances are not perhaps exceptions at all, but simply applications of the rules in their most general sense. Such rules apply not only to those men who engage in sexual intercourse with other men; they apply equally to men who have sex only with women. The noise of stigma is the clatter of a malicious gossip that targets others' vulnerabilities. Thus, if a man fails to maintain the upper hand in his relations with women, his demeanour might well be judged 'passive', and he would be stigmatized, by degrees, as a *cabrón* (cuckold), *maricón* (effeminate man), and *cochón*. Whoever fails to maintain an aggressively masculine front will be teased, ridiculed, and, ultimately, stigmatized. In this regard, accusations that one is a *cochón* are bandied about in an almost random manner: as a jest between friends, as an incitement between rivals, as a violent insult between enemies. Cats that fail to catch mice, dogs that fail to bark, boys who fail to fight, and men who fail in their pursuit of a woman: all are reproached with the term. And sometimes, against all this background noise, the charge is levelled as an earnest accusation. That is the peculiar and extravagant power of the stigmatizing category: like a 'prison-house of language', it indeed confines those to whom it is most strictly applied; but ambiguously used, it conjures a terror that rules all men, all actions, all relationships.

Conclusion: the *cochón*, machismo, and the politics of gender

A rule is best preserved in its infractions. And a structure, a system of practices, is most readily defined, not by what is central to it, but by what is apparently marginal to it. The *cochón*, by violating the standards of appropriate male behaviour, defines the conception of appropriate masculinity in Nicaragua. His passivity, as the opposite of activity, defines the latter (even as it is defined by the former). His status constitutes the ultimate sanction within a political economy of the body, its practices, its instrumentalities.

The *cochón* occupies the space and defines the nexus of all that is denigrated in men and among men. His presence allows the construction of another nexus, where the symbolic capital of masculinity is accumulated. In the cultural code of machismo, a series of couplings deploy themselves and define reality: masculinity/femininity, activity/passivity, violence/abuse, domination/subordination. Decoupling such a chain of associations would have to entail a political programme far more radical than anything AMNLAE proposed or the Sandinistas actually tried.

Very much to the point: when I interviewed Nicaraguan men on the New Family Laws (with their stipulation that paternity entail economic responsibility, both inside and outside marriage) and their intention (to minimize irresponsible sex, irresponsible parenting, and familial dislocation), my informants very frequently took recourse to the same standard constructs. First, the interrogative: 'What do the Sandinistas want from us? That we should all become *cochones*?' And then, the tautological: 'A man has to be a man.' That is, a man is defined by what he is not (a *cochón*).

From one angle, the distinction between men and women might seem enough to keep machismo's dynamics in play. Not so. For men do not 'fall' to the status of women when they fail to maintain their pre-defined masculinity; they become something else: not quite men, not quite women. It could be said, then, that they fall both further and less far than women's station. *Less far*, because for some purposes and in some contexts, despite his stigma, a *cochón* can usually maintain some masculine prerogatives. *Further*, because a woman is not stigmatized for being a woman, *per se*, not even for being a strong woman whose demeanour violates certain gender norms. One is, however, stigmatized for being less than a man.

It might moreover seem tempting to understand the sexual stigma of the *cochón* as a direct extension of the logic of gender onto the realm of sexuality: as man is to woman, so the *hombre-hombre* is to the *cochón*. This equation partly holds, but is not quite adequate. While it is clear that the *cochón*'s denigration is cast in strongly gendered terms, it is also cast in excess of those terms: as failure, inadequacy, weakness, and defeat.[14] Such meanings can scarcely be directly attributed to Nicaragua's traditional conceptions of womanhood, which celebrates a cult of elevated motherhood. This 'excess' marks all that is ingredient in the production of manhood. Not simply the opposite of femininity, masculinity proper is itself the locus of important distinctions.

The arguments I have been developing here attempt to demonstrate the connections between gender and sexuality without theoretically collapsing the two. This model also represents an attempt to understand the concrete connections between micropolitics and macropolitics, between sexuality and the state.

Did the Sandinista revolution fail because it failed to emancipate *cochones*? Not *per se*, and that is not the argument that I would like to make. Did the revolution decline because it deferred a revolution in gender roles? Again, to put it that way would be an exaggeration. In the aftermath of the 1990 electoral defeat, some have argued in effect that the revolution failed because it was not radical enough (see Gonzalez, 1990; Randall, 1992). Such arguments are not convincing. An agenda of legal and social reforms were already underway. More militancy on such issues, under the circumstances, probably would have been more divisive. More divisions, in the context of war and crisis, would probably have shortened the life of the revolution. While the results of legal and social reforms were ambiguous at best, a decade is scarcely long enough to break family habits, change the meaning of gender, and overhaul the sexual economy.

The argument that I would construct goes more like this: the war, the embargo, and the crisis were all felt most intimately in Nicaraguan family life: increasing gender conflicts, accelerated rates of male abandonment, the surplus impoverishment of women and children ... And how could one speak meaningfully of 'working-class solidarity' while its families remained divided by an oppressive culture of machismo, and were at war within themselves? The fabric of personal life, already tattered and patched together at best, unravelled. And with it, a revolution.

It is in this context that the stigma of the *cochón* and the practices of homosexuality were relevant to the larger course of history. For the structure of family life and the nature of gender cannot be understood – or altered – without reference to homosexuality. Homosexual intercourse and homosexual stigma play a clear and major role in the construction of appropriate gender for men. Their force on the male body is both differentiating and disciplinary. And machismo's ultimate reinforcement is the sanction: that one might be seen as, or become stigmatized as, or become, a *cochón*, if one fails to maintain one's proper masculinity as defined by machismo. If the New Family Laws, the project of the New Man, and attempts at rolling back the culture of machismo have largely failed, this is because such attempts at cultural reconstruction left undeconstructed the grounding oppositions of the system, and thus left machismo's driving engine largely untouched.

However, I do not wish to conclude by making that system appear all-powerful. The role of theory should never be to bolt every window and bar every escape hatch from such a prison-house.

No less than any other system of arbitrary power, privilege, and exploitation, machismo's routine operation generates innumerable resistances, evasions, and conflicts (Certeau, 1984). Among men, these have not yet been as systematically mobilized as they have been among women, though the slow emergence after 1990 of an open gay liberation movement in Managua would seem to mark an important turning point in Nicaragua's political culture.

But even in a public world defined by power and cruelty, there are private worlds that turn on love. I have already said that in their personal relations, some couples – even couples that define themselves as consisting of an *hombre-hombre* and a *cochón* – conduct their affairs in a humane and tender way. These relationships violate the rules of the system, subvert its operation, play with its meanings, and elaborate new possibilities, even to the point of rendering null the opposition between 'hombre-hombre' and 'cochón'. In private transactions, then, the political economy of machismo is routinely subverted. Should such private arrangements ever be aired in open discussion, they would constitute a radical challenge to the stability of the system.

On the public occasion of *carnaval*, and in other carnivalesque festivities, the official body is travestied and a rebellious libidinal body is liberated. The political economy of machismo is transgressed, and its values are rudely reversed.[15] Queers are not the only ones who enjoy the antics of *carnaval*; everyone becomes a bit queer. It might be countered that carnival time comes but once a year, or that it affords only a momentary reprieve from the strictures of everyday life, and that is true. And carnival is, after all, only play. But play is not a trivial matter. Carnival play is very different from those serious games that make boys into men. It models new perceptions, alternative bodies, utopian realities. This spirit of play has been growing and developing inside carnival for the better part of five centuries. And when that spirit of play escapes *carnaval*, it will remake the world.

Acknowledgements

Some sections of this essay are drawn from my book *Life is Hard: Machismo, Danger and the Intimacy of Power in Nicaragua* (1992). This paper developed over the course of time from talks given in several places: Modern Times Bookstore in San Francisco; the Evergreen State College in Olympia, Washington; the departments of anthropology at the University of California, Columbia University, and Yale University. It was formally presented as part of the 'Gender Power' panel at the 1993 conference on International Perspectives in Sex Research held in Rio de Janeiro. I am grateful to all of the above audiences for their helpful criticisms. Specific thanks are in order to Samual Colón, Elaine Combs-Schilling, John Gagnon, Paul Kutsche, Rachel Moore, Stephen O. Murray, Richard Parker, Jim Quesada, Nancy Scheper-Hughes, and Michael Taussig. It is too late to thank the ardent Nicaraguanist and tireless gay activist Tede Matthews, who died of AIDS in 1993. His work, networking, and sense of humour were all invaluable resources for several political communities. We miss him, and I dedicate this essay to his memory.

Notes

1 For a thorough overview of the economic consequences of war and embargo, see Conroy, 1990. See also Walker, 1987.
2 See Dirección de Orientación y Protección Familiar, 1983; IHCA, 1984; Molyneux, 1985; Collinson, 1990.
3 Dirección de Orientación y Protección Familiar, 1983; IHCA, 1984; Borge, 1985; Molyneux, 1985; Dirección Nacional, FSLN, 1987.

4 See Lancaster, 1992, pp. 283–93. See also Stacey's (1990) and Ginsburg's (1984, 1989) parallels regarding evangelicals, women, and the religious right in the United States.

5 Critiques include Valentine, 1968; Leacock, 1971; and Rigdon, 1988. For a more recent discussion of the resurgence of 'culture of poverty' theory implicit in many discussions of the 'black underclass', see Reed, 1991.

6 See Adams, 1956, p. 892; Adams, 1957, pp. 189–95, 457–8; Anderson, 1971, p. 13; Brown, 1975.

7 Boswell's (1992) position is nuanced; he prefers the term 'realist' to 'essentialist', and avoids speculating on the 'causes' of sexual preference. However, Ruse's (1988) gay-friendly sociobiology proposes a genetic anchor with hormonal wiring for the essential sexual orientations. The flurry of recent brain studies and twin studies attests to the popularity of such vulgar essentialist groundings. The media have sagely announced with each study 'compelling new evidence' that homosexuality is genetically fixed or biologically shaped (Burr, 1993), although the research methods employed in these studies were poorly conceived, and their findings have been ambiguous at best (see Rist, 1992; Fausto-Sterling, 1992, pp. 245–56). For sophisticated developments of the so-called 'constructionist' position, see Halperin, 1990; see also Weeks, 1977, 1981, 1985; and Ponse, 1978.

8 See also Stewart, 1984; Hennessy, 1993.

9 Yet it must be remembered that all theory is metaphorical. The work of theory, like that of metaphor, is to construct models. Models, by design, work by analogy: they draw out connections between two (or more) different things, based on resemblances (of elements, characteristics, activities, or effects) held in common between them.

10 I am touching here on arguments that I have offered elsewhere. For a fuller review, see Lancaster, 1992, pp. 19–21, 223–4, 280–2, 319 n. 3–4.

11 Male power, it would seem, is a largely homosocial phenomenon. If we take homosociality – of secret societies, male cults, men's clubs, the military, sports – as homosexual desire sublimated, then the role of the homosocial in structuring both the heterosexual and male power deserves a distinctly queer reading. Lévi-Strauss' (1969) classical analysis of kinship argues that men structure political alliances between themselves through the exchange of women; in this version, political society emerged as a bonded male–male relationship mediated by women. Rubin (1975) took this account of kinship as the point of departure for a critical understanding of male power and female powerlessness. Sedgwick (1985, 1990), too, understands the patriarchy as a social inheritance passed from one generation of men to the next through the cultivation of male homosocial power, structured by the sublimation of overt homosexual desire (see also Castiglia, 1988). And Sanday (1990, pp. 12–14) understands gang rape as both an instrument of male dominance and a method of male bonding, conducted precisely through a homoerotic medium where homosexual desire is simultaneously expressed and repressed.

12 See also Carrier, 1976a, 1976b; Parker, 1985; Adam, 1989 and Almaguer, 1991.

13 A pun, but an appropriate one. The term *cochón* apparently derives from the Spanish term for 'pig'. Plainly, the term is meant to dehumanize; it most likely emerged by analogy with the prone-receptive position in intercourse. At the micro level (in a sexual relationship), one man maintains his masculinity by assuming the insertive role in intercourse; at the macro level (in society at large), the circulation of stigma and its assignment to a well-demarcated minority of men creates the 'surplus' value of masculinity, which is distributed to the unlabelled men.

14 See Loizons and Papataxiarchis's (1991, pp. 227–8) similar argument regarding the stigma attached to the receptive partner in homosexual intercourse in contemporary Greece.

15 See Davis, 1978; Bakhtin, 1984; Lancaster, 1988, pp. 38–54; 1992, pp. 233, 251–2; Parker, 1991.

References

ADAM, B. (1989) 'Homosexuality without a gay world: pasivos y activos en Nicaragua', *Out/Look*, 1, pp. 74–82.

ADAMS, R.N. (1956) 'Cultural components of Central America', *American Anthropologist*, 58, pp. 881–907.

—— (1957) *Cultural Surveys of Panama-Nicaragua-Guatemala-El Salvador-Honduras*, Scientific Publications, 33, Washington, DC, Pan American Sanitary Bureau, Regional Office of the World Health Organization.

ALMAGUER, T. (1991) 'Chicano men: a cartography of homosexual identity and behaviour', *Differences: A Journal of Feminist Cultural Studies*, 3, pp. 75–100.

ALTMAN, D. (1972) *Homosexual Oppression & Liberation*, New York: Outerbridge & Dienstfrey.

—— (1982) *The Homosexualization of America*, Boston, MA: Beacon Press.

ANDERSON, T.P. (1971) *Matanza: El Salvador's Communist Revolt of 1932*, Lincoln: University of Nebraska Press.

BAKHTIN, M. (1981) *The Dialogic Imagination: Four Essays*, Austin: University of Texas Press.

—— (1984) *Rabelais and His World*, Bloomington: Indiana University Press.

BORGE, T. (1985) 'Women and the Nicaraguan revolution', in MARCUS, B. (ed.) *Nicaragua: The Sandinista Revolution: Speeches by Sandinista Leaders*, New York: Pathfinder Press.

BOSWELL, J. (1992) 'Concepts, experience, and sexuality', in STEIN, E. (ed.) *Forms of Desire: Sexual Orientation and the Social Constructionist Controversy*, New York and London: Routledge.

BOURDIEU, P. (1977) *Outline of a Theory of Practice*, Cambridge: Cambridge University Press.

BROWN, N.O. (1990) *Love's Body*, Berkeley and Los Angeles: University of California Press.

BROWN, S.E. (1975) 'Love unites them and hunger separates them: poor women in the Dominican Republic', in REITER, R.R. (ed.) *Toward an Anthropology of Women*, New York: Monthly Review Press.

BURR, C. (1993) 'Homosexuality and biology', *The Atlantic*, 271, March, pp. 47–65.

BUTLER, J. (1990) *Gender Trouble: Feminism and the Subversion of Identity*, New York and London: Routledge.

CARRIER, J.M. (1976a) 'Cultural factors affecting urban Mexican male homosexual behaviour', *Archives of Sexual Behaviour*, 5, pp. 103–24.

—— (1976b) 'Family attitudes and Mexican male homosexuality', *Urban Life*, 5, pp. 359–76.

CASTIGLIA, C. (1988) 'Rebel without a closet: homosexuality and Hollywood', *Critical Texts*, 5, pp. 31–5.

CERTEAU, M. (1984) *The Practice of Everyday Life*, Berkeley and Los Angeles: University of California Press.

CHODOROW, N. (1974) 'Family structure and feminine personality', in ROSALDO, M.Z. and LAMPHERE, L. (eds) *Woman, Culture, and Society*, Stanford: Stanford University Press.

—— (1978) *The Reproduction of Mothering: Psychoanalysis and the Psychology of Gender*, Berkeley and Los Angeles: University of California Press.

COLLINSON, H. (ed.) (1990) *Women and Revolution in Nicaragua*, London: Zed Books.

COMAROFF, J. (1985) *Body of Power, Spirit of Resistance: The Culture and History of a South African People*, Chicago: University of Chicago Press.

—— and COMAROFF, J. (1991) *Of Revelation and Revolution: Christianity, Colonialism, and Consciousness in South Africa*, Vol. 1, Chicago: University of Chicago Press.

COMBS-SCHILLING, M.E. (1989) *Sacred Performances: Islam, Sexuality and Sacrifice*, New York: Columbia University Press.

CONROY, M.E. (1990) 'The political economy of the 1990 Nicaraguan elections', *International Journal of Political Economy*, fall, pp. 5–33.

DAVIS, N.Z. (1978) 'Women on top: symbolic sexual inversion and political disorder in early modern Europe', in BABCOCK, B.A. (ed.) *The Reversible World: Symbolic Inversion in Art and Society*, Ithaca, NY: Cornell University Press.

DIRECCIÓN DE ORIENTACIÓN Y PROTECCIÓN FAMILIAR (1983) *Informe sobre la familia en Nicaragua*, Managua: Instituto Nicaraguense de Seguridad Social y Bienestar, Oficina de la Mujer, Secretaría de la Junta del Gobierno de Reconstrucción Nacional.

DIRECCIÓN NACIONAL, FSLN (1987) *El FSLN y la Mujer*, Managua: Editorial Vanguardia.

DWORKIN, A. (1987) *Intercourse*, New York: Free Press.

—— (1989) *Pornography: Men Possessing Women*, New York: Dutton.

FAUSTO-STERLING, A. (1992) *Myths of Gender: Biological Theories about Women and Men*, revised edition, New York: Basic Books.

FOUCAULT, M. (1980) *The History of Sexuality, Vol. 1: An Introduction*, New York: Random House, Vintage Books.

GILMORE, D.D. (1990) *Manhood in the Making: Cultural Concepts of Masculinity*, New Haven, CT: Yale University Press.

GINSBURG, F. (1984) 'The body politic: the defence of sexual restriction by anti-abortion activists', in VANCE, C.S. (ed.) *Pleasure and Danger: Exploring Female Sexuality*, New York and London: Routledge.

—— (1989) *Contested Lives: The Abortion Debate in America*, Berkeley and Los Angeles: University of California Press.

GOFFMAN, E. (1959) *The Presentation of Self in Everyday Life*, New York: Doubleday.

GONZALEZ, M. (1990) *Nicaragua: What Went Wrong?*, London: Bookmarks.

HALPERIN, D.M. (1990) *One Hundred Years of Homosexuality*, New York and London: Routledge.

HARAWAY, D. (1989) *Primate Visions: Gender, Race, and Nature in the World of Modern Science*, New York: Routledge.

—— (1990) 'A manifesto for cyborgs: science, technology, and socialist feminism in the 1980s', in NICHOLSON, L.J. (ed.) *Feminism/Postmodernism*, New York and London: Routledge.

—— (1991) *Simians, Cyborgs, and Women: The Reinvention of Nature*, New York and London: Routledge.

HENNESSY, R. (1993) *Materialist Feminism and the Politics of Discourse*, New York and London: Routledge.

HERDT, G.H. (1981) *Guardians of the Flutes: Idioms of Masculinity*, New York: McGraw-Hill.

—— (1982) 'Fetish and fantasy in Sambia initiation', in HERDT, G.H. (ed.) *Rituals of Manhood: Male Initiation in Papua New Guinea*, Berkeley and Los Angeles: University of California Press.

IHCA (INSTITUTO HISTORICO CENTROAMERICANO) (1984) 'La familia Nicaraguense en el proceso de cambio', *Envio*, April, pp. 1–12.

—— (1988) 'Sandinistas surviving in a percentage game', *Envio*, December, pp. 10–23.

JAMESON, F. (1991) *Postmodernism; or, The Cultural Logic of Late Capitalism*, Durham, NC: Duke University Press.

LACQUER, T.W. (1990) *Making Sex: Body and Gender from the Greeks to Freud*, Cambridge, MA: Harvard University Press.

—— (1992) 'Sexual desire and the market economy during the industrial revolution', in STANTON, D.C. (ed.) *Discourses of Sexuality: From Aristotle to AIDS*, Ann Arbor: University of Michigan Press.

LANCASTER, R.N. (1988) *Thanks to God and the Revolution: Popular Religion and Class Consciousness in the New Nicaragua*, New York: Columbia University Press.

—— (1991) 'Skin color, race, and racism in Nicaragua', *Ethnology*, 34, pp. 339–53.

—— (1992) *Life is Hard: Machismo, Danger, and the Intimacy of Power in Nicaragua*, Berkeley and Los Angeles: University of California Press.

LEACOCK, E. (1971) *The Culture of Poverty: A Critique*, New York: Simon and Schuster.

LÉVI-STRAUSS, C. (1969) *The Elementary Structures of Kinship*, Boston, MA: Beacon.

LEWIS, O. (1966) 'The culture of poverty', *Scientific American*, 215, 4, pp. 3–10.

LOIZONS, P. and PAPATAXIARCHIS, E. (1991) 'Gender, sexuality, and person in Greek culture', in LOIZONS, P and PAPATAXIARCHIS, E. (eds) *Contested Identities: Gender and Kinship in Modern Greece*, Princeton: Princeton University Press.

LUKÁCS, G. (1971) *History and Class Consciousness: Studies in Marxist Dialectics*, London: Merlin Press.

MACKINNON, C. (1987) *Feminism Unmodified*, Cambridge, MA: Harvard University Press.

—— (1989) *Toward a Feminist Theory of the State*, Cambridge, MA: Harvard University Press.

MARCUSE, H. (1966) *Eros and Civilization: A Philosophical Inquiry into Freud*, Boston, MA: Beacon Press.

MARX, K. (1967) *Capital, Vol. 1: A Critical Analysis of Capitalist Production*, New York: International Publishers.

—— and ENGELS, F. (1964) *The German Ideology*, Moscow: Progress Publishers.

MOLYNEUX, M. (1985) 'Mobilization without emancipation? Women's interests, the state and revolution in Nicaragua', in FAGAN, R.R. *et al.* (eds) *Transition and Development*, New York: Monthly Review Press.

PARKER, R.G. (1985) 'Masculinity, femininity and homosexuality: on the anthropological interpretation of sexual meanings in Brazil', *Journal of Homosexuality*, 11, pp. 155–63.

—— (1991) *Bodies, Pleasures and Passions: Sexual Cultural in Contemporary Brazil*, Boston, MA: Beacon Press.

PONSE, B. (1978) *Identities in the Lesbian World: The Social Construction of Self*, Westport, CT: Greenwood Press.

RANDALL, M. (1992) *Gathering Rage: The Failure of Twentieth Century Revolutions to Develop a Feminist Agenda*, New York: Monthly Review Press.

REED, A.L. (1991) 'The underclass myth', *The Progressive*, 55, August, pp. 18–20.

RIGDON, S.M. (1988) *The Culture Façade: Art, Science, and Politics in the Work of Oscar Lewis*, Urbana: University of Illinois Press.

RIST, D.Y. (1992) 'Sex on the brain: are homosexuals born that way?', *The Nation*, 255, pp. 424–9.

RUBIN, G. (1975) 'The traffic in women: notes on the political economy of sex', in REITER, R.R. (ed.) *Toward an Anthropology of Women*, New York: Monthly Review Press.

—— (1984) 'Thinking sex: notes for a radical theory of the politics of sexuality', in VANCE, C.S. (ed.) *Pleasure and Danger: Exploring Female Sexuality*, London: Routledge and Kegan Paul.

RUSE, M. (1988) *Homosexuality: A Philosophical Inquiry*, Oxford: Basil Blackwell.

SANDAY, P.R. (1990) *Fraternity Gang Rape: Sex, Brotherhood, and Privilege on Campus*, New York: New York University Press.

SARTRE, J.P. (1963) *Search for a Method*, New York: Knopf.

SCHEPER-HUGHES, N. (1979) *Saints, Scholars and Schizophrenics: Mental Illness in Rural Ireland*, Berkeley and Los Angeles: University of California Press.

—— (1992) *Death Without Weeping: The Violence of Everyday Life in Brazil*, Berkeley and Los Angeles: University of California Press.

—— and LOCK, M. (1987) 'The mindful body: a prolegomenon to future work in medical anthropology', *Medical Anthropology Quarterly*, (n.s.) 1, pp. 6–41.

SEDGWICK, E.K. (1985) *Between Men: English Literature and Male Homosocial Desire*, New York: Columbia University Press.

—— (1990) *Epistemology of the Closet*, Berkeley and Los Angeles: University of California Press.

STACEY, J. (1990) *Brave New Families: Stories of Domestic Upheaval in Late Twentieth Century America*, New York: Basic.

STEWART, S. (1984) *On Longing*, Baltimore, MD: Johns Hopkins University Press.

VALENTINE, C.A. (1968) *Culture and Poverty: A Critique and Counter-Proposal*, Chicago: University of Chicago Press.

VOLOŠINOV, V.N. (1993) *Marxism and the Philosophy of Language*, Cambridge, MA: Harvard University Press.

WALKER, T.W. (ed.) (1987) *Reagan versus the Sandinistas: The Undeclared War on Nicaragua*, Boulder, CO: Westview.

WEEKS, J. (1977) *Coming Out: Homosexual Politics in Britain from the Nineteenth Century to the Present*, London: Quartet.

—— (1981) *Sex, Politics, and Society: The Regulation of Sexuality since 1800*, New York: Longman.

—— (1985) *Sexuality and its Discontents: Meanings, Myths, and Modern Sexualities*, London: Routledge and Kegan Paul.

Part 3
From gender to sexuality

8   Discourse, desire and sexual deviance

Some problems in a history of homosexuality

Jeffrey Weeks [1981]

The publication by the Kinsey Institute of the book *Homosexualities* underlines what is likely to become a truism in the next few years: that we can no longer speak of a single homosexual category as if it embraced the wide range of same sex experiences in our society (Bell and Weinberg, 1978). But recognition of this, tardy as it has been, calls into question a much wider project: that of providing a universal theory and consequently a 'history' of homosexuality. The distinction originally made by sociologists (and slowly being taken up by historians) between homosexual behaviours, roles and identities, or between homosexual desire and 'homosexuality' as a social and psychological category (Hocquenghem, 1978), is one that challenges fundamentally the coherence of the theme and poses major questions for the historian. This paper addresses some of these problems, first, by examining approaches that have helped construct our concepts of homosexuality, second, by tracing the actual evolution of the category of homosexuality, third, by exploring some of the theoretical approaches that have attempted to explain its emergence and, finally, by charting some of the problems that confront the modern researcher studying 'homosexuality'.

Approaches

It has been widely recognized for almost a century that attitudes towards homosexual behaviour are culturally specific, and have varied enormously across different cultures and through various historical periods. Two closely related and virtually reinforcing sources for this awareness can be pinpointed: first, the pioneering work of sexologists such as Magnus Hirschfeld, Iwan Bloch, Havelock Ellis and others, whose labelling, categorizing and taxonomic zeal led them, partially at least, outside their own culture, and, second, the work of anthropologists and ethnographers who attempted to chart the varieties of sexual behaviour and who supplied the data on which the sexologists relied. The actual interest and zeal in the pursuit of sex was, of course, a product of their own culture's preoccupations, and the resulting findings often displayed an acute 'ethnocentric bias' (Trumbach, 1977, p. 1), particularly with regard to homosexuality, but this early work has had a long resonance. The three most influential English-language cross-cultural studies – that of the traveller Sir Richard Burton in the 1880s (1888), the work of Edward Westermarck in the 1900s (1906), and the Human Area Files of Ford and Beach in the 1950s (1952) – have deeply affected perceptions of homosexuality in their respective generations. Unfortunately, awareness of different cultural patterns has been used to reinforce rather than confront our own culture-bound conceptions.

Three phases in the construction of a history of homosexuality are discernible. The first, manifested in the works of the early sexologists as well as the propagandists like Edward

Carpenter (1914), attempted above all to demonstrate the trans-historical existence, and indeed value, of homosexuality as a distinct sexual experience. All the major works of writers such as Havelock Ellis (1936) had clear-cut historical sections; some, like Iwan Bloch's (1938), were substantive historical works. Writers during this phase were above all anxious to establish the parameters of homosexuality, what distinguished it from other forms of sexuality, what history suggested for its aetiology and social worth, the changing cultural values accorded to it, and the great figures – in politics, art, literature – one could associate with the experience. These efforts, taking the form of naturalistic recordings of what was seen as a relatively minor but significant social experience, were actually profoundly constructing of modern concepts of homosexuality. They provided a good deal of the data on which later writers depended even as they reworked them, and a hagiographical sub-school produced a multitude of texts on the great homosexuals of the past, 'great queens of history'; its most recent manifestation is found in the egregious essay of A.L. Rowse, *Homosexuals in History* (1977).

The second phase, most usefully associated with the reformist endeavours of the 1950s and 1960s, took as unproblematic the framework established by the pioneers. Homosexuality was a distinct social experience; the task was to detail it. The result was a new series of texts, some of which, such as H. Montgomery Hyde's various essays, synthesized in *The Other Love* in 1970, brought together a good deal of empirical material even as they failed to theorize its contradictions adequately.

As a major aspect of the revival of historical interest was the various campaigns to change the law and public attitudes, both in Europe and America, the historical studies inevitably concentrated on issues relevant to these. The assumed distinction, derived from nineteenth-century sexological literature, between 'perversion' (a product of moral weakness) and 'inversion' (constitutional and hence unavoidable), which D.S. Bailey adumbrates in *Homosexuality and the Western Christian Tradition* (1955), was highly significant for debates in the churches. The influential essay on English legal attitudes by Francois Lafitte, 'Homosexuality and the Law', was designed to indicate that laws that were so arbitrarily, indeed accidentally, imposed could as easily be removed (Lafitte, 1958–59). Donald Webster Cory's various works of the 1950s, such as *The Homosexual Outlook* (1953), sought to underline the values of the homosexual experience. Employing the statistical information provided by Kinsey, the cross-cultural evidence of Ford and Beach, and the ethnographic studies of people such as Evelyn Hooker, historians were directed towards the commonness of the homosexual experience in history and began to trace some of the forces that shaped public attitudes.

A third phase, overlapping with the second but more vocal in tone, can be seen as the direct product of the emergence of more radical gay movements in the late 1960s and 1970s in Europe and North America. Here the emphasis was on reasserting the values of a lost experience, stressing the positive value of homosexuality and locating the sources of its social oppression. A major early emphasis was on recovering the pre-history of the gay movement itself, particularly in Germany, the USA and Britain (Ford and Beach, 1952; Katz, 1976; Lauritsen and Thorstad, 1974; Steakley, 1975). Stretching beyond this was a search for what one might term 'ethnicity', the lineaments and validation of a minority experience that history had denied. But the actual work of research posed new problems, which threatened to burst out of the bounds established within the previous half century. This is admirably demonstrated in Jonathan Katz's splendid documentary *Gay American History* (1976). But rather than exploring its virtues, I want to pick out two points that seem to me to pose fresh problems. The first concerns the title. It seems to me that to use a modern self-labelling term, 'gay', itself a product of contemporary political struggles, to define an ever-changing concept over a period of 400 years suggests a constant homosexual essence which the evidence presented in the book itself suggests is just not there. Katz in fact recognizes this very clearly. He makes the vital point that the 'concept of homosexuality must be historicized', and hopes that the book will revolutionize the traditional concept of homosexuality.

> The problem of the historical researcher is thus to study and establish the character and meaning of each manifestation of same sex relations within a specific time and society ... All homosexuality is situational.
>
> (Katz, 1976, pp. 6–7)

This is absolutely correct and is the measure of the break between this type of history and, say, A.L. Rowse's extravaganza. But to talk at the same time of our history as if homosexuals were a distinct, fixed minority suggests a slightly contradictory attitude. It poses a major theoretical problem on which the gay movement has had little to say until recently.

A second problem arises from this, concerning attitudes to lesbianism. Katz very commendably has, unlike most of his predecessors, attempted to give equal space to both male and female homosexuality, and although this is impossible in some sections, overall he succeeds. But this again suggests a problematic of a constant racial-sexual identity which Katz explicitly rejects theoretically. Lesbianism and male homosexuality in fact have quite different, if inevitably interconnected, social histories, related to the social evolution of distinct gender identities; there is a danger that this fundamental, if difficult, point will be obscured by discussing them as if they were part of the same experience. These points will be taken up later.

Certainly there has been a considerable extension of interest in the history of homosexuality over the past decade, and as well as the general works, a number of essays and monographs have appeared, most of which accept readily the cultural specificity of attitudes and concepts. Nevertheless considerable contradictions recur. A.D. Harvey in a study of buggery prosecutions at the beginning of the nineteenth century has noted that:

> It is too commonly forgotten how far the incidence of homosexual behaviour varies from age to age and from culture to culture. ... In fact it is only very crudely true that there are homosexuals in every period and in every society. Societies which accept homosexual behaviour as normal almost certainly have a higher proportion of men who have experimented with homosexual activity than societies which regard homosexuality as abnormal but tolerate it, and societies which grudgingly tolerate homosexuality probably have a higher incidence of homosexual activity than societies where it is viciously persecuted.
>
> (Harvey, 1978, p. 944)

But Harvey, despite making this highly significant point, goes on to speak of 'homosexuals' as if they realized a trans-historical nature. He writes of the Home Secretary complaining in 1808 that Hyde Park and St James' Park were 'being used as a resort for homosexuals', apparently oblivious of the absence of such a term until the later part of the century. The actual term the Home Secretary used is extremely important in assessing his perception of the situation and the type of people involved, and the evidence suggests a problematic of public nuisance rather than a modern concept of the homosexual person.[1]

Similarly Randolph Trumbach, in what is a very valuable study of London 'sodomites' in the eighteenth century, despite a long and carefully argued discussion of different cross-cultural patterns, writes as if the homosexual sub-culture had a natural existence serving the eternal social needs (or at least eternal in the West) of a fixed minority of people (Trumbach, 1977, p. 23). But there is plentiful evidence that the sub-culture changed considerably over time, partly at least dependent on factors such as urbanization, and can one really speak of the courtly or theatrical sub-cultures of the early seventeenth century as if they were the same as the modern sub-cultures of New York or San Francisco?

Implicit in Trumbach's essay is an alternative view that profoundly challenges such assumptions. He notes 'only one significant change' in attitudes during the Christian millennia: 'Beginning in the late 19th century it was no longer the act that was stigmatised, but the state of mind' (Trumbach, 1977, p. 9). But this, I would argue, is the crucial change, indicating a massive shift in attitude, giving rise to what is distinctively new in our culture: the categorization of homosexuality as a separate condition and the correlative emergence of a homosexual identity.

I would argue that we should employ cross-cultural and historical evidence not only to chart changing *attitudes* but to challenge the very concept of a single trans-historical notion of homosexuality. In different cultures (and at different historical moments or conjunctures within the same culture) very different meanings are given to same-sex activity both by society at large and by the individual participants. The physical acts might be similar, but the social construction of meanings around them are profoundly different. The social integration of forms of pedagogic homosexual relations in ancient Greece have no continuity with contemporary notions of a homosexual identity (Dover, 1978). To put it another way, the various possibilities of what Hocquenghem calls homosexual desire, or what more neutrally might be termed homosexual behaviours, which seem from historical evidence to be a permanent and ineradicable aspect of human sexual possibilities, are variously constructed in different cultures as an aspect of wider gender and sexual regulation. If this is the case, it is pointless discussing questions such as, what are the origins of homosexual oppression, or what is the nature of the homosexual taboo, as if there was a single, causative factor. The crucial question must be: what are the conditions for the emergence of this particular form of regulation of sexual behaviour in this particular society? Transferred to our own history, this must involve an exploration of what Mary McIntosh (1968) pin-pointed as the significant problem: the emergence of the notion that homosexuality is a condition peculiar to some people and not others.

A historical study of homosexuality over the past two centuries or so must therefore have as its focus three closely related questions: the social conditions for the emergence of the category of homosexuality and its construction as the unification of disparate experiences, the relation of this categorization to other socio-sexual categorizations, and the relationship of this categorization to those defined, not simply 'described' or labelled but 'invented' by it, in particular historical circumstances.

Evolution

The historical evidence points to the latter part of the nineteenth century as the crucial period in the conceptualization of homosexuality as the distinguishing characteristic of a particular type of person, the 'invert' or 'homosexual', and the corresponding development of a new awareness of self amongst some 'homosexuals' (Weeks, 1977). From the mid-nineteenth century there is a bubbling of debate, notation and classification, associated with names such as Casper, Tardieu, Ulrichs, Westphal, Krafft-Ebing, Havelock Ellis, Magnus Hirschfeld, Moll, Freud, all of whom sought to define, and hence psychologically or medically to construct, new categorizations. Westphal's description of the 'contrary sexual instinct' in the 1870s may be taken as the crucial formative moment, for out of it grew the notion of 'sexual inversion', the dominant formulation until the 1950s.

The word 'homosexuality' itself was not invented until 1869 (by the Hungarian Benkert von Kertbeny) and did not enter English usage until the 1880s and 1890s, and then largely as a result of the work of Havelock Ellis. I suggest that the widespread adoption of these neologisms during this period marks as crucial a turning point in attitudes to homosexuality as the adoption of 'gay' as a self-description of homosexuals in the 1970s. It indicated not just a changing usage but the emergence of a whole new set of assumptions. And in Britain (as also in Germany and elsewhere) the reconceptualization and categorization (at first medical and later social) coincided with the development of new legal and ideological sanctions, particularly against male homosexuality.

Until 1885 the only law dealing *directly* with homosexual behaviour in England was that relating to buggery, and legally, at least, little distinction was made between buggery between man and woman, man and beast and man and man, though the majority of prosecutions were directed at men for homosexual offences. This had been a capital crime from the 1530s, when the incorporation of traditional ecclesiastical sanctions into law had been part of the decisive assumption by the state of many of the powers of the medieval church. Prosecutions under this law had fluctuated, partly because of changing rules on evidence, partly through other social pressures. There seems, for instance, to have been a higher incidence of prosecutions (and executions) in times of war; penalties were particularly harsh in cases affecting the discipline of the armed services, particularly the navy (Radzinowicz, 1968; Gilbert, 1974, 1976, 1977). 'Sodomite' (denoting contact between men) became the typical epithet of abuse for the sexual deviant.

The legal classification and the epithet had, however, an uncertain status and was often used loosely to describe various forms of non-reproductive sex. There was therefore a crucial distinction between traditional concepts of buggery and modern concepts of homosexuality. The former was seen as a potentiality in all sinful nature, unless severely execrated and judicially punished; homosexuality, however, is seen as the characteristic of a particular type of person, a type whose specific characteristics (inability to whistle, penchant for the colour green, adoration of mother or father, age of sexual maturation, 'promiscuity', etc.) have been exhaustively and inconclusively detailed in many twentieth-century textbooks. It became a major task of psychology in the present century to attempt to explain the aetiology of this homosexual 'condition' (McIntosh, 1968). The early articles on homosexuality in the 1880s and 1890s treated the subject as if they were entering a strange continent. An eminent doctor, Sir George Savage, described in the *Journal of Mental Science* the homosexual case histories of a young man and woman and wondered if 'this perversion is as rare as it appears', while Havelock Ellis was to claim that he was the first to record any homosexual cases unconnected with prison or asylums. The sodomite, as Michel Foucault has put it (1979), was a temporary aberration; the homosexual belongs to a species, and social science during this century has made various – if by and large unsuccessful – efforts to explore this phenomenon.

These changing concepts do not mean, of course, that those who engaged in a predominantly homosexual life style did not regard themselves as somehow different until the late nineteenth century, and there is evidence for sub-cultural formation around certain monarchs and in the theatre for centuries. But there is much stronger evidence for the emergence of a distinctive male homosexual sub-culture in London and one or two other cities from the late seventeenth century, often characterized by transvestism and gender-role inversion; and by the early nineteenth century there was a recognition in the courts that homosexuality represented a condition different from the norm (McIntosh, 1968; Trumbach, 1977). By the mid-nineteenth century, it seems the male homosexual sub-culture at least had characteristics not dissimilar to the modern, with recognized cruising places and homosexual haunts, ritualized sexual contact and a distinctive argot and 'style'. But there is also abundant evidence until late into the nineteenth century of practices which by modern standards would be regarded as highly sexually compromising. Lawrence Stone (1977) describes how Oxbridge male students often slept with male students with no sexual connotations until comparatively late in the eighteenth century, while Smith-Rosenberg (1975) has described the intimate – and seemingly non-sexualized – relations between women in the nineteenth century.

Nevertheless, even as late as the 1870s there was considerable doubt in the minds of the police, the medical profession and the judiciary about the nature and extent of homosexual offences. When the transvestites Boulton and Park were brought to trial in 1871 for conspiracy to commit buggery, there was considerable police confusion about the nature of the alleged offences, the medical profession differed over the relevance of the evidence relating to anal intercourse, the counsel seemed never to have worked on similar cases before, the 'scientific' literature cited from British sources was nugatory, while the court was either ignorant of the French sources or ready to despise them. The Attorney General suggested that it was fortunate that there was 'very little learning or knowledge upon this subject in this country', while a defence counsel attacked 'the new found treasures of French literature upon the subject which thank God is still foreign to the libraries of British surgeons'.[2] Boulton and Park were eventually acquitted, despite an overwhelming mass of evidence, including correspondence, that today would be regarded as highly compromising.

The latter part of the nineteenth century, however, saw a variety of concerns that helped to focus awareness: the controversy about 'immorality' in public schools, various sexual scandals, a new legal situation, the beginnings of a 'scientific' discussion of homosexuality and the emergence of the 'medical model'. The subject, as Edward Carpenter put it at the time, 'has great actuality and is pressing upon us from all sides' (Carpenter, 1908, p. 9). It appears likely that it was in this developing context that some of those with homosexual inclinations began to perceive themselves as 'inverts', 'homosexuals', 'Uranians', a crucial stage in the prolonged and uneven process whereby homosexuality began to take on a recognizably modern configuration. And although the evidence cited here has been largely British, this development was widespread throughout Western Europe and America.

The changing legal and ideological situations were crucial markers in this development. The 1861 Offences Against the Person Act removed the death penalty for buggery (which had not been used since the 1830s), replacing it by sentences of between ten years and life. But in 1885 the famous Labouchere Amendment to the Criminal Law Amendment Act made all male homosexual activities (acts of 'gross indecency') illegal, punishable by up to two years' hard labour. And in 1898 the laws on importuning for 'immoral purposes' were tightened up and effectively applied to male homosexuals (this was clarified by the Criminal Law Amendment Act of 1912 with respect to England and Wales – Scotland has different provisions). Both were significant extensions of the legal controls on male homosexuality, whatever their origins or intentions (Smith, 1976; Bristow, 1977; Weeks, 1977, p. 2). Though formally less severe than capital punishments for sodomy, the new legal situation is likely to have ground harder on a much wider circle of people, particularly as it was dramatized in a series of sensational scandals, culminating in the trials of Oscar Wilde, which had the function of drawing a sharp dividing line between permissible and tabooed forms of behaviour. The Wilde scandal in particular was a vital moment in the creation of a male homosexual identity (Ellis, 1936, p. 392). It must be noted, however, that the new legal situation did not apply to women, and the attempt in 1921 to extend the 1885 provisions to women failed, in part at least on the grounds that publicity would only serve to make more women aware of homosexuality (Weeks, 1977, p. 107). But the different legal situation alone does not explain the different social resonances of male and female homosexuality. Much more likely, this must be related to the complexly developing social structuring of male and female sexualities.

The emergence of a psychological and medical model of homosexuality was intimately connected with the legal situation. The most commonly quoted European writers on homosexuality in the mid-nineteenth century were Casper and Tardieu, the leading medico-legal experts of Germany and France respectively. Both, as Arno Karlen has put it, were 'chiefly concerned with whether the disgusting breed of perverts could be physically identified for courts, and whether they should be held legally responsible for their acts' (Karlen, 1971, p. 185). The same problem was apparent in Britain. According to Magnus Hirschfeld, most of the 1000 or so works on homosexuality that appeared between 1898 and 1908 were directed, in part at least, at the legal profession. Even J.A. Symond's privately printed pamphlet *A Problem in Modern Ethics* (1983 [orig. 1883]) declared itself to be addressed 'especially to Medical psychologists and jurists', while Havelock Ellis's *Sexual Inversion* (1936 [orig. 1897]) was attacked for not being published by a medical press and for being too popular in tone. The medicalization of homosexuality – a transition from notions of sin to concepts of sickness or mental illness – was a vitally significant move, even though its application was uneven. Around it the poles of scientific discourse ranged for decades: was homosexuality congenital or acquired, ineradicable or susceptible to cure, to be quietly if unenthusiastically accepted as unavoidable (even the liberal Havelock Ellis felt it necessary to warn his invert reader not to 'set himself in violent opposition' to his society) or to be resisted with all the force of one's Christian will? In the discussions of the 1950s and 1960s these were crucial issues: was it right, it was sometimes wondered, to lock an alcoholic up in a brewery; should those who suffered from an incurable (or at best unfortunate) condition be punished? Old notions of the immorality or sinfulness of homosexuality did not die in the nineteenth century; they still survive, unfortunately, in many dark corners. But from the nineteenth century they were inextricably entangled with 'scientific' theories that formed the boundaries within which homosexuals had to begin to define themselves.

The challenge to essentialism

Clearly the emergence of the homosexual category was not arbitrary or accidental. The scientific and medical speculation can be seen in one sense as a product of the characteristic nineteenth-century process whereby the traditionally execrated (and monolithic) crimes against nature – linking up, for instance, homosexuality with masturbation and mechanical birth control (Bullough and Voght, 1973) – are differentiated into discrete deviations whose aetiologies are mapped out in late nineteenth- and early twentieth-century works (Ellis, 1936; Hirschfeld, 1938, 1946; Krafft-Ebing, 1965). In another series of relationships the emergence of the concept of the homosexual can be seen as corresponding to and complexly linked with the classification and articulation of a variety of social categories: the redefinitions of childhood and adolescence, the hysterical woman, the congenitally inclined prostitute (or indeed, in the work of Ellis and others, the congenital criminal as well) and linked to the contemporaneous debate and ideological definition of the role of housewife and mother.[3] On the other hand, the categorization was never simply an imposition of a new definition; it was the result of various pressures and forces, in which new concepts merged into older definitions.

It is striking that the social purity campaigners of the 1880s saw both prostitution and male homosexuality as products of undifferentiated male lust (Weeks, 1977, p. 17), and equally significant, if generally unremarked, that the major enactments affecting male homosexuality from the 1880s (the Labouchere Amendment, the 1898 Vagrancy Act) were primarily concerned with female prostitution. Indeed as late as the 1950s it was still seen as logical to set up a single government committee – the Wolfenden Committee – to study both prostitution and male homosexuality. It is clear, however, that the emergence of the homosexual category and the changing focus of the definition of homosexual behaviour are intimately related to wider changes. The problem is to find means of explaining and theorizing these changes without falling into the twin traps of a naive empiricism or a reductive materialism. The former would assume that what was happening was simply a discovery of pre-existing phenomena, a problematic which, as we have suggested, has little historical validity; the latter poses the danger of seeing the restrictive definitions of homosexual behaviours as a necessary effect of a pre-existing causative complex (usually 'capitalism'). Given the absence in orthodox Marxism of any theorization of sexuality and gender that is able to cope with the actual historical phenomena, the tendency has been to graft a form of functionalism on to historical materialism, which, while it suggests useful connections which might be worth exploring, simultaneously produces historical descriptions that are often difficult to fit with more empirical substantiation.

Most attempts to explain this more closely have relied on variations of role theory. Male homosexuality has been seen as a threat to the ensemble of assumptions about male sexuality and a perceived challenge to the male heterosexual role within capitalism.

> In Britain sexual intercourse has been contained within marriage which has been presented as the ultimate form of sexual maturity ... the heterosexual nuclear family assists a system like capitalism because it produces and socialises the young in certain values ... the maintenance of the nuclear family with its role-specific behaviour creates an apparent consensus concerning sexual normalcy.
>
> (Brake, 1976, p. 178)

So that:

> Any ambiguity such as transvestism, hermaphrodism, transsexuality, or homosexuality is moulded into 'normal' appropriate gender behaviour or is relegated to the categories of sick, dangerous or pathological. The actor is forced to slot into patterns of behaviour appropriate to heterosexual gender roles.
>
> (Brake, 1976, p. 176)

The result is the emergence of a specific male 'homosexual role', a specialized, despised and punished role which 'keeps the bulk of society pure in rather the same way that the similar treatment of some kinds of criminal helps keep the rest of society law abiding' (McIntosh, 1968, p. 184). Such a role has two effects: first, it helps to provide a clear-cut threshold between permissible and impermissible behaviour, and, second, it helps to segregate those labelled as deviant from others, and thus contains and limits their behaviour patterns. In the same way, a homosexual sub-culture, which is the correlative of the development of a specialized role, provides both access to the socially outlawed need (sex) and contains the deviant. Male homosexuals can thus be conceptualized as those excluded from the sexual family, and as potential scapegoats whose oppression can keep the family members in line.

The notion of a homosexual role in this posing of it has certain difficulties. It is, for example, a negative role, not one that is socially sustained. It also assumes a unilinear fit between the socially created role and the identity that it delineates, whereas all the evidence indicates that this is problematical. It also suggests an intentionality in the creation of the role that again is historically dubious. But beyond this are other related problems in the functionalist model. It apparently assumes that the family acts as a unilinear funnel for the channelling of socially necessary sexual identities and responds automatically to the needs of society (or in the Marxist functionalist model, capitalism). It assumes, in other words, that the family can be simply defined as a unitary form (the 'nuclear family') that acts in a determined way on society's members, and at the same time it takes for granted a sexual essence that can be organized through this institution.[4] Neither is true.

Mark Poster has recently suggested that 'historians and social scientists in general have gone astray by viewing the family as a unitary phenomenon which has undergone some type of linear transformation' (1978, p. xvii). He argues instead that the history of the family is discontinuous, evolving several distinct family structures, each with its own emotional pattern. What this points to is the *construction* of different family forms in different historical periods and with different class effects. A functionalist model which sees the family as an essential and necessary agent of social control and with the role of ensuring efficient reproduction ignores both the constant ineffectiveness of the family in doing so and the immense class variations in family forms.

But even more problematic are the assumptions classically made about the nature of sexuality, assumptions current both in traditionalist and in Left thought (and particularly evident in the writings of the Freudian Left: Reich, Fromm, Marcuse). They also have the undoubted strength of the appearance of common sense: in this view sex is conceived of as an overpowering, instinctive force, whose characteristics are built into the biology of the human animal, which shapes human institutions and whose will must express itself, either in the form of direct sexual expression or, if blocked, in the form of perversion or neurosis. Krafft-Ebing expressed an orthodox view in the late nineteenth century when he described sex as a 'natural instinct', which 'with all conquering force and might demands fulfilment' (1965, p. 1). The clear presupposition here is that the sex drive is basically male in character, with the female conceived of as a passive receptacle. More sophisticated versions of what Gagnon and Simon have termed the 'drive reduction' model (1973) recur in twentieth-century thought. It is ambiguously there in parts of Freud's work, though the careful distinction he draws between 'instinct' and 'drive' has often been lost, both by commentators and translators. But it is unambiguously present in the writings of his epigones. Thus Rattray Taylor in his neo-Freudian interpretation of *Sex in History*:

> The history of civilisation is the history of a long warfare between the dangerous and powerful forces of the id, and the various systems of taboos and inhibitions which man has erected to control them.
>
> (Taylor, 1964, n.p.n.)

Here we have a clear notion of a 'basic biological mandate' that presses on, and so must be firmly controlled by the cultural and social matrix (Gagnon and Simon, 1973, p. 11). What is peculiar about this model is that is has been adopted both by Marxists, who in other regards have firmly rejected the notion of 'natural man', and by taxonomists, such as Kinsey, whose findings have revealed a wide variety of sexual experiences. With regard to homosexuality, the instinctual model has seen it either as a more or less pathological deviation, a failure of socially necessary repression, as the effect of the morally restrictive organization of sexual morality, or, more romantically but no less ahistorically, as the 'great refusal' (Marcuse, 1969) of sexual normality in the capitalist organization of sexuality.[5]

Against this, Gagnon and Simon have argued that sexuality is subject to 'socio-cultural moulding to a degree surpassed by few other forms of human behaviour' (1973, p. 26), and in so arguing they are building both on a century of sex research and on a century of 'decentring' natural man. Marx's formulation of historical materialism and Freud's discovery of the unconscious have been the major contributions to what over the past few decades, in structuralism, anthropology, psychoanalysis and Marxism, has been a major theoretical effort to challenge the unitary subject in social theory. 'Sexuality' has in many ways been most resistant to this challenge, precisely because its power seems to derive from our natural being, but there have recently been three sustained challenges to sexual essentialism from three quite different theoretical approaches: the interactionist (associated with the work of Gagnon and Simon), the psychoanalytic (associated with the re-interpretation of Freud initiated by Jacques Lacan) and the discursive, taking as its starting point the work of Michel Foucault. They have quite different epistemological starting points and different objects of study – the social sources of human conduct, the unconscious and power – but between them they have posed formidable challenges to our received notions of sexuality, challenges which have already been reflected in the presentation of this paper.[6]

Despite their different approaches and in the end different aims, their work converges on several important issues. First, they all reject sex as an autonomous realm, a natural force with specific effects, a rebellious energy that the 'social' controls. In the work of Gagnon and Simon, it seems to be suggested that nothing is intrinsically sexual, or rather that anything can be sexualized (though what creates the notion of 'sexuality' is itself never answered). In Lacan's 'recovery' of Freud, it is the law of the father, the castration fear and the pained entry into the symbolic order – the order of language – at the Oedipal moment that instigates desire (cf. Mitchell, 1974). It is the expression of a fundamental absence, which can never be fulfilled, the desire to be the other, the father, which is both alienated and insatiable: alienated because the child can only express its desire by means of language that itself constitutes its submission to the father, and insatiable because it is desire for a symbolic position that is itself arbiter of the possibilities for the expression of desire. The law of the father therefore constitutes both desire and the lack on which it is predicated.

In Foucault's work 'sexuality' is seen as a historical apparatus, and 'sex' is a 'complex idea that was formed within the deployment of sexuality'.

> *Sexuality* must not be thought of as a kind of natural given which power tries to hold in check, or as an obscure domain which knowledge gradually tries to uncover. It is the name that can be given to a historical construct: not a furtive reality that is difficult to grasp, but a great surface network in which the stimulation of bodies, the intensification of pleasures, the incitement to discourse, the formation of special knowledges, the strengthening of controls and resistances, are linked to one another, in accordance with a few major strategies of knowledge and power.
>
> (Foucault, 1979, pp. 105–6)

It is not fully clear what are the elements on which these social constructs of sexuality play. In the neo-psychoanalytic school there is certainly rejection of the concept of a pool of natural instincts that are distorted by society, but nevertheless there seems to be an acceptance of permanent drives; and the situation is complicated by what must be termed an essentialist and trans-historical reading of Oedipus, which seems to be essential for any culture, or in Juliet Mitchell's version, 'patriarchal' culture.[7] Gagnon and Simon and Plummer (1975) seem to accept the existence of a pool of possibilities on which 'sexuality' draws, and in this they do not seem far removed from Foucault's version that 'sexuality' plays upon 'bodies, organs, somatic localizations, functions, anatamophysiological systems, sensations, and pleasures', which have no intrinsic unity or 'laws' of their own (Foucault, 1979, p. 153).

Second, then, what links the anti-essentialist critique is a recognition of the social sources of sexual definitions. In the feminist appropriation of Lacan this can be seen as a result of patriarchal structures and the differential entry into the symbolic of the human male and female. But this poses massive theoretical problems, particularly in the attempt at a materialist position. The problem here is that the trans-historical perception of the Oedipal crisis and the consequent focusing of sex and gender already presuppose the existence of a unified notion of sexuality which we are suggesting is historically specific. Both the interactionists and Foucault make this clear. Gagnon and Simon suggest that:

> It is possible that, given the historical nature of human societies we are victim to the needs of earlier social orders. To earlier societies it may not have been a need to constrain severely the powerful sexual impulse in order to maintain social stability or limit inherently anti-social force, *but rather a matter of having to invent an importance for sexuality.* This would not only assure a high level of reproductive activity but also provide socially available rewards unlimited by natural resources, rewards that promote conforming behaviour in sectors of social life far more important than the sexual.
>
> (Gagnon and Simon, 1973, p. 17, my italics)

Foucault makes much clearer a historical specification and locates the rise of the sexuality apparatus in the eighteenth century, linked with specific historical processes. As a consequence of this, a third point of contact lies in the rejection, both by the interactionists and Foucault, of the notion that the history of sexuality can fruitfully be seen in terms of 'repression'. Foucault, as Zinner has put it:

> ... offers four major arguments against the repression hypothesis. (1) it is based on an outmoded model of power; (2) it leads to a narrow construction of the family's function; (3) it is class specific and applies historically to bourgeois sexuality; and (4) it often results in a one-sided conception of how authority interacts with sexuality – a negative rather than a positive conception.
>
> (Zinner, 1978, pp. 215–16)

Again Gagnon and Simon have been less historically specific, but both interactionists and Foucault tend to the view that sexuality is organized not by repression but through definition and regulation. More specifically, regulation is organized though the creation of sexual categories – homosexual, paedophile, transvestite and so on. In the case of Gagnon and Simon and those influenced by them (for example, Plummer) the theoretical framework derives both from Meadean social psychology, which sees the individual as having a developing personality that is created in an interaction with others, and from labelling theories of deviance. In the case of Foucault it derives from his belief that it is through discourse that our relation to reality is organized – or rather, language structures the real – and in particular Foucault analyses discourse 'as an act of violence imposed upon things' (Zinner, 1978, p. 219).

Fourth, however, in all three tendencies there is a curious relationship to history. Symbolic interactionism, by stressing the subjective and the impact of particular labelling events, has almost invariably displayed an ahistorical bias. The psychoanalytical school, almost by definition, has based itself on supra-historical assumptions which have been almost valueless in conjunctural analyses. Foucault stresses that his work is basically aimed at constructing a 'genealogy', the locating of the 'traces' of the present; it is basically a history of the present. So while the interactional adherent by and large has stressed the contingent and personalist, the tendency in the others is towards a form of structuralism in which 'history cannot be a study of man but only of determinate structures of social relations of which men and women are "bearers"' (History Workshop, 1978).

It is this ambiguous relationship of the critique of essentialism to traditional historical work which has made it seem difficult to absorb unproblematically any one of the particular approaches. Nevertheless, each in quite different ways ultimately poses problems which any historical approach to homosexuality must confront, particularly in the difficult relationship of historical structuration to individualized meanings. A close examination of the historical implications of the various approaches will illustrate this.

Constructing the homosexual

The dominant theoretical framework in Britain and the USA has derived from 'symbolic interactionism'. Here ideas are not treated in terms of their historical roots or practical effectiveness, but are seen as forming the background to every social process so that social processes are treated essentially in terms of ideas, and it is through ideas that we construct social reality itself. Most of the important work that has informed the theoretical study of homosexuality in Britain has derived from symbolic interactionism (for example, Kenneth Plummer's *Sexual Stigma* [1975], which is the major British study of how homosexual meanings are acquired). In this theory sexual meanings are constructed in social interaction: a homosexual identity is not inherent, but is socially created. This has had a vitally important clarifying influence, and has, as we have seen, broken with lay ideas of sex as a goal-directed instinct. Linked to labelling theories of deviance, it has been a valuable tool for exploring the effects of public stigmatizations and their impact on sub-cultural formation.

But interactionism has been unable fully to theorize the sexual variations that it can so ably describe; nor has it conceptualized the relations between possible sexual patterns and other social variables. Although it recognizes the disparities of power between various groups and the importance of the power to label, it has often had difficulties in theorizing questions of structural power and authority. Nor has it been willing, in the field of sexuality, to investigate the question of determination. It is unable to theorize why, despite the endless possibilities of sexualization it suggests, the genitals continue to be the focus of sexual imagination, nor why there are, at various times, shifts in the location of the sexual taboos. And there is a political consequence too, for if meanings are entirely developed in social interaction, an act of collective will can transform them; this leads, as Mary McIntosh has suggested, to a politics of 'collective voluntarism'. Both in theory and practice it has ignored the historical location of sexual taboos. Interactionism therefore stops precisely at the point where theorization seems essential: at the point of historical determination and ideological structuring in the creation of subjectivity.

It is for this reason that recently, particularly amongst feminists, interest has begun to switch to a reassessment of Freud and psychoanalysis with a view to employing it as a tool for developing a theoretical understanding of patriarchy. It is becoming apparent that if the emergence of a distinct homosexual identity is linked to the evolution of the family, then within this it is the role of the male – theorized in terms of the symbolic role of the phallus and the law of the father – that is of central significance. This, it is suggested, will allow the space to begin to understand the relationship between gender and sex (for it is in the family that the anatomical differences between the sexes acquire their social significance) and also to begin to uncover the specific history of female sexuality, within which the social history of lesbianism must ultimately be located. The focal point for most of the preliminary discussion has been Juliet Mitchell's *Psychoanalysis and Feminism* (1974), which takes as its starting point the work of Lacan, Althusser and Lévi-Strauss and which, as it was recently put by a sympathetic critic:

> ... opens the way to a re-evaluation of psychoanalysis as a theory which can provide scientific knowledge of the way in which patriarchal ideology is maintained through the foundation of psychological 'masculinity' and 'femininity'.
>
> (Albury, 1976, p. 7)

But though the question of sexuality (and its role in the creation of sexed and gendered subjects) has now been strategically linked to the whole problematic of patriarchy, there has been no effort to theorize the question of sexual variation.

The tendency of thought that Juliet Mitchell represents can be criticized on a number of grounds. Politically she seems to accept that separation of the struggle against patriarchy from the struggle against capitalism which most socialist feminist work has in theory attempted to overcome. Historically she appears to accept the universality of the Oedipal experience. A historical materialist when analysing capitalist social relations, she readily accepts idealist notions of the primal father when discussing the origins of patriarchy. Theoretically in her universalizing of the Oedipal processes she comes close to accepting drive as autonomous, pre-individual and again trans-historical and transcultural. It is a peculiar feature of recent radical thought that while stressing the conjunctural forces which partly at least shape the political, social and ideological, and while stressing the historical construction of subjectivity, it has nevertheless at the same time implicitly fallen back on a form of psychic determinism which it nominally rejects.

It is this which gives a particular interest to the recent appearance in English translation of Guy Hocquenghem's *Homosexual Desire* (1978 [first published in France as *Le Désir Homosexuel* in 1972]). The essay is located in the general area generated by the Lacanian reinterpretation of Freud, linguistic theory and the question of ideology, but its specific debt is to Gilles Deleuze and Felix Guattari, their work *L'Anti Oedipe*, their critique of Freudian (and Lacanian) categories and their subsequent theory of 'desire' and their espousal of schizoanalysis (Deleuze and Guattari, 1977). As in our argument, Hocquenghem recognizes the culturally specific function of the concept of 'the homosexual'; Hocquenghem makes references to Foucault and he points to what he calls the 'growing imperialism' of society, which seeks to attribute a social status to everything, even the unclassified. The result has been that homosexuality has been ever more closely defined (see Weeks, 1978).

Hocquenghem argues that 'homosexual desire', indeed like heterosexual, is an arbitrary division of the flux of desire, which in itself is polyvocal and undifferentiated, so that the notion of exclusive homosexuality is a 'fallacy of the imaginary', a misrecognition and ideological misperception. But despite this, homosexuality has a vivid social presence, and this is because it expresses an aspect of desire which appears nowhere else. For the direct manifestation of homosexual desire opposes the relations of roles and identities necessarily imposed by the Oedipus complex in order to ensure the reproduction of society. Capitalism, in its necessary employment of Oedipalization to control the tendency to decoding, manufactures 'homosexuals' just as it produces proletarians, and what is manufactured is a psychologically repressive category. He argues that the principal ideological means of thinking about homosexuality are ultimately, though not mechanically, connected with the advance of Western capitalism. They amount to a perverse 're-territorialization', a massive effort to regain social control, in a world tending towards disorder and decoding. As a result the establishment of homosexuality as a separate category goes hand in hand with its repression. On the one hand, we have the creation of a minority of 'homosexuals', on the other, the transformation in the majority of the repressed homosexual elements of desire into the desire to repress. Hence sublimated homosexuality is the basis of the paranoia about homosexuality which pervades social behaviour, which in turn is a guarantee of the survival of the Oedipal relations, the victory of the law of the father. Hocquenghem argues that only one organ is allowed in the Oedipal triangle, what Deleuze and Guattari call the 'despotic signifier', the phallus. And as money is the true universal reference point for capitalism, so the phallus is the reference point for heterosexism. The phallus determines, whether by absence or presence, the girl's penis envy, the boy's castration anxiety; it draws on libidinal energy in the same way as money draws on labour. And as this comment underlines, this Oedipalization is itself a product of capitalism and not, as the Lacanian school might argue, a law of culture or of all patriarchal societies.

Without going into further details several difficulties emerge. The first relates to the whole question of homosexual paranoia – reminiscent in many ways of the recent discussion of homophobia in Britain and the USA (Weinberg, 1973). The idea that repression of homosexuality in modern society is a product of suppressed homosexuality comes at times very close to a hydraulic theory of sexuality, which both symbolic interactionism and Lacanian interpretations of Freud have ostensibly rejected. It is not a sufficient explanatory principle simply to reverse the idea that homosexuality is a paranoia, peddled by the medical profession in the present century, into the idea that hostile attitudes to homosexuality are themselves paranoid. Nor does the theory help explain the real, if limited, liberalization of attitudes that has taken place in some Western countries or the range of attitudes that are empirically known to exist in different countries and even in different families.

Second, following from this, there is the still unanswered problem of why some individuals become 'homosexual' and others do not. The use of the concept of Oedipalization restores some notion of social determinacy that symbolic interactionism lacks, but, by corollary, its use loses any sense of the relevance of the specific family pressures, the educational and labelling processes, the media images that reinforce the identity and the individual shaping of meaning. Third, there is the ambiguous relationship of capitalism to patriarchy. If Mitchell can be rightly criticized for creating two separate areas for political struggle, the economic (against capitalism) and the ideological (against patriarchy), then Hocquenghem can be criticized for collapsing them together.

Finally, there is Hocquenghem's failure to explore the different modalities of lesbianism. It is important to note that what Hocquenghem is discussing is essentially male homosexuality, for in Hocquenghem's view, although the law of the father dominates both the male and the female, it is to the authority of the father in reproduction (both of the species and of Oedipalization itself) that homosexuality poses the major challenge; as Deleuze and Guattari note, male homosexuality, far from being a product of the Oedipus complex, as some Freudians imply, itself constitutes a totally different mode of social relationships, no longer vertical, but horizontal. Lesbianism, by implication, assumes its significance as a challenge to the secondary position accorded to female sexuality in capitalist society. It is not so much lesbianism as female sexuality that society denies. But Hocquenghem quite fails to pursue the point, which is central if we are to grasp the formation of sexual meanings. Despite these objections, however, Hocquenghem's essay raises important questions, some of which will be taken up below.

Whereas Hocquenghem, following Deleuze and Guattari, is intent on developing a philosophy of desire, Foucault, though much influenced by and having influence on this tendency, is more concerned in his later works with delineating a theory of power and the complex interplay between power and discourses. Foucault's work marks a break with conventional views of power. Power is not unitary, it does not reside in the state, it is not a thing to hold.

> By power, I do not mean 'Power' as a group of institutions and mechanisms that ensure the subservience of the citizens of a given state. By power, I do not mean, either, a mode of subjugation which, in contrast to violence, has the form of the rule. Finally, I do not have in mind a general system of domination exerted by one group over another … these are only the terminal forms power takes. It seems to me that power must be understood in the first instance as the multiplicity of force relations, immanent in the sphere in which they operate and which constitute their own organisation; as the process which, through ceaseless struggles and confrontations transforms, strengthens, or reverses them; as the support which these force relations find in one another, thus forming a chain or a system, or on the contrary, the disfunctions and contradictions which isolate them from one another; and lastly, as the strategies in which they take effect, whose general design or institutional crystallization is embodied in the state apparatus, in the formulation of the law, in the various social hegemonies.
>
> (Foucault, 1979, pp. 92–3)

The problem with this theory of power is that by breaking with a reductive or negative view, power 'remains almost as a process, without specification within different instances' (Coward, 1978, p. 20). And although he is unwilling to specify in advance any privileged source of power, there nevertheless underlies his work what might be termed a 'philosophical monism' (Zinner, 1978, p. 220), a conception of a will to power (and hence his complex linkage with Nietzsche) forever expanding and bursting forth in the form of the will to know. It is the complexes of power/knowledge that Foucault explores in his essay on *The History of Sexuality*; the original French version of its 'Introduction' has the title 'La volonté de savoir', 'The will to knowledge', which makes his concerns transparent:

> Things are accorded the weight of creation, while the human subject becomes a mere appendage – the speaker, the knower, the listener, the transmitter – and above all the spectator of the passage of discourse.
>
> (Zinner, 1978, p. 220)

It is through discourse that the complex of power/knowledge is realized. Foucault is not interested in the history of mind but in the history of discourse:

> The question which I ask is not of codes but of events: the law of existence of the statements, that which has rendered them possible – these and none other in their place: the conditions of their singular emergence; their correlations with other previous or simultaneous events, discursive or not. The question, however, I try to answer without referring

to the consciousness, obscure or explicit, of speaking subjects; without relating the facts
of discourse to the will – perhaps involuntary – of their authors.

(Foucault, 1978b, p. 14)

What he is suggesting is that the relationship between symbol and symbolized is not only
referential but productive. The order of language produces its own material forms and desires
as much as the physical possibilities. But there is no single hidden hand of history, no
complex causative complex, no pre-ordained goal, no final truth of human history.
Discourses produce their own truths as the possibilities of seeing the world in fresh ways
emerge.

The history of sexuality therefore becomes a history of our discourses about sexuality. And
the Western experience of sex, he argues, is not the inhibition of discourse but a constant, and
historically changing, deployment of discourses on sex, and this ever-expanding discursive
explosion is part of a complex growth of control over individuals, partly though the apparatus
of sexuality. Power is articulated through discourse: it invests, creates, produces. 'Power as
form of productivity forms the subject rather than simply imposing itself; power is desiring
rather than constraining' (D'Amico, 1978, p. 179).

But behind the vast explosion of discourses on sexuality since the eighteenth century, there
is no single unifying strategy valid for the whole of society. And in particular, breaking with
an orthodox Marxist problematic, he denies that it can be simply interpreted in terms of problems of 'reproduction'. In the 'Introduction' to *The History of Sexuality* (which is a methodological excursus, rather than a complete 'history') Foucault suggests four strategic unities,
linking together a host of practices and techniques, which formed specific mechanics of
knowledge and power centring on sex: a hysterization of women's bodies, a pedagogization
of children's sex, a socialization of procreative behaviour, a psychiatrization of perverse pleasures. And four figures emerged from these preoccupations, four objects of knowledge, four
subjects subjected, targets of and anchorages for the categories that were being
simultaneously investigated and regulated: the hysterical woman, the masturbating child,
the Malthusian couple and the perversive adult. The thrust of these discursive creations is
control, control not through denial or prohibition, but through production, through imposing
a grid of definition on the possibilities of the body.

The deployment of sexuality has its reasons for being, not in reproducing itself, but in
proliferating, innovating, annexing, creating, and penetrating bodies in an increasingly
detailed way, and in controlling populations in an increasingly comprehensive way.

(Foucault, 1979, p. 107)

This is obviously related to Foucault's analysis of the genealogy of the disciplinary society, a
society of surveillance and control, in *Discipline and Punish* (Foucault, 1977a) and to his
argument that power proceeds not in the traditional model of sovereignty but through admin-
istering and fostering life.

The old power of death that symbolised sovereign power was now carefully supplanted
by the administration of bodies and the calculated management of life.

(Foucault, 1979, pp. 139–40)

The obvious question is why. Foucault's 'radical nominalism' rejects the question of causation, but he quite clearly perceives the significance of extra-discursive references. In *I, Pierre*

Riviere, the French revolution is perceived as having profound resonances (Foucault, 1978a). In *The History of Sexuality*, as in *Discipline and Punish*, he refers to the profound changes of the eighteenth century:

> What occurred in the eighteenth century in some western countries, an event bound up with the development of capitalism, was … nothing less than the entry of life into history.
>
> (Foucault, 1979, p. 141)

And in the emergence of 'bio-power', Foucault's characteristic term of 'modern' social forms, sexuality becomes a key element. For sex, argues Foucault, is the pivot of two axes along which the whole technology of life developed; it was the point of entry to the body, to the harnessing, identification and distribution of forces over the body, and it was the entry to control and regulation of populations. 'Sex was a means of access both to the life of the body and the life of the species' (Foucault, 1979, p. 146). As a result, sex becomes a crucial target of power organized around the management of life, rather than the sovereign threat of death which organizes 'pre-modern' societies.

Foucault stresses not the historical cause of events but the conditions for the emergence of discourses and practices. Nevertheless there appears to be a strong functionalist tendency in his work. 'Social control' is no longer a product of a materially motivated ruling class but the concept of subjection within discourse seems as ultimately enveloping a concept.

'Where there is power, there is resistance', he argues, but nevertheless, and because of this, 'resistance is never in a position of exteriority in relation to power' (Foucault, 1979, p. 95). Indeed the very existence of power relies on a multiplicity of points of resistance, which play the role of 'adversary, target, support, or handle in power relations'. Foucault apparently envisages the power of social explosions in forcing new ways of seeing: the great social changes (industrial capitalism?) of the eighteenth and nineteenth centuries, the French Revolution, the possibilities opened up by the 'événements' of 1968. But one reading of his work would suggest that without such explosions, techniques of discipline and surveillance, strategies of power/knowledge leave us always, already, trapped.

But an alternative reading is possible. First of all there is the possibility of struggles over definition. This can be seen both in struggles over definitions of female sexuality and over the various and subtle forms of control of homosexuality.

> There is no question that the appearance in nineteenth century psychiatry, jurisprudence, and literature of a whole series of discourses on the species and subspecies of homosexuality, inversion, pederasty, and 'psychic hermaphrodism' made possible a strong advance of social controls into this area of 'perversity'; but it also made possible the formation of a 'reverse' discourse: homosexuality began to speak on its own behalf, to demand that its legitimacy or 'naturality' be acknowledged, often in the same vocabulary, using the same categories by which it was radically disqualified.
>
> (Foucault, 1979, p. 101)

This reverse affirmation is the sub-text of the history of the homosexual rights movement; it points to the significance of the definitional struggle *and* to its limitations. Hence Foucault's comment:

> I believe that the movements labelled 'sexual liberation' ought to be understood as movements of affirmation starting with sexuality. Which means two things: they are

movements that start with sexuality, with the apparatus of sexuality in the midst of which we're caught, and which make it function to the limit; but, at the same time, they are in motion relative to it, disengaging themselves and surmounting it.

(Foucault, 1977b, p. 155)

The ramifications of this 'surmounting' are not clear, but it is apparent that both the evolution of homosexual meanings and identities is not complete or 'scientifically' established and that homosexuals are, possibly for the first time, self-consciously participating as a group in that evolution.

The other point of high importance in Foucault's work is the emphasis on the genesis of particular institutions: of prisons, the clinic, medical and psychiatric practices that both produce and regulate the objects of knowledge. Appreciation of this emphasis will draw us away from such questions as: what is the relationship between the mode of production and this form of sexuality? Instead we can concentrate on the practices that actually constitute social and sexual categories and ensure their controlling impact. But, in turn, to do this we need to recognize that discourses do not arbitrarily emerge from the flux of possibilities, nor are discourses our only contact with the real: they have their conditions of existence and their effects in concrete, historical, social, economic and ideological situations.

Perspectives and projects

We are now in a sounder position to indicate more effective lines of historical research, or rather to pose the questions to which the historians of sexuality need to address themselves. They are effectively in two parts. First, what were the conditions for the emergence of the homosexual category (or indeed other sexual categories), the complex of factors which fixed the possibilities of homosexual behaviours into a system of defining concepts? Second, what were and are the factors which define the individual acceptance or rejection of categorizations? This is a question that many might regard as invalid but which seems to us of critical importance in determining the impact of control and regulation.

Conditions

Foucault and others have stressed the growing importance of the 'norm' since the eighteenth century.

> Another consequence of this development of bio-power was the growing importance assumed by the action of the norm at the expense of the juridical system of the law.
>
> (Foucault, 1979, p. 149)

A power whose task is to take charge of life needs continuous regulatory and corrective mechanisms. It has to qualify, measure, appraise and hierarchize: 'it affects distributions around the norms'. This is not far removed from a more commonplace observation that the development of liberal ('individualistic') society in the nineteenth century led to an increase of conventionality, or to discussions of ideological 'interpellations' in the construction of hegemonic forms (Laclau, 1977); but the examination of the 'norm' does point effectively to the centrality since the nineteenth century of the norm of the monogamous, heterosexual family. The uncertain status of sodomy points to the fact that before the nineteenth century, the codes governing sexual practices – canonical, pastoral, civil – all centred on non-reproductive relations. Sodomy was part of a continuum of non-procreative practices, often more serious than rape precisely because it was barren. But these regulations were not extra-marital; they entered the marriage bed, were directly about non-reproductive sex in conjugality, whatever the effectiveness of enforcement. From the nineteenth century the regulations are increasingly of non-conjugal relations: from incest and childhood sex to homosexuality. As sexuality is increasingly privatized, seen as the characteristic of the personal sphere, as its public manifestations are challenged (in terms that speak all the time of sex while denying it), so deviant forms of sex become subject to more closely defined *public* regulation. The family norm is strengthened by a series of extra-marital regulations, which refer back all the time to its normality and morality. This is, of course, underlined by a whole series of other developments, from the enforcement of the Poor Laws and the Factory Acts to the Welfare State support of particular household models in the twentieth century. To repeat a point made earlier, the specification, and hence greater regulation, of homosexual behaviour is closely interconnected with the revaluation and construction of the bourgeois family, not necessarily as a conscious effort to support or sustain the family but because, as Plummer has put it:

> The family as a social institution does not of itself condemn homosexuality, but through its mere existence it implicitly provides a model that renders the homosexual experience invalid.
>
> (Plummer, 1975, p. 210)

But if we accept this outline as a fruitful guideline for research we need, second, to stress its class specificities. For if 'sexuality' and its derivative sexual categorizations are social constructs, then they are constructions within specific class milieux, whatever the impact of their 'diffusion' or reappropriation. We need to explore, in much greater depth than before, the class application of the homosexual categorizations. The common interest among many early twentieth-century middle-class, self-defined homosexuals with the male working class, conceived of as relatively indifferent to homosexual behaviour, is a highly significant element in the homosexual sub-culture.

There was in fact a notable predominance of upper-middle-class values. Perhaps on one level only middle-class men had a sufficient sense of a 'personal life' through which to develop a homosexual identity (Zaretsky, 1976). The stress that is evident among male homosexual writers on cross-class liaisons and on youth (typically the representative idealized relationship is between an upper-middle-class man and a working-class youth) is striking, and not dissimilar, it may be noted in passing, to certain middle-class heterosexual patterns of the nineteenth century and earlier. See for example, the anonymous author, usually known as Walter, of the nineteenth-century sexual chronicle *My Secret Life* (Anonymous, c.1880). The impossibility of same-class liaisons is a constant theme of homosexual literature, demonstrating the strong elements of guilt (class and sexual) that pervade the male identity. But it also illustrates a pattern of what can be called 'sexual colonialism', which saw the working-class youth or soldier as a source of 'trade', often coinciding uneasily with an idealization of the reconciling effect of cross-class liaisons.

But if the idealization of working-class youth was one major theme, the attitude of these working-class men themselves is less easy to trace. They appear in all the major scandals (for example, the Wilde trial, the Cleveland Street scandal) but their self-conceptions are almost impossible to disinter. We may hypothesize that the spread of a homosexual consciousness was much less strong among working-class men than middle-class – for obvious family and social factors – even though the law in Britain (on, for example, importuning) probably affected more working-class than middle-class men. We can also note the evidence regarding the patterns of male prostitution as, for example, in the Brigade of Guards, a European-wide phenomenon. Most of the so far sparse evidence on male prostitution suggests a reluctance on the part of the 'prostitute' to define himself as homosexual (Weeks, 1980).

A third point relates to this, concerning the gender specificity of homosexual behaviour. The lesbian sense of self has been much less pronounced than the male homosexual and the sub-cultural development exiguous. If the Wilde trial was a major labelling event for men, the comparable event for lesbianism, the trial of Radclyffe Hall's lesbian novel, *The Well of Loneliness*, was much less devastating in its impact, and a generation later. Even science, so anxious to detail the characteristics of male homosexuals, largely ignored lesbianism.

These factors underline the fact that what is needed is not so much a monist explanation for the emergence of a 'homosexual identity' as a differential social history of male homosexuality and lesbianism. But this in turn demands an awareness of the construction of specific gender definitions, and their relationship to sexual identities. Gagnon and Simon have noted that:

> … the patterns of overt sexual behaviour on the part of homosexual females tend to resemble those of heterosexual females and to differ radically from the sexual patterns of both heterosexual and homosexual males.
>
> (Gagnon and Simon, 1973, p. 180)

The impact on lesbianism of, for example, the discourses on (basically male) homosexuality has never been explored.

Fourth, this underscores again the need to explore the various practices that create the terrain or space in which behaviour is constructed. There is a long historical tradition, as we have seen, of exploring legal regulation, but its impact in constructing categories has never been considered. The role of the medicalization of sexual deviance has also been tentatively explored, but it is only now that its complexly differentiated impact is being traced. Equally important are the various forms of ideological representations of homosexual behaviour, whether through the press or through the dramatizing effects of major rituals of public condemnation, such as the Oscar Wilde trial in the 1890s.

Fifth, there is an absence of any study of the political appropriation of concepts of sexual perversity, although there is a great deal of empirical evidence from the nineteenth century to the present that sexual deviance had a significant place in sexual-political discourse. This indicates the need for a close attention to specific conjunctures of sexual politics and to the social forces at work in constructing political alliances around crimes of morality. The role of sexual respectability in helping to cement the dominant power bloc in the nineteenth century and the relevance of sexual liberalism in constructing the social democratic hegemony of the 1960s in Britain and elsewhere are examples in point (Gray, 1977; Hall *et al.*, 1978).

What this schematic sketch suggests is the importance of locating sexual categorization within a complex of discourses and practices, but also at the same time it is important to reject descriptions that ignore the importance of external referents. The agitation for legal regulation, the impact of medicalization and the stereotyping of media representation all have sources in perceptions of the world and in complex power situations. One may mention, for example, the network of fears over moral decay, imperial decline and public vice behind the 1885 Criminal Law Amendment Act or the Cold War fears that form the background to the establishment of the Wolfenden Committee in 1954. Or, with regard to the growth of a medical model, we cannot disregard the significance of the growing professionalization of medicine in the nineteenth century, its ideological and material links with upper-middle-class male society and its consequent role in defining sexuality as well as 'sexual perversions'. So although it would be wrong to see the regulation of homosexual behaviour as a simple effect of capitalist development, it is intricately linked to wider changes within the growth of a highly industrialized, bourgeois society.

Identities

All ideologies, Althusser has argued, work by interpellating ('hailing') particular subjects, and the ideological discourses that establish the categories of sexual perversity address particular types of persons. They also, as Foucault suggests, create the possibility of reversals within the discourses: where there is power, there is resistance. Foucault is here offering a space for the self-creation of a homosexual identity, but what is absent is any interest in why some are able to respond or recognize themselves in the interpellation and others are not (Johnson, 1979, p. 75).

There are major problems in this area for which our guidelines are tentative. There is abundant evidence that individual, self-defined homosexuals see their sexuality as deeply rooted, and often manifest at a very early age. This would, on the surface at least, seem to deny that interaction with significant others creates the desire (as opposed to the identity), hence undermining a purely voluntarist position. On the other hand, the notion of a deeply structured homosexual component is equally questionable, if for no other reason than that all the evidence of historical variations contradicts it. Labelling theory has been quite able to accept the distinctions we are making, for example, between primary and secondary deviation.

> Primary deviation, as contrasted with secondary, is polygenetic, arising out of a variety of social, cultural, psychological, and adventitious or recurring combinations ... secondary deviance refers to a special class of socially defined responses which people make to problems created by the societal reaction to their deviance ... The secondary deviant, as opposed to his actions, is a person whose life and identity are organised around the facts of deviance.
>
> (Lemert, 1967, p. 40)

This is a valuable distinction stressing the real (and hitherto ignored) importance of social labelling, but it ignores precisely those historical (and hence variable) factors which structure the differences. To put it another way, if the homosexual component is not a factor present only in a fixed minority of people, but on the contrary an aspect of the body's sexual possibilities, what social and cultural forces are at work which ensure its dominance in some people, whereas in others the heterosexual element is apparently as strong and determined? Social labelling is obviously central in making the divide between 'normal' and 'deviant', but what shapes the components at the level of the human animal?

This must lead us again to ask whether we can rescue any lessons from psychoanalytical speculations. A recent attempt to reinterpret Freud's analysis of Little Hans throws some light on this question. Mia Campioni and Liz Gross appear to accept the arguments of Deleuze and Guattari (and Foucault) that Freud's work was simultaneously a recognition of, and another form of control over, the organization of desire under capitalism (Campioni and Gross, 1978). The function of Oedipus is thus to organize sexuality into properly different gender roles to accord both with patriarchal norms and a society that privileges sexuality.

> The purpose of concentrating on the case of Little Hans is to reveal the precise mecha-
> nisms whereby a system of representation (ideology), correlative with existing social
> structures, is inscribed upon the child within the constraints of relations specified by the
> family ... the process by which Hans is inserted into his patriarchal heritage gives us an
> indication of this process's mechanisms – at least in the case of male socialization. ...
> Moreover, the case allows us to clarify the strategies by which the child is inscribed into
> the power relations that stratify society, and to discover that this occurs by means of the
> sexualization of privileged erogenous zones. It is by the privileging of sexual zones,
> desires and objects, and by their social control through psychical defence mechanisms, in
> particular repression, that class and patriarchal social values are instilled in the child
> which are constructive of his or her very identity. Sexualization is the means both of the
> production and the limitation of desire, and therefore is also the locus of the control of
> desire. Sexual desire provides the socio-political structure with a specific site for power
> relations (relations of domination and subordination in general) to be exercised.
>
> (Campioni and Gross, 1978, p. 103)

At the beginning of Hans' case what is most apparent are the overwhelming number of objects and aims of his eroticism. Over the two years of the analysis this sexuality is channelled into the forms of masculine sexuality demanded by familial ideology, and in this we can see, dramatically at work in Freud's analysis and the father's work as agent, the actual imposition of the Oedipal network by the psychoanalytical institution, a paradigm of its controlling role in the twentieth century.

Several points come out of this which are worth underlining. First, this re-analysis does not assume the family is a natural, biological entity with single effects. On the contrary, it is seen as historically constituted and a consequent intersection of various developments, including the development of childhood and the social differentiation of women and men. Second, the analysis does not assume the naturalness of heterosexuality. Instead it relates its privileging precisely to the construction of masculinity and femininity within the monogamous (and socially constituted) family. Third, it does not see the Oedipus complex as in any way universal. Not only is it historically specific, but it is also class specific. Fourth, the analysis suggests that the child's development is neither natural nor internal to the family unit. The young human animal, with all his or her potentialities, is structured within a family, which all the time is a combination of social processes, and by constant reference to the social other.

It is within this context that psychological masculinity and femininity are structured at the level of the emotions. It seems likely that the possibilities of heterosexuality and homosexuality as socially structured limitations on the flux of potentialities are developed in this nexus in the process of emotional socialization. The emotion thus draws on sexuality rather than being created by it.

But what is created, this would suggest, is not an identity but a propensity. It is the whole series of social interactions, encounters with peers, educational processes, rituals of exclusion, labelling events, chance encounters, political identifications, and so on, which structure the sexual identities. They are not pre-given in nature; probably like the propensities themselves they are social creations, though at different levels in the formation of psychological individuality. This again suggests a rich field for historical explorations: the conditions for the growth of sub-cultural formations (urbanization, response to social pressure, etc.), the degree of sub-cultural participation, the role of sub-cultural involvement in the fixing of sexual identities, the impact of legal and ideological regulation, the political responses to the sub-culture, both from within the homosexual community and without, and the possibilities for transformations.

Conclusion

What has been offered here is neither a prescription for correct research procedures nor a collection of dogmatic answers, but a posing of important and fundamentally *historical* questions which the historians of sexuality have generally ignored. Earlier in the paper, the problem was posed on two levels: the level of the social categorization and the level of the *individual*, subjective construction of meaning. Until very recently, as Mary McIntosh pointed out, the latter level was exclusively concentrated on, to the extent that the question of aetiology dominated. Since then, particularly with the rise of sociological studies, the social has rightly been emphasized. What I am now tentatively suggesting is that we must see both as aspects of the same process, which is above all a historical process. Social processes construct subjectivities not just as 'categories' but at the level of individual desires. This perception, rather than the search for epistemological purity, should be the starting point for future social and historical studies of 'homosexuality' and indeed of 'sexuality' in general.

Notes

1 See, for example, Public Record Office, HO 79/1 66: Lord Hawkesbury to Lord Sydney, 8 November 1808.
2 Public Record Office: transcript of Regina v. Boulton and Others, 1871, DDP4/6, Day 1, p. 82; Day 3, p. 299.
3 On youth, see Gillis (1974); Gorham (1978); and on housework and motherhood, see Oakley (1976) and Davin (1978).
4 For comments on this theme, see Adams and Minson (1978), Coward (1978), Kuhn (1978, pp. 61–2).
5 For Wilhelm Reich's comments on homosexuality, see Reich, 1970. 'It can be reduced only by establishing all necessary prerequisites for a natural love life among the masses' [n.p.n.]. For a useful comment on the historical context of Reich's views, see Mitchell, 1974, p. 141. A similar leftist view that homosexuality was a 'symptom of arrested or distorted development' can be seen in Craig, 1934, p. 129. Herbert Marcuse's views are to be found in *Eros and Civilization* (1969). Reich, *The Sexual Revolution* (1970), expresses a viewpoint that homosexuality is a product of capitalist distortion of the libido.
6 Compare Plummer's slightly different account in the SSRC Report (Plummer, 1979).
7 Campioni and Gross (1978, p. 100) in their paper on 'Little Hans: The Production of Oedipus' propose a useful critique of Mitchell. See also Hall's point: 'Surely, we must say that, without further work, further historical specification, the mechanisms of the Oedipus in the discourse both of Freud and Lacan are universalist, trans-historical and therefore "essentialist" ... the concepts elaborated by Freud (and reworked by Lacan) cannot, in their in-general and universalist form, enter the theoretical space of historical materialism, without further specification and elaboration – specification at the level at which the concepts of historical materialism operate' (Hall, 1978, pp. 118–19).

References

ADAMS, R. and MINSON, J. (1978) 'The "subject" of feminism', *M/F*, 2, pp. 43–61.
ALBURY, R. (1976) 'Two readings of Freud', *Working Papers in Sex, Science and Culture*, 1, pp. 4–9.
ANONYMOUS (c.1880) *My Secret Life*, 11 vols, privately printed, Amsterdam.
BAILEY, D.S. (1955) *Homosexuality and the Western Christian Tradition*, London: Longman.
BELL, A.P. and WEINBERG, M.S. (1978) *Homosexualities: A Study of Diversity Among Men and Women*, London: Mitchell Beazley.
BLOCH, I. (1938) *Sexual Life in England, Past and Present*, London: Francis Adler.
BRAKE, M. (1976) 'I may be queer but at least I'm a man: male hegemony and ascribed "v" achieved gender', in BARKER, D.L. and ALLEN, S. (eds) *Sexual Divisions and Society*, London: Tavistock.
BRISTOW, E.J. (1977) *Vice and Vigilance: Purity Movements in Britain since 1700*, Dublin: Gill and Macmillan.

BULLOUGH, V.L. and VOGHT, M. (1973) 'Homosexuality and its confusion with the "secret sin" in pre-Freudian America', *Journal of the History of Medicine*, 27(2), pp. 143–55.

BURTON, R. (1888) *A Plain and Literal Translation of the Arabian Nights Entertainment with Terminal Essay*, Benares: Kamashastra Society.

CAMPIONI, M. and GROSS, L. (1978) 'Little Hans: the production of Oedipus', in FOSS, P. and MORRIS, M. (eds) *Language, Sexuality and Subversion*, Darlington, Australia: Ferral Publications.

CARPENTER, E. (1908) *The Intermediate Sex*, London: Allen & Unwin.

—— (1914) *Intermediate Types Among Primitive Folk*, London: Allen & Unwin.

CORY, D.W. (1953) *The Homosexual Outlook: A Subjective Approach*, New York: Nevill.

COWARD, R. (1978) 'Sexual liberation and the family', *M/F*, 1, pp. 7–24.

CRAIG, A. (1934) *Sex and Revolution*, London: Allen and Unwin.

D'AMICO, R. (1978) 'Review of Foucault', *Telos*, 36, pp. 169–83.

DAVIN, A. (1978) 'Imperialism and motherhood', *History Workshop*, 5, pp. 9–65.

DELEUZE, G. and GUATTARI, F. (1977) *Anti-Oedipus: Capitalism and Schizophrenia*, New York: Viking Press.

DOVER, K.G. (1978) *Greek Homosexuality*, London: Duckworth.

ELLIS, H. (1936) *Studies in the Psychology of Sex, vol. 2: Sexual Inversion*, New York: Random House.

FORD, C.S. and BEACH, F. (1952) *Patterns of Sexual Behaviour*, London: Methuen.

FOUCAULT, M. (1977a) *Discipline and Punish: The Birth of the Prison*, London: Allen and Lane.

—— (1977b) 'Power and sex: an interview with Michel Foucault', *Telos*, 32, summer, pp. 152–61.

—— (1978a) *I, Pierre Riviere*, Brighton: Harvester.

—— (1978b) 'Politics and the study of discourse', *Ideology and Consiousness*, 3, spring, pp. 7–26.

—— (1979) *The History of Sexuality, vol. 1, An Introduction*, London: Allen and Lane.

GAGNON, J.H. and SIMON, W.S. (1973) *Sexual Conduct: The Social Sources of Human Sexuality*, Chicago: Aldine.

GILBERT, A.N. (1974) 'The Africaine court martial', *Journal of Homosexuality*, 1, pp. 111–22.

—— (1976) 'Buggery and the British Navy, 1700–1861', *Journal of Social History*, 10, pp. 72–98.

—— (1977) 'Social deviance and disaster during the Napoleonic Wars', *Albion*, 9, pp. 98–113.

GILLIS, J. (1974) *Youth and History*, New York: Academic Press.

GORHAM, D. (1978) 'The "maiden tribute of modern Babylon" re-examined: child prostitution and the idea of childhood in late Victorian England', *Victorian Studies*, 21, pp. 353–79.

GRAY, R. (1977) 'Bourgeois hegemony in Victorian Britain', in BLOOMFELD, J. (ed.) *Class, Hegemony and Party*, London: Lawrence and Wishart.

HALL, R. (1928) *The Well of Loneliness*, London: Hogarth Press.

HALL, S. (1978) 'Some problems with the ideology/subject couplet', *Ideology & Consciousness*, 3, pp. 113–21.

——, CHRITCHER, C., JEFFERSON, T., CLARKE, J. and ROBERTS, B. (1978) *Policing the Crisis: Mugging, the State and Law and Order*, Basingstoke: Macmillan.

HARVEY, A.D. (1978) 'Prosecutions for sodomy in England at the beginning of the nineteenth century', *The Historical Journal*, 21, pp. 939–48.

HIRSCHFELD, M. (1938) *Sexual Anomalies and Perversions*, New York: Encyclopaedia Press.

—— (1946) *Sexual Anomalies and Perversions*, revised edition, New York: Encyclopaedia Press.

HISTORY WORKSHOP (1978) 'Editorial: history and theory', *History Workshop*, 6, pp. 1–6.

HOCQUENGHEM, G. (1978) *Homosexual Desire*, London: Allison & Busby.

HYDE, M. (1970) *The Other Love: An Historical and Contemporary Survey of Homosexuality in Britain*, London: Heinemann.

JOHNSON, R. (1979) 'Histories of culture/theories of ideology: notes on an impasse', in BARRETT, M. (ed.), *Ideology and Cultural Production*, London: Croon Helm.

KARLEN, A. (1971) *Sexuality and Homosexuality: The Complete Account of Male and Female Sexual Behaviour and Deviation with Case Histories*, London: MacDonald.

KATZ, J. (1976) *Gay American History: Lesbians and Gay Men in the USA*, New York: Thomas & Crowell.

KRAFFT-EBING, R. VON (1965) *Psychopathia Sexualis: A Medico-Forensic Study*, New York: G.P. Putnam's & Sons.

KUHN, A. (1978) 'Structures of patriarchy and capital in the family', in KUHN, A. and WOLPE, A.M. (eds) *Feminism and Materialism*, London: Routledge and Kegan Paul.

LACLAU, E. (1977) *Politics and Ideology in Marxist Theory*, London: New Left Books.

LAFITTE, F. (1958–59) 'Homosexuality and the law', *British Journal of Delinquency*, 9, pp. 8–19.

LAURITSEN, J. and THORSTAD, D. (1974) *The Early Homosexual Rights Movement (1864–1935)*, New York: Times Change Press.

LEMERT, E. (1967) *Human Deviance, Social Problems and Social Control*, New Jersey: Prentice-Hall.

MCINTOSH, M. (1968) 'The homosexual role', *Social Problems*, 16, pp. 182–92.

MARCUSE, H. (1969) *Eros and Civilization*, London: Sphere.

MITCHELL, J. (1974) *Psychoanalysis and Feminism*, London: Allen Lane.

OAKLEY, A. (1976) *Housewife*, Harmondsworth: Penguin.

PLUMMER, K. (1975) *Sexual Stigma: An Interactionist Account*, London: Routledge and Kegan Paul.

—— (1979) *Symbolic Interactionism and Sexual Differentation: An Empirical Investigation*, unpublished report to SSRC.

POSTER, M. (1978) *Critical Theory of the Family*, London: Pluto Press.

RADZINOWICZ, L. (1968) *A History of English Criminal Law, vol. 4: Grappling for Control*, London: Stevens & Sons.

REICH, W. (1970) *The Sexual Revolution*, New York: Strauss and Giroux.

ROWSE, A.L. (1977) *Homosexuals in History: A Study of Ambivalence in Society, Literature and the Arts*, London: Weidenfeld & Nicolson.

SMITH, F.B. (1976) 'Labouchere's amendment to the Criminal Law Amendment Act', *Historical Studies*, 17, pp. 165–75.

SMITH-ROSENBERG, C. (1975) 'The female world of love and ritual: relations between women in nineteenth century America', *Signs*, 1, pp. 1–29.

STEAKLEY, J.D. (1975) *The Homosexual Emancipation Movement in Germany*, New York: Arno Press.

STONE, L. (1977) *The Family, Sex and Marriage*, London: Weidenfeld & Nicolson.

SYMONDS, J.A. (1983) *A Problem in Greek Ethics and Other Writings*, New York: Pagan Press.

TAYLOR, G.R. (1964) *Sex in History*, London: Panther.

TRUMBACH, R. (1977) 'London's sodomites: homosexual behaviour and Western culture in the 18th century', *Journal of Social History*, 11, pp. 1–33.

WEEKS, J. (1977) *Coming Out: Homosexual Politics in Britain from the 19th Century to the Present*, London: Quartet.

—— (1978) 'Preface', in HOCQUENGHEM, G., *Homosexual Desire*, London: Allison & Busby.

—— (1980) 'Inverts, perverts and mary annes: male prostitution and the regulation of homosexuality in England in the 19th and early 20th centuries', *Journal of Homosexuality*, 6 [n.p.n.].

WEINBERG, G. (1973) *Society and the Healthy Homosexual*, New York: Anchor.

WESTERMARCK, E. (1906) *The Origin and Development of the Moral Ideas*, Basingstoke: Macmillan.

ZARETSKY, E. (1976) *Capitalism, the Family and Personal Life*, London: Pluto Press.

ZINNER, J. (1978) 'Review of *La Volonté de Savoir*', *Telos*, 36, pp. 215–25.

9 Thinking sex

Notes for a radical theory of the politics of sexuality

Gayle S. Rubin [1984]

The sex wars

> Asked his advice, Dr. J. Guerin affirmed that, after all other treatments had failed, he had succeeded in curing young girls affected by the vice of onanism by burning the clitoris with a hot iron ... I apply the hot point three times to each of the large labia and another on the clitoris ... After the first operation, from forty to fifty times a day, the number of voluptuous spasms was reduced to three or four ... We believe, then, that in cases similar to those submitted to your consideration, one should not hesitate to resort to the hot iron, and at an early hour, in order to combat clitoral and vaginal onanism in the little girls.
>
> (Zambaco, 1981, pp. 31, 36)

The time has come to think about sex. To some, sexuality may seem to be an unimportant topic, a frivolous diversion from the more critical problems of poverty, war, disease, racism, famine, or nuclear annihilation. But it is precisely at times such as these, when we live with the possibility of unthinkable destruction, that people are likely to become dangerously crazy about sexuality. Contemporary conflicts over sexual values and erotic conduct have much in common with the religious disputes of earlier centuries. They acquire immense symbolic weight. Disputes over sexual behaviour often become the vehicles for displacing social anxieties, and discharging their attendant emotional intensity. Consequently, sexuality should be treated with special respect in times of great social stress.

The realm of sexuality also has its own internal politics, inequities, and modes of oppression. As with other aspects of human behaviour, the concrete institutional forms of sexuality at any given time and place are products of human activity. They are imbued with conflicts of interest and political manoeuvre, both deliberate and incidental. In that sense, sex is always political. But there are also historical periods in which sexuality is more sharply contested and more overtly politicized. In such periods, the domain of erotic life is, in effect, renegotiated.

In England and the United States, the late nineteenth century was one such era. During that time, powerful social movements focused on 'vices' of all sorts. There were educational and political campaigns to encourage chastity, to eliminate prostitution, and to discourage masturbation, especially among the young. Morality crusaders attacked obscene literature, nude paintings, music halls, abortion, birth-control information, and public dancing (see Gordon and Dubois, 1983; Marcus, 1974; Ryan, 1979; Walkowitz, 1980, 1982; Weeks, 1981). The consolidation of Victorian morality, and its apparatus of social, medical, and legal enforcement, was the outcome of a long period of struggle whose results have been bitterly contested ever since.

The consequences of these great nineteenth-century moral paroxysms are still with us. They have left a deep imprint on attitudes about sex, medical practice, child-rearing, parental anxieties, police conduct, and sex law.

The idea that masturbation is an unhealthy practice is part of that heritage. During the nineteenth century, it was commonly thought that 'premature' interest in sex, sexual excitement, and, above all, sexual release, would impair the health and maturation of a child. Theorists differed on the actual consequences of sexual precocity. Some thought it led to insanity, while others merely predicted stunted growth. To protect the young from premature arousal, parents tied children down at night so they would not touch themselves; doctors excised the clitorises of onanistic little girls (see Barker-Benfield, 1976; Marcus, 1974; Weeks, 1981; Zambaco, 1981). Although the more gruesome techniques have been abandoned, the attitudes that produced them persist. The notion that sex *per se* is harmful to the young has been chiselled into extensive social and legal structures designed to insulate minors from sexual knowledge and experience.

Much of the sex law currently on the books also dates from the nineteenth-century morality crusades. The first federal anti-obscenity law in the United States was passed in 1873. The Comstock Act named for Anthony Comstock – an ancestral anti-porn activist and the founder of the New York Society for the Suppression of Vice – made it a federal crime to make, advertise, sell, possess, send through the mails, or import books or pictures deemed obscene. The law also banned contraceptive or abortifacient drugs and devices and information about them (Beserra, Franklin and Clevenger, 1977). In the wake of the federal statute, most states passed their own anti-obscenity laws.

The Supreme Court began to whittle down both federal and state Comstock laws during the 1950s. By 1975, the prohibition of materials used for, and information about, contraception and abortion had been ruled unconstitutional. However, although the obscenity provisions have been modified, their fundamental constitutionality has been upheld. Thus it remains a crime to make, sell, mail, or import material which has no purpose other than sexual arousal (Beserra, Franklin and Clevenger, 1977).

Although sodomy statutes date from older strata of the law, when elements of canon law were adopted into civil codes, most of the laws used to arrest homosexuals and prostitutes come out of the Victorian campaigns against 'white slavery'. These campaigns produced the myriad prohibitions against solicitation, lewd behaviour, loitering for immoral purposes, age offences, and brothels and bawdy houses.

In her discussion of the British 'white slave' scare, historian Judith Walkowitz observes that: 'Recent research delineates the vast discrepancy between lurid journalistic accounts and the reality of prostitution. Evidence of widespread entrapment of British girls in London and abroad is slim' (Walkowitz, 1980, p. 83).[1] However, public furore over this ostensible problem

> forced the passage of the Criminal Law Amendment Act of 1885, a particularly nasty and pernicious piece of omnibus legislation. The 1885 Act raised the age of consent for girls from 13 to 16, but it also gave police far greater summary jurisdiction over poor working-class women and children … it contained a clause making indecent acts between consenting male adults a crime, thus forming the basis of legal prosecution of male homosexuals in Britain until 1967 … the clauses of the new bill were mainly enforced against working-class women, and regulated adult rather than youthful sexual behaviour.
>
> (Walkowitz, 1982, p. 85)

In the United States, the Mann Act, also known as the White Slave Traffic Act, was passed in 1910. Subsequently, every state in the union passed anti-prostitution legislation (Beserra, Franklin and Clevenger, 1977).

In the 1950s, in the United States, major shifts in the organization of sexuality took place. Instead of focusing on prostitution or masturbation, the anxieties of the 1950s condensed most specifically around the image of the 'homosexual menace' and the dubious spectre of the 'sex offender'. Just before and after World War II, the 'sex offender' became an object of public fear and scrutiny. Many states and cities, including Massachusetts, New Hampshire, New Jersey, New York State, New York City, and Michigan, launched investigations to gather information about this menace to public safety (Commonwealth of Massachusetts, 1947; State of New Hampshire, 1949; City of New York, 1939; State of New York, 1950; Hartwell, 1950; State of Michigan, 1951). The term 'sex offender' sometimes applied to rapists, sometimes to 'child molesters', and eventually functioned as a code for homosexuals. In its bureaucratic, medical, and popular versions, the sex offender discourse tended to blur distinctions between violent sexual assault and illegal but consensual acts such as sodomy. The criminal justice system incorporated these concepts when an epidemic of sexual psychopath laws swept through state legislatures (Freedman, 1983). These laws gave the psychological professions increased police powers over homosexuals and other sexual 'deviants'.

From the late 1940s until the early 1960s, erotic communities whose activities did not fit the postwar American dream drew intense persecution. Homosexuals were, along with communists, the objects of federal witch hunts and purges. Congressional investigations, executive orders, and sensational exposés in the media aimed to root out homosexuals employed by the government. Thousands lost their jobs, and restrictions on federal employment of homosexuals persist to this day (Bérubé, 1981a, 1981b; D'Emilio, 1983; Katz, 1976). The FBI began systematic surveillance and harassment of homosexuals, which lasted at least into the 1970s (D'Emilio, 1983; Bérubé, personal communication).

Many states and large cities conducted their own investigations, and the federal witch hunts were reflected in a variety of local crackdowns. In Boise, Idaho, in 1955, a schoolteacher sat down to breakfast with his morning paper and read that the vice-president of the Idaho First National Bank had been arrested on felony sodomy charges; the local prosecutor said that he intended to eliminate all homosexuality from the community. The teacher never finished his breakfast. 'He jumped up from his seat, pulled out his suitcases, packed as fast as he could, got into his car, and drove straight to San Francisco ... The cold eggs, coffee, and toast remained on his table for two days before someone from his school came by to see what had happened' (Gerassi, 1968, p. 14).[2]

In San Francisco, police and media waged war on homosexuals throughout the 1950s. Police raided bars, patrolled cruising areas, conducted street sweeps, and trumpeted their intention of driving the queers out of San Francisco (Bérubé, personal communication; D'Emilio, 1981, 1983). Crackdowns against gay individuals, bars, and social areas occurred throughout the country. Although anti-homosexual crusades are the best-documented examples of erotic repression in the 1950s, future research should reveal similar patterns of increased harassment against pornographic materials, prostitutes, and erotic deviants of all sorts. Research is needed to determine the full scope of both police persecution and regulatory reform.[3]

The current period bears some uncomfortable similarities to the 1880s and the 1950s. The 1977 campaign to repeal the Dade County, Florida, gay rights ordinance inaugurated a new wave of violence, state persecution, and legal initiatives directed against minority sexual populations and the commercial sex industry. For the last six years, the United States and Canada have undergone an extensive sexual repression in the political, not the psychological, sense. In the spring of 1977, a few weeks before the Dade County vote, the news media were suddenly full of reports of raids on gay cruising areas, arrests for prostitution, and investigations into the manufacture and distribution of pornographic materials. Since then, police activity against the gay community has increased exponentially. The gay press has documented hundreds of arrests, from the libraries of Boston to the streets of Houston and the beaches of San Francisco. Even the large, organized, and relatively powerful urban gay communities have been unable to stop these depredations. Gay bars and bath houses have been busted with alarming frequency, and police have gotten bolder. In one especially dramatic incident, police in Toronto raided all four of the city's gay baths. They broke into cubicles with crowbars and hauled almost 300 men out into the winter streets, clad in their bath towels. Even 'liberated' San Francisco has not been immune. There have been proceedings against several bars, countless arrests in the parks, and, in the fall of 1981, police arrested over 400 people in a series of sweeps of Polk Street, one of the thorough-fares of local gay nightlife. Queerbashing has become a significant recreational activity for young urban males. They come into gay neighbourhoods armed with baseball bats and looking for trouble, knowing that the adults in their lives either secretly approve or will look the other way.

The police crackdown has not been limited to homosexuals. Since 1977, enforcement of existing laws against prostitution and obscenity has been stepped up. Moreover, states and munic-ipalities have been passing new and tighter regulations on commercial sex. Restrictive ordinances have been passed, zoning laws altered, licensing and safety codes amended, sentences increased, and evidentiary requirements relaxed. This subtle legal codification of more stringent controls over adult sexual behaviour has gone largely unnoticed outside of the gay press.

For over a century, no tactic for stirring up erotic hysteria has been as reliable as the appeal to protect children. The current wave of erotic terror has reached deepest into those areas bordered in some way, if only symbolically, by the sexuality of the young. The motto of the Dade County repeal campaign was 'Save Our Children' from alleged homosexual recruit-ment. In February 1977, shortly before the Dade County vote, a sudden concern with 'child pornography' swept the national media. In May, the *Chicago Tribune* ran a lurid four-day series with three-inch headlines, which claimed to expose a national vice ring organized to lure young boys into prostitution and pornography.[4] Newspapers across the country ran similar stories, most of them worthy of the *National Enquirer*. By the end of May, a congres-sional investigation was underway. Within weeks, the federal government had enacted a sweeping bill against 'child pornography' and many of the states followed with bills of their own. These laws have reestablished restrictions on sexual materials that had been relaxed by some of the important Supreme Court decisions. For instance, the Court ruled that neither nudity nor sexual activity *per se* was obscene. But the child pornography laws define as obscene any depiction of minors who are nude or engaged in sexual activity. This means that photographs of naked children in anthropology textbooks and many of the ethnographic movies shown in college classes are technically illegal in several states. In fact, the instructors are liable to an additional felony charge for showing such images to each student under the age of 18. Although the Supreme Court has also ruled that it is a constitutional right to possess obscene material for private use, some child pornography laws prohibit even the private possession of any sexual material involving minors.

The laws produced by the child-porn panic are ill-conceived and misdirected. They repre-sent far-reaching alterations in the regulation of sexual behaviour and abrogate important sexual civil liberties. But hardly anyone noticed as they swept through Congress and state legislatures. With the exception of the North American Man/Boy Love Association and American Civil Liberties Union, no one raised a peep of protest.[5]

A new and even tougher federal child-pornography bill has just reached House–Senate conference. It removes any requirement that prosecutors must prove that alleged child pornography was distributed for commercial sale. Once this bill becomes law, a person merely possessing a nude snapshot of a 17-year-old lover or friend may go to jail for fifteen years, and be fined $100,000. This bill passed the House 400 to 1.[6]

The experiences of art photographer Jacqueline Livingston exemplify the climate created by the child-porn panic. An assistant professor of photography at Cornell University, Livingston was fired in 1978 after exhibiting pictures of male nudes that included photographs of her seven-year-old son masturbating. *Ms. Magazine, Chrysalis,* and *Art News* all refused to run ads for Livingston's posters of male nudes. At one point, Kodak confiscated some of her film, and for several months Livingston lived with the threat of prosecution under the child-pornography laws. The Tompkins Country Department of Social Services investigated her fitness as a parent. Livingston's posters have been collected by the Museum of Modern Art, the Metropolitan, and other major museums. But she has paid a high cost in harassment and anxiety for her efforts to capture on film the uncensored male body at different ages (Stambolian, 1980, 1983).

It is easy to see someone like Livingston as a victim of the child-porn wars. It is harder for most people to sympathize with actual boy-lovers. Like communists and homosexuals in the 1950s, boy-lovers are so stigmatized that it is difficult to find defenders for their civil liberties, let alone for their erotic orientation. Consequently, the police have feasted on them. Local police, the FBI, and watchdog postal inspectors have joined to build a huge apparatus whose sole aim is to wipe out the community of men who love underaged youth. In twenty years or so, when some of the smoke has cleared, it will be much easier to show that these men have been the victims of a savage and undeserved witch hunt. A lot of people will be embarrassed by their collaboration with this persecution, but it will be too late to do much good for those men who have spent their lives in prison.

While the misery of boy-lovers affects very few, the other long-term legacy of the Dade County repeal affects almost everyone. The success of the anti-gay campaign ignited long-simmering passions of the American right, and sparked an extensive movement to compress the boundaries of acceptable sexual behaviour.

Right-wing ideology linking non-familial sex with communism and political weakness is nothing new. During the McCarthy period, Alfred Kinsey and his Institute for Sex Research were attacked for weakening the moral fibre of Americans and rendering them more vulnerable to communist influence. After congressional investigations and bad publicity, Kinsey's Rockefeller grant was terminated in 1954 (Gebhard, 1976).

Around 1969, the extreme right discovered the Sex Information and Education Council of the United States (SIECUS). In books and pamphlets, such as *The Sex Education Racket: Pornography in the Schools* and *SIECUS: Corrupter of Youth,* the right attacked SIECUS and sex education as communist plots to destroy the family and sap the national will (Courtney, 1969; Drake, 1969). Another pamphlet, *Pavlov's Children (They May Be Yours)* (n.a., 1969), claims that the United Nations Educational, Scientific and Cultural Organization (UNESCO) is in cahoots with SIECUS to undermine religious taboos, to promote the acceptance of abnormal sexual relations, to downgrade absolute moral standards, and to 'destroy racial cohesion', by exposing white people (especially white women) to the alleged 'lower' sexual standards of black people.

New Right and neo-conservative ideology has updated these themes, and leans heavily on linking 'immoral' sexual behaviour to putative declines in American power. In 1977, Norman Podhoretz wrote an essay blaming homosexuals for the alleged inability of the

United States to stand up to the Russians (Podhoretz, 1977). He thus neatly linked 'the anti-gay fight in the domestic arena and the anti-Communist battles in foreign policy' (Wolfe and Sanders, 1979).

Right-wing opposition to sex education, homosexuality, pornography, abortion, and pre-marital sex moved from the extreme fringes to the political centre-stage after 1977, when right-wing strategists and fundamentalist religious crusaders discovered that these issues had mass appeal. Sexual reaction played a significant role in the right's electoral success in 1980 (Breslin, 1981; Gordon and Hunter, 1977–78; Gregory-Lewis, 1977a, 1977b, 1977c; Kopkind, 1977; Petchesky, 1981). Organizations such as the Moral Majority and Citizens for Decency have acquired mass followings, immense financial resources, and unanticipated clout. The Equal Rights Amendment has been defeated, legislation has been passed that mandates new restrictions on abortion, and funding for programmes such as Planned Parenthood and sex education has been slashed. Laws and regulations making it more difficult for teenage girls to obtain contraceptives or abortions have been promulgated. Sexual backlash was exploited in successful attacks on the Women's Studies Program at California State University at Long Beach.

The most ambitious right-wing legislative initiative has been the Family Protection Act (FPA), introduced in Congress in 1979. The Family Protection Act is a broad assault on feminism, homosexuals, non-traditional families, and teenage sexual privacy (Brown, 1981). The Family Protection Act has not and probably will not pass, but conservative members of Congress continue to pursue its agenda in a more piecemeal fashion. Perhaps the most glaring sign of the times is the Adolescent Family Life Program. Also known as the Teen Chastity Program, it gets some 15 million federal dollars to encourage teenagers to refrain from sexual intercourse, and to discourage them from using contraceptives if they do have sex, and from having abortions if they get pregnant. In the last few years, there have been countless local confrontations over gay rights, sex education, abortion rights, adult bookstores, and public school curricula. It is unlikely that the anti-sex backlash is over, or that it has even peaked. Unless something changes dramatically, it is likely that the next few years will bring more of the same.

Periods such as the 1880s in England, and the 1950s in the United States, recodify the relations of sexuality. The struggles that were fought leave a residue in the form of laws, social practices, and ideologies which then affect the way in which sexuality is experienced long after the immediate conflicts have faded. All the signs indicate that the present era is another of those watersheds in the politics of sex. The settlements that emerge from the 1980s will have an impact far into the future. It is therefore imperative to understand what is going on and what is at stake in order to make informed decisions about what policies to support and oppose.

It is difficult to make such decisions in the absence of a coherent and intelligent body of radical thought about sex. Unfortunately, progressive political analysis of sexuality is relatively underdeveloped. Much of what is available from the feminist movement has simply added to the mystification that shrouds the subject. There is an urgent need to develop radical perspectives on sexuality.

Paradoxically, an explosion of exciting scholarship and political writing about sex has been generated in these bleak years. In the 1950s, the early gay rights movement began and prospered while the bars were being raided and anti-gay laws were being passed. In the last six years, new erotic communities, political alliances, and analyses have been developed in the midst of the repression. In this essay, I will propose elements of a descriptive and conceptual framework for thinking about sex and its politics. I hope to contribute to the pressing task of creating an accurate, humane, and genuinely liberatory body of thought about sexuality.

Sexual thoughts

> 'You see, Tim', Phillip said suddenly, 'your argument isn't reasonable. Suppose I granted your first point that homosexuality is justifiable in certain instances and under certain controls. Then there is the catch: where does justification end and degeneracy begin? Society must condemn to protect. Permit even the intellectual homosexual a place of respect and the first bar is down. Then comes the next and the next until the sadist, the flagellist, the criminally insane demand their places, and society ceases to exist. So I ask again: where is the line drawn? Where does degeneracy begin if not at the beginning of individual freedom in such matters?'
>
> [Fragment from a discussion between two gay men
> trying to decide if they may love each other (Barr, 1950, p. 310)]

A radical theory of sex must identify, describe, explain, and denounce erotic injustice and sexual oppression. Such a theory needs refined conceptual tools which can grasp the subject and hold it in view. It must build rich descriptions of sexuality as it exists in society and history. It requires a convincing critical language that can convey the barbarity of sexual persecution.

Several persistent features of thought about sex inhibit the development of such a theory. These assumptions are so pervasive in Western culture that they are rarely questioned. Thus, they tend to reappear in different political contexts, acquiring new rhetorical expressions but reproducing fundamental axioms.

One such axiom is sexual essentialism – the idea that sex is a natural force that exists prior to social life and shapes institutions. Sexual essentialism is embedded in the folk wisdoms of Western societies, which consider sex to be eternally unchanging, asocial, and transhistorical. Dominated for over a century by medicine, psychiatry, and psychology, the academic study of sex has reproduced essentialism. These fields classify sex as a property of individuals. It may reside in their hormones or their psyches. It may be construed as physiological or psychological. But within these ethnoscientific categories, sexuality has no history and no significant social determinants.

During the last five years, a sophisticated historical and theoretical scholarship has challenged sexual essentialism both explicitly and implicitly. Gay history, particularly the work of Jeffrey Weeks, has led this assault by showing that homosexuality as we know it is a relatively modern institutional complex.[7] Many historians have come to see the contemporary institutional forms of heterosexuality as an even more recent development (Hansen, 1979). An important contributor to the new scholarship is Judith Walkowitz, whose research has demonstrated the extent to which prostitution was transformed around the turn of the century. She provides meticulous descriptions of how the interplay of social forces such as ideology, fear, political agitation, legal reform, and medical practice can change the structure of sexual behaviour and alter its consequences (Walkowitz, 1980, 1982).

Michel Foucault's *The History of Sexuality* (1978) has been the most influential and emblematic text of the new scholarship on sex. Foucault criticizes the traditional understanding of sexuality as a natural libido yearning to break free of social constraint. He argues that desires are not pre-existing biological entities, but rather that they are constituted in the course of historically specific social practices. He emphasizes the generative aspects of the social organization of sex rather than its repressive elements by pointing out that new sexualities are constantly produced. And he points to a major discontinuity between kinship-based systems of sexuality and more modern forms.

The new scholarship on sexual behaviour has given sex a history and created a constructivist alternative to sexual essentialism. Underlying this body of work is an assumption that sexuality is constituted in society and history, not biologically orda[...]. This does not mean the biological capacities are not prerequisites for human sexuality. It do[...] mean that human sexuality is not comprehensible in purely biological terms. Human organ- isms with human brains are necessary for human cultures, but no examination of the body or its parts can explain the nature and variety of human social systems. The belly's hunger gives no clues as to the complexities of cuisine. The body, the brain, the genitalia, and the capacity for language are necessary for human sexuality. But they do not determine its content, its experiences, or its institutional forms. Moreover, we never encounter the body unmediated by the meanings that cultures give to it. To paraphrase Lévi-Strauss, my position on the relation- ship between biology and sexuality is a 'Kantianism without a transcendental libido'.[9]

It is impossible to think with any clarity about the politics of race or gender as long as these are thought of as biological entities rather than as social constructs. Similarly, sexuality is impervious to political analysis as long as it is primarily conceived as a biological phenom- enon or an aspect of individual psychology. Sexuality is as much a human product as are diets, methods of transportation, systems of etiquette, forms of labour, types of entertainment, processes of production, and modes of oppression. Once sex is understood in terms of social analysis and historical understanding, a more realistic politics of sex becomes possible. One may then think of sexual politics in terms of such phenomena as populations, neighbour- hoods, settlement patterns, migration, urban conflict, epidemiology, and police technology. These are more fruitful categories of thought than the more traditional ones of sin, disease, neurosis, pathology, decadence, pollution, or the decline and fall of empires.

By detailing the relationships between stigmatized erotic populations and the social forces that regulate them, work such as that of Allan Bérubé, John D'Emilio, Jeffrey Weeks, and Judith Walkowitz contains implicit categories of political analysis and criticism. Neverthe- less, the constructivist perspective has displayed some political weaknesses. This has been most evident in misconstructions of Foucault's position.

Because of his emphasis on the ways that sexuality is produced, Foucault has been vulner- able to interpretations that deny or minimize the reality of sexual repression in the more polit- ical sense. Foucault makes it abundantly clear that he is not denying the existence of sexual repression so much as inscribing it within a large dynamic (Foucault, 1978, p. 11). Sexuality in Western societies has been structured within an extremely punitive social framework, and has been subjected to very real formal and informal controls. It is necessary to recognize repressive phenomena without resorting to the essentialist assumptions of the language of libido. It is important to hold repressive sexual practices in focus, even while situating them within a different totality and a more refined terminology (Weeks, 1981, p. 9).

Most radical thought about sex has been embedded within a model of the instincts and their restraints. Concepts of sexual oppression have been lodged within that more biological understanding of sexuality. It is often easier to fall back on the notion of a natural libido subjected to inhumane repression than to reformulate concepts of sexual injustice within a more constructivist framework. But it is essential that we do so. We need a radical critique of sexual arrangements that has the conceptual elegance of Foucault and the evocative passion of Reich.

The new scholarship on sex has brought a welcome insistence that sexual terms be restricted to their proper historical and social contexts, and a cautionary scepticism towards sweeping generalizations. But it is important to be able to indicate groupings of erotic behav- iour and general trends within erotic discourse. In addition to sexual essentialism, there are at least five other ideological formations whose grip on sexual thought is so strong that to fail to discuss them is to remain enmeshed within them. These are sex negativity, the fallacy of

hierarchical valuation of sex acts, the domino theory of sexual peril, and
of benign sexual variation.

most important is sex negativity. Western cultures generally consider sex
structive, negative force (Weeks, 1981, p. 22). Most Christian tradition,
that sex is inherently sinful. It may be redeemed if performed within
ve purposes and if the pleasurable aspects are not enjoyed too much. In
the assumption that the genitalia are an intrinsically inferior part of the
body, much lower and less holy than the mind, the 'soul', the 'heart', or even the upper part of
the digestive system (the status of the excretory organs is close to that of the genitalia).[10] Such
notions have by now acquired a life of their own and no longer depend solely on religion for
their perseverance.

This culture always treats sex with suspicion. It construes and judges almost any sexual
practice in terms of its worst possible expression. Sex is presumed guilty until proven innocent. Virtually all erotic behaviour is considered bad unless a specific reason to exempt it has
been established. The most acceptable excuses are marriage, reproduction, and love. Sometimes scientific curiosity, aesthetic experience, or a long-term intimate relationship may
serve. But the exercise of erotic capacity, intelligence, curiosity, or creativity all require
pretexts that are unnecessary for other pleasures, such as the enjoyment of food, fiction, or
astronomy.

What I call the fallacy of misplaced scale is a corollary of sex negativity. Susan Sontag
once commented that since Christianity focused 'on sexual behaviour as the root of virtue,
everything pertaining to sex has been a "special case" in our culture' (Sontag, 1969, p. 46).
Sex law has incorporated the religious attitude that heretical sex is an especially heinous sin
that deserves the harshest punishments. Throughout much of European and American
history, a single act of consensual anal penetration was grounds for execution. In some states,
sodomy still carries twenty-year prison sentences. Outside the law, sex is also a marked category. Small differences in value or behaviour are often experienced as cosmic threats.
Although people can be intolerant, silly, or pushy about what constitutes proper diet, differences in menu rarely provoke the kinds of rage, anxiety, and sheer terror that routinely
accompany differences in erotic taste. Sexual acts are burdened with an excess of
significance.

Modern Western societies appraise sex acts according to a hierarchical system of sexual
value. Marital, reproductive heterosexuals are alone at the top erotic pyramid. Clamouring
below are unmarried monogamous heterosexuals in couples, followed by most other heterosexuals. Solitary sex floats ambiguously. The powerful nineteenth-century stigma on masturbation lingers in less potent, modified forms, such as the idea that masturbation is an
inferior substitute for partnered encounters. Stable, long-term lesbian and gay male couples
are verging on respectability, but bar dykes and promiscuous gay men are hovering just above
the groups at the very bottom of the pyramid. The most despised sexual castes currently
include transsexuals, transvestites, fetishists, sadomasochists, sex workers such as prostitutes
and porn models, and the lowliest of all, those whose eroticism transgresses generational
boundaries.

Individuals whose behaviour stands high in this hierarchy are rewarded with certified
mental health, respectability, legality, social and physical mobility, institutional support, and
material benefits. As sexual behaviours or occupations fall lower on the scale, the individuals
who practise them are subjected to a presumption of mental illness, disreputability, criminality, restricted social and physical mobility, loss of institutional support, and economic
sanctions.

Extreme and punitive stigma maintains some sexual behaviours as low status and is an effective sanction against those who engage in them. The intensity of this stigma is rooted in Western religious traditions. But most of its contemporary content derives from medical and psychiatric opprobrium.

The old religious taboos were primarily based on kinship forms of social organization. They were meant to deter inappropriate unions and to provide proper kin. Sex laws derived from Biblical pronouncements were aimed at preventing the acquisition of the wrong kinds of affinal partners: consanguineous kin (incest), the same gender (homosexuality), or the wrong species (bestiality). When medicine and psychiatry acquired extensive powers over sexuality, they were less concerned with unsuitable mates than with unfit forms of desire. If taboos against incest best characterized kinship systems of sexual organization, then the shift to an emphasis on taboos against masturbation was more apposite to the newer systems organized around qualities of erotic experience (Foucault, 1978, pp. 106–7).

Medicine and psychiatry multiplied the categories of sexual misconduct. The section on psychosexual disorders in the *Diagnostic and Statistical Manual of Mental and Physical Disorders* (*DSM*) of the American Psychiatric Association (APA) is a fairly reliable map of the current moral hierarchy of sexual activities. The APA list is much more elaborate than the traditional condemnations of whoring, sodomy, and adultery. The most recent edition, *DSM-III*, removed homosexuality from the roster of mental disorders after a long political struggle. But fetishism, sadism, masochism, transsexuality, transvestism, exhibitionism, voyeurism, and paedophilia are quite firmly entrenched as psychological malfunctions (American Psychiatric Association, 1980). Books are still being written about the genesis, aetiology, treatment, and cure of these assorted 'pathologies'.

Psychiatric condemnation of sexual behaviours invokes concepts of mental and emotional inferiority rather than categories of sexual sin. Low-status sex practices are vilified as mental diseases or symptoms of defective personality integration. In addition, psychological terms conflate difficulties of psycho-dynamic functioning with modes of erotic conduct. They equate sexual masochism with self-destructive personality patterns, sexual sadism with emotional aggression, and homoeroticism with immaturity. These terminological muddles have become powerful stereotypes that are indiscriminately applied to individuals on the basis of their sexual orientations.

Popular culture is permeated with ideas that erotic variety is dangerous, unhealthy, depraved, and a menace to everything from small children to national security. Popular sexual ideology is a noxious stew made up of ideas of sexual sin, concepts of psychological inferiority, anti-communism, mob hysteria, accusations of witchcraft, and xenophobia. The mass media nourish these attitudes with relentless propaganda. I would call this system of erotic stigma the last socially respectable form of prejudice if the old forms did not show such obstinate vitality, and new ones did not continually become apparent.

All these hierarchies of sexual value – religious, psychiatric, and popular – function in much the same ways as do ideological systems of racism, ethnocentrism, and religious chauvinism. They rationalize the well-being of the sexually privileged and the adversity of the sexual rabble.

Figure 9.1 diagrams a general version of the sexual value system. According to this system, sexuality that is 'good', 'normal', and 'natural' should ideally be heterosexual, marital, monogamous, reproductive, and non-commercial. It should be coupled, relational, within the same generation, and occur at home. It should not involve pornography, fetish objects, sex toys of any sort, or roles other than male and female. Any sex that violates these rules is 'bad', 'abnormal', or 'unnatural'. Bad sex may be homosexual, unmarried, promiscuous, non-procreative, or commercial. It may be masturbatory or take place at orgies, may be casual, may cross generational lines, and may take place in 'public', or at least in the bushes or the baths. It may involve the use of pornography, fetish objects, sex toys, or unusual roles (see Figure 9.1).

Figure 9.2 diagrams another aspect of the sexual hierarchy: the need to draw and maintain an imaginary line between good and bad sex. Most of the discourses on sex, be they religious, psychiatric, popular, or political, delimit a very small portion of human sexual capacity as sanctifiable, safe, healthy, mature, legal, or politically correct. The 'line' distinguishes these from all other erotic behaviours, which are understood to be the work of the devil, dangerous, psychopathological, infantile, or politically reprehensible. Arguments are then conducted over 'where to draw the line', and to determine what other activities, if any, may be permitted to cross over into acceptability.

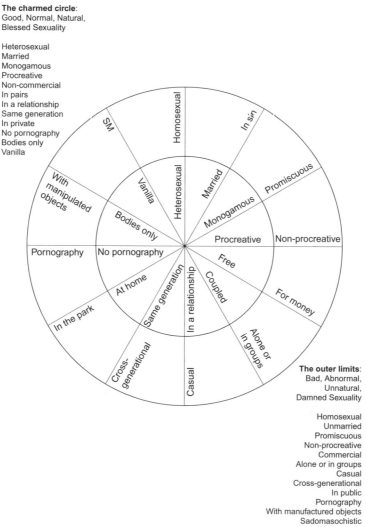

Figure 9.1 The sex hierarchy: the charmed circle vs. the outer limits

All these models assume a domino theory of sexual peril. The line appears to stand between sexual order and chaos. It expresses the fear that if anything is permitted to cross this erotic DMZ, the barrier against scary sex will crumble and something unspeakable will skitter across.

Most systems of sexual judgement – religious, psychological, feminist, or socialist – attempt to determine on which side of the line a particular act falls. Only sex acts on the good side of the line are accorded moral complexity. For instance, heterosexual encounters may be sublime or disgusting, free or forced, healing or destructive, romantic or mercenary. As long as it does not violate other rules, heterosexuality is acknowledged to exhibit the full range of human experience. In contrast, all sex acts on the bad side of the line are considered utterly repulsive and devoid of all emotional nuance. The further from the line a sex act is, the more it is depicted as a uniformly bad experience.

As a result of the sex conflicts of the last decade, some behaviour near the border is inching across it. Unmarried couples living together, masturbation, and some forms of homosexuality are moving in the direction of respectability (see Figure 9.2). Most homosexuality is still on the bad side of the line. But if it is coupled and monogamous, the society is beginning to recognize that it includes the full range of human interaction. Promiscuous homosexuality, sadomasochism, fetishism, transsexuality, and cross-generational encounters are still viewed as unmodulated horrors incapable of involving affection, love, free choice, kindness, or transcendence.

This kind of sexual morality has more in common with ideologies of racism than with true ethics. It grants virtue to the dominant groups, and relegates vice to the underprivileged. A democratic morality should judge sexual acts by the way partners treat one another, the level of mutual consideration, the presence or absence of coercion, and quantity and quality of the pleasures they provide. Whether sex acts are gay or straight, coupled or in groups, naked or in underwear, commercial or free, with or without video, should not be ethical concerns.

It is difficult to develop a pluralistic sexual ethics without a concept of benign sexual variation. Variation is a fundamental property of all life, from the simplest biological organisms to the most complex human social formations. Yet sexuality is supposed to conform to a single

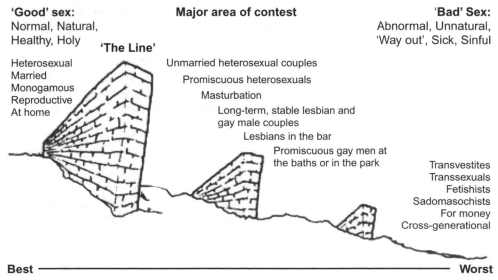

Figure 9.2 The sex hierarchy: the struggle over where to the draw the line

standard. One of the most tenacious ideas about sex is that there is one best way to do it, and that everyone should do it that way.

Most people find it difficult to grasp that whatever they like to do sexually will be thoroughly repulsive to someone else, and that whatever repels them sexually will be the most treasured delight of someone, somewhere. One need not like or perform a particular sex act in order to recognize that someone else will, and that this difference does not indicate a lack of good taste, mental health, or intelligence in either party. Most people mistake their sexual preferences for a universal system that will or should work for everyone.

This notion of a single ideal sexuality characterizes most systems of thought about sex. For religion, the ideal is procreative marriage. For psychology, it is mature heterosexuality. Although its content varies, the format of a single sexual standard is continually reconstituted within other rhetorical frameworks, including feminism and socialism. It is just as objectionable to insist that everyone should be lesbian, non-monogamous, or kinky, as to believe that everyone should be heterosexual, married, or vanilla – though the latter set of opinions are backed by considerably more coercive power than the former.

Progressives who would be ashamed to display cultural chauvinism in other areas routinely exhibit it towards sexual differences. We have learned to cherish different cultures as unique expressions of human inventiveness rather than as the inferior or disgusting habits of savages. We need a similarly anthropological understanding of different sexual cultures.

Empirical sex research is the one field that does incorporate a positive concept of sexual variation. Alfred Kinsey approached the study of sex with the same uninhibited curiosity he had previously applied to examining a species of wasp. His scientific detachment gave his work a refreshing neutrality that enraged moralists and caused immense controversy (Kinsey *et al.*, 1948, 1953). Among Kinsey's successors, John Gagnon and William Simon have pioneered the application of sociological understandings to erotic variety (Gagnon and Simon, 1967, 1970; Gagnon, 1977). Even some of the older sexology is useful. Although his work is imbued with unappetizing eugenic beliefs, Havelock Ellis was an acute and sympathetic observer. His monumental *Studies in the Psychology of Sex* is resplendent with detail (Ellis, 1936).

Much political writing on sexuality reveals complete ignorance of both classical sexology and modern sex research. Perhaps this is because so few colleges and universities bother to teach human sexuality, and because so much stigma adheres even to scholarly investigation of sex. Neither sexology nor sex research has been immune to the prevailing sexual value system. Both contain assumptions and information which should not be accepted uncritically. But sexology and sex research provide abundant detail, a welcome posture of calm, and a well-developed ability to treat sexual variety as something that exists rather than as something to be exterminated. These fields can provide an empirical grounding for a radical theory of sexuality more useful than the combination of psychoanalysis and feminist first principles to which so many texts resort.

Sexual transformation

As defined by the ancient civil or canonical codes, sodomy was a category of forbidden acts; their perpetrator was nothing more than the juridical subject of them. The nineteenth-century homosexual became a personage, a past, a case history, and a childhood, in addition to being a type of life, a life form, and a morphology, with an indiscreet anatomy and possibly a mysterious physiology ... The sodomite had been a temporary aberration; the homosexual was now a species (Foucault, 1978, p. 43).

In spite of many continuities with ancestral forms, modern sexual arrangements have a distinctive character which sets them apart from preexisting systems. In Western Europe and the United States, industrialization and urbanization reshaped the traditional rural and peasant populations into a new urban industrial and service workforce. It generated new forms of state apparatus, reorganized family relations, altered gender roles, made possible new forms of identity, produced new varieties of social inequality, and created new formats for political and ideological conflict. It also gave rise to a new sexual system characterized by distinct types of sexual persons, populations, stratification, and political conflict.

The writings of nineteenth-century sexology suggest the appearance of a kind of erotic speciation. However outlandish their explanations, the early sexologists were witnessing the emergence of new kinds of erotic individuals and their aggregation into rudimentary communities. The modern sexual system contains sets of these sexual populations, stratified by the operation of an ideological and social hierarchy. Differences in social value create friction among these groups, who engage in political contest to alter or maintain their place in the ranking. Contemporary sexual politics should be reconceptualized in terms of the emergence and on-going development of this system, its social relations, the ideologies that interpret it, and its characteristic modes of conflict.

Homosexuality is the best example of this process of erotic speciation. Homosexual behaviour is always present among humans. But in different societies and epochs it may be rewarded or punished, required or forbidden, a temporary experience or a life-long vocation. In some New Guinea societies, for example, homosexual activities are obligatory for all males. Homosexual acts are considered utterly masculine, roles are based on age, and partners are determined by kinship status (Baal, 1966; Herdt, 1981; Kelly, 1976; Rubin, 1974, 1982; Williams, 1936). Although these men engage in extensive homosexual and paedophile behaviour, they are neither homosexuals nor pederasts.

Nor was the sixteenth-century sodomite a homosexual. In 1631, Mervyn Touchet, Earl of Castlehaven, was tried and executed for sodomy. It is clear from the proceedings that the Earl was not understood by himself or anyone else to be a particular kind of sexual individual. 'While from the twentieth-century viewpoint Lord Castlehaven obviously suffered from psychosexual problems requiring the services of an analyst, from the seventeenth-century viewpoint he had deliberately broken the Law of God and the Laws of England, and required the simpler services of an executioner' (Bingham, 1971, p. 465). The Earl did not slip into his tightest doublet and waltz down to the nearest gay tavern to mingle with his fellow sodomists. He stayed in his manor house and buggered his servants. Gay self-awareness, gay pubs, the sense of group commonality, and even the term homosexual were not part of the Earl's universe.

The New Guinea bachelor and the sodomite nobleman are only tangentially related to a modern gay man, who may migrate from rural Colorado to San Francisco in order to live in a gay neighbourhood, work in a gay business, and participate in an elaborate experience that includes a self-conscious identity, group solidarity, a literature, a press, and a high level of political activity. In modern, Western, industrial societies, homosexuality has acquired much of the institutional structure of an ethnic group (Murray, 1979).

The relocation of homoeroticism into these quasi-ethnic, nucleated, sexually constituted communities is to some extent a consequence of the transfers of population brought by industrialization. As labourers migrated to work in cities, there were increased opportunities for voluntary communities to form. Homosexually inclined women and men, who would have been vulnerable and isolated in most pre-industrial villages, began to congregate in small corners of the big cities. Most large nineteenth-century cities in Western Europe and North

America had areas where men could cruise for other men. Lesbian communities seem to have coalesced more slowly and on a smaller scale. Nevertheless, by the 1890s, there were several cafes in Paris near the Place Pigalle that catered to a lesbian clientele, and it is likely that there were similar places in the other major capitals of Western Europe.

Areas like these acquired bad reputations, which alerted other interested individuals of their existence and location. In the United States, lesbian and gay male territories were well established in New York, Chicago, San Francisco, and Los Angeles in the 1950s. Sexually motivated migration to places such as Greenwich Village had become a sizable sociological phenomenon. By the late 1970s, sexual migration was occurring on a scale so significant that it began to have a recognizable impact on urban politics in the United States, with San Francisco being the most notable and notorious example.[11]

Prostitution has undergone a similar metamorphosis. Prostitution began to change from a temporary job to a more permanent occupation as a result of nineteenth-century agitation, legal reform, and police persecution. Prostitutes, who had been part of the general working-class population, became increasingly isolated as members of an outcast group (Walkowitz, 1980). Prostitutes and other sex workers differ from homosexuals and other sexual minorities. Sex work is an occupation, while sexual deviation is an erotic preference. Nevertheless, they share some common features of social organization. Like homosexuals, prostitutes are a criminal sexual population stigmatized on the basis of sexual activity. Prostitutes and male homosexuals are the primary prey of vice police everywhere.[12] Like gay men, prostitutes occupy well-demarcated urban territories and battle with police to defend and maintain those territories. The legal persecution of both populations is justified by an elaborate ideology that classifies them as dangerous and inferior undesirables who are not entitled to be left in peace.

Besides organizing homosexuals and prostitutes into localized populations, the 'modernization of sex' has generated a system of continual sexual ethnogenesis. Other populations of erotic dissidents – commonly known as the 'perversions' or the 'paraphilias' – also began to coalesce. Sexualities keep marching out of the *Diagnostic and Statistical Manual* and on to the pages of social history. At present, several other groups are trying to emulate the successes of homosexuals. Bisexuals, sadomasochists, individuals who prefer cross-generational encounters, transsexuals, and transvestites are all in various states of community formation and identity acquisition. The perversions are not proliferating as much as they are attempting to acquire social space, small businesses, political resources, and a measure of relief from the penalties for sexual heresy.

Sexual stratification

> An entire sub-race was born, different – despite certain kinship ties – from the libertines of the past. From the end of the eighteenth century to our own, they circulated through the pores of society; they were always hounded, but not always by laws; were often locked up, but not always in prisons; were sick perhaps, but scandalous, dangerous victims, prey to a strange evil that also bore the name of vice and sometimes crime. They were children wise beyond their years, precocious little girls, ambiguous schoolboys, dubious servants and educators, cruel or maniacal husbands, solitary collectors, ramblers with bizarre impulses; they haunted the houses of correction, the penal colonies, the tribunals, and the asylums; they carried their infamy to the doctors and their sickness to the judges. This was the numberless family of perverts who were on friendly terms with delinquents and akin to madmen.
>
> (Foucault, 1978, p. 40)

The industrial transformation of Western Europe and North America brought about new forms of social stratification. The resultant inequalities of class are well known and have been explored in detail by a century of scholarship. The construction of modern systems of racism and ethnic injustice has been well documented and critically assessed. Feminist thought has analysed the prevailing organization of gender oppression. But although specific erotic groups, such as militant homosexuals and sex workers, have agitated against their own mistreatment, there has been no equivalent attempt to locate particular varieties of sexual persecution within a more general system of sexual stratification. Nevertheless, such a system exists, and in its contemporary form it is a consequence of Western industrialization.

Sex law is the most adamantine instrument of sexual stratification and erotic persecution. The state routinely intervenes in sexual behaviour at a level that would not be tolerated in other areas of social life. Most people are unaware of the extent of sex law, the quantity and qualities of illegal sexual behaviour, and the punitive character of legal sanctions. Although federal agencies may be involved in obscenity and prostitution cases, most sex laws are enacted at the state and municipal level, and enforcement is largely in the hands of local police. Thus, there is a tremendous amount of variation in the laws applicable to any given locale. Moreover, enforcement of sex laws varies dramatically with the local political climate. In spite of this legal thicket, one can make some tentative and qualified generalizations. My discussion of sex law does not apply to laws against sexual coercion, sexual assault, or rape. It does pertain to the myriad prohibitions on consensual sex and the 'status' offences such as statutory rape.

Sex law is harsh. The penalties for violating sex statutes are universally out of proportion to any social or individual harm. A single act of consensual but illicit sex, such as placing one's lips upon the genitalia of an enthusiastic partner, is punished in many states with more severity than rape, battery, or murder. Each such genital kiss, each lewd caress, is a separate crime. It is therefore painfully easy to commit multiple felonies in the course of a single evening of illegal passion. Once someone is convicted of a sex violation, a second performance of the same act is grounds for prosecution as a repeat offender, in which case penalties will be even more severe. In some states, individuals have become repeat felons for having engaged in homosexual love-making on two separate occasions. Once an erotic activity has been proscribed by sex law, the full power of the state enforces conformity to the values embodied in those laws. Sex laws are notoriously easy to pass, as legislators are loath to be soft on vice. Once on the books, they are extremely difficult to dislodge.

Sex law is not a perfect reflection of the prevailing moral evaluations of sexual conduct. Sexual variation *per se* is more specifically policed by the mental-health professions, popular ideology, and extra-legal social practice. Some of the most detested erotic behaviours, such as fetishism and sadomasochism, are not as closely or completely regulated by the criminal justice system as somewhat less stigmatized practices, such as homosexuality. Areas of sexual behaviour come under the purview of the law when they become objects of social concern and political uproar. Each sex scare or morality campaign deposits new regulations as a kind of fossil record of its passage. The legal sediment is thickest – and sex law has its greatest potency – in areas involving obscenity, money, minors, and homosexuality.

Obscenity laws enforce a powerful taboo against direct representation of erotic activities. Current emphasis on the ways in which sexuality has become a focus of social attention should not be misused to undermine a critique of this prohibition. It is one thing to create sexual discourse in the form of psychoanalysis, or in the course of a morality crusade. It is quite another to depict sex acts or genitalia graphically. The first is socially permissible in a way the second is not. Sexual speech is forced into reticence, euphemism, and indirection.

Freedom of speech about sex is a glaring exception to the protections of the First Amendment, which is not even considered applicable to purely sexual statements.

The anti-obscenity laws also form part of a group of statutes that make almost all sexual commerce illegal. Sex law incorporates a very strong prohibition against mixing sex and money, except via marriage. In addition to the obscenity statutes, other laws impinging on sexual commerce include anti-prostitution laws, alcoholic-beverage regulations, and ordinances governing the location and operation of 'adult' businesses. The sex industry and the gay economy have both managed to circumvent some of this legislation, but that process has not been easy or simple. The underlying criminality of sex-oriented business keeps it marginal, underdeveloped, and distorted. Sex businesses can only operate in legal loopholes. This tends to keep investment down and to divert commercial activity towards the goal of staying out of jail rather than delivery of goods and services. It also renders sex workers more vulnerable to exploitation and bad working conditions. If sex commerce were legal, sex workers would be more able to organize and agitate for higher pay, better conditions, greater control, and less stigma.

Whatever one thinks of the limitations of capitalist commerce, such an extreme exclusion from the market process would hardly be socially acceptable in other areas of activity. Imagine, for example, that the exchange of money for medical care, pharmacological advice, or psychological counselling were illegal. Medical practice would take place in a much less satisfactory fashion if doctors, nurses, druggists, and therapists could be hauled off to jail at the whim of the local 'health squad'. But that is essentially the situation of prostitutes, sex workers, and sex entrepreneurs.

Marx himself considered the capitalist market a revolutionary, if limited, force. He argued that capitalism was progressive in its dissolution of pre-capitalist superstition, prejudice, and the bonds of traditional modes of life. 'Hence the great civilizing influence of capital, its production of a state of society compared with which all earlier stages appear to be merely local progress and idolatry of nature' (Marx, 1971, p. 94). Keeping sex from realizing the positive effects of the market economy hardly makes it socialist.

The law is especially ferocious in maintaining the boundary between childhood 'innocence' and 'adult' sexuality. Rather than recognizing the sexuality of the young, and attempting to provide for it in a caring and responsible manner, our culture denies and punishes erotic interest and activity by anyone under the local age of consent. The amount of law devoted to protecting young people from premature exposure to sexuality is breathtaking.

The primary mechanism for insuring the separation of sexual generations is age of consent laws. These laws make no distinction between the most brutal rape and the most gentle romance. A 20-year-old convicted of sexual contact with a 17-year-old will face a severe sentence in virtually every state, regardless of the nature of the relationship (Norton, 1981).[13] Nor are minors permitted access to 'adult' sexuality in other forms. They are forbidden to see books, movies, or television in which sexuality is 'too' graphically portrayed. It is legal for young people to see hideous depictions of violence, but not to see explicit pictures of genitalia. Sexually active young people are frequently incarcerated in juvenile homes, or otherwise punished for their 'precocity'.

Adults who deviate too much from conventional standards of sexual conduct are often denied contact with the young, even their own. Custody laws permit the state to steal the children of anyone whose erotic activities appear questionable to a judge presiding over family court matters. Countless lesbians, gay men, prostitutes, swingers, sex workers, and 'promiscuous' women have been declared unfit parents under such provisions. Members of the teaching professions are closely monitored for signs of sexual misconduct. In most states, certification laws require that teachers arrested for sex offences lose their jobs and credentials. In some cases, a teacher may be fired merely because an unconventional lifestyle becomes known to school officials. Moral turpitude is one of the few legal grounds for revoking academic tenure (Beserra, Franklin and Clevenger, 1977, pp. 165–7). The more influence one has over the next generation, the less latitude one is permitted in behaviour and opinion. The coercive power of the law ensures the transmission of conservative sexual values with these kinds of controls over parenting and teaching.

The only adult sexual behaviour that is legal in every state is the placement of the penis in the vagina in wedlock. Consenting adults statutes ameliorate this situation in fewer than half the states. Most states impose severe criminal penalties on consensual sodomy, homosexual contact short of sodomy, adultery, seduction, and adult incest. Sodomy laws vary a great deal. In some states, they apply equally to homosexual and heterosexual partners and regardless of marital status. Some state courts have ruled that married couples have the right to commit sodomy in private. Only homosexual sodomy is illegal in some states. Some sodomy statutes prohibit both anal sex and oral–genital contact. In other states, sodomy applies only to anal penetration, and oral sex is covered under separate statutes (Beserra *et al.*, 1973, pp. 163–8).[14]

Laws like these criminalize sexual behaviour that is freely chosen and avidly sought. The ideology embodied in them reflects the value hierarchies discussed above. That is, some sex acts are considered to be so intrinsically vile that no one should be allowed under any circumstance to perform them. The fact that individuals consent to or even prefer them is taken to be additional evidence of depravity. This system of sex law is similar to legalized racism. State prohibition of same-sex contact, anal penetration, and oral sex make homosexuals a criminal group denied the privileges of full citizenship. With such laws, prosecution is persecution. Even when the laws are not strictly enforced, as is usually the case, the members of criminalized sexual communities remain vulnerable to the possibility of arbitrary arrest, or to periods in which they become the objects of social panic. When those occur, the laws are in place and police action is swift. Even sporadic enforcement serves to remind individuals that they are members of a subject population. The occasional arrest for sodomy, lewd behaviour, solicitation, or oral sex keeps everyone else afraid, nervous, and circumspect.

The state also upholds the sexual hierarchy through bureaucratic regulation. Immigration policy still prohibits the admission of homosexuals (and other sexual 'deviates') into the United States. Military regulations bar homosexuals from serving in the armed forces. The fact that gay people cannot legally marry means that they cannot enjoy the same legal rights as heterosexuals in many matters, including inheritance, taxation, protection from testimony in court, and the acquisition of citizenship for foreign partners. These are but a few of the ways that the state reflects and maintains the social relations of sexuality. The law buttresses structures of power, codes of behaviour, and forms of prejudice. At their worst, sex law and sex regulation are simply sexual apartheid.

Although the legal apparatus of sex is staggering, most everyday social control is extralegal. Less formal, but very effective social sanctions are imposed on members of 'inferior' sexual populations.

In her marvellous ethnographic study of gay life in the 1960s, Esther Newton observed that the homosexual population was divided into what she called the 'overts' and 'coverts'. 'The overts live their entire working lives within the context of the [gay] community; the coverts live their *entire nonworking* lives within it' (Newton, 1972, p. 21, emphasis in the original). At the time of Newton's study, the gay community provided far fewer jobs than it does now, and the non-gay work world was almost completely intolerant of homosexuality. There were some fortunate individuals who could be openly gay and earn decent salaries. But the vast majority of homosexuals had to choose between honest poverty and the strain of maintaining a false identity.

Though this situation has changed a great deal, discrimination against gay people is still rampant. For the bulk of the gay population, being out on the job is still impossible. Generally, the more important and higher paid the job, the less the society will tolerate overt erotic deviance. If it is difficult for gay people to find employment where they do not have to pretend, it is doubly and triply so for more exotically sexed individuals. Sadomasochists leave their fetish clothes at home, and know that they must be especially careful to conceal their real identities. An exposed paedophile would probably be stoned out of the office. Having to maintain such absolute secrecy is a considerable burden. Even those who are content to be secretive may be exposed by some accidental event. Individuals who are erotically unconventional risk being unemployable or unable to pursue their chosen careers.

Public officials and anyone who occupies a position of social consequence are especially vulnerable. A sex scandal is the surest method for hounding someone out of office or destroying a political career. The fact that important people are expected to conform to the strictest standards of erotic conduct discourages sex perverts of all kinds from seeking such positions. Instead, erotic dissidents are channelled into positions that have less impact on the mainstream of social activity and opinion.

The expansion of the gay economy in the last decade has provided some employment alternatives and some relief from job discrimination against homosexuals. But most of the jobs provided by the gay economy are low-status and low-paying. Bartenders, bathhouse attendants, and disc jockeys are not bank officers or corporate executives. Many of the sexual migrants who flock to places like San Francisco are downwardly mobile. They face intense competition for choice positions. The influx of sexual migrants provides a pool of cheap and exploitable labour for many of the city's businesses, both gay and straight.

Families play a crucial role in enforcing sexual conformity. Much social pressure is brought to bear to deny erotic dissidents the comforts and resources that families provide. Popular ideology holds that families are not supposed to produce or harbour erotic nonconformity. Many families respond by trying to reform, punish, or exile sexually offending members. Many sexual migrants have been thrown out by their families, and many others are fleeing from the threat of institutionalization. Any random collection of homosexuals, sex workers, or miscellaneous perverts can provide heartstopping stories of rejection and mistreatment by horrified families. Christmas is the great family holiday in the United States and consequently it is a time of considerable tension in the gay community. Half the inhabitants go off to their families of origin; many of those who remain in the gay ghettos cannot do so, and relive their anger and grief.

In addition to economic penalties and strain on family relations, the stigma of erotic dissidence creates friction at all other levels of everyday life. The general public helps to penalize erotic non-conformity when, according to the values they have been taught, landlords refuse housing, neighbours call in the police, and hoodlums commit sanctioned battery. The ideologies of erotic inferiority and sexual danger decrease the power of sex perverts and sex workers in social encounters of all kinds. They have less protection from unscrupulous or criminal behaviour, less access to police protection, and less recourse to the courts. Dealings with institutions and bureaucracies – hospital, police coroners, banks, public officials – are more difficult.

Sex is a vector of oppression. The system of sexual oppression cuts across other modes of social inequality, sorting out individuals and groups according to its own intrinsic dynamics. It is not reducible to, or understandable in terms of, class, race, ethnicity, or gender. Wealth, white skin, male gender, and ethnic privileges can mitigate the effects of sexual stratification. A rich, white male pervert will generally be less affected than a poor, black, female pervert. But even the most privileged are not immune to sexual oppression. Some of the consequences of the system of sexual hierarchy are mere nuisances. Others are quite grave. In its most serious manifestations, the sexual system is a Kafkaesque nightmare in which unlucky victims become herds of human cattle whose identification, surveillance, apprehension, treatment, incarceration, and punishment produce jobs and self-satisfaction for thousands of vice police, prison officials, psychiatrists, and social workers.[15]

Sexual conflicts

> The moral panic crystallizes widespread fears and anxieties, and often deals with them not by seeking the real causes of the problems and conditions which they demonstrate but by displacing them on to 'Folk Devils' in an identified social group (often the 'immoral' or 'degenerate'). Sexuality has had a peculiar centrality in such panics, and sexual 'deviants' have been omnipresent scapegoats.
>
> (Weeks, 1981, p. 14)

The sexual system is not a monolithic, omnipotent structure. There are continuous battles over the definitions, evaluations, arrangements, privileges, and costs of sexual behaviour. Political struggle over sex assumes characteristic forms.

Sexual ideology plays a crucial role in sexual experience. Consequently, definitions and evaluations of sexual conduct are objects of bitter contest. The confrontations between early gay liberation and the psychiatric establishment are the best example of this kind of fight, but there are constant skirmishes. Recurrent battles take place between the primary producers of sexual ideology – the churches, the family, the shrinks, and the media – and the groups whose experience they name, distort, and endanger.

The legal regulation of sexual conduct is another battleground. Lysander Spooner dissected the system of state-sanctioned moral coercion over a century ago in a text inspired primarily by the temperance campaigns. In *Vices Are Not Crimes: A Vindication of Moral Liberty*, Spooner argued that government should protect its citizens against crime, but that it is foolish, unjust, and tyrannical to legislate against vice. He discusses rationalizations still heard today in defence of legalized moralism – that 'vices' (Spooner is referring to drink, but homosexuality, prostitution, or recreational drug use may be substituted) lead to crimes, and should therefore be prevented; that those who practise 'vice' are *non compos mentis* and should therefore be protected from their self-destruction by state-accomplished ruin; and that children must be protected from supposedly harmful knowledge (Spooner, 1977). The discourse on victimless crimes has not changed much. Legal struggle over sex law will continue until basic freedoms of sexual action and expression are guaranteed. This requires the repeal of all sex laws except those few that deal with actual, not statutory, coercion; and it entails the abolition of vice squads, whose job it is to enforce legislated morality.

In addition to the definitional and legal wars, there are less obvious forms of sexual political conflict which I call the territorial and border wars. The processes by which erotic minorities form communities and the forces that seek to inhibit them lead to struggles over the nature and boundaries of sexual zones.

Dissident sexuality is rarer and more closely monitored in small towns and rural areas. Consequently, metropolitan life continually beckons to young perverts. Sexual migration creates concentrated pools of potential partners, friends, and associates. It enables individuals to create adult, kin-like networks in which to live. But there are many barriers which sexual migrants have to overcome.

According to the mainstream media and popular prejudice, the marginal sexual worlds are bleak and dangerous. They are portrayed as impoverished, ugly, and inhabited by psychopaths and criminals. New migrants must be sufficiently motivated to resist the impact of such discouraging images. Attempts to counter negative propaganda with more realistic information generally meet with censorship, and there are continuous ideological struggles over which representations of sexual communities make it into the popular media.

Information on how to find, occupy, and live in the marginal sexual worlds is also suppressed. Navigational guides are scarce and inaccurate. In the past, fragments of rumour, distorted gossip, and bad publicity were the most available clues to the location of underground erotic communities. During the late 1960s and early 1970s, better information became available. Now groups like the Moral Majority want to rebuild the ideological walls around the sexual undergrounds and make transit in and out of them as difficult as possible.

Migration is expensive. Transportation costs, moving expenses, and the necessity of finding new jobs and housing are economic difficulties that sexual migrants must overcome. These are especially imposing barriers to the young, who are often the most desperate to move. There are, however, routes into the erotic communities that mark trails through the propaganda thicket and provide some economic shelter along the way. Higher education can be a route for young people from affluent backgrounds. In spite of serious limitations, the information on sexual behaviour at most colleges and universities is better than elsewhere, and most colleges and universities shelter small erotic networks of all sorts.

For poorer kids, the military is often the easiest way to get the hell out of wherever they are. Military prohibitions against homosexuality make this a perilous route. Although young queers continually attempt to use the armed forces to get out of intolerable hometown situations and closer to functional gay communities, they face the hazards of exposure, court martial, and dishonourable discharge.

Once in the cities, erotic populations tend to nucleate and to occupy some regular, visible territory. Churches and other anti-vice forces constantly put pressure on local authorities to contain such areas, reduce their visibility, or to drive their inhabitants out of town. There are periodic crackdowns in which local vice squads are unleashed on the populations they control. Gay men, prostitutes, and sometimes transvestites are sufficiently territorial and numerous to engage in intense battles with the cops over particular streets, parks, and alleys. Such border wars are usually inconclusive, but they result in many casualties.

For most of this century, the sexual underworlds have been marginal and impoverished, their residents subjected to stress and exploitation. The spectacular success of gay entrepreneurs in creating a variegated gay economy has altered the quality of life within the gay ghetto. The level of material comfort and social elaboration achieved by the gay community in the last fifteen years is unprecedented. But it is important to recall what happened to similar miracles. The growth of the black population in New York in the early part of the twentieth century led to the Harlem Renaissance, but that period of creativity was doused by the Depression. The relative prosperity and cultural florescence of the ghetto may be equally fragile. Like blacks who fled the South for the metropolitan North, homosexuals may have merely traded rural problems for urban ones.

Gay pioneers occupied neighbourhoods that were centrally located but run down. Consequently, they border poor neighbourhoods. Gays, especially low-income gays, end up competing with other low-income groups for the limited supply of cheap and moderate housing. In San Francisco, competition for low-cost housing has exacerbated both racism and homophobia, and is one source of the epidemic of street violence against homosexuals. Instead of being isolated and invisible in rural settings, city gays are now numerous and obvious targets for urban frustrations.

In San Francisco, unbridled construction of downtown skyscrapers and high-cost condominiums is causing affordable housing to evaporate. Megabuck construction is creating pressure on all city residents. Poor gay renters are visible in low-income neighbourhoods; multimillionaire contractors are not. The spectre of the 'homosexual invasion' is a convenient scapegoat, which deflects attention from the banks, the planning commission, the political establishment, and the big developers. In San Francisco, the well-being of the gay community has become embroiled in the high-stakes politics of urban real estate.

Downtown expansion affects all the territorial erotic underworlds. In both San Francisco and New York, high investment construction and urban renewal have intruded on the main areas of prostitution, pornography, and leather bars. Developers are salivating over Times Square, the Tenderloin, what is left of North Beach, and South of Market. Anti-sex ideology, obscenity law, prostitution regulations, and the alcoholic beverage codes are all being used to dislodge seedy adult business, sex workers, and leathermen. Within ten years, most of these areas will have been bulldozed and made safe for convention centres, international hotels, corporate headquarters, and housing for the rich.

The most important and consequential kind of sex conflict is what Jeffrey Weeks has termed the 'moral panic'. Moral panics are the 'political moment' of sex, in which diffuse attitudes are channelled into political action and from there into social change.[16] The white-slavery hysteria of the 1880s, the anti-homosexual campaigns of the 1950s, and the child pornography panic of the late 1970s were typical moral panics.

Because sexuality in Western societies is so mystified, the wars over it are often fought at oblique angles, aimed at phony targets, conducted with misplaced passions, and are highly, intensely symbolic. Sexual activities often function as signifiers for personal and social apprehensions to which they have no intrinsic connection. During a moral panic such fears attach to some unfortunate sexual activity or population. The media become ablaze with indignation, the public behaves like a rabid mob, the police are activated, and the state enacts new laws and regulations. When the furor has passed, some innocent erotic group has been decimated, and the state has extended its power into new areas of erotic behaviour.

The system of sexual stratification provides easy victims who lack the power to defend themselves, and a preexisting apparatus for controlling their movements and curtailing their freedoms. The stigma against sexual dissidents renders them morally defenceless. Every moral panic has consequences on two levels. The target population suffers most, but everyone is affected by the social and legal changes.

Moral panics rarely alleviate any real problem, because they are aimed at chimeras and signifiers. They draw on the pre-existing discursive structure which invents victims in order to justify treating 'vices' as crimes. The criminalization of innocuous behaviours such as homosexuality, prostitution, obscenity, or recreational drug use, is rationalized by portraying them as menaces to health and safety, women and children, national security, the family, or civilization itself. Even when an activity is acknowledged to be harmless, it may be banned because it is alleged to 'lead' to something ostensibly worse (another manifestation of the domino theory).[17] Great and mighty edifices have been built on the basis of such phantasms. Generally, the outbreak of a moral panic is preceded by an intensification of such scapegoating.

It is always risky to prophesy. But it does not take much prescience to detect potential moral panics in two current developments: the attacks on sadomasochists by a segment of the feminist movement, and the right's increasing use of AIDS to incite virulent homophobia.

Feminist anti-pornography ideology has always contained an implied, and sometimes overt, indictment of sadomasochism. The pictures of sucking and fucking that comprise the bulk of pornography may be unnerving to those who are not familiar with them. But it is hard to make a convincing case that such images are violent. All of the early anti-porn slide shows used a highly selective sample of S/M imagery to sell a very flimsy analysis. Taken out of context, such images are often shocking. This shock value was mercilessly exploited to scare audiences into accepting the anti-porn perspective.

A great deal of anti-porn propaganda implies sadomasochism is the underlying and essential 'truth' towards which all pornography tends. Porn is thought to lead to S/M porn which in turn is alleged to lead to rape. This is a just-so story that revitalizes the notion that sex perverts commit sex crimes, not normal people. There is no evidence that the readers of S/M erotica or practising sadomasochists commit a disproportionate number of sex crimes. Anti-porn literature scapegoats an unpopular sexual minority and its reading material for social problems they do not create.

The use of S/M imagery in anti-porn discourse is inflammatory. It implies that the way to make the world safe for women is to get rid of sadomasochism. The use of S/M images in the movie *Not a Love Story* was on a moral par with the use of depictions of black men raping white women, or of drooling old Jews pawing young Aryan girls, to incite racist or anti-Semitic frenzy.

Feminist rhetoric has a distressing tendency to reappear in reactionary contexts. For example, in 1980 and 1981, Pope John Paul II delivered a series of pronouncements reaffirming his commitment to the most conservative and Pauline understandings of human sexuality. In condemning divorce, abortion, trial marriage, pornography, prostitution, birth control, unbridled hedonism, and lust, the pope employed a great deal of feminist rhetoric about sexual objectification. Sounding like lesbian feminist polemicist Julia Penelope, His Holiness explained that 'considering anyone in a lustful way makes that person a sexual object rather than a human being worthy of dignity'.[18]

The right wing opposes pornography and has already adopted elements of feminist anti-porn rhetoric. The anti-S/M discourse developed in the women's movement could easily become a vehicle for a moral witch hunt. It provides a ready-made defenceless target population. It provides a rationale for the recriminalization of sexual materials that have escaped the reach of current obscenity laws. It would be especially easy to pass laws against S/M erotica resembling the child pornography laws. The ostensible purpose of such laws would be to reduce violence by banning so-called violent porn. A focused campaign against the leather menace might also result in the passage of laws to criminalize S/M behaviour that is not currently illegal. The ultimate result of such a moral panic would be the legalized violation of a community of harmless perverts. It is dubious that such a sexual witch hunt would make any appreciable contribution towards reducing violence against women.

An AIDS panic is even more probable. When fears of incurable disease mingle with sexual terror, the resulting brew is extremely volatile. A century ago, attempts to control syphilis led to the passage of the Contagious Diseases Acts in England. The Acts were based on erroneous medical theories and did nothing to halt the spread of the disease. But they did make life miserable for the hundreds of women who were incarcerated, subjected to forcible vaginal examination, and stigmatized for life as prostitutes (Walkowitz, 1980; Weeks, 1981).

Whatever happens, AIDS will have far-reaching consequences on sex in general, and on homosexuality in particular. The disease will have a significant impact on the choices gay people make. Fewer will migrate to the gay meccas out of fear of the disease. Those who already reside in the ghettos will avoid situations they fear will expose them. The gay economy, and political apparatus it supports, may prove to be evanescent. Fear of AIDS has already affected sexual ideology. Just when homosexuals have had some success in throwing off the taint of mental disease, gay people find themselves metaphorically welded to an image of lethal physical deterioration. The syndrome, its peculiar qualities, and its transmissibility are being used to reinforce old fears that sexual activity, homosexuality, and promiscuity led to disease and death.

AIDS is both a personal tragedy for those who contract the syndrome and a calamity for the gay community. Homophobes have gleefully hastened to turn this tragedy against its victims. One columnist has suggested that AIDS has always existed, that the Biblical prohibitions on sodomy were designed to protect people from AIDS, and that AIDS is therefore an appropriate punishment for violating the Levitical codes. Using fear of infection as a rationale, local right-wingers attempted to ban the gay rodeo from Reno, Nevada. A recent issue of the *Moral Majority Report* featured a picture of a 'typical' white family of four wearing surgical masks. The headline read: 'AIDS: HOMOSEXUAL DISEASES THREATEN AMERICAN FAMILIES'.[19] Phyllis Schlafly has recently issued a pamphlet arguing that passage of the Equal Rights Amendment would make it impossible to 'legally protect ourselves against AIDS and other diseases carried by homosexuals' (cited in Bush, 1983, p. 60). Current right-wing literature calls for shutting down the gay baths, for a legal ban on homosexual employment in food-handling occupations, and for state-mandated prohibitions on blood donations by gay people. Such policies would require the government to identify all homosexuals and impose easily recognizable legal and social markers on them.

It is bad enough that the gay community must deal with the medical misfortune of having been the population in which a deadly disease first became widespread and visible. It is worse to have to deal with the social consequences as well. Even before the AIDS scare, Greece passed a law that enables police to arrest suspected homosexuals and force them to submit to an examination for venereal disease. It is likely that until AIDS and its methods of transmission are understood, there will be all sorts of proposals to control it by punishing the gay community and by attacking its institutions. When the cause of Legionnaires' Disease was unknown, there were no calls to quarantine members of the American Legion or to shut down their meeting halls. The Contagious Diseases Acts in England did little to control syphilis, but they caused a great deal of suffering for the women who came under their purview. The history of panic that has accompanied new epidemics, and of the casualties incurred by their scapegoats, should make everyone pause and consider with extreme scepticism any attempts to justify anti-gay policy initiatives on the basis of AIDS.

The limits of feminism

> We know that in an overwhelmingly large number of cases, sex crime is associated with pornography. We know that sex criminals read it, are clearly influenced by it. I believe that, if we can eliminate the distribution of such items among impressionable children, we shall greatly reduce our frightening sex-crime rate.
>
> (J. Edgar Hoover, cited in Hyde, 1965, p. 31)

In the absence of a more articulated radical theory of sex, most progressives have turned to feminism for guidance. But the relationship between feminism and sex is complex. Because sexuality is a nexus of relationships between genders, much of the oppression of women is borne by, mediated through, and constituted within, sexuality. Feminism has always been vitally interested in sex. But there have been two strains of feminist thought on the subject. One tendency has criticized the restrictions on women's sexual behaviour and denounced the high costs imposed on women for being sexually active. This tradition of feminist sexual thought has called for a sexual liberation that would work for women as well as for men. The second tendency has considered sexual liberalization to be inherently a mere extension of male privilege. This tradition resonates with conservative, anti-sexual discourse. With the advent of the anti-pornography movement, it achieved temporary hegemony over feminist analysis.

The anti-pornography movement and its texts have been the most extensive expression of this discourse.[20] In addition, proponents of this viewpoint have condemned virtually every variant of sexual expression as anti-feminist. Within this framework, monogamous lesbianism that occurs within long-term, intimate relationships and which does not involve playing with polarized roles, has replaced married, procreative heterosexuality at the top of the value hierarchy. Heterosexuality has been demoted to somewhere in the middle. Apart from this change, everything else looks more or less familiar. The lower depths are occupied by the usual groups and behaviours: prostitution, transsexuality, sadomasochism, and cross-generational activities (Barry, 1979, 1982; Linden *et al.*, 1982; Raymond, 1979; Rush, 1980). Most gay male conduct, all casual sex, promiscuity, and lesbian behaviour that does involve roles or kink or non-monogamy are also censured.[21] Even sexual fantasy during masturbation is denounced as a phallocentric holdover (Penelope, 1980).

This discourse on sexuality is less a sexology than a demonology. It presents most sexual behaviour in the worst possible light. Its descriptions of erotic conduct always use the worst available example as if it were representative. It presents the most disgusting pornography, the most exploited forms of prostitution, and the least palatable or most shocking manifestations of sexual variation. This rhetorical tactic consistently misrepresents human sexuality in all its forms. The picture of human sexuality that emerges from this literature is unremittingly ugly.

In addition, this anti-porn rhetoric is a massive exercise in scapegoating. It criticizes non-routine acts of love rather than routine acts of oppression, exploitation, or violence. This demon sexology directs legitimate anger at women's lack of personal safety against innocent individuals, practices, and communities. Anti-porn propaganda often implies that sexism originates within the commercial sex industry and subsequently infects the rest of society. This is sociologically nonsensical. The sex industry is hardly a feminist utopia. It reflects the sexism that exists in the society as a whole. We need to analyse and oppose the manifestations of gender inequality specific to the sex industry. But this is not the same as attempting to wipe out commercial sex.

Similarly, erotic minorities such as sadomasochists and transsexuals are as likely to exhibit sexist attitudes or behaviour as any other politically random social grouping. But to claim that they are inherently anti-feminist is sheer fantasy. A good deal of current feminist literature attributes the oppression of women to graphic representations of sex, prostitution, sex education, sadomasochism, male homosexuality, and transsexualism. Whatever happened to the family, religion, education, child-rearing practices, the media, the state, psychiatry, job discrimination, and unequal pay?

Finally, this so-called feminist discourse recreates a very conservative sexual morality. For over a century, battles have been waged over just how much shame, distress, and punishment should be incurred by sexual activity. The conservative tradition has promoted opposition to pornography, prostitution, homosexuality, all erotic variation, sex education, sex research, abortion, and contraception. The opposing, pro-sex tradition has included individuals such as Havelock Ellis, Magnus Hirschfeld, Alfred Kinsey, and Victoria Woodhull, as well as the sex-education movement, organizations of militant prostitutes and homosexuals, the reproductive rights movement, and organizations such as the Sexual Reform League of the 1960s. This motley collection of sex reformers, sex educators, and sexual militants has mixed records on both sexual and feminist issues. But surely they are closer to the spirit of modern feminism than are moral crusaders, the social purity movement, and anti-vice organizations. Nevertheless, the current feminist sexual demonology generally elevates the anti-vice crusaders to positions of ancestral honour, while condemning the more liberatory tradition as anti-feminist. In an essay that exemplifies some of these trends, Sheila Jeffreys blames Havelock Ellis, Edward Carpenter, Alexandra Kollantai, 'believers in the joy of sex of every possible political persuasion', and the 1929 congress of the World League for Sex Reform for making 'a great contribution to the defeat of militant feminism' (Jeffreys, 1981, p. 26).[22]

The anti-pornography movement and its avatars have claimed to speak for all feminism. Fortunately, they do not. Sexual liberation has been and continues to be a feminist goal. The women's movement may have produced some of the most retrogressive sexual thinking this side of the Vatican. But it has also produced an exciting, innovative, and articulate defence of sexual pleasure and erotic justice. This 'pro-sex' feminism has been spearheaded by lesbians whose sexuality does not conform to movement standards of purity (primarily lesbian sadomasochists and butch/femme dykes), by unapologetic heterosexuals, and by women who adhere to classic radical feminism rather than to the revisionist celebrations of femininity that have become so common.[23] Although the anti-porn forces have attempted to weed anyone who disagrees with them out of the movement, the fact remains that feminist thought about sex is profoundly polarized (Orlando, 1982b; Willis, 1982).

Whenever there is polarization, there is an unhappy tendency to think the truth lies somewhere in between. Ellen Willis has commented sarcastically that 'the feminist bias is that women are equal to men and the male chauvinist bias is that women are inferior. The unbiased view is that the truth lies somewhere in between' (Willis, 1982, p. 146).[24] The most recent development in the feminist sex wars is the emergence of a 'middle' that seeks to evade the dangers of anti-porn fascism, on the one hand, and a supposed 'anything goes' libertarianism, on the other.[25] Although it is hard to criticize a position that is not yet fully formed, I want to draw attention to some incipient problems.

The emergent middle is based on a false characterization of the poles of debate, construing both sides as equally extremist. According to B. Ruby Rich, 'the desire for a language of sexuality has led feminists into locations (pornography, sadomasochism) too narrow or overdetermined for a fruitful discussion. Debate has collapsed into a rumble' (Rich, 1983, p. 76). True, the fights between Women Against Pornography (WAP) and lesbian sadomasochists have resembled gang warfare. But the responsibility for this lies primarily with the anti-porn movement, and its refusal to engage in principled discussion. S/M lesbians have been forced into a struggle to maintain their membership in the movement, and to defend themselves against slander. No major spokeswoman for lesbian S/M has argued for any kind of S/M supremacy, or advocated that everyone should be a sadomasochist. In addition to self-defence, S/M lesbians have called for appreciation for erotic diversity and more open discussion of sexuality (Samois, 1979, 1982; Califia, 1980e, 1981a). Trying to find a middle course between WAP and Samois is a bit like saying that the truth about homosexuality lies somewhere between the positions of the Moral Majority and those of the gay movement.

In political life, it is all too easy to marginalize radicals, and to attempt to buy acceptance for a moderate position by portraying others as extremists. Liberals have done this for years to communists. Sexual radicals have opened up the sex debates. It is shameful to deny their contribution, misrepresent their positions, and further their stigmatization.

In contrast to cultural feminists, who simply want to purge sexual dissidents, the sexual moderates are willing to defend the rights of erotic non-conformists to political participation. Yet this defence of political rights is linked to an implicit system of ideological condescension. The argument has two major parts. The first is an accusation that sexual dissidents have not paid close enough attention to the meaning, sources, or historical construction of their sexuality. This emphasis on meaning appears to function in much the same way that the question of aetiology has functioned in discussions of homosexuality. That is, homosexuality, sadomasochism, prostitution, or boy-love are taken to be mysterious and problematic in some way that more respectable sexualities are not. The search for a cause is a search for something that could change so that these 'problematic' eroticisms would simply not occur. Sexual militants have replied to such exercises that although the question of aetiology or cause is of intellectual interest, it is not high on the political agenda and that, moreover, the privileging of such questions is itself a regressive political choice.

The second part of the 'moderate' position focuses on questions of consent. Sexual radicals of all varieties have demanded the legal and social legitimation of consenting sexual behaviour. Feminists have criticized them for ostensibly finessing questions about 'the limits of consent' and 'structural constraints' on consent (Orlando, 1983; Wilson, 1983, especially pp. 35–41). Although there are deep problems with the political discourse of consent, and although there are certainly structural constraints on sexual choice, this criticism has been consistently misapplied in the sex debates. It does not take into account the very specific semantic content that consent has in sex law and sex practice.

As I mentioned earlier, a great deal of sex law does not distinguish between consensual and coercive behaviour. Only rape law contains such a distinction. Rape law is based on the assumption, correct in my view, that heterosexual activity may be freely chosen or forcibly coerced. One has the legal right to engage in heterosexual behaviour as long as it does not fall under the purview of other statutes and as long as it is agreeable to both parties.

This is not the case for most other sexual acts. Sodomy laws, as I mentioned above, are based on the assumption that the forbidden acts are an 'abominable and detestable crime against nature'. Criminality is intrinsic to the acts themselves, no matter what the desires of the participants. 'Unlike rape, sodomy or an unnatural or perverted sexual act may be committed between two persons both of whom consent, and, regardless of which is the aggressor, both may be prosecuted.'[26] Before the consenting adults statute was passed in California in 1976, lesbian lovers could have been prosecuted for committing oral copulation. If both participants were capable of consent, both were equally guilty (Beserra *et al.*, 1973, pp. 163–5).[27]

Adult incest statutes operate in a similar fashion. Contrary to popular mythology, the incest statutes have little to do with protecting children from rape by close relatives. The incest statutes themselves prohibit marriage or sexual intercourse between adults who are closely related. Prosecutions are rare, but two were reported recently. In 1979, a 19-year-old Marine met his 42-year-old mother, from whom he had been separated at birth. The two fell in love and got married. They were charged and found guilty of incest, which under Virginia law carries a maximum ten-year sentence. During their trial, the Marine testified, 'I love her very much. I feel that two people who love each other should be able to live together.'[28] In another case, a brother and sister who had been raised separately met and decided to get married. They were arrested and pleaded guilty to felony incest in return for probation. A condition of probation was that they not live together as husband and wife. Had they not accepted, they would have faced twenty years in prison (Norton, 1981, p. 18). In a famous S/M case, a man was convicted of aggravated assault for a whipping administered in an S/M scene. There was no complaining victim. The session had been filmed and he was prosecuted on the basis of the film. The man appealed his conviction by arguing that he had been involved in a consensual sexual encounter and had assaulted no one. In rejecting his appeal, the court ruled that one may not consent to an assault or battery 'except in a situation involving ordinary physical contact or blows incident to sports such as football, boxing, or wrestling'.[29] The court went on to note that the 'consent of a person without legal capacity to give consent, such as a child or insane person, is ineffective', and that 'It is a matter of common knowledge that a normal person in full possession of his mental faculties does not freely consent to the use, upon himself, of force likely to produce great bodily injury.'[30] Therefore, anyone who would consent to a whipping would be presumed *non compos mentis* and legally incapable of consenting. S/M sex generally involves a much lower level of force than the average football game, and results in far fewer injuries than most sports. But the court ruled that football players are sane, whereas masochists are not.

Sodomy laws, adult incest laws, and legal interpretations such as the one above clearly interfere with consensual behaviour and impose criminal penalties on it. Within the law, consent is a privilege enjoyed only by those who engage in the highest-status sexual behaviour. Those who enjoy low-status sexual behaviour do not have the legal right to engage in it. In addition, economic sanctions, family pressures, erotic stigma, social discrimination, negative ideology, and the paucity of information about erotic behaviour, all serve to make it difficult for people to make unconventional sexual choices. There certainly are structural constraints that impede free sexual choice, but they hardly operate to coerce anyone into being a pervert. On the contrary, they operate to coerce everyone towards normality.

The 'brainwash theory' explains erotic diversity by assuming that some sexual acts are so disgusting that no one would willingly perform them. Therefore, the reasoning goes, anyone who does so must have been forced or fooled. Even constructivist sexual theory has been pressed into the service of explaining away why otherwise rational individuals might engage in variant sexual behaviour. Another position that is not yet fully formed uses the ideas of Foucault and Weeks to imply that the 'perversions' are an especially unsavoury or problematic aspect of the construction of modern sexuality (Valverde, 1980; Wilson, 1983, p. 38). This is yet another version of the notion that sexual dissidents are victims of the subtle machinations of the social system. Weeks and Foucault would not accept such an interpretation, since they consider all sexuality to be constructed, the conventional no less than the deviant.

Psychology is the last resort of those who refuse to acknowledge that sexual dissidents are as conscious and free as any other group of sexual actors. If deviants are not responding to the manipulations of the social system, then perhaps the source of their incomprehensible choices can be found in a bad childhood, unsuccessful socialization, or inadequate identity formation. In her essay on erotic domination, Jessica Benjamin draws upon psychoanalysis and philosophy to explain why what she calls 'sadomasochism' is alienated, distorted, unsatisfactory, numb, purposeless, and an attempt to 'relieve an original effort at differentiation that failed' (Benjamin, 1983, p. 292).[31] This essay substitutes a psycho-philosophical inferiority for the more usual means of devaluing dissident eroticism. One reviewer has already construed Benjamin's argument as showing that sadomasochism is merely an 'obsessive replay of the infant power struggle' (Ehrenreich, 1983, p. 247).

The position which defends the political rights of perverts but which seeks to understand their 'alienated' sexuality is certainly preferable to the WAP-style blood-baths. But for the most part, the sexual moderates have not confronted their discomfort with erotic choices that differ from their own. Erotic chauvinism cannot be redeemed by tarting it up in Marxist drag, sophisticated constructivist theory, or retro-psychobabble.

Whichever feminist position on sexuality – right, left, or centre – eventually attains dominance, the existence of such a rich discussion is evidence that the feminist movement will always be a source of interesting thought about sex. Nevertheless, I want to challenge the assumption that feminism is or should be the privileged site of a theory of sexuality. Feminism is the theory of gender oppression. To assume automatically that this makes it the theory of sexual oppression is to fail to distinguish between gender, on the one hand, and erotic desire, on the other.

In the English language, the word 'sex' has two very different meanings. It means gender and gender identity, as in 'the female sex' or 'the male sex'. But sex also refers to sexual activity, lust, intercourse, and arousal, as in 'to have sex'. This semantic merging reflects a cultural assumption that sexuality is reducible to sexual intercourse and that it is a function of the relations between women and men. The cultural fusion of gender with sexuality has given rise to the idea that a theory of sexuality may be derived directly out of a theory of gender.

In an earlier essay, 'The Traffic in Women', I used the concept of sex/gender system, defined as a 'set of arrangements by which a society transforms biological sexuality into products of human activity' (Rubin, 1975, p. 159). I went on to argue that 'Sex as we know it – gender identity, sexual desire and fantasy, concepts of childhood – is itself a social product' (1975, p. 66). In that essay, I did not distinguish between lust and gender, treating both as modalities of the same underlying social process.

'The Traffic in Women' was inspired by the literature on kin-based systems of social organization. It appeared to me at the time that gender and desire were systematically intertwined in such social formations. This may or may not be an accurate assessment of the relationship between sex and gender in tribal organizations. But it is surely not an adequate formulation for sexuality in Western industrial societies. As Foucault has pointed out, a system of sexuality has emerged out of earlier kinship forms and has acquired significant autonomy.

> Particularly from the eighteenth century onward, Western societies created and deployed a new apparatus which was superimposed on the previous one, and which, without completely supplanting the latter, helped to reduce its importance. I am speaking of the deployment of sexuality ... For the first [kinship], what is pertinent is the link between partners and definite statutes; the second [sexuality] is concerned with the sensations of the body, the quality of pleasures, and the nature of impressions.
>
> (Foucault, 1978, p. 106)

The development of this sexual system has taken place in the context of gender relations. Part of the modern ideology of sex is that lust is the province of men, purity that of women. It is no accident that pornography and perversions have been considered part of the male domain. In the sex industry, women have been excluded from most production and consumption, and allowed to participate primarily as workers. In order to participate in the 'perversions', women have had to overcome serious limitations on their social mobility, their economic resources, and their sexual freedoms. Gender affects the operation of the sexual system, and the sexual system has had gender-specific manifestations. But although sex and gender are related, they are not the same thing, and they form the basis of two distinct arenas of social practice.

In contrast to my perspective in 'The Traffic in Women', I am now arguing that it is essential to separate gender and sexuality analytically to reflect more accurately their separate social existence. This goes against the grain of much contemporary feminist thought, which treats sexuality as a derivation of gender. For instance, lesbian feminist ideology has mostly analysed the oppression of lesbians in terms of the oppression of women. However, lesbians are also oppressed as queers and perverts, by the operation of sexual, not gender, stratification. Although it pains many lesbians to think about it, the fact is that lesbians have shared many of the sociological features and suffered from many of the same social penalties as have gay men, sadomasochists, transvestites, and prostitutes.

Catherine MacKinnon has made the most explicit theoretical attempt to subsume sexuality under feminist thought. According to MacKinnon, 'Sexuality is to feminism what work is to marxism … the moulding, direction, and expression of sexuality organizes society into two sexes, women and men' (MacKinnon, 1982, pp. 5–16). This analytic strategy in turn rests on a decision to 'use sex and gender relatively interchangeably' (MacKinnon, 1983, p. 635). It is this definitional fusion that I want to challenge.

There is an instructive analogy in the history of the differentiation of contemporary feminist thought from Marxism. Marxism is probably the most supple and powerful conceptual system extant for analysing social inequality. But attempts to make Marxism the sole explanatory system for all social inequalities have been dismal exercises. Marxism is most successful in the areas of social life for which it was originally developed – class relations under capitalism.

In the early days of the contemporary women's movement, a theoretical conflict took place over the applicability of Marxism to gender stratification. Since Marxist theory is relatively powerful, it does in fact detect important and interesting aspects of gender oppression. It works best for those issues of gender most closely related to issues of class and the organization of labour. The issues more specific to the social structure of gender were not amenable to Marxist analysis.

The relationship between feminism and a radical theory of sexual oppression is similar. Feminist conceptual tools were developed to detect and analyse gender-based hierarchies. To the extent that these overlap with erotic stratifications, feminist theory has some explanatory power. But as issues become less those of gender and more those of sexuality, feminist analysis becomes misleading and often irrelevant. Feminist thought simply lacks angles of vision that can fully encompass the social organization of sexuality. The criteria of relevance in feminist thought do not allow it to see or assess critical power relations in the area of sexuality.

In the long run, feminism's critique of gender hierarchy must be incorporated into a radical theory of sex, and the critique of sexual oppression should enrich feminism. But an autonomous theory and politics specific to sexuality must be developed.

It is a mistake to substitute feminism for Marxism as the last word in social theory. Feminism is no more capable than Marxism of being the ultimate and complete account of all social inequality. Nor is feminism the residual theory which can take care of everything to which Marx did not attend. These critical tools were fashioned to handle very specific areas of social activity. Other areas of social life, their forms of power, and their characteristic modes of oppression, need their own conceptual implements. In this essay, I have argued for theoretical as well as sexual pluralism.

Conclusion

> … these pleasures which we lightly call physical …
>
> (Colette, 1982, p. 72)

Like gender, sexuality is political. It is organized into systems of power, which reward and encourage some individuals and activities, while punishing and suppressing others. Like the capitalist organization of labour and its distribution of rewards and powers, the modern sexual system has been the object of political struggle since it emerged and as it has evolved. But if the disputes between labour and capital are mystified, sexual conflicts are completely camouflaged.

The legislative restructuring that took place at the end of the nineteenth century and in the early decades of the twentieth was a refracted response to the emergence of the modern erotic system. During that period, new erotic communities formed. It became possible to be a male homosexual or a lesbian in a way it had not been previously. Mass-produced erotica became available, and the possibilities for sexual commerce expanded. The first homosexual rights organizations were formed, and the first analyses of sexual oppression were articulated (Lauritsen and Thorstad, 1974).

The repression of the 1950s was in part a backlash to the expansion of sexual communities and possibilities which took place during World War Two (Bérubé, 1981a, 1981b; D'Emilio, 1983). During the 1950s, gay rights organizations were established, the Kinsey reports were published, and lesbian literature flourished. The 1950s were a formative as well as a repressive era.

The current right-wing sexual counter-offensive is in part a reaction to the sexual liberalization of the 1960s and early 1970s. Moreover, it has brought about a unified and self-conscious coalition of sexual radicals. In one sense, what is now occurring is the emergence of a new sexual movement, aware of new issues and seeking a new theoretical basis. The sex wars out on the streets have been partly responsible for provoking a new intellectual focus on sexuality. The sexual system is shifting once again, and we are seeing many symptoms of its change.

In Western culture, sex is taken all too seriously. A person is not considered immoral, is not sent to prison, and is not expelled from her or his family, for enjoying spicy cuisine. But an individual may go through all this and more for enjoying shoe leather. Ultimately, of what possible social significance is it if a person likes to masturbate over a shoe? It may even be non-consensual, but since we do not ask permission of our shoes to wear them, it hardly seems necessary to obtain dispensation to come on them.

If sex is taken too seriously, sexual persecution is not taken seriously enough. There is systematic mistreatment of individuals and communities on the basis of erotic taste or behaviour. There are serious penalties for belonging to the various sexual occupational castes. The sexuality of the young is denied, adult sexuality is often treated like a variety of nuclear waste, and the graphic representation of sex takes place in a mire of legal and social circumlocution. Specific populations bear the brunt of the current system of erotic power, but their persecution upholds a system that affects everyone.

The 1980s have already been a time of great sexual suffering. They have also been a time of ferment and new possibility. It is up to all of us to try to prevent more barbarism and to encourage erotic creativity. Those who consider themselves progressive need to examine their preconceptions, update their sexual educations, and acquaint themselves with the existence and operation of sexual hierarchy. It is time to recognize the political dimensions of erotic life.

Acknowledgements

It is always a treat to get to the point in a chapter when I can thank those who contributed to its realization. Many of my ideas about the formation of sexual communities first occurred to me during a course given by Charles Tilly on 'The Urbanization of Europe from 1500–1900'. Few courses could ever provide as much excitement, stimulation, and conceptual richness as did that one. Daniel Tsang alerted me to the significance of the events of 1977 and taught me to pay attention to sex law. Pat Califia deepened my appreciation for human sexual variety and taught me to respect the much-maligned fields of sex research and sex education. Jeff Escoffier shared his powerful grasp of gay history and sociology, and I have especially benefited from his insights into the gay economy. Allan Bérubé's work in progress on gay history has enabled me to think with more clarity about the dynamics of sexual oppression. Conversations with Ellen Dubois, Amber Hollibaugh, Mary Ryan, Judy Stacey, Kay Trimberger, Rayna Rapp, and Martha Vicinus have influenced the direction of my thinking.

I am very grateful to Cynthia Astuto for advice and research on legal matters, and to David Sachs, book dealer extraordinary, for pointing out the right-wing pamphlet literature on sex. I am grateful to Allan Bérubé, Ralph Bruno, Estelle Freedman, Kent Gerard, Barbara Kerr, Michael Shively, Carole Vance, Bill Walker, and Judy Walkowitz for miscellaneous references and factual information. I cannot begin to express my gratitude to those who read and commented on versions of this paper: Jeanne Bergman, Sally Binford, Lynn Eden, Laura Engelstein, Jeff Escoffier, Carole Vance, and Ellen Willis. Mark Leger both edited and performed acts of secretarial heroism in preparing the manuscript. Marybeth Nelson provided emergency graphics assistance.

I owe special thanks to two friends whose care mitigated the strains of writing. E.S. kept my back operational and guided me firmly through some monumental bouts of writer's block. Cynthia Astuto's many kindnesses and unwavering support enabled me to keep working at an absurd pace for many weeks.

None of these individuals should be held responsible for my opinions, but I am grateful to them all for inspiration, information, and assistance.

A note on definitions

Throughout this essay, I use terms such as homosexual, sex worker, and pervert. I use 'homosexual' to refer to both women and men. If I want to be more specific, I use terms such as 'lesbian' or 'gay male'. 'Sex worker' is intended to be more inclusive than 'prostitute', in order to encompass the many jobs of the sex industry. Sex worker includes erotic dancers, strippers, porn models, nude women who will talk to a customer via telephone hook-up and can be seen but not touched, phone partners, and the various other employees of sex businesses such as receptionists, janitors and barkers. Obviously, it also includes prostitutes, hustlers, and 'male models'. I use the term 'pervert' as a shorthand for all the stigmatized sexual orientations. It is used to cover male and female homosexuality as well but as these become less disreputable, the term has increasingly referred to the other 'deviations'. Terms such as 'pervert' and 'deviant' have, in general use, a connotation of disapproval, disgust, and dislike. I am using these terms in a denotative fashion, and do not intend them to convey any disapproval on my part.

Notes

1 Walkowitz's entire discussion of the *Maiden Tribute of Modern Babylon* and its aftermath (1982, pp. 83–5) is illuminating.
2 I am indebted to Allan Bérubé for calling my attention to this incident.
3 The following examples suggest avenues for additional research. A local crackdown at the University of Michigan is documented in Tsang (1977a, 1977b). At the University of Michigan, the number of faculty dismissed for alleged homosexuality appears to rival the number fired for alleged communist tendencies. It would be interesting to have figures comparing the number of professors who lost their positions during this period due to sexual and political offences. On regulatory reform, many states

passed laws during this period prohibiting the sale of alcoholic beverages to 'known sex perverts' or providing that bars that catered to 'sex perverts' be closed. Such a law was passed in California in 1955, and declared unconstitutional by the state Supreme Court in 1959 (Allan Bérubé, personal communication). It would be of great interest to know exactly which states passed such statutes, the dates of their enactment, the discussion that preceded them, and how many are still on the books. On the persecution of other erotic populations, evidence indicates that John Willie and Irving Klaw, the two premier producers and distributors of bondage erotica in the United States from the late 1940s through the early 1960s, encountered frequent police harassment and that Klaw, at least, was affected by a congressional investigation conducted by the Kefauver Committee. I am indebted to personal communication from J.B. Rund for information on the careers of Willie and Klaw. Published sources are scarce, but see Willie (1974); Rund (1977, 1978, 1979). It would be useful to have more systematic information on legal shifts and police activity affecting non-gay erotic dissidence.

4 'Chicago is center of national child porno ring: the child predators', 'Child sex: square in new town tells it all', 'U.S. orders hearings on child pornography: Rodino calls sex racket an "outrage"', 'Hunt six men, twenty boys in crackdown', *Chicago Tribune*, 16 May 1977; 'Dentist seized in child sex raid: Carey to open probe', 'How ruses lure victims to child pornographers', *Chicago Tribune*, 1977; 'Child pornographers thrive on legal confusion', 'U.S. raids hit porn sellers', *Chicago Tribune*, 1977.

5 For more information on the 'Kiddie porn panic' see Califia (1980c, 1980d); Mitzel (1980); Rubin (1981). On the issue of cross-generational relationships, see also Moody (1980), O'Carroll (1980), Tsang (1981), and Wilson (1981).

6 'House passes tough bill on child porn', *San Francisco Chronicle*, 15 November 1983, p. 14.

7 This insight was first articulated by Mary McIntosh (1968); the idea has been developed in Jeffrey Weeks (1977, 1981); see also D'Emilio (1983) and Rubin (1979).

8 A very useful discussion of these issues can be found in Robert Padgug (1979).

9 Lévi-Strauss (1970). In this conversation, Lévi-Strauss calls his position 'a Kantianism without a transcendental subject'.

10 See, for example, 'Pope praises couples for self-control', *San Francisco Chronicle*, 13 October 1980; 'Pope says sexual arousal isn't a sin if it's ethical', *San Francisco Chronicle*, 6 November 1980; 'Pope condemns "carnal lust" as abuse of human freedom', *San Francisco Chronicle*, 15 January 1981; 'Pope again hits abortion, birth control', *San Francisco Chronicle*, 16 January 1981; and 'Sexuality, not sex in heaven', *San Francisco Chronicle*, 3 December 1981. See also footnote 18 below.

11 For further elaboration of these processes, see: Bérubé (1981a); D'Emilio (1981, 1983); Foucault (1978); Katz (1976); Weeks (1977, 1981).

12 Vice cops also harass all sex businesses, be these gay bars, gay baths, adult book stores, the producers and distribution of commercial erotica, or swing clubs.

13 This article (Norton, 1981) is a superb summary of much current sex law and should be required reading for anyone interested in sex.

14 This earlier edition of the Sex Code of California preceded the 1976 consenting adults statute and consequently gives a better overview of sodomy laws.

15 D'Emilio (1983, pp. 40–53) has an excellent discussion of gay oppression in the 1950s, which covers many of the areas I have mentioned. The dynamics he describes, however, are operative in modified forms for other erotic populations, and in other periods. The specific model of gay oppression needs to be generalized to apply, with appropriate modifications, to other sexual groups.

16 I have adopted this terminology from the very useful discussion in Weeks, 1981, pp. 14–15.

17 See Spooner, 1977, pp. 25–9. Feminist anti-porn discourse fits right into the tradition of justifying attempts at moral control by claiming that such action will protect women and children from violence.

18 'Pope's talk on sexual spontaneity', *San Francisco Chronicle*, 13 November 1980, p. 8; see also footnote 10 above. Julia Penelope argues that 'we do not need anything that labels itself purely sexual' and that 'fantasy, as an aspect of sexuality, may be a phallocentric "need" from which we are not yet free … ' in Penelope, 1980, p. 103.

19 *Moral Majority Report*, July 1983. I am indebted to Allan Bérubé for calling my attention to this image.

20 See for example Lederer (1980); Dworkin (1981). The *Newspage* of San Francisco's Women Against Violence in Pornography and Media and the *Newsreport* of New York Women Against Pornography are excellent sources.

21 Gearhart (1979); Rich (1979, p. 225). (On the other hand, there is homosexual patriarchal culture, a culture created by homosexual men, reflecting such male stereotypes as dominance and submission as modes of relationship, and separation of sex from emotional involvement – a culture tainted by profound hatred for women. The male 'gay' culture has offered lesbians the imitation role-stereotypes of 'butch' and 'femme', 'active' and 'passive', cruising, sadomasochism, and the violent, self-destructive world of 'gay bars': Pasternack, 1983; Rich, 1983.)

22 A further elaboration of this tendency can be found in Pasternack, 1983.

23 Califia (1980a, 1980b, 1980c, 1980d, 1980e, 1981b, 1982a, 1982b, 1983a, 1983b, 1983c); English, Hollibaugh, and Rubin (1981a, 1981b); Hollibaugh (1983); Holz (1983); O'Dair (1983); Orlando (1982a); Russ (1982); Samois (1979, 1982); Sundhal (1983); Wechsler (1981a, 1981b); Willis (1981). For an excellent overview of the history of the ideological shifts in feminism that have affected the sex debates, see Echols (1983).

24 I am indebted to Jeanne Bergman for calling my attention to this quote.

25 See for example, Benjamin (1983, p. 297) and Rich (1983).

26 Taylor v. State, 214 Md. 156, 165, 133 A. 2d 414, 418. This quote is from a dissenting opinion, but it is a statement of prevailing law.

27 See note 14 above.

28 'Marine and Mom Guilty of Incest', *San Francisco Chronicle*, 16 November 1979, p. 16.

29 People v. Samuels, 250 Cal. App. 2d 501, 513, 58 Cal. Rptr. 439, 447 (1967).

30 People v. Samuels, 250 Cal. App. 2d at 513–14, 58 Cal. Rptr. at 447.

31 But see also pp. 286, 291–7.

References

[N.A.], (1969) *Pavlov's Children (They May Be Yours)*, Los Angeles: Impact Publishers.

ALDERFER, H., JAKER, B. and NELSON, M. (1982) *Diary of a Conference on Sexuality*, New York: Faculty Press.

AMERICAN PSYCHIATRIC ASSOCIATION (1980) *Diagnostic and Statistical Manual of Mental and Physical Disorders*, Third Edition, Washington, DC: American Psychiatric Association.

BAAL, J.V. (1966) *Dema*, The Hague: Nijhoff.

BARKER-BENFIELD, G.J. (1976) *The Horrors of the Half-Known Life*, New York: Harper Colophon.

BARR, J. (1950) *Quatrefoil*, New York: Greenberg.

BARRY, K. (1979) *Female Sexual Slavery*, Englewood Cliffs, NJ: Prentice-Hall.

—— (1982) 'Sadomasochism: the new backlash to feminism', *Trivia*, 1, fall, [n.p.n.].

BENJAMIN, J. (1983) 'Master and slave: the fantasy of erotic domination', in SNITOW, A., STANSELL, C. and THOMPSON, S. (eds) *Powers of Desire*, New York: Monthly Review Press.

BÉRUBÉ, A. (1981a) 'Behind the spectre of San Francisco', *Body Politic*, April, [n.p.n.].

—— (1981b) 'Marching to a different drummer', *Advocate*, 15 October, [n.p.n.].

BESERRA, S.S., FRANKLIN, S.G. and CLEVENGER, N. (eds) (1977) *Sex Code of California*, Sacramento: Planned Parenthood Affiliates of California.

——, JEWEL, N.M., MATTHEWS, M.W. and GATOV, E.R. (eds) (1973) *Sex Code of California*, Public Education and Research Committee of California.

BINGHAM, C. (1971) 'Seventeenth-century attitudes toward deviant sex', *Journal of Interdisciplinary History*, spring, pp. 447–68.

BRESLIN, J. (1981) 'The moral majority in your motel room', *San Francisco Chronicle*, 22 January, p. 41.

BROWN, R. (1981) 'Blueprint for a moral America', *Nation*, 23 May, [n.p.n.].

BUSH, L. (1983) 'Capitol report', *Advocate*, 8 December, [n.p.n.].

CALIFIA, P. (1980a) 'Among us, against us – the new puritans', *Advocate*, 17 April, [n.p.n.].

—— (1980b) 'Feminism vs. sex: a new conservative wave', *Advocate*, 21 February, [n.p.n.].

—— (1980c) 'The great kiddy porn scare of '77 and its aftermath', *Advocate*, 16 October, [n.p.n.].

—— (1980d) 'A thorny issue splits a movement', *Advocate*, 30 October, [n.p.n.].

—— (1980e) *Sapphistry*, Tallahassee: Naiad.

—— (1981a) 'Feminism and sadomasochism', *Co-Evolution Quarterly*, 33, spring, [n.p.n.].

—— (1981b) 'What is gay liberation?', *Advocate*, 25 June, [n.p.n.].

184   *Gayle S. Rubin*

—— (1982a) 'Public sex', *Advocate*, 30 September, [n.p.n.].
—— (1982b) 'Response to Dorchen Leidholdt', *New Women's Times*, October, [n.p.n.].
—— (1983a) 'Doing it together: gay men, lesbians and sex', *Advocate*, 7 July, [n.p.n.].
—— (1983b) 'Gender-bending', *Advocate*, 15 September, [n.p.n.].
—— (1983c) 'The sex industry', *Advocate*, 13 October, [n.p.n.].
CITY OF NEW YORK (1939) *Report of the Mayor's Committee for the Study of Sex Offenses*.
COLETTE, S.G. (1982) *The Ripening Seed*, translated and cited in ALDERFER, H., JAKER, B. and NELSON, M., *Diary of a Conference on Sexuality*, New York: Faculty Press.
COMMONWEALTH OF MASSACHUSETTS (1947) *Preliminary Report of the Special Commission Investigating the Prevalence of Sex Crimes*.
COURTNEY, P. (1969) *The Sex Education Racket: Pornography in the Schools (An Exposé)*, New Orleans: Free Men Speak.
D'EMILIO, J. (1981) 'Gay politics, gay community: San Francisco's experience', *Socialist Review*, 55, pp. 77–104.
—— (1983) *Sexual Politics, Sexual Communities: The Making of the Homosexual Minority in the United States, 1940–1970*, Chicago: University of Chicago Press.
DRAKE, G.V. (1969) *SIECUS: Corrupter of Youth*, Tulsa, OK: Christian Crusade Publications.
DWORKIN, A. (1981) *Pornography*, New York: Perigee.
ECHOLS, A. (1983) 'Cultural feminism: feminist capitalism and the anti-pornography movement', *Social Text*, 7, spring/summer, pp. 34–53.
EHRENREICH, B. (1983) 'What is this thing called sex?', *Nation*, 24 September, p. 247.
ELLIS, H. (1936) *Studies in the Psychology of Sex*, 2 vols, New York: Random House.
ENGLISH, D., HOLLIBAUGH, A. and RUBIN, G. (1981a) 'Talking sex', *Socialist Review*, July–August, [n.p.n.].
—— (1981b) 'Sex issue', *Heresies*, 12, [n.p.n.].
FOUCAULT, M. (1978) *The History of Sexuality, Volume 1: An Introduction*, New York: Pantheon.
FREEDMAN, E.B. (1983) '"Uncontrolled desire": the threat of the sexual psychopath in America, 1935–60', paper presented at the Annual Meeting of the American Historical Association, San Francisco, December.
GAGNON, J. (1977) *Human Sexualities*, Glenview: Scott, Foresman.
—— and SIMON, W. (eds) (1967) *Sexual Deviance*, New York: Harper & Row.
—— (1970) *The Sexual Scene*, Chicago: Transaction Books, Aldine.
GEARHART, S. (1979) 'An open letter to the voters in district 5 and San Francisco's gay community' [no publication details available].
GEBHARD, P.H. (1976) 'The institute,' in WEINBERG, M.S. (ed.) *Sex Research: Studies From the Kinsey Institute*, New York: Oxford University Press.
GERASSI, J. (1968) *The Boys of Boise*, New York: Collier.
GORDON, L. and DUBOIS, E. (1983) 'Seeking ecstasy on the battlefield: danger and pleasure in nineteenth century feminist sexual thought', *Feminist Studies*, 9, pp. 7–26.
—— and HUNTER, A. (1977–78) 'Sex, family, and the new right', *Radical America*, [no issue no.], pp. 9–26.
GREGORY-LEWIS, S. (1977a) 'Right wing finds new organizing tactic', *Advocate*, 23 June, [n.p.n.].
—— (1977b) 'The neo-right political apparatus', *Advocate*, 8 February, [n.p.n.].
—— (1977c) 'Unraveling the anti-gay network', *Advocate*, 7 September, [n.p.n.].
HANSEN, B. (1979) 'The historical construction of homosexuality', *Radical History Review*, 20, pp. 66–73.
HARTWELL, S. (1950) *A Citizen's Handbook of Sexual Abnormalities and the Mental Hygiene Approach to Their Prevention*, State of Michigan.
HERDT, G. (1981) *Guardians of the Flutes*, New York: McGraw-Hill.
HOLLIBAUGH, A. (1983) 'The erotophobic voice of women: building a movement for the nineteenth century', *New York Native*, 26 September–9 October, [n.p.n.].
HOLZ, M. (1983) 'Porn: turn on or put down, some thoughts on sexuality', *Processed World*, 7, spring, [n.p.n.].

HYDE, H.M. (1965) *A History of Pornography*, New York: Dell.

JEFFREYS, S. (1981) 'The spinster and her enemies: sexuality and the last wave of feminism', *Scarlet Woman*, 13, July, [n.p.n.].

KATZ, J. (1976) *Gay American History*, New York: Thomas Y. Crowell.

KELLY, R. (1976) 'Witchcraft and sexual relations', in BROWN, P. and BUCHBINDER, G. (eds) *Man and Woman in the New Guinea Highlands*, Washington, DC: American Anthropological Association.

KINSEY, A., POMEROY, W. and MARTIN, C. (1948) *Sexual Behavior in the Human Male*, Philadelphia, PA: W.B. Saunders.

——, POMEROY, W., MARTIN, C. and GEBHARD, P. (1953) *Sexual Behavior in the Human Female*, Philadelphia, PA: W.B. Saunders.

KOPKIND, A. (1977) 'America's new right', *New Times*, 30 September, [n.p.n.].

LAURITSEN, J. and THORSTAD, D. (1974) *The Early Homosexual Rights Movement in Germany*, New York: Times Change Press.

LEDERER, L. (ed.) (1980) *Take Back the Night*, New York: William Morrow.

LÉVI-STRAUSS, C. (1970) 'A confrontation', *New Left Review*, 62, July–August, [n.p.n.].

LINDEN, R.R., PAGANO, D.R., RUSSELL, D.E.H. and STARR, S.L. (eds) (1982) *Against Sadomasochism*, East Palo Alto, CA: Frog in the Well.

MCINTOSH, M. (1968) 'The homosexual role', *Social Problems*, 16, pp. 182–92.

MACKINNON, C. (1982) 'Feminism, marxism, method and the state: an agenda for theory', *Signs*, 7, pp. 515–44.

—— (1983) 'Feminism, marxism, method and the state: toward feminist jurisprudence', *Signs*, 8(4), pp. 635–58.

MARCUS, S. (1974) *The Other Victorians*, New York: New American Library.

MARX, K. (1971) *The Grundrisse*, New York: Harper Torchbooks.

MITZEL (1980) *The Boston Sex Scandal*, Boston, MA: Glad Day Books.

MOODY, R. (1980) *Indecent Assault*, London: Word Is Out Press.

MORAL MAJORITY (1983) *Moral Majority Report*, July, [no publication details available].

MURRAY, S.O. (1979) 'The institutional elaboration of a quasi-ethnic community', *International Review of Modern Sociology*, 9(2), pp. 165–78.

NEWTON, E. (1972) *Mother Camp: Female Impersonators in America*, Englewood Cliffs, NJ: Prentice Hall.

NORTON, C. (1981) 'Sex in America', *Inquiry*, 5 October, [n.p.n.].

O'CARROLL, T. (1980) *Paedophilia: The Radical Case*, London: Peter Owen.

O'DAIR, B. (1983) 'Sex, love and desire: feminists struggle over the portrayal of sex', *Alternative Media*, spring, [n.p.n.].

ORLANDO, L. (1982a) 'Bad girls and "good" politics', *Village Voice*, Literary Supplement, December, [n.p.n.].

—— (1982b) 'Lust at last! Spandex invades the academy', *Gay Community News*, 15 May, [n.p.n.].

—— (1983) 'Power plays: coming to terms with lesbian S/M', *Village Voice*, 26 July, [n.p.n.].

PADGUG, R. (1979) 'Sexual matters: on conceptualizing sexuality in history', *Radical History Review*, 20, pp. 3–23.

PASTERNACK, J. (1983) 'The strangest bedfellows: lesbian feminism and the sexual revolution', *WomanNews*, October, [n.p.n.].

PENELOPE, J. (1980) 'And now for the really hard questions', *Sinister Wisdom*, 15, fall, [n.p.n.].

PETCHESKY, R.P. (1981) 'Anti-abortion, anti-feminism, and the rise of the new right', *Feminist Studies*, 7(2), pp. 206–46.

PODHORETZ, N. (1977) 'The culture of appeasement', *Harper's*, October, [n.p.n.].

RAYMOND, J. (1979) *The Transsexual Empire*, Boston, MA: Beacon.

RICH, A. (1979) *On Lies, Secrets, and Silence*, New York: W.W. Norton.

—— (1983) 'Compulsory heterosexuality and lesbian existence', in SNITOW, A., STANSELL, C. and THOMPSON, S. (eds) *Powers of Desire: The Politics of Sexuality*, New York: Monthly Review Press.

RICH, B.R. (1983) 'Review of Powers of Desire', *In These Times*, 16–22 November.

RUBIN, G. (1974) 'Coconuts: aspects of male/female relationships in New Guinea', unpublished manuscript.

—— (1975) 'The traffic in women: notes on the political economy of sex', in REITER, R. (ed.) *Toward an Anthropology of Women*, New York: Monthly Review Press.

—— (1979) 'Introduction', in VIVIEN, R., *A Woman Appeared to Me*, Weatherby Lake: Naiad Press.

—— (1981) 'Sexual politics, the new right and the sexual fringe', in TSANG, D. (ed.) *The Age Taboo*, Boston, MA: Alyson.

—— (1982) 'Guardians of the Flutes', *Advocate*, 23 December, [n.p.n.].

RUND, J.B. (1977) 'Preface', *Bizarre Commix*, vol. 8, New York: Belier Press.

—— (1978) 'Preface', *Bizarre Fotos*, vol. 1, New York: Belier Press.

—— (1979) 'Preface', *Bizarre Katalogs*, New York: Belier Press.

RUSH, F. (1980) *The Best Kept Secret*, New York: McGraw-Hill.

RUSS, J. (1982) 'Being against pornography', *Thirteenth Moon*, 6(1–2), [n.p.n.].

RYAN, M. (1979) 'The power of women's networks: a case study of female moral reform in America', *Feminist Studies*, 5(1), pp. 66–85.

SAMOIS (1979) *What Color Is Your Handkerchief?*, Berkeley, CA: Samois.

—— (1982) *Coming to Power*, Boston, MA: Alyson.

SONTAG, S. (1969) *Styles of Radical Will*, New York: Farrar, Straus, & Giroux.

SPOONER, L. (1977) *Vices Are Not Crimes: A Vindication of Moral Liberty*, Cupertino, CA: Tanstaafl Press.

STAMBOLIAN, G. (1980) 'Creating the new man: a conversation with Jacqueline Livingston', *Christopher Street*, May, [n.p.n.].

—— (1983) 'Jacqueline Livingston', *Clothed With the Sun*, 3(1), May, [n.p.n.].

STATE OF MICHIGAN (1951) *Report of the Governor's Study Commission on the Deviated Criminal Sex Offender*.

STATE OF NEW HAMPSHIRE (1949) *Report of the Interim Commission of The State of New Hampshire to Study the Cause and Prevention of Serious Sex Crimes*.

STATE OF NEW YORK (1950) *Report to the Governor on a Study of 102 Sex Offenders at Sing Sing Prison*.

SUNDHAL, D. (1983) 'Stripping for a living', *Advocate*, 13 October, [n.p.n.].

TSANG, D. (1977a) 'Gay Ann Arbor purges', *Midwest Gay Academic Journal*, 1(1), [n.p.n.].

—— (1977b) 'Ann Arbor purges, part 2', *Midwest Gay Academic Journal*, 1(2), [n.p.n.].

—— (ed.) (1981) *The Age Taboo*, Boston, MA: Alyson Publications.

VALVERDE, M. (1980) 'Feminism meets fist-fucking: getting lost in lesbian S & M', *Body Politic*, February, [n.p.n.].

WALKOWITZ, J.R. (1980) *Prostitution and Victorian Society*, Cambridge: Cambridge University Press.

—— (1982) 'Male vice and feminist virtue: feminism and the politics of prostitution in nineteenth-century Britain', *History Workshop Journal*, 13, spring, pp. 77–93.

WECHSLER, N. (1981a) 'Interview with Pat Califia and Gayle Rubin, part I', *Gay Community News*, 18 July, [n.p.n.].

—— (1981b) 'Interview with Pat Califia and Gayle Rubin, part II', *Gay Community News*, 15 August, [n.p.n.].

WEEKS, J. (1977) *Coming Out: Homosexual Politics in Britain from the Nineteenth Century to the Present*, New York: Quartet.

—— (1981) *Sex, Politics and Society: The Regulation of Sexuality since 1800*, New York: Longman.

WILLIAMS, F.E. (1936) *Papuans of the Trans-Fly*, Oxford: Clarendon.

WILLIE, J. (1974) *The Adventures of Sweet Gwendoline*, New York: Belier Press.

WILLIS, E. (1981) *Beginning to See the Light*, New York: Knopf.

—— (1982) 'Who is feminist? An open letter to Robin Morgan', *Village Voice*, Literary Supplement, December, [n.p.n.].

WILSON, E. (1983) 'The context of "between pleasure and danger": The Barnard Conference on Sexuality', *Feminist Review*, 13, spring, pp. 35–41.

WILSON, P. (1981) *The Man They Called A Monster*, New South Wales: Cassell Australia.

WOLFE, A. and SANDERS, J. (1979) 'Resurgent cold war ideology: the case of the Committee on the Present Danger', in FAGEN, R. (ed.) *Capitalism and the State in US–Latin American Relations*, Stanford, CA: Stanford University Press.

ZAMBACO, D. (1981) 'Onanism and nervous disorders in two girls', in PERALDI, F. (ed.) *Polysexuality, Semiotext(e)*, 4(1), [n.p.n.].

10 'The unclean motion of the generative parts'

Frameworks in Western thought on sexuality

R. W. Connell and Gary W. Dowsett [1992]

Sexuality is a major theme in our culture, from the surf video to the opera stage to the papal encyclical. It is, accordingly, one of the major themes of the human sciences, and figures as weighty as Darwin and Freud have made major contributions to it. Social research has, over the last hundred years, produced crucially important evidence for the understanding of sexuality. But social *theory* has been slow to grapple with the issue, to give it the sophisticated attention that has been devoted to questions of production or of communication.

We are convinced that an adequate social theory of sexuality is essential for progress on 'applied' issues, such as the design of research on the social transmission of human immunodeficiency virus (HIV). This chapter attempts a mapping exercise, sorting out the major intellectual frameworks that have governed Western thinking about sexuality. We discuss first the religious and scientific nativism that dominated the field into the twentieth century, the problems this approach ran into, and the rise of social construction approaches to sexuality. We discuss the impasse that social constructionism has reached. In the final part of the chapter we sketch the outline of an approach which can move past these difficulties.

Governing such a large issue in a short time necessitates taking a fairly broad approach. But we hope to give enough of the key details to show the practical significance of theoretical frameworks.

Nativism

At the bedrock of our culture's thinking about sexuality is the assumption that a given pattern of sexuality is native to the human constitution. We will call this position 'nativism'. It has much in common with what others call 'essentialism', but we want to stress the assumption about origin. Whether laid down by God, achieved by evolution, or settled by the hormones, the nativist assumption is that sexuality is fundamentally *pre-social*. Whatever society does, in attempts to control, channel or restrict, cannot alter the fundamentals of sexuality.

Until quite recently in Western culture nativism was mainly expressed in religious terms. In the ascetic Christian tradition sexuality was read as 'lust'. It was part of the old Adam, an aspect of fallen humanity to be wrestled with and defeated. As Saint Augustine, no stranger to the pleasures of the flesh, put it:

> Although therefore there may be many lusts, yet when we read the word 'lust' alone without mention of the object, we commonly take it for the unclean motion of the generative parts. For this holds sway in the whole body, moving the whole man, without and within, with such a mixture of mental emotion and carnal appetite that hence is the highest bodily pleasure of all produced: so that in the very moment of consummation, it

overwhelms almost all of the light and power of cogitation … Justly is man ashamed of this lust, and justly are those members (which lust moves or suppresses against our wills, as it lusts) called shameful.

(Augustine, 1945 [426 orig.], pp. xvi–xvii)

This outlook was institutionalized in monasticism. (Augustine himself was involved in the very early days of the monastic movement.) Chastity as an ideal spread beyond the monasteries. Thus an attack on married priests was a major feature of Pope Gregory VII's church reforms in the eleventh century. In a process that prefigures a more recent sexual politics, sexuality became an arena for the assertion of other agendas. The attack on priestly marriage occurred in the context of an assertion of the centralized power of the papacy and its attempts to control the priesthood more generally (Greenberg, 1988, pp. 290–2).

Resistance to asceticism, a reassertion of the flesh, correspondingly arose in the form of anticlericalism and irreligious humour. The classic expressions were the songs of the wandering scholars and the bawdy tales of the *Decameron*. As the medieval Archpoet put it in his *Confession* (1952 [1160 orig.]):

Wounded to the quick am I
By a young girl's beauty:
She's beyond my touching? Well,
Can't the mind do duty?

Hard beyond all hardness, this
Mastering of Nature:
Who shall say his heart is clean,
Near so fair a creature?

Young are we, so hard a law,
How should we obey it?
And our bodies, they are young,
Shall they have no say in't?

Sit you down amid the fire,
Will the fire not burn you?
To Pavia come, will you
Just as chaste return you?

Yet another strand in Christian thought affirmed the flesh in the service of God. No less a figure than Martin Luther, the married monk, stands for this view. The mainstream Protestant concept of Christian marriage has offered a picture of legitimate lust, flowing in channels divinely ordained. Here, sexuality was not condemned as such but divided between the territory of God and the terrain of the Devil. In this splitting we can see the remote roots of the image of the sexual 'other' which has haunted the modern Western imagination from Don Juan, the villain of Mozart's operatic stage, to 'Patient Zero', the media villain of the HIV epidemic in the United States (Shilts, 1987).

In the later nineteenth century religious nativism began to be displaced as our culture's main account of sexuality. What replaced it was scientific nativism. Darwin's *Descent of Man*, published in 1874, marks the shift. This offered a detailed account of 'sexual selection' which Darwin now emphasized alongside 'natural selection' as a mechanism of evolution.

Sexual attraction was firmly located in the order of nature and indeed given a steering role in organic evolution.

Only twelve years later Krafft-Ebing in Austria published *Psychopathia Sexualis*, the marker of scientific nativism applied to humans. This was essentially a scientization of the image of the 'sexual other'. Using medical and legal records Krafft-Ebing catalogued and classified, like a horrified butterfly collector, the many types of sexual degeneracy. His catch-all explanation of sexual otherness was 'hereditary taint'. As well as deploying a natural science rhetoric he attempted to deploy natural science methods. For instance, in his case study of the 'Countess in male attire' he attempted anthropometries. After measuring everything from her ear/chin line (26.5 cm) to her vagina, which was too narrow for the 'insertion of a membrum virile', he concluded her congenital sexual inversion 'expressed itself, anthropologically, in anomalies of the development of the body, depending on great hereditary taint' (Krafft-Ebing, 1965 [1886 orig.], pp. 437–8).

The type of scientificity was redefined, but the basic claim could only be reinforced, when sexology moved out of a forensic into a clinical context. The Western *scientia sexualis*, which Foucault (1978, p. 57) has tellingly contrasted with the erotic lore of other cultures, reached its first climax when Freud's key volumes appeared in 1900 and 1905, and Ellis's in 1897. Freud developed a flexible but profound therapeutic and research technique; he produced also a detailed developmental model of human sexuality, bringing childhood sexuality into focus. His most influential arguments demonstrated the protean character of sexual motivation and the significance of sexuality for human psychology generally. Ellis added a more sympathetic documentation of the range of sexual practices and the forms of life that might be built around them.

Across the Atlantic, the monuments of American sexology in the twentieth century sustained the claim to scientificity. Kinsey was a zoologist by training (a specialist in gall wasps), and regarded his massive interview studies of human sexuality as an extension of biology. When the twin storms of fundamentalist religious denunciation and media salacity broke over his head, it was to his identity as a scientist that Kinsey clung for salvation (Pomeroy, 1972). (It is worth remembering, in the light of current debates about research funding in Australia, that Kinsey *did* have his research grants cut off after his work had become politically embarrassing.) Masters and Johnson, working in a school of medicine, had a more clinical style and claimed to be even more nativist than Kinsey:

> Although the Kinsey work has become a landmark of sociologic investigation [certainly not how Kinsey saw it], it was not designed to interpret physiologic or psychologic response to sexual stimulation. [In fact Kinsey's group did such research but kept it secret.] Those *fundamentals of human sexual behaviour* [our emphasis] cannot be established until two questions are answered: What physical reactions develop as the human male and female respond to effective sexual stimulation? Why do men and women behave as they do when responding to effective sexual stimulation?
>
> (Masters and Johnson, 1966, pp. 3–4)

The irony of attempting to answer these universally stated questions by a study of 382 female and 312 male white heterosexual upper-status midwestern urban Americans in their twenties and thirties has not been lost on critics. Nevertheless, Masters and Johnson produced a result that has a claim to be the only research finding in all sexology that has no social significance at all. During sexual excitement the vaginal walls of their female subjects changed colour, and changed back again ten or fifteen minutes later (Masters and Johnson, 1966, pp. 75, 79). The only social question of interest here is why someone would be watching.

The work on homosexuality by the same research group highlights the extent to which social relationships and social meanings are excised in the pursuit of scientificity. For instance, the foreplay of heterosexual and homosexual couples, fellatio/cunnilingus, masturbation, anal intercourse and other activities are compared as if these were purely technical performances (Masters and Johnson, 1970). That anal intercourse, for one, is relationally quite a different matter for heterosexual and homosexual couples in American culture is an issue that does not arise.

With Masters and Johnson scientific nativism, considered as a paradigm or research programme in the sense of Kuhn (1962) and Lakatos (1970), is in full collapse. Far from offering an expanding programme of investigation, a way of talking about sexuality in its fullness, such research is only able to operate by fencing off a small corner of the field. It may call this corner the 'fundamentals', but this is rhetoric. The research itself does not provide a path by which we may account for 'the rest' in terms of these fundamentals. Within a few years two veterans of Kinsey's institute, Gagnon and Simon, would point to the 'noncumulative' character of research in naturalistic sexology and commit themselves to a decisively different framework based on a kind of sociology (Gagnon and Simon, 1974, p. 7).

The flaws in scientific nativism are clear enough in retrospect. It has never come to terms with one of the key bodies of evidence on human sexuality built up in the last hundred years, the anthropologists' documentation of massive cross-cultural variation in sexual practice (Marshall and Suggs, 1971). It has not even been able to account for sexual variation within its own culture – despite many futile studies attempting to find a physiological basis for male or female homosexuality (Wakeling, 1979). What Freud called 'object choice' remains a mystery to sexology. The guiding metaphor of scientific nativism, that the body and its natural processes provide a 'base' or 'foundation' which determines the superstructure of social relations, in fundamental ways misrepresents the relationships between bodies and social processes. This issue is taken up again in the final section.

The nativist discourse is curiously silent on two issues which pervade representations of sexuality in literature, art and music: desire and pleasure. The closest that nativism comes to the concept of desire is the idea of a sex 'drive' or, in Freud's term, 'libido'. This is a force compelling effects, an urge or impulse to behaviour – a more or less uncontrollable one in some accounts going back to Augustine's. It is difficult to connect this to the kind of experience recalled by our poets and writers, that sharp intake of breath as light falls unexpectedly on a breast or buttock, or the memory of a first kiss:

> at first
> a feeling like
> silk, then
> a slight motion
> of lip on lip
> and breathing
> I take your
> lower lip
> into my mouth,
> delight
> in its blood-round
> softness, re-
> lease it, we kiss,
> your tongue

explores; for
the first time
it touches mine:
tip and surface,
root and vein,
our eyes open.

(Peters, 1973)

Pleasure is equally remote in a discourse of nerve endings, engorged vesicles, muscular spasm. The imaginative dimension in enjoyment, the creative search for erotic pleasures, is put firmly in its place:

> Epstein (1960) argued that some of the behaviours of fetishists resemble the symptoms of temporal lobe dysfunction … [However] He has advanced no physiological evidence to directly point to temporal lobe dysfunction in fetishists.
>
> (Lester, 1975, pp. 162–3)

Again the approach is curiously lacking in a grasp of, or even reference to, human experience. Scientific nativism has lost its grasp of the most important subject-matter. Even de Sade, in his extraordinary catalogues of libertinage and violence, managed to survey sexual capacity, diversity and perversity with considerable attention to pleasure (de Sade, 1966 [1785 orig.]).

Though nativism is dead as a scientific programme, it remains powerful as social ideology. Here religion and natural science are in unexpected alliance to support social 'common sense': boys need to sow their wild oats, rapists may be caught but rape cannot be stopped, girls naturally want to look beautiful and to have babies, lesbianism is unnatural … The half-scientific, half-demonological concept of 'the pervert' is an active one, as current politics shows. Consider the persistent attempts of New South Wales politicians in 1989–90 (continuing at the time of writing) to mobilize hatred of 'child molesters' in the aftermath of the legal vindication of the accused in the so-called 'Mr Bubbles' case.

A less dramatic but telling example of nativist ideology is the treatment of transsexuals in the prison system. Though placing male-to-female transsexuals in a men's prison places them at acute risk of rape and bashing, it has proved difficult to get official agreement to place them in women's prisons. The chromosomes rule; more exactly, a biological warrant is found for pre-existing social ideology.

'Frame' theories: the social construction of sexuality

The view that sexuality is shaped by society was stated with particular clarity by Gagnon and Simon (1974), who developed the image of sexual conduct as the enactment of social 'scripts':

> It is the authors' contention … that all human sexual behaviour is socially scripted behaviour. The sources of sexual arousal are to be found in socio-cultural definitions, and it is extremely difficult to conceive of any type of human sexual activity without this definitional aspect … It is not the physical aspects of sexuality but the social aspects that generate the arousal and organize the action.
>
> (Gagnon and Simon, 1974, p. 262)

Such a viewpoint had been developing for a good while before it was so clearly stated. Indeed its origins go back at least to Freud. Freud's general framework was solidly nativist. He saw himself as a natural scientist and physician, he took a reductionist view of psychology, and his conception of the sexual drive or instinct was developed on the analogy of physiological needs. Yet Freud's psychiatric practice, his case studies, and his specific theorization of psychosexual development (particularly in the *Three Essays* of 1905), all undermined the reductionist framework.

Though most discussions of Freud's sexual science emphasize the abstract theory, we would emphasize the case studies, the core of psychoanalysis as he saw it. With astonishing delicacy – given his cultural context – Freud documented the role played by social relationships, especially those within the family, in the shaping of the sexual-emotional life of his patients. Here was the first, and in some ways still the most powerful, evidence for some crucially important conclusions. Freud demonstrated that actual sexualities are not received as a package from biology; that adult sexuality is arrived at by a highly variable and observable process of construction, not by an 'unfolding' of the natural; and that social process is deeply implicated in this construction.

Freud's oscillation between nativist presumptions and constructionist insights has remained characteristic of psychoanalysis, and psychoanalytic sociology, ever since. Conservative medical psychoanalysis has leaned more to the nativist side, and psychoanalytic radicals have leaned more to the constructionist, but the tension has remained. Thus Reich (1972), who had a more vivid understanding than any other psychoanalytic theorist of the pressures placed by class oppression on working-class sexuality, never abandoned his belief in the naturalness of heterosexuality. Dinnerstein (1976), by contrast, sees heterosexuality as necessarily abrasive and discordant, as a result of its construction through the gendered parenting practices that pervade Western societies. Marcuse (1968) developed a classic analysis of the social bases of the bodily organization of sexual pleasure, the pressures leading towards genital primacy and the focusing of sexuality on procreation. Yet he was so convinced of the importance of the organic basis of sexual desire that he found in it the fulcrum for resistance to the repressive social dynamic of advanced capitalism.

A similar ambivalence can be found in classic anthropological works on sexuality. After psychoanalysis, ethnography became during the twentieth century the most important body of evidence requiring a social theory of sexuality. Ethnographers brought back to the European and American intelligentsia accounts of sexual customs so varied but so comprehensible that it was impossible to regard them simply as exotica, as primitivism, or as simple variants on the European pattern. As the Newtonian universe shrank the Earth from being the focus of creation to being merely one of a number of bodies following gravitational laws, so ethnography shrank Western culture from the status of norm, or historic pinnacle, to being one among a large number of comparable cultures which simply had different ways of handling questions of sex.

Yet the ethnographers, confronted with the spectacular variety of sexual custom, persisted in a search for a natural order beneath it. Malinowski, both a pioneer ethnographer of sexuality and a major anthropological theorist, clearly illustrates this. His famous study of the Trobriand Islanders, *The Sexual Life of Savages* (1929), was praised by Ellis as the first serious ethnography of sexuality, placing sexual practices in their full cultural context. It is indeed a richer cultural analysis than anything about *European* sexuality written at the time. But at a theoretical level, in *Sex and Repression in Savage Society* (1927), Malinowski was already hovering between a nativist conception of instinct and a theory of the shaping of emotion by a 'sociological mechanism'. Sexuality appears in this text on the border between nature and culture. As Malinowski's functionalist theory of culture matured, the nativist underpinnings became more explicit. The account of institutions was now based on a statement of the 'biological foundations of culture'. The sequence 'sex appetite → conjugation → detumescence' was one of eleven 'permanent vital sequences incorporated in all cultures'. Kinship institutions were the cultural response to a social need for reproduction (1960 [1944], pp. 75–103). The various sexual customs were thus particular ways in which cultures solved common problems of naturally given human need, each making sense within the *Gestalt* of its own culture. The culture provided context for the resolution of natural need.

Gagnon and Simon's sociology of sex pushed further the tradition that we will call 'frame' theories of sexuality. Gagnon and Simon's version is an adaptation of role theory, the approach in sociology that locates the constraints on behaviour in the stereotyped expectations held by other social actors (Connell, 1979). Individuals internalize these normative expectations or enact them under the threat of social sanctions; in Gagnon and Simon's metaphor, they follow social scripts. Much of the *Sexual Conduct* is a heroic attempt to spell out the scripts. Most notable is the grand script of a lifelong sexual career in contemporary Western culture (1974, pp. 99–103). Gagnon and Simon also attempt to decipher the scripts for homosexual women and men, for youth, for prostitutes and for prisoners.

Read as radical in its day, this now appears a curiously unfocused exercise. The reason is that Gagnon and Simon's framework provides no *social* account of what links the diverse scripts together, what makes them all 'sexuality'. Nor is the unity within a script very clear. The framework does not account for progress along the career path, how we are moved from stage to stage. One eventually realizes that this self-consciously social account has a non-social centre. What defines a matter as 'sexual' is in fact the biology of arousal and reproduction. Gagnon and Simon's sociology does not displace Masters and Johnson's natural history. It provides a social frame for their subject matter. The corner has become a centre; and the scope of the frame is defined by a backward movement from that centre.

Foucault's theorizing provides a social account of the unity of 'sexuality', and in that regard is the pinnacle of the social framing account. As a cultural historian and post-structuralist philosopher, Foucault came from a very different intellectual background from Gagnon and Simon. But he insists as strongly on rejecting nativism and asserting the social. 'The social' here is more concrete than a set of social expectations or scripts. It is a set of historically describable discourses which, operating in professions and state apparatuses, *constitute* 'sexuality' as an object of knowledge and social concern:

> Sexuality must not be thought of as a kind of natural given which power tries to hold in check, or as an obscure domain which knowledge tries gradually to uncover. It is the name that can be given to a historical construct: not a furtive reality that is difficult to grasp, but a great surface network in which the stimulation of bodies, the intensification of pleasures, the incitement to discourse, the formation of special knowledges, the strengthening of controls and resistances, are linked to one another, in accordance with a few major strategies of knowledge and power.
>
> (Foucault, 1978, pp. 105–6)

Foucault is particularly scathing about the 'repressive hypothesis' as a guide to the history of sexuality. Against the view of deepening repression and silence about sexuality as modern capitalism developed, he argues that this was precisely the era when discourses of sexuality multiplied, the social incitement to talk about the secrets of sex grew. 'Sexuality' was created as a social fact, a realm for the operation of power (in the sense of social control).

Establishing that control involved an effort to classify and define. The very science of sexuality which its pioneers – most eloquently Ellis – saw as a means of human progress and emancipation, was to Foucault a means of control. The sexual types of which it spoke were constituted as the objects of new strategies of knowledge and control. Foucault's now celebrated list includes the masturbating child, the perverse (principally homosexual) man, the hysterical woman, and the 'Malthusian' couple (Foucault, 1978, pp. 103–5). Here Foucault's argument connects with the important body of historical research which has traced the emergence of 'the homosexual' as a category in Western culture in historically recent times (e.g. Weeks, 1977; Bray, 1982). The term 'homosexual' itself was coined in the 1860s.

It is significant that this picture of sexuality did not come out of sexology. Rather it came out of a long research programme in cultural history in which Foucault had traced the growth of other systems of knowledge, surveillance and control, notably criminology and the prison, medicine and the clinic, psychiatry and the asylum (Foucault, 1973a, 1973b, 1977). Focusing closely on systems of control, Foucault left little space for what it is that is being controlled.

'Bodies', certainly; but bodies that seem marked by an unusual passivity in the face of these technologies of power and knowledge. Critics of Foucault have asked where the resistance comes from, if his picture of history is not to be a black night of domination more total than even Marcuse (1968) imagined. Foucault (1978, p. 95) replied that resistance arises at every point in a network of power. But this remains a metaphysical claim in the absence of a substantive account of the generation, articulation and historical organization of resistance. And that Foucault does not supply. Indeed he dismissed the issue with a gibe at the Marcusian idea of a 'great refusal' (Foucault, 1978, p. 96).

Though Foucault's account of the social frame is markedly more realistic and historically sophisticated than Gagnon and Simon's, there is as great a problem about what holds it together. Foucault's concept of the 'deployment of sexuality' as a strategy of power (1978, p. 106) avoids making the definition of the social process of sexuality dependent on a malleable native 'human sexual response', but it does make the definition dependent on a 'will to knowledge' and a will to power whose social base, location and dynamics remain vague. Where Foucault begins to specify this (1978, pp. 122–7), he does so in surprisingly conventional class terms, as a strategy of bourgeois class formation as well as hegemony. He acknowledged that the (French) working class long escaped the effects of the deployment of sexuality.

Foucault's sudden shift to the language of class is symptomatic of a crisis in social framing theories. Moving away from the physiological concept of sexuality to a focus on the discourses that socially define it leaves an increasingly empty 'frame'. Yet this movement has found no way of conceptualizing the social in terms of sexuality itself. Instead it is obliged to introduce structural and dynamic concepts (class, hegemony, discourse, state) already defined in reference to other historical processes. Sexuality as an object of knowledge and as an object of politics seems to crumble as we look.

The problems this creates are well illustrated by the theoretical difficulties of gay liberation. Deconstructionist ideas, including those of Foucault, had a considerable impact on gay theorists, among them the distinguished British historian Weeks (1985, 1986). Deconstructionist framing theory seemed to give powerful support to themes already important in gay analyses of sexuality. It pointed to the social bases of concepts of normality and deviance, to the pervasiveness of social control, and to the role of professions such as medicine in sustaining control over 'deviants'. The category of 'homosexuality' itself could be seen to be socially constructed by penal laws and medical interpretations.

Here the problems begin. For according to this argument, to claim an identity as a homosexual is to claim a place in a system of social regulation. Yet 'homosexual identity' is the logical basis of homosexual solidarity and the gay movement itself. To resist the identity means to dismantle the movement, leaving no place from which to contest the regulatory power.

The political implications of social construction theory and the deconstructionist reaction to issues of identity were vigorously debated from the end of the 1970s (e.g. Johnston, 1981; Sargent, 1983). The sense that gay theory had somehow become inimical to gay politics was summed up in reactions recorded in Vance's (1989) useful review of social construction theory: 'deconstruct heterosexuality first!' and 'I'll deconstruct when they deconstruct'. This intellectual climate was perhaps among the centrifugal forces and divergent strategies among homosexual men which, as Pollak (1988) has noted in his study of homosexuals and HIV/AIDS in France, made it more difficult to organize a collective response to the epidemic.

One of the basic problems in social framing theory is the lack of a definition of sexuality outside the act of scripting or controlling. As Vance puts it:

> … to the extent that social construction theory grants that sexual acts, identities and even desire are mediated by cultural and historical factors, the object of the study – sexuality – becomes evanescent and threatens to disappear.
>
> (Vance, 1989, p. 21)

It is understandable that an appeal to nativism may result. There has recently been a revival of a more essentialist position in lesbian and gay analyses of homosexuality (e.g. Williams, 1986, ch. 12; Wieringa, 1989). Basic forms of sexuality are seen as constant, to some degree, across cultures and periods.

Such a response is given urgency by the attacks on homosexual rights and on recent political gains that have followed the HIV epidemic. HIV infection is an intensely personal and organic condition. Cruel notions of 'innocent' victims versus the others who are infected, or ideas for criminal sanctions to control the epidemic, are reminders of medico-legal sanctions on homosexuality defeated only in the recent past. A neo-essentialist position offers a kind of defence against moral blame. It authenticates experience, particularly body sensations and sexual and emotional responses at the individual level. But by retreating to the individual for basic explanations it loses vital purchase on the social.

If it is not to lapse into a kind of nativism, or into a paradoxical liquidation of the object of knowledge and of social practice, the social analysis of sexuality needs a qualitatively different approach from role theory or deconstructionism. We can say, broadly, what kind of theory is required. It is necessary to find ways of understanding the imbrication of bodies and histories, giving full weight to bodily experience without treating the body as the container of an ahistorical essence of sexuality. It is necessary to find ways of understanding social relations as themselves sexual, not merely as framing sexuality from outside. And it is necessary to understand the coherence and constraint within such relationships. Where role theory collapses structure into action, we need a conceptualization of social structure in the domain of sexual practice.

From the social construction of sexuality to the sexual construction of society

To resolve the political dilemma of deconstruction in the face of the enemy, and the conceptual problem of the absent centre in social constructionism, are two problems that require the same approach. Rather than moving back towards nativism, we need to move further into the social, developing an account of sexuality which is *fully* social and can stand on its own as social analysis.

Not even Freud, for all his emphasis on Eros, developed a concept of sexuality as social structure. When he tried to sociologize psychoanalysis (notably in *Civilization and its Discontents*) the social constraint upon Eros came from vaguely specified imperatives of technological development and social order (1953 [1930 orig.]). The breakthrough came with 'second-wave' feminism and gay liberation – and then it came with a rush. Within ten years a whole battery of linked, though by no means equivalent, concepts had been proposed.

Millett's (1972) concept of 'sexual politics' struck to the heart of the matter, announcing from the start that questions about sexuality were questions about power. Her book explored the way sexual relationships in the work of certain novelists become a form of domination of women by men. We might now take a more complex view of the relation between text and practice. But the insight into power, which Millett shared with others in the first years of the women's liberation movement (Willis, 1984), is still basic.

In the first years of the gay liberation movement the point was taken further. Sexuality involves relations of power within genders as well as between them. Though using a similar terminology of oppression (Altman, 1972; Johnston, 1981), the focus here was on differences of identity as much as on relations of subordination. The idea of multiple sexualities with a complex of social relationships between them readily follows from this. The 1970s indeed saw a multiplication of sexual personae in gay and lesbian milieux, from androgynes and drag queens to leather dykes and clones. But diversity did not mean disintegration. These presentations of sexuality were also involved in the construction of modern visible gay communities, which appear to people outside as homogeneous.

Since the new feminism took some years to come to terms with lesbianism, these two arguments did not immediately merge. They were eventually brought together in a striking way by Rich (1980), who turned the social construction of deviance argument on its head and argued the social construction of heterosexuality. 'Compulsory heterosexuality', she proposed, was a political institution, requiring women to be sexually available to men and sustaining their dependence on men. Rich contrasted this with a 'lesbian continuum' of relationships among women independent of men, including erotic relationships but also friendship, work, child care and so on. Her handling of the theme is ahistorical, but the idea is useful in dramatizing the scale on which social relationships may be organized through sexuality.

A significantly different approach to sexuality was taken in Mitchell's now somewhat neglected *Woman's Estate* (1971), under the influence of structuralist Marxism. Mitchell was concerned to distinguish the different sites of women's oppression, on the assumption that relationships in different sites might follow different historical trajectories and give rise to differently configured political struggles. 'Sexuality' figured in her theorizing as one of the four 'structures' of women's oppression, alongside production, reproduction and the socialization of children.

It is not difficult to see the logical incoherence of this framework, and Mitchell herself did not persist with it for long. Yet the moment is important. This text is where sexuality is *named* as a domain of social structure in its own right, alongside and interacting with other social structures, and requiring its own mapping as structure.

Curiously, Mitchell's (1974) second essay in structural analysis was a considerable retreat from this prospect of a structural history of sexuality. The model of 'structure' was now drawn from Lévi-Strauss's essentially ahistorical anthropology. Sexuality became the means by which persons are inserted into kinship and gender structures. The analysis of affect was greatly expanded, but separated from the analysis of structure. Mitchell's later work moved back towards orthodox psychoanalysis.

In a key paper by Rubin the idea of sexuality as social structure received a clear definition:

> ... they [Freud and Lévi-Strauss] provide conceptual tools with which one can build descriptions of the part of social life which is the locus of the oppression of women, of sexual minorities, and of certain aspects of human personality within individuals. I call that part of life the 'sex/gender system', for lack of a more elegant term. As a preliminary definition, a 'sex/gender system' is a set of arrangements by which a society transforms biological sexuality into products of human activity, and in which these transformed sexual needs are satisfied.
>
> (Rubin, 1975, p. 159)

Though Rubin maintains a concept of biological capacity and need, she is emphatic that actual sexuality is historically produced:

> Sex as we know it – gender identity, sexual desire and fantasy, concepts of childhood – is itself a social product. We need to understand the relations of its production.
>
> (Rubin, 1975, p. 166)

As this phrasing suggests, the content of the 'sex/gender system' is twofold. On the one hand there is the socially produced *domain* of practice. On the other hand are the *social relations* organizing that *domain*, which take different structural forms in different societies or periods of history. Rubin (1975, pp. 177, 204–10) draws much from Lévi-Strauss here, but also argues for going beyond kinship to a 'political economy of sexual systems' drawing on Marxist concepts about production systems.

The territory opened up by this conceptual work in the 1970s has been developed in three bodies of research, which inflect in slightly different ways the basic idea of social relations constituted in or through sexuality. The first pursues the political economy of sex through studies of sexuality in workplaces. A notable example is Pringle's (1988) study of secretaries. Pringle demonstrates that sexuality is not an optional extra in office life, nor something that starts and finishes with the Christmas cocktail party. It is intricately interwoven with routine labour processes in a quite inescapable way. Sexuality is part of the way boss/secretary relationships are *constituted*.

One of the most striking things in Pringle's book is the demonstration that this holds whether or not there is the kind of behaviour that Kinsey would count as a sexual act, or a court would count as sexual harassment. And it holds regardless of the gender of the boss (though with a female boss the configuration of sexuality is different). Sexual pleasure and unpleasure are part of the ordinary motivational structure of office life. A similar conclusion pushed Hearn and Parkin (1987), working on what they call 'organization sexuality', to reconsider their initial understanding of the topic:

> We have found it necessary to broaden our definition in at least two ways: firstly, to see sexuality as an ordinary and frequent public process rather than an extraordinary and predominantly private process; and secondly, to see sexuality as an aspect and part of an allpervasive body politics rather than a separate and discrete set of practices. Thus the term sexuality is used here specifically to refer to the social expression of or social relations to physical, bodily desires, real or imagined, by or for others or for oneself.
>
> (Hearn and Parkin, 1987, pp. 57–8)

The theme of 'imagined' relations is central to the second body of work on the symbolic dimension of sexuality. This takes off from the fertile encounter of semiotics and psychoanalysis in the work of Kristeva and others. Previous work on media and culture had debated the way sexuality is governed by discourse (a familiar example is the debates about the effects of pornography – Lockhart *et al.*, 1970). What was at issue now was the way sexuality is constitutive of symbolism and language.

Kristeva herself (1984) saw the very possibility of language as rooted in psychosexual development. If true this would open the whole domain of human communication to analysis in terms of sexual social relations. By extension, sexual theory would be required to understand all the decentred social forms spoken of by post-modernists to whom 'the social bond is linguistic' (Lyotard, 1984).

More specifically there is a semiotics of sexuality, in which relationships of acceptance and expulsion, identity and difference, possession and domination, are established (e.g. Burgin, Donald and Kaplan, 1986). Much feminist work on sexual 'difference' (Eisenstein and Jardine, 1980) operates at the level of symbolism and meanings, where sexual differences are sharp, rather than at the level of personality and interpersonal practice, where differences are much slighter than is usually believed (Epstein, 1988).

The process of constructing sexual meanings is particularly clearly shown by recent work on the cultural dimensions of the HIV epidemic – an 'epidemic of signification' as Treichler (1988) wittily put it. In what Watney (1988) calls 'the spectacle of AIDS' we can see at a particular historical moment how social relations of dominance are asserted through the generation of sexual meanings.

The third body of research reworks the terrain once visited by Malinowski and Mead. Mead (1949) classically formulated the cross-cultural study of sex and gender as a standard human nature finding varied cultural expression. Mead argued that the making of the 'social personalities of the two sexes' was a social process, a matter of a cultural template being placed over the natural variability of temperament (Mead, 1935). But her argument became deeply confused about the role of innate differences – which she was convinced existed both within and between the sexes – and their interaction with the *Gestalt* of a culture. Ultimately Mead wished to proclaim the common humanity underlying cultural difference – a radical enough message in the era of Fascism and late colonialism – and this had the effect of domesticating her ethnography and tying her to a philosophical nativism.

By contrast the new anthropology of sexuality has emphasized the genuine alienness of other cultures' sexual arrangements. Herdt (1981), in the study that has done more than any other to establish this approach, describes a Papua New Guinea culture that violates the cross-cultural assumption of heterosexuality as norm and homosexuality as minority practice. In this culture homosexual practice is virtually universal among men, and is not only tolerated but ritually insisted upon at certain stages of the life cycle. In a range of other Melanesian cultures too, it can be shown that same-sex erotic contact is socially required in certain contexts, is part of the routine ritual work of the society (Herdt, 1984).

To use the category of 'the homosexual' to describe the people involved, or 'homosexuality' as a name for their practice, would be to impose an alien frame of reference that would make nonsense of the behaviour as situated, meaningful practice. Similarly Parker, Guimarães and Struchner (1989) have argued, in the context of the HIV epidemic, that North American notions of 'homosexuality' are inappropriate as a basis for health promotion strategies for Brazilian men who have sex with men. HIV/AIDS prevention models developed in Europe and North America equally misconstrue male-to-male sex in South-east Asia. This point applies to Australia, where assumptions are often made in research and education that all men who have sex with men are 'gay' or 'homosexual' and a standard meaning is read into those terms.

We learn from these anthropological accounts that the structures of sexual relationships, and the social categories constituted through them, are not uniform from one society to another. They are historically produced. In the ethnographer's telescope we can see more dramatically, because of the alienness of the categories and the practices, something that is also true of our own society. Erotic contact is part of a process of relationship-making, of society-making. The Czech philosopher Kosik (1976) nicely described human praxis as 'onto-formative', constitutive of the reality we live in. This is true of sexuality as social practice also.

In this section we have attempted to move beyond the idea of structure as a determining frame which is characteristic of both structuralist and post-structuralist approaches; beyond even the idea of a frame in motion. Sexuality is more than a domain in which history is enacted. It is constitutive of history itself. Society does not simply construct sexuality, society is constructed sexually. Once this is accepted we cannot be content with images of moulding, regulating, controlling. We must think of sexuality in terms of historically dynamic patternings of practice and relationship, which have considerable scope and power.

Growth points for theory

The previous section attempted to state the logical shape of the next step in theory, and outlined the bodies of research requiring it. We now turn to some of the problems the construction of such an approach faces. The theoretical work of the last two decades has established the need for, and the possibility of, an analysis of the structure of relationships constituted through sexual practice. But it has certainly not arrived at anything like agreement on what this structure is. Two main possibilities exist.

First, an account of structure in sexuality can be built on the approach in social theory that emphasizes the mutual implication of structure and practice, but does not reject a structuralist account of structure *per se* (cf. Giddens, 1984). Thus Connell (1987, pp. 111–16) offers an account of sexuality centring on the social relation of emotional attachment. This account suggests that in our culture a highly visible structure, characterized by gender oppositions and couple relationships, coexists with a 'shadow' structure detectable in the ambivalence of major relationships. This ambivalence is a theme developed by Dinnerstein (1976) in particular.

An alternative approach moves away from this concept of structure to analyse the social as the intersection and interplay of a multiplicity of discourses, symbolic systems or language games (Weedon, 1987). This would lead to a more fragmented and multi-levelled account of sexualities (e.g. Coward, 1984). This approach yields some gain in the capacity to grasp large-scale issues such as those involved in the impact of Western on non-Western sexual cultures.

One of the main advantages that social construction theories of sexuality had over nativism and individualism is that they offered a way of accounting for the sexual categories present at a particular moment in history (which nativism takes to be pre-ordained) and for the sexual options available in a given setting to the individual (which profoundly shape the choice, however free the act of choosing may be). Fascinating historical work has been done on the making of such categories as the homosexual man (McIntosh, 1968; Weeks, 1977; Bray, 1982), the prostitute (Walkowitz, 1980; Allen, 1990), the housewife (Game and Pringle, 1979).

The sophistication of this historical work has not, however, been matched by a theoretical capacity to analyse the process by which new sexual categories are generated. This lack is disturbing, since history has not quite come to an end. We can see in the culture around us, beyond the signs of changing styles in sexuality, evidence of the production of whole new categories.

The *transsexual* is clearly being produced as a new social category, despite the fervent wish of most people in it to disappear into the taken-for-granted categories of 'woman' or 'man' (Bolin, 1988). A clear indication is the emergence of a market for the services of trans-sexual prostitutes (Perkins, 1983). The *paedophile* is also perhaps on the way from being a category in forensic psychiatry to being a character in popular culture. The word itself is now used in journalism, presupposing a much wider recognition of the sexual 'type' than could have been presumed even ten years ago. Indeed the title is being claimed by paedophiles themselves (O'Carroll, 1982); both to separate themselves from homosexuals, and also to claim, in a classic sexual-liberation-inspired way, the contested ground from those who would regulate them, namely the state.

In HIV/AIDS policy the production of categories takes the form of a medical discourse of 'risk groups'. The conceptual muddle produced by blurring practices into groups can be seen in the monthly *Australian HIV Surveillance Reports*, where there is an HIV transmission category entitled 'Homosexual/Bisexual'. Logically there is no such thing as bisexual trans-mission of HIV, unless a man is having simultaneous anal and/or vaginal intercourse with a man and a woman, both of them are already infected, and they infect him at the same moment!

The key to an understanding of the production of categories is a concept of collective agency. 'Agency' is most commonly thought of as a property of the individual person. The couples 'agency/determination', 'practice/structure' are thus assimilated to the opposition 'individual/society'.

Yet agency in sexual matters is often a question of the historical creation and mobilization of collectivities. Witness the mobilization of women's agency in relation to sexuality (marriage and contraception for instance) around the turn of the century traced by Magarey (1985). A more recent example is the mobilization of homosexual men achieved by the gay liberation movement in the 1970s, and the 'safe sex' movement itself in the 1980s.

Collectivities may of course mean institutions, as well as social movements. Thus one may recognize the historical effect of a company, a market, or the state. The case of HIV/AIDS 'risk groups' illustrates the effect of the institutions of medicine and their ways of catego-rizing the world. The idea of multiple collectivities – as distinct from multiple subjectivities or even intersubjectivity – allows far more room for politics in the operation of structure. Regulation and contestation become more observable and, in one sense, more concrete.

An irony of social framing theory is its tendency to lose the body. In much argumentation about sexuality, the body and relationships fall apart, or are opposed as natural to social. The key to the difficulty is the implicit equation of 'body' and 'nature'. As long as that equation holds, then the fuller the recognition of the bodily dimension in sexuality – whether in eroti-cism, violence, male/female bodily difference – the stronger the push towards nativism. The tendency is clear in some feminist argument about sexual violence. Argument that empha-sizes the social tends to be bloodless, to lose the sweat and passion. This can be seen in role theory, in semiotics, and in structural analysis.

It is only with a concept of *the body as social* that the problem can be overcome. Such a concept has been worked out in relation to gender (Kessler and McKenna, 1978; Connell, 1987, pp. 66–88). The very limited biological differences of sex are appropriated by a social process that constructs gender oppositions as taken-for-granted facts of life, naturalizes them, and even transforms the body in pursuit of a social logic. This process is dramatically shown in the social history of fashion (Wilson, 1987).

Keat (1986) makes a similar point in showing that Reich and Foucault, far from being polar opposites, in fact share a position on this issue. The relationship of biological to social processes, Keat argues, does not occur at a boundary between 'the body' and 'society'. It is internal to the human body itself. Bodily processes such as muscular tensions, physical attitudes, etc., are already social. Turner's (1984, p. 190) concept of 'body practices' emphasizes the collective and cultural aspect of this (and perhaps over-emphasizes the intentional).

In relation to sexuality this approach will emphasize such issues as the construction of sexual desirability (the social meanings of age, among other things, being important here); the control of fertility (for instance recent feminist work on the social meaning of *in vitro* fertilization); the social structuring of arousal ('Never the time, the place / And the loved one all together!'); the collective dimension in body self-images and body fantasies (as illustrated by Glassner's (1988) research on the industry that has grown up in the United States around appearance and fitness).

This approach has some disturbing consequences for methodology in the social sciences. The effect of abstraction in research practices, especially in quantification and experimentation, is to eliminate whole, functioning bodies as components of social-scientific knowledge. In terms of research on sexuality, this has the odd and important effect that fucking is treated as an act of cognition. In this sense it is capable of incorporation into language and therefore is able to be reflected on and represented abstractly. It can be studied in the accounts of individuals as an assemblage of sexual events. Inventories of sexual practices such as those retrieved in sexual diary keeping (Davies, 1990) provide a striking example of the schematization of sexuality that results. Our argument would suggest the crucial importance of research methods open to an understanding of embodiment, the choreography of sex, the tactics of sensation, the manoeuvres of desire.

Finally, we need to consider the political implications of the theoretical re-focusing being proposed. A driving force in the theoretical work of the 1960s and 1970s was the idea of sexual liberation. This concept combined two ideas: the lifting of social prohibitions on sexual behaviour (as in the journalistic notion of 'permissiveness'), and the dismantling of the power of one social group over another. In the 1970s, in the work of gay activists and theorists influenced by radical readings of Freud (Altman, 1972; Mieli, 1980), this approached the idea of a general social revolution fuelled by sex as a kind of erotic explosive. It was a considerable comedown from this to the Foucauldian notions of sexuality as an effect of power and of gay sexual identity as a product of 'regulation'. Social framing theories helped the critique of nativist models of deviance, but they did not point towards positive goals for change.

It now seems clear that the prospect of sexual revolution (and gay liberation) became transformed in practice as well as in theory in the developing modern gay communities. It modulated into a pursuit of the self in sex, a claim to sexual rights, exercised in the institutionalized sex-on-premises venues and in a growing sense of gay community. A more conspicuous manifestation was the reclaiming of masculinity by gay men, that colonization of masculine imagery and style, which simultaneously undermined classic masculine pretence. The irony of this colonization was not lost on gay men themselves (Bersani, 1988). Gay liberation was not alone during the 1970s and 1980s in this softening of agendas. Segal (1987) traces the internal conflicts in British feminism that led to a shift from the defence of erotic freedom in the face of an essentially nativist emphasis on sexual difference.

The agenda of gay liberation was not completely lost, nor reduced to civil liberties. It remained sufficiently available to challenge the early responses to the HIV epidemic, which called for homosexual celibacy, and was able to produce the idea of 'safe sex' as we now know it. Safe sex and later programmes which mobilize its erotic and transgressive character (Gordon, n.d.; Dowsett, 1990) are examples of the importance of this early recognition of power in sexuality.

A fully social concept of sexuality, of the kind discussed in the previous section, would revive the concept of sexual liberation. But the concept would take a different form from the idea of an erotic explosion. Rather it would have to do with the democratization of the social relationships constituted through sexuality.

As in the earlier argument, homosexuality may play a leading role in this, but for a different reason. It is significant not so much as the site of the severest repression, but as the milieu of the most egalitarian sexual relationships currently available as models in our culture. The high degree of reciprocity in gay men's sexual practice (documented in Connell and Kippax, 1990) suggests one path forward.

The need for a revitalized liberation agenda becomes more urgent with regard to the negotiation of safe sex in the face of the HIV epidemic. Part of the success of gay men's responses to sexual behaviour change is, arguably, due to this reciprocity. Kippax *et al.* (1990) have argued that HIV/AIDS prevention strategies designed for heterosexuals may not be able to rely on the same negotiation, given the structure of power relations in heterosexuality, which disadvantage women. Liberation in sexual relationships is thus not only an expressive demand. It is crucially connected with the struggle for *equality* between social groups.

References

ALLEN, J.A. (1990) *Sex and Secrets: Crimes Involving Australian Women since 1880*, Melbourne: Oxford University Press.
ALTMAN, D. (1972) *Homosexual Oppression and Liberation*, Sydney: Angus and Robertson.
ARCHPOET (1952 [1160 orig.]) 'Confession', in WADDELL, H. (ed.) *Medieval Latin Lyrics*, Harmondsworth: Penguin.
AUGUSTINE, (1945 [426 orig.]) *The City of God XIV*, London: J.M. Dent and Sons.
BERSANI, L. (1988) 'Is the rectum a grave?', in CRIMP, D. (ed.) *AIDS: Cultural Analysis, Cultural Activism*, Cambridge, MA: MIT Press.
BOLIN, A. (1988) *In Search of Eve: Transsexual Rights of Passage*, Massachusetts: Bergin and Garvey.
BRAY, A. (1982) *Homosexuality in Renaissance England*, London: Gay Men's Press.
BURGIN, V., DONALD, J. and KAPLAN, C. (1986) *Formations of Fantasy*, London: Methuen.
CONNELL, R.W. (1987) *Gender and Power*, Sydney: Allen and Unwin.
—— (1987) 'The concept of role and what to do with it', *Australian and New Zealand Journal of Sociology*, 15(3), pp. 7–17.
—— and KIPPAX, S. (1990) 'Sexuality and the AIDS crisis: patterns of pleasure and practice in an Australian sample of gay and bisexual men', *The Journal of Sex Research*, 27(2), pp. 167–98.
COWARD, R. (1984) *Female Desire*, London: Paladin.
DARWIN, C. (1874) *Descent of Man*, London, John Murray.
DAVIES, P. (1990) 'Patterns in homosexual relations: the use of the diary method', *Project SIGMA Working Paper 17*, Cardiff: University College, Social Research Unit.
DINNERSTEIN, D. (1976) *The Mermaid and the Minotaur*, New York: Harper and Row.
DOWSETT, G.W. (1990) 'Reaching men who have sex with men in Australia: an overview of AIDS education, community intervention and community attachment strategies', *Australian Journal of Social Issues*, 25(3), pp. 186–98.
EISENSTEIN, H. and JARDINE A. (1980) *The Future of Difference*, Boston, MA: G.K. Hall.
EPSTEIN, C.F. (1988) *Deceptive Distinctions: Sex, Gender and the Social Order*, New Haven, CT: Yale University Press.

FOUCAULT, M. (1973a) *Madness and Civilization: A History of Insanity in the Age of Reason*, New York: Vintage Books.

—— (1973b) *The Birth of the Clinic*, New York: Pantheon.

—— (1977) *Discipline and Punish*, New York: Vintage Books.

—— (1978) *The History of Sexuality, vol. 1: An Introduction*, Harmondsworth: Penguin.

FREUD, S. (1953 [1900 orig.]) 'The interpretation of dreams', in *Complete Psychological Works*, Standard Edition, vols 4 and 5, London: Hogarth.

—— (1953 [1905 orig.]) 'Three essays on the theory of sexuality', in *Complete Psychological Works*, Standard Edition, vol. 7, London: Hogarth.

—— (1953 [1930 orig.]) 'Civilization and its discontents', in *Complete Psychological Works*, Standard Edition, vol. 21, London: Hogarth.

GAGNON, J.H. and SIMON, H. (1974) *Sexual Conduct: The Social Sources of Human Sexuality*, London: Hutchinson.

GAME, A. and PRINGLE, R. (1979) 'Sexuality and the suburban dream', *Australian and New Zealand Journal of Sociology*, 15(2), pp. 4–15.

GIDDENS, A. (1984) *The Constitution of Society*, Cambridge: Polity Press.

GLASSNER, B. (1988) *Bodies: Why We Look the Way We Do (And How We Feel About It)*, New York: Putnam.

GORDON, P. (n.d.) *Safe Sex Education Workshops for Gay and Bisexual Men*. A Review, London, unpublished.

GREENBERG, D.F. (1988) *The Construction of Homosexuality*, Chicago: University of Chicago Press.

HEARN, J. and PARKIN, W. (1987) *Sex at Work: The Power and Paradox of Organization Sexuality*, Brighton: Wheatsheaf Books.

HERDT, G. (1981) *Guardians of the Flutes*, New York: McGraw-Hill.

—— (ed.) (1984) *Ritualized Homosexuality in Melanesia*, Berkeley: University of California Press.

JOHNSTON, C. (1981) 'Review of M. Mieli, Homosexuality and Liberation', *Gay Information*, 5, pp. 20–1.

KEAT, R. (1986) 'The human body in social theory: Reich, Foucault and the repressive hypothesis', *Radical Philosophy*, 42, pp. 24–32.

KESSLER, S.J. and MCKENNA, W. (1978) *Gender: An Ethnomethodological Approach*, New York: Wiley.

KIPPAX, S., CRAWFORD, J., WALDBY, C. and BENTON, P. (1990) 'Women negotiating heterosex: implications for AIDS prevention', *Women's Studies International Forum*, 13(6), pp. 533–42.

KOSIK, K. (1976) *Dialetics of the Concrete: A Study of the Problems of Man and World*, Dordrecht: D. Reidel Publishing Company.

KRAFFT-EBING, R. von (1965 [1886 orig.]) *Psychopathia Sexualis*, 12th edition, New York: Paperback Library.

KRISTEVA, J. (1984) *Revolution in Poetic Language*, New York: Columbia University Press.

KUHN, T.S. (1962) *The Structure of Scientific Revolutions*, Chicago: University of Chicago Press.

LAKATOS, I. (1970) 'Falsification and the methodology of scientific research programmes', in LAKATOS, I. and MUSGRAVE, A. (eds) *Criticism and the Growth of Knowledge*, Cambridge: Cambridge University Press.

LESTER, D. (1975) *Unusual Sexual Behaviour*, Springfield: Charles C. Thomas.

LOCKHART, W.B. *et al.* [The Presidential Commission on Obscenity and Pornography] (1970) *The Report of the Commission on Obscenity*, Washington, DC: US Government Printing Office.

LYOTARD, J. (1984) *The Postmodern Condition: A Report on Knowledge*, Manchester: Manchester University Press.

MCINTOSH, M. (1968) 'The homosexual role', *Social Problems*, 16(2), pp. 182–92.

MAGAREY, S. (1985) 'Conditions for the emergence of an activist feminist movement in Australia in the nineteenth century', paper to the annual conference of Sociological Association of Australia and New Zealand, Brisbane.

MALINOWSKI, B. (1927) *Sex and Repression in Savage Society*, Chicago: Meridian Books.

—— (1929) *The Sexual Life of Savages in North-western Melanesia*, New York: Brace & World.

MARCUSE, H. (1968) *One Dimensional Man*, London: Sphere Books.

MARSHALL, D.S. and SUGGS, R.C. (eds) (1971) *Human Sexual Behaviour: Variations in the Ethnographic Spectrum*, New York: Basic Books.

MASTERS, W.H. and JOHNSON, V.E. (1966) *Human Sexual Response*, Boston, MA: Little, Brown.

—— (1970) *Homosexuality in Perspective*, Boston, MA: Little, Brown.

MEAD, M. (1935) *Sex and Temperament in Three Primitive Societies*, New York: Morrow.

—— (1949) *Male and Female: A Study of the Sexes in a Changing World*, London: Gollancz.

MIELI, M. (1980) *Homosexuality and Liberation: Elements of a Gay Critique*, London: Gay Men's Press.

MILLETT, K. (1972) *Sexual Politics*, London: Abacus.

MITCHELL, J. (1971) *Woman's Estate*, Harmondsworth: Penguin.

—— (1974) *Psychoanalysis and Feminism: Freud, Reich, Laing and Women*, New York: Vintage Books.

O'CARROLL, T. (1982) *Paedophilia: The Radical Case*, Boston, MA: Alyson.

PARKER, R., GUIMARÃES, C.D. and STRUCHNER, C.D. (1989) 'The impact of AIDS health promotion for gay and bisexual men in Rio de Janeiro, Brazil', paper to WHO Workshop on AIDS Health Promotion Activities Directed towards Gay and Bisexual Men, Geneva, May.

PERKINS, R. (1983) *The 'Drag Queen' Scene: Transsexuals in King's Cross*, Sydney: Allen and Unwin.

PETERS, R. (1973) 'The first kiss', in YOUNG, I. (ed.) *The Male Muse: A Gay Anthology*, New York: The Crossing Press.

POLLAK, M. (1988) *Les Homosexuels et le SIDA: sociologie d'une épidémie*, Paris: A.M. Métailié.

POMEROY, W.B. (1972) *Dr Kinsey and the Institute for Sex Research*, New York: Harper and Row.

PRINGLE, R. (1988) *Secretaries Talk: Sexuality, Power and Work*, Sydney: Allen and Unwin.

REICH, W. (1972) *Sexpol: Essays 1929–1934*, BAXANDALL, L. (ed.), New York: Vintage.

RICH, A. (1980) 'Compulsory heterosexuality and lesbian existence', *Signs*, 5(4), pp. 631–60.

RUBIN, G. (1975) 'The traffic in women: notes on the "political economy" of sex,' in REITER, R., *Toward an Anthropology of Women*, New York: Monthly Review Press.

DE SADE, M. (1966 [1785 orig.]) *120 Days of Sodom*, in WAINHOUSE, A. and SEAVER, R. (eds) *The Marquis de Sade. The 120 Days of Sodom and Other Writings*, New York: Grove.

SARGENT, D. (1983) 'Reformulating (homo)sexual politics: radical theory and practice in the gay movement', in ALLEN, J.A. and PATTON, P. (eds) *Beyond Marxism?: Interventions After Marx*, Sydney: Intervention Publications.

SEGAL, L. (1987) 'Sensual uncertainty or why the clitoris is not enough', in CARTLEDGE, S. and RYAN, J. (eds) *Sex and Love: New Thoughts on Old Contradictions*, London: The Women's Press.

SHILTS, R. (1987) *And the Band Played On*, New York: St Martin's Press.

TREICHLER, P. (1988) 'AIDS, homophobia and biomedical discourse: an epidemic of signification', in CRIMP, D. (ed.) *AIDS: Cultural Analysis, Cultural Activism*, Cambridge, MA: MIT Press.

TURNER, B.S. (1984) *The Body and Society*, Oxford: Blackwell.

VANCE, C. (1989) 'Social construction theory: problems in the history of sexuality', in ALTMAN, D. *et al.* (eds) *Homosexuality, Which Homosexuality?*, London: Gay Men's Press.

WAKELING, A. (1979) 'A general psychiatric approach to sexual deviation', in ROSEN, I. (ed.) *Sexual Deviation*, 2nd edition, Oxford: Oxford University Press.

WALKOWITZ, J.R. (1980) *Prostitution and Victorian Society: Women, Class, and the State*, Cambridge: Cambridge University Press.

WATNEY, S. (1988) 'The Spectacle of AIDS', in CRIMP, D. (ed.) *AIDS: Cultural Analysis, Cultural Activism*, Cambridge, MA: MIT Press.

WEEDON, C. (1987) *Feminist Practice and Poststructuralist Theory*, Oxford: Blackwell.

WEEKS, J. (1977) *Coming Out: Homosexual Politics in Britain from the 19th Century to the Present*, London: Quartet.

206   *R. W. Connell and Gary W. Dowsett*

—— (1985) *Sexuality and Its Discontents: Meanings, Myths and Modern Sexualities*, London: Routledge and Kegan Paul.

—— (1986) *Sexuality*, London: Horwood and Tavistock.

WIERINGA, S. (1989) 'An anthropological critique of constructionism: berdaches and butches', in ALTMAN, D. *et al.* (eds) *Homosexuality, Which Homosexuality?*, London: Gay Men's Press.

WILLIAMS, W. (1986) *The Spirit and the Flesh: Sexual Diversity in American Indian Culture*, Boston, MA: Beacon Press.

WILLIS, E. (1984) 'Radical feminism and feminist radicalism', in SAYRES, S. (ed.) *The 60s Without Apology*, Minneapolis: University of Minnesota Press/Social Text.

WILSON, E. (1987) *Adorned in Dreams: Fashion and Modernity*, Berkeley and Los Angeles: University of California Press.

Part 4

Sexual identities/sexual communities

11 Compulsory heterosexuality and lesbian existence

Adrienne Rich [1982/1986]

Foreword [1982]

I want to say a little about the way 'Compulsory Heterosexuality' was originally conceived and the context in which we are now living. It was written in part to challenge the erasure of lesbian existence from so much of scholarly feminist literature, an erasure which I felt (and feel) to be not just anti-lesbian, but anti-feminist in its consequences, and to distort the experience of heterosexual women as well. It was not written to widen divisions but to encourage heterosexual feminists to examine heterosexuality as a political institution which disempowers women – and to change it. I also hoped that other lesbians would feel the depth and breadth of woman identification and woman bonding that has run like a continuous though stifled theme through the heterosexual experience, and that this would become increasingly a politically activating impulse, not simply a validation of personal lives. I wanted the essay to suggest new kinds of criticism, to incite new questions in classrooms and academic journals, and to sketch, at least, some bridge over the gap between *lesbian* and *feminist*. I wanted, at the very least, for feminists to find it less possible to read, write, or teach from a perspective of unexamined heterocentricity.

Within the three years since I wrote 'Compulsory Heterosexuality' – with this energy of hope and desire – the pressures to conform in a society increasingly conservative in mood have become more intense. The New Right's messages to women have been, precisely, that we are the emotional and sexual property of men, and that the autonomy and equality of women threaten family, religion, and state. The institutions by which women have traditionally been controlled – patriarchal motherhood, economic exploitation, the nuclear family, compulsory heterosexuality – are being strengthened by legislation, religious fiat, media imagery, and efforts at censorship. In a worsening economy, the single mother trying to support her children confronts the feminization of poverty which Joyce Miller of the National Coalition of Labor Union Women has named one of the major issues of the 1980s. The lesbian, unless in disguise, faces discrimination in hiring and harassment and violence in the street. Even within feminist-inspired institutions such as battered-women's shelters and Women's Studies programmes, open lesbians are fired and others warned to stay in the closet. The retreat into sameness-assimilation for those who can manage it is the most passive and debilitating of responses to political repression, economic insecurity, and a renewed open season on difference.

I want to note that documentation of male violence against women – within the home especially – has been accumulating rapidly in this period. At the same time, in the realm of literature which depicts woman bonding and woman identification as essential for female survival, a steady stream of writing and criticism has been coming from women of colour in general and lesbians of colour in particular – the latter group being even more profoundly erased in academic feminist scholarship by the double bias of racism and homophobia.[1]

There has recently been an intensified debate on female sexuality among feminists and lesbians, with lines often furiously and bitterly drawn, with *sadomasochism* and *pornography* as key words which are variously defined according to who is talking. The depth of women's rage and fear regarding sexuality and its relation to power and pain is real, even when the dialogue sounds simplistic, self-righteous, or like parallel monologues.

Because of all these developments, there are parts of this essay that I would word differently, qualify, or expand if I were writing it today. But I continue to think that heterosexual feminists will draw political strength for change from taking a critical stance toward the ideology which *demands* heterosexuality, and that lesbians cannot assume that we are untouched by that ideology and the institutions founded upon it. There is nothing about such a critique that requires us to think of ourselves as victims, as having been brainwashed or totally powerless. Coercion and compulsion are among the conditions in which women have learned to recognize our strength. Resistance is a major theme in this essay and in the study of women's lives, if we know what we are looking for.

I

> Biologically men have only one innate orientation – a sexual one that draws them to women – while women have two innate orientations, sexual toward men and reproductive toward their young.
>
> (Rossi, 1976)

> I was a woman terribly vulnerable, critical, using femaleness as a sort of standard or yardstick to measure and discard men. Yes – something like that. I was an Anna who invited defeat from men without ever being conscious of it. (But I am conscious of it. And being conscious of it means I shall leave it all behind me and become – but what?) I was stuck fast in an emotion common to women of our time, that can turn them bitter, or Lesbian, or solitary. Yes, that Anna during that time was …
>
> (Lessing, 1977, p. 480)

The bias of compulsory heterosexuality, through which lesbian experience is perceived on a scale ranging from deviant to abhorrent or simply rendered invisible, could be illustrated from many texts other than the two just preceding. The assumption made by Rossi, that women are 'innately' sexually oriented only toward men, and that made by Lessing, that the lesbian is simply acting out of her bitterness toward men, are by no means theirs alone; these assumptions are widely current in literature and in the social sciences.

I am concerned here with two other matters as well: first, how and why women's choice of women as passionate comrades, life partners, co-workers, lovers, community has been crushed, invalidated, forced into hiding and disguise; and second, the virtual or total neglect of lesbian existence in a wide range of writings, including feminist scholarship. Obviously there is a connection here. I believe that much feminist theory and criticism is stranded on this shoal.

My organizing impulse is the belief that it is not enough for feminist thought that specifically lesbian texts exist. Any theory or cultural/political creation that treats lesbian existence as a marginal or less 'natural' phenomenon, as mere 'sexual preference', or as the mirror image of either heterosexual or male homosexual relations is profoundly weakened thereby, whatever its other contributions. Feminist theory can no longer afford merely to voice a toleration of 'lesbianism' as an 'alternative life style' or make token allusion to lesbians. A feminist critique of compulsory heterosexual orientation for women is long overdue. In this exploratory paper, I shall try to show why.

I will begin by way of examples, briefly discussing four books that have appeared in the last few years, written from different viewpoints and political orientations, but all presenting themselves, and favourably reviewed, as feminist (see Chodorow, 1978; Dinnerstein, 1976; Ehrenreich and English, 1978; Miller, 1976). All take as a basic assumption that the social relations of the sexes are disordered and extremely problematic, if not disabling, for women; all seek paths toward change. I have learned more from some of these books than from others, but on this I am clear: each one might have been more accurate, more powerful, more truly a force for change had the author dealt with lesbian existence as a reality and as a source of knowledge and power available to women, or with the institution of heterosexuality itself as a beachhead of male dominance.[2] In none of them is the question ever raised as to whether, in a different context or other things being equal, women would *choose* heterosexual coupling and marriage; heterosexuality is presumed the 'sexual preference' of 'most women', either implicitly or explicitly. In none of these books, which concern themselves with mothering, sex roles, relationships, and societal prescriptions for women, is compulsory heterosexuality ever examined as an institution powerfully affecting all these, or the idea of 'preference' or 'innate orientation' even indirectly questioned.

In *For Her Own Good: 150 Years of the Experts' Advice to Women* by Barbara Ehrenreich and Deirdre English, the authors' superb pamphlets, *Witches, Midwives and Nurses: A History of Women Healers* and *Complaints and Disorders: The Sexual Politics of Sickness*, are developed into a provocative and complex study. Their thesis in this book is that the advice given to American women by male health professionals, particularly in the areas of marital sex, maternity, and child care, has echoed the dictates of the economic marketplace and the role capitalism has needed women to play in production and/or reproduction. Women have become the consumer victims of various cures, therapies, and normative judgements in different periods (including the prescription to middle-class women to embody and preserve the sacredness of the home – the 'scientific' romanticization of the home itself). None of the advice from the 'experts' has been either particularly scientific or women-oriented; it has reflected male needs, male fantasies about women, and male interest in controlling women particularly in the realms of sexuality and motherhood – fused with the requirements of industrial capitalism. So much of this book is so devastatingly informative and is written with such lucid feminist wit, that I kept waiting as I read for the basic proscription against lesbianism to be examined. It never was.

This can hardly be for lack of information. Jonathan Katz's *Gay American History* (1976) tells us that as early as 1656 the New Haven Colony prescribed the death penalty for lesbians. Katz provides many suggestive and informative documents on the 'treatment' (or torture) of lesbians by the medical profession in the nineteenth and twentieth centuries. Recent work by the historian Nancy Sahli (1979) documents the crackdown on intense female friendships among college women at the turn of the present century. The ironic title *For Her Own Good* might have referred first and foremost to the economic imperative to heterosexuality and marriage and to the sanctions imposed against single women and widows – both of whom have been and still are viewed as deviant. Yet, in this often enlightening Marxist-feminist overview of male prescriptions for female sanity and health, the economics of prescriptive heterosexuality go unexamined.[3]

Of the three psychoanalytically based books, one, Jean Baker Miller's *Toward a New Psychology of Women*, is written as if lesbians simply do not exist, even as marginal beings.

Given Miller's title, I find this astonishing. However, the favourable reviews the book has received in feminist journals, including *Signs* and *Spokeswoman*, suggest that Miller's heterocentric assumptions are widely shared. In *The Mermaid and the Minotaur: Sexual Arrangements and the Human Malaise*, Dorothy Dinnerstein makes an impassioned argument for the sharing of parenting between women and men and for an end to what she perceives as the male/female symbiosis of 'gender arrangements', which she feels are leading the species further into violence and self-extinction. Apart from other problems that I have with this book (including her silence on the institutional and random terrorism men have practised on women – and children – throughout history [see Barry, 1979; Brownmiller, 1975; Daly, 1978; Griffin, 1978; Russell and van der Ven, 1976; and *Aegis: Magazine on Ending Violence against Women*, n.d.),[4] and her obsession with psychology to the neglect of economic and other material realities that help to create psychological reality], I find Dinnerstein's view of the relations between women and men as 'a collaboration to keep history mad' utterly ahistorical. She means by this a collaboration to perpetuate social relations which are hostile, exploitative, and destructive to life itself. She sees women and men as equal partners in the making of 'sexual arrangements', seemingly unaware of the repeated struggles of women to resist oppression (their own and that of others) and to change their condition. She ignores, specifically, the history of women who – as witches, *femmes seules*, marriage resisters, spinsters, autonomous widows, and/or lesbians – have managed on varying levels *not* to collaborate. It is this history, precisely, from which feminists have so much to learn and on which there is overall such blanketing silence. Dinnerstein acknowledges at the end of her book that 'female separatism', though 'on a large scale and in the long run wildly impractical', has something to teach us: 'Separate, women could in principle set out to learn from scratch – undeflected by the opportunities to evade this task that men's presence has so far offered – what intact self-creative humanness is' (Dinnerstein, 1976, p. 272). Phrases like 'intact self-creative humanness' obscure the question of what the many forms of female separatism have actually been addressing. The fact is that women in every culture and throughout history *have* undertaken the task of independent, nonheterosexual, woman-connected existence, to the extent made possible by their context, often in the belief that they were the 'only ones' ever to have done so. They have undertaken it even though few women have been in an economic position to resist marriage altogether, and even though attacks against unmarried women have ranged from aspersion and mockery to deliberate gynocide, including the burning and torturing of millions of widows and spinsters during the witch persecutions of the fifteenth, sixteenth, and seventeenth centuries in Europe.

Nancy Chodorow does come close to the edge of an acknowledgement of lesbian existence. Like Dinnerstein, Chodorow believes that the fact that women, and women only, are responsible for child care in the sexual division of labour has led to an entire social organization of gender inequality, and that men as well as women must become primary carers for children if that inequality is to change. In the process of examining, from a psychoanalytic perspective, how mothering by women affects the psychological development of girl and boy children, she offers documentation that men are 'emotionally secondary' in women's lives, that 'women have a richer, ongoing inner world to fall back on … men do not become as emotionally important to women as women do to men' (Chodorow, 1978, pp. 197–8). This would carry into the late-twentieth-century Smith-Rosenberg's findings about eighteenth- and nineteenth-century women's emotional focus on women. 'Emotionally important' can, of course, refer to anger as well as to love, or to that intense mixture of the two often found in women's relationships with women – one aspect of what I have come to call the 'double life of women' (see below). Chodorow concludes that because women have women as mothers, 'the mother remains a primary internal object [*sic*] to the girl, so that heterosexual relationships are on the model of a nonexclusive, second relationship for her, whereas for the boy they re-create an exclusive, primary relationship'. According to Chodorow, women 'have learned to deny the limitations of masculine lovers for both psychological and practical reasons' (1978, pp. 198–9).

But the practical reasons (like witch burnings, male control of law, theology, and science, or economic nonviability within the sexual division of labour) are glossed over. Chodorow's account barely glances at the constraints and sanctions which historically have enforced or ensured the coupling of women with men and obstructed or penalized women's coupling or allying in independent groups with other women. She dismisses lesbian existence with the comment that 'lesbian relationships do tend to re-create mother–daughter emotions and connections, but most women are heterosexual' (implied: more mature, having developed beyond the mother–daughter connection?). She then adds: 'This heterosexual preference and taboos on homosexuality, in addition to objective economic dependence on men, make the option of primary sexual bonds with other women unlikely – though more prevalent in recent years' (1978, p. 200). The significance of that qualification seems irresistible, but Chodorow does not explore it further. Is she saying that lesbian existence has become more *visible* in recent years (in certain groups), that economic and other pressures have changed (under capitalism, socialism, or both), and that consequently more women are rejecting the heterosexual 'choice'? She argues that women want children because their heterosexual relationships lack richness and intensity, that in having a child a woman seeks to re-create her own intense relationship with her mother. It seems to me that on the basis of her own findings, Chodorow leads us implicitly to conclude that heterosexuality is *not* a 'preference' for women, that, for one thing, it fragments the erotic from the emotional in a way that women find impoverishing and painful. Yet her book participates in mandating it. Neglecting the covert socializations and the overt forces which have channelled women into marriage and heterosexual romance, pressures ranging from the selling of daughters to the silences of literature to the images of the television screen, she, like Dinnerstein, is stuck with trying to reform a man-made institution – compulsory heterosexuality – as if, despite profound emotional impulses and complementarities drawing women toward women, there is a mystical/biological heterosexual inclination, a 'preference' or 'choice' which draws women toward men.

Moreover, it is understood that this 'preference' does not need to be explained unless through the tortuous theory of the female Oedipus complex or the necessity for species reproduction. It is lesbian sexuality which (usually, and incorrectly, 'included' under male homosexuality) is seen as requiring explanation. This assumption of female heterosexuality seems to me in itself remarkable: it is an enormous assumption to have glided so silently into the foundations of our thought.

The extension of this assumption is the frequently heard assertion that in a world of genuine equality, where men are nonoppressive and nurturing, everyone would be bisexual Such a notion blurs and sentimentalizes the actualities within which women have experienced sexuality; it is a liberal leap across the tasks and struggles of here and now, the continuing process of sexual definition which will generate its own possibilities and choices. (It also assumes that women who have chosen women have done so simply because men are oppressive and emotionally unavailable, which still fails to account for women who continue to pursue relationships with oppressive and/or emotionally unsatisfying men.) I am suggesting that heterosexuality, like motherhood, needs to be recognized and studied as a *political institution* – even, or especially, by those individuals who feel they are, in their personal experience, the precursors of a new social relation between the sexes.

II

If women are the earliest sources of emotional caring and physical nurture for both female and male children, it would seem logical, from a feminist perspective at least, to pose the following questions: whether the search for love and tenderness in both sexes does not originally lead toward women; *why in fact women would ever redirect that search*; why species survival, the means of impregnation, and emotional/erotic relationships should ever have become so rigidly identified with each other; and why such violent strictures should be found necessary to enforce women's total emotional, erotic loyalty and subservience to men. I doubt that enough feminist scholars and theorists have taken the pains to acknowledge the societal forces which wrench women's emotional and erotic energies away from themselves and other women and from woman-identified values. These forces, as I shall try to show, range from literal physical enslavement to the disguising and distorting of possible options.

I do not assume that mothering by women is a 'sufficient cause' of lesbian existence. But the issue of mothering by women has been much in the air of late, usually accompanied by the view that increased parenting by men would minimize antagonism between the sexes and equalize the sexual imbalance of power of males over females. These discussions are carried on without reference to compulsory heterosexuality as a phenomenon, *let alone* as an ideology. I do not wish to psychologize here, but rather to identify sources of male power. I believe large numbers of men could, in fact, undertake child care on a large scale without radically altering the balance of male power in a male-identified society.

In her essay 'The Origin of the Family' (1975), Kathleen Gough lists eight characteristics of male power in archaic and contemporary societies which I would like to use as a framework: 'men's ability to deny women sexuality or to force it upon them; to command or exploit their labour to control their produce; to control or rob them of their children; to confine them physically and prevent their movement; to use them as objects in male transactions; to cramp their creativeness; or to withhold from them large areas of the society's knowledge and cultural attainments' (Gough, 1975, pp. 69–70). (Gough does not perceive these power characteristics as specifically enforcing heterosexuality, only as producing sexual inequality.) Below, Gough's words appear in italics; the elaboration of each of her categories, in brackets, is my own.

Characteristics of male power include *the power of men*

1   *to deny women* [their own] *sexuality* – [by means of clitoridectomy and infibulation; chastity belts; punishment, including death, for female adultery; punishment, including death, for lesbian sexuality; psychoanalytic denial of the clitoris; strictures against masturbation; denial of maternal and postmenopausal sensuality; unnecessary hysterectomy; pseudolesbian images in the media and literature; closing of archives and destruction of documents relating to lesbian existence]

2   *or to force it* [male sexuality] *upon them* – [by means of rape (including marital rape) and wife beating; father–daughter, brother–sister incest; the socialization of women to feel that male sexual 'drive' amounts to a right (Barry, 1979, pp. 216–19); idealization of heterosexual romance in art, literature, the media, advertising, etc.; child marriage; arranged marriage, prostitution; the harem; psychoanalytic doctrines of frigidity and vaginal orgasm; pornographic depictions of women responding pleasurably to sexual violence and humiliation (a subliminal message being that sadistic heterosexuality is more 'normal' than sensuality between women)]

3   *to command or exploit their labour to control their produce* – [by means of the institutions of marriage and motherhood as unpaid production; the horizontal segregation of women in paid employment; the decoy of the upwardly mobile token woman; male control of abortion, contraception, sterilization, and childbirth; pimping; female infanticide, which robs mothers of daughters and contributes to generalized devaluation of women]

4   *to control or rob them of their children* – [by means of father right and 'legal kidnapping' (Demeter, 1977, pp. xx, 126–8); enforced sterilization; systematized infanticide; seizure of children from lesbian mothers by the courts; the malpractice of male obstetrics; use of the mother as 'token torturer' (Daly, 1978, pp. 139–41, 163–5) in genital mutilation or in binding the daughter's feet (or mind) to fit her for marriage]

5   *to confine them physically and prevent their movement* – [by means of rape as terrorism, keeping women off the streets; purdah; foot binding; atrophying of women's athletic capabilities; high heels and 'feminine' dress codes in fashion; the veil; sexual harassment on the streets; horizontal segregation of women in employment; prescriptions for 'full-time' mothering at home; enforced economic dependence of wives]

6   *to use them as objects in male transactions* – [use of women as 'gifts'; bride price; pimping; arranged marriage; use of women as entertainers to facilitate male deals – e.g., wife-hostess, cocktail waitress required to dress for male sexual titillation, call girls, 'bunnies', geisha, *kisaeng* prostitutes, secretaries]

7   *to cramp their creativeness* – [witch persecutions as campaigns against midwives and female healers, and as pogrom against independent, 'unassimilated' women (see Ehrenreich and English, 1973; Dworkin, 1974); definition of male pursuits as more valuable than female within any culture, so that cultural values become the embodiment of male subjectivity; restriction of female self-fulfilment to marriage and motherhood; sexual exploitation of women by male artists and teachers; the social and economic disruption of women's creative aspirations (see Woolf, 1929, 1966; Olsen, 1978; Cliff, 1979); erasure of female tradition (see Daly, 1973; Olsen, 1978)]

8   *to withhold from them large areas of the society's knowledge and cultural attainments* – [by means of noneducation of females; the 'Great Silence' regarding women and particularly lesbian existence in history and culture (Daly, 1973, p. 93); sex-role tracking which deflects women from science, technology, and other 'masculine' pursuits; male social/ professional bonding which excludes women; discrimination against women in the professions]

These are some of the methods by which male power is manifested and maintained. Looking at the schema, what surely impresses itself is the fact that we are confronting not a simple maintenance of inequality and property possession, but a pervasive cluster of forces, ranging from physical brutality to control of consciousness, which suggests that an enormous potential counter-force is having to be restrained.

Some of the forms by which male power manifests itself are more easily recognizable as enforcing heterosexuality on women than are others. Yet each one I have listed adds to the cluster of forces within which women have been convinced that marriage and sexual orientation toward men are inevitable – even if unsatisfying or oppressive – components of their lives. The chastity belt; child marriage; erasure of lesbian existence (except as exotic and perverse) in art, literature, film; idealization of heterosexual romance and marriage – these are some fairly obvious forms of compulsion, the first two exemplifying physical force, the second two control of consciousness. While clitoridectomy has been assailed by feminists as a form of woman torture (Hosken, 1979; Russell and van der Ven, 1976),[5] Kathleen Barry first pointed out that it is not simply a way of turning the young girl into a 'marriageable' woman through brutal surgery. It intends that women in the intimate proximity of polygynous marriage will not form sexual relationships with each other, that – from a male, genital fetishist perspective – female erotic connections, even in a sex-segregated situation, will be literally excised (Barry, 1979, pp. 163–4).

The function of pornography as an influence on consciousness is a major public issue of our time, when a multibillion-dollar industry has the power to disseminate increasingly sadistic, women-degrading visual images. But even so-called soft-core pornography and advertising depict women as objects of sexual appetite devoid of emotional context, without individual meaning or personality – essentially as a sexual commodity to be consumed by males. (So-called lesbian pornography, created for the male voyeuristic eye, is equally devoid of emotional context or individual personality.) The most pernicious message relayed by pornography is that women are natural sexual prey to men and love it, that sexuality and violence are congruent, and that for women sex is essentially masochistic, humiliation plea-surable, physical abuse erotic. But along with this message comes another, not always recog-nized: that enforced submission and the use of cruelty, if played out in heterosexual pairing, is sexually 'normal', while sensuality between women, including erotic mutuality and respect, is 'queer', 'sick', and either pornographic in itself or not very exciting compared with the sexuality of whips and bondage.[6] Pornography does not simply create a climate in which sex and violence are interchangeable; *it widens the range of behaviour considered acceptable from men in heterosexual intercourse* – behaviour which reiteratively strips women of their autonomy, dignity, and sexual potential, including the potential of loving and being loved by women in mutuality and integrity.

In her brilliant study *Sexual Harassment of Working Women: A Case of Sex Discrimina-tion*, Catharine A. MacKinnon delineates the intersection of compulsory heterosexuality and economics. Under capitalism, women are horizontally segregated by gender and occupy a structurally inferior position in the workplace. This is hardly news, but MacKinnon raises the question why, even if capitalism 'requires some collection of individuals to occupy low-status, low-paying positions … such persons must be biologically female', and goes on to point out that 'the fact that male employers often do not hire qualified women, *even when they could pay them less than men* suggests that more than the profit motive is implicated' [emphasis added] (MacKinnon, 1979, pp. 15–16). She cites a wealth of material documenting the fact that women are not only segregated in low-paying service jobs (as secretaries, domes-tics, nurses, typists, telephone operators, child-care workers, waitresses), but that 'sexualiza-tion of the woman' is part of the job. Central and intrinsic to the economic realities of women's lives is the requirement that women will 'market sexual attractiveness to men, who tend to hold the economic power and position to enforce their predilections'. And MacKinnon documents that 'sexual harassment perpetuates the interlocked structure by which women have been kept sexually in thrall to men at the bottom of the labour market. Two forces of American society converge: men's control over women's sexuality and capi-tal's control over employees' work lives' (1979, p. 174). Thus, women in the workplace are at the mercy of sex as power in a vicious circle. Economically disadvantaged, women – whether waitresses or professors – endure sexual harassment to keep their jobs and learn to behave in a complaisantly and ingratiatingly heterosexual manner because they discover this is their true qualification for employment, whatever the job description. And, MacKinnon notes, the woman who too decisively resists sexual overtures in the workplace is accused of being 'dried up' and sexless, or lesbian. This raises a specific difference between the experiences of lesbians and homosexual men. A lesbian, closeted on her job because of heterosexist prejudice, is not simply forced into denying the truth of her outside relationships or private life. Her job depends on her pretending to be not merely heterosexual, but a heterosexual *woman* in terms of dressing and playing the feminine, deferential role required of 'real women'.

MacKinnon raises radical questions as to the qualitative differences between sexual harassment, rape, and ordinary heterosexual intercourse. ('As one accused rapist put it, he hadn't used "any more force than is usual for males during the preliminaries".') She criticizes Susan Brownmiller (1975) for separating rape from the mainstream of daily life and for her unexamined premise that 'rape is violence, intercourse is sexuality', removing rape from the sexual sphere altogether. Most crucially she argues that 'taking rape from the realm of "the sexual", placing it in the realm of "the violent", allows one to be against it without raising any questions about the extent to which the institution of heterosexuality has defined force as a normal part of "the preliminaries"' (MacKinnon, 1979, p. 219).[7] 'Never is it asked whether, under conditions of male supremacy, the notion of "consent" has any meaning' (1979, p. 298).

The fact is that the workplace, among other social institutions, is a place where women have learned to accept male violation of their psychic and physical boundaries as the price of survival; where women have been educated – no less than by romantic literature or by pornography – to perceive themselves as sexual prey. A woman seeking to escape such casual violations along with economic disadvantage may well turn to marriage as a form of hoped-for protection, while bringing into marriage neither social nor economic power, thus entering that institution also from a disadvantaged position. MacKinnon finally asks:

> What if inequality is built into the social conceptions of male and female sexuality, of masculinity and femininity, of sexiness and heterosexual attractiveness? Incidents of sexual harassment suggest that male sexual desire itself may be aroused by female vulnerability ... Men feel they can take advantage, so they want to, so they do. Examination of sexual harassment, precisely because the episodes appear commonplace, forces one to confront the fact that sexual intercourse normally occurs between economic (as well as physical) unequals ... the apparent legal requirement that violations of women's sexuality appear out of the ordinary before they will be punished helps prevent women from defining the ordinary conditions of their own consent.
>
> (MacKinnon, 1979, p. 220)

Given the nature and extent of heterosexual pressures – the daily 'eroticisation of women's subordination', as MacKinnon phrases it (1979, p. 221) – I question the more or less psychoanalytic perspective (suggested by such writers as Karen Horney, H.R. Hayes, Wolfgang Lederer, and, most recently, Dorothy Dinnerstein) that the male need to control women sexually results from some primal male 'fear of women' and of women's sexual insatiability. It seems more probable that men really fear not that they will have women's sexual appetites forced on them or that women want to smother and devour them, but that women could be indifferent to them altogether, that men could be allowed sexual and emotional – therefore economic – access to women *only* on women's terms, otherwise being left on the periphery of the matrix.

The means of assuring male sexual access to women have recently received searching investigation by Kathleen Barry (1979).[8] She documents extensive and appalling evidence for the existence, on a very large scale, of international female slavery, the institution once known as 'white slavery' but which in fact has involved, and at this very moment involves, women of every race and class. In the theoretical analysis derived from her research, Barry makes the connection between all enforced conditions under which women live subject to men: prostitution, marital rape, father–daughter and brother–sister incest, wife beating, pornography, bride price, the selling of daughters, purdah, and genital mutilation. She sees the rape paradigm – where the victim of sexual assault is held responsible for her own victimization – as leading to the rationalization and acceptance of other forms of enslavement where the woman is presumed to have 'chosen' her fate, to embrace it passively, or to have courted it perversely, through rash or unchaste behaviour. On the contrary, Barry maintains, 'female sexual slavery is present in *all* situations where women or girls cannot change the conditions of their existence; where regardless of how they got into those conditions, e.g., social pressure, economic hardship, misplaced trust, or the longing for affection, they cannot get out; and where they are subject to sexual violence and exploitation' (Barry, 1979, p. 33). She provides a spectrum of concrete examples, not only as to the existence of a widespread international traffic in women, but also as to how this operates – whether in the form of a 'Minnesota pipeline' funnelling blonde, blue-eyed Midwestern runaways to Times Square, or the purchasing of young women out of rural poverty in Latin America or Southeast Asia, or the providing of *maisons d'abattage* for migrant workers in the eighteenth arrondissement of Paris. Instead of 'blaming the victim' or trying to diagnose her presumed pathology, Barry turns her floodlight on the pathology of sex colonization itself, the ideology of 'cultural sadism' represented by the pornography industry and by the overall identification of women primarily as 'sexual beings whose responsibility is the sexual service of men' (1979, p. 103).

Barry delineates what she names a 'sexual domination perspective' through whose lens sexual abuse and terrorism of women by men has been rendered almost invisible by treating it as natural and inevitable. From its point of view, women are expendable as long as the sexual and emotional needs of the male can be satisfied. To replace this perspective of domination with a universal standard of basic freedom for women from gender-specific violence, from constraints on movement, and from male right of sexual and emotional access is the political purpose of her book. Like Mary Daly in *Gyn/Ecology*, Barry rejects structuralist and other cultural-relativist rationalizations for sexual torture and anti-woman violence. In her opening chapter, she asks of her readers that they refuse all handy escapes into ignorance and denial. 'The only way we can come out of hiding, break through our paralysing defences, is to know it all – the full extent of sexual violence and domination of women. ... In *knowing*, in facing directly, we can learn to chart our course out of this oppression, by envisioning and creating a world which will preclude sexual slavery' (1979, p. 5).

> Until we name the practice, give conceptual definition and form to it, illustrate its life over time and in space, those who are its most obvious victims will also not be able to name it or define their experience.

But women are all, in different ways and to different degrees, its victims; and part of the problem with naming and conceptualizing female sexual slavery is, as Barry (1979, p. 100) clearly sees, compulsory heterosexuality.[9] Compulsory heterosexuality simplifies the task of the procurer and pimp in worldwide prostitution rings and 'eros centres', while, in the privacy of the home, it leads the daughter to 'accept' incest/rape by her father, the mother to deny that it is happening, the battered wife to stay on with an abusive husband. 'Befriending or love' is a major tactic of the procurer, whose job it is to turn the runaway or the confused young girl over to the pimp for seasoning. The ideology of heterosexual romance, beamed at her from childhood out of fairy tales, television, films, advertising, popular songs, wedding pageantry, is a tool ready to the procurer's hand and one which he does not hesitate to use, as Barry documents. Early female indoctrination in 'love' as an emotion may be largely a Western concept; but a more universal ideology concerns the primacy and uncontrollability of the male sexual drive. This is one of many insights offered by Barry's work:

> As sexual power is learned by adolescent boys through the social experience of their sex drive, so do girls learn that the locus of sexual power is male. Given the importance placed on the male sex drive in the socialization of girls as well as boys, early adolescence is probably the first significant phase of male identification in a girl's life and development ... As a young girl becomes aware of her own increasing sexual feelings ... she turns away from her heretofore primary relationships with girlfriends. As they become secondary to her, recede in importance in her life, her own identity also assumes a secondary role and she grows into male identification.
>
> (Barry, 1979, p. 218)

We still need to ask why some women never, even temporarily, turn away from 'heretofore primary relationships' with other females. And why does male identification – the casting of one's social, political, and intellectual allegiances with men – exist among lifelong sexual lesbians? Barry's hypothesis throws us among new questions, but it clarifies the diversity of forms in which compulsory heterosexuality presents itself. In the mystique of the overpowering, all-conquering male sex drive, the penis-with-a-life-of-its-own, is rooted in the law of male sex right to women, which justifies prostitution as a universal cultural assumption on the one hand, while defending sexual slavery within the family on the basis of 'family privacy and cultural uniqueness' on the other (Barry, 1979, p. 140). The adolescent male sex drive, which, as both young women and men are taught, once triggered cannot take responsibility for itself or take no for an answer, becomes, according to Barry, the norm and rationale for adult male sexual behaviour: a condition of *arrested sexual development*. Women learn to accept as natural the inevitability of this 'drive' because they receive it as dogma. Hence, marital rape; hence, the Japanese wife resignedly packing her husband's suitcase for a weekend in the *kisaeng* brothels of Taiwan; hence, the psychological as well as economic imbalance of power between husband and wife, male employer and female worker, father and daughter, male professor and female student.

The effect of male identification means

> internalizing the values of the colonizer and actively participating in carrying out the colonization of one's self and one's sex ... Male identification is the act whereby women place men above women, including themselves, in credibility, status, and importance in most situations, regardless of comparative quality the women may bring to the situation ... Interaction with women is seen as a lesser form of relating on every level.
>
> (Barry, 1979, p. 172)

What deserves further exploration is the doublethink many women engage in and from which no woman is permanently and utterly free. However woman-to-woman relationships, female support networks, a female and feminist value system are relied on and cherished, indoctrination in male credibility and status can still create synapses in thought, denials of feeling, wishful thinking, a profound sexual and intellectual confusion.[10] I quote here from a letter I received the day I was writing this passage: 'I have had very bad relationships with men – I am now in the midst of a very painful separation. I am trying to find my strength through women – without my friends, I could not survive'. How many times a day do women speak words like these or think them or write them, and how often does the synapse reassert itself?

Barry summarizes her findings:

> Considering the arrested sexual development that is understood to be normal in the male population, and considering the numbers of men who are pimps, procurers, members of slavery gangs, corrupt officials participating in this traffic, owners, operators, employees of brothels and lodging and entertainment facilities, pornography purveyors, associated with prostitution, wife beaters, child molesters, incest perpetrators, Johns (tricks) and rapists, one cannot but be momentarily stunned by the enormous male population engaging in female sexual slavery. The huge number of men engaged in these practices should be cause for declaration of an international emergency, a crisis in sexual violence. But what should be cause for alarm is instead accepted as normal sexual intercourse.
>
> (Barry, 1979, p. 220)

Susan Cavin, in a rich and provocative, if highly speculative, dissertation, suggests that patriarchy becomes possible when the original female band, which includes children but ejects adolescent males, becomes invaded and outnumbered by males; that not patriarchal marriage, but the rape of the mother by son, becomes the first act of male domination. The entering wedge, or leverage, which allows this to happen is not just a simple change in sex ratios; it is also the mother–child bond, manipulated by adolescent males in order to remain within the matrix past the age of exclusion. Maternal affection is used to establish male right of sexual access, which, however, must ever after be held by force (or through control of consciousness) since the original deep adult bonding is that of woman for woman (Cavin, 1978).[11] I find this hypothesis extremely suggestive, since one form of false consciousness which serves compulsory heterosexuality is the maintenance of a mother–son relationship between women and men, including the demand that women provide maternal solace, nonjudgmental nurturing, and compassion for their harassers, rapists, and batterers (as well as for men who passively vampirize them).

But whatever its origins, when we look hard and clearly at the extent and elaboration of measures designed to keep women within a male sexual purlieu, it becomes an inescapable question whether the issue feminists have to address is not simple 'gender inequality' nor the domination of culture by males nor mere 'taboos against homosexuality', but the enforcement of heterosexuality for women as a means of assuring male right of physical, economic, and emotional access.[12] One of many means of enforcement is, of course, the rendering invisible of the lesbian possibility, an engulfed continent which rises fragmentedly into view from time to time only to become submerged again. Feminist research and theory that contribute to lesbian invisibility or marginality are actually working against the liberation and empowerment of women as a group.[13]

The assumption that 'most women are innately heterosexual' stands as a theoretical and political stumbling block for feminism. It remains a tenable assumption partly because lesbian existence has been written out of history or catalogued under disease, partly because it has been treated as exceptional rather than intrinsic, partly because to acknowledge that for women heterosexuality may not be a 'preference' at all but something that has had to be imposed, managed, organized, propagandized, and maintained by force is an immense step to take if you consider yourself freely and 'innately' heterosexual. Yet the failure to examine heterosexuality as an institution is like failing to admit that the economic system called capitalism or the caste system of racism is maintained by a variety of forces, including both physical violence and false consciousness. To take the step of questioning heterosexuality as a 'preference' or 'choice' for women – and to do the intellectual and emotional work that follows – will call for a special quality of courage in heterosexually identified feminists, but I think the rewards will be great: a freeing-up of thinking, the exploring of new paths, the shattering of another great silence, new clarity in personal relationships.

III

I have chosen to use the terms *lesbian existence* and *lesbian continuum* because the word lesbianism has a clinical and limiting ring. Lesbian existence suggests both the fact of the historical presence of lesbians and our continuing creation of the meaning of that existence. I mean the term *lesbian continuum* to include a range – through each woman's life and throughout history – of woman-identified experience, not simply the fact that a woman has had or consciously desired genital sexual experience with another woman. If we expand it to embrace many more forms of primary intensity between and among women, including the sharing of a rich inner life, the bonding against male tyranny, the giving and receiving of practical and political support, if we can also hear it in such associations as *marriage resistance* and the 'haggard' behaviour identified by Mary Daly (obsolete meanings: 'intractable', 'willful', 'wanton', and 'unchaste', 'a woman reluctant to yield to wooing' [Daly, 1978, p. 15]) we begin to grasp breadths of female history and psychology which have lain out of reach as a consequence of limited, mostly clinical, definitions of *lesbianism*.

Lesbian existence comprises both the breaking of a taboo and the rejection of a compulsory way of life. It is also a direct or indirect attack on male right of access to women. But it is more than these, although we may first begin to perceive it as a form of naysaying to patriarchy, an act of resistance. It has, of course, included isolation, self-hatred, breakdown, alcoholism, suicide, and intrawoman violence; we romanticize at our peril what it means to love and act against the grain, and under heavy penalties; and lesbian existence has been lived (unlike, say, Jewish, or Catholic existence) without access to any knowledge of a tradition, a continuity, a social underpinning. The destruction of records and memorabilia and letters documenting the realities of lesbian existence must be taken very seriously as a means of keeping heterosexuality compulsory for women, since what has been kept from our knowledge is joy, sensuality, courage, and community, as well as guilt, self-betrayal, and pain.[14]

Lesbians have historically been deprived of a political existence through 'inclusion' as female versions of male homosexuality. To equate lesbian existence with male homosexuality because each is stigmatized is to erase female reality once again. Part of the history of lesbian existence is, obviously, to be found where lesbians, lacking a coherent female community, have shared a kind of social life and common cause with homosexual men. But there are differences: woman's lack of economic and cultural privilege relative to men; qualitative differences in female and male relationships – for example, the patterns of anonymous sex among male homosexuals, and the pronounced ageism in male homosexual standards of sexual attractiveness. I perceive the lesbian experience as being, like motherhood, a profoundly *female* experience, with particular oppressions, meanings, and potentialities we cannot comprehend as long as we simply bracket it with other sexually stigmatized existences. Just as the term *parenting* serves to conceal the particular and significant reality of being a parent who is actually a mother, the term *gay* may serve the purpose of blurring the very outlines we need to discern, which are of crucial value for feminism and for the freedom of women as a group.[15]

As the term lesbian has been held to limiting, clinical associations in its patriarchal definition, female friendship and comradeship have been set apart from the erotic, thus limiting the erotic itself. But as we deepen and broaden the range of what we define as lesbian existence, as we delineate a lesbian continuum, we begin to discover the erotic in female terms: as that which is unconfined to any single part of the body or solely to the body itself; as an energy not only diffuse but, as Audre Lorde has described it, omnipresent in 'the sharing of joy, whether physical, emotional, psychic', and in the sharing of work; as the empowering joy which 'makes us less willing to accept powerlessness, or those other supplied states of being which are not native to me, such as resignation, despair, self-effacement, depression, self-denial' (Lorde, 1984b). In another context, writing of women and work, I quoted the autobiographical passage in which the poet H.D. described how her friend Bryher supported her in persisting with the visionary experience which was to shape her mature work:

> I knew that this experience, this writing-on-the-wall before me, could not be shared with anyone except the girl who stood so bravely there beside me. This girl said without hesitation, 'Go on.' It was she really who had the detachment and integrity of the Pytheness of Delphi. But it was I, battered and dissociated ... who was seeing the pictures, and who was reading the writing or granted the inner vision. Or perhaps, in some sense, we were 'seeing' it together, for without her, admittedly, I could not have gone on.
>
> (Rich, 1979a, p. 209; H.D., 1971, pp. 50–4)

If we consider the possibility that all women – from the infant suckling at her mother's breast, to the grown woman experiencing orgasmic sensations while suckling her own child, perhaps recalling her mother's milk smell in her own, to two women, like Virginia Woolf's Chloe and Olivia, who share a laboratory (Woolf, 1929, p. 126), to the woman dying at ninety, touched and handled by women – exist on a lesbian continuum, we can see ourselves as moving in and out of this continuum, whether we identify ourselves as lesbian or not.

We can then connect aspects of woman identification as diverse as the impudent, intimate girl friendships of eight- or nine-year-olds and the banding together of those women of the twelfth and fifteenth centuries known as Beguines who 'shared houses, rented to one another, bequeathed houses to their room-mates ... in cheap subdivided houses in the artisans' area of town', who 'practice Christian virtue on their own, dressing and living simply and not associating with men', 'who earned their livings as spinsters, bakers, nurses, or ran schools for young girls, and who managed – until the Church forced them to disperse – to live independent both of marriage and of conventual restrictions' (Clark, 1975). It allows us to connect these women with the more celebrated 'Lesbians' of the women's school around Sappho of the seventh century BC, with the secret sororities and economic networks reported among African women, and with the Chinese marriage-resistance sisterhoods – communities of women who refused marriage or who, if married, often refused to consummate their marriages and soon left their husbands, the only women in China who were not footbound and who, Agnes Smedley tells us, welcomed the births of daughters and organized successful women's strikes in the silk mills.[16] It allows us to connect and compare disparate individual instances of marriage resistance: for example, the strategies available to Emily Dickinson, a nineteenth-century white woman genius, with the strategies available to Zora Neale Hurston, a twentieth-century black woman genius. Dickinson never married, had tenuous intellectual friendships with men, lived self-convented in her genteel father's house in Amherst, and wrote a lifetime of passionate letters to her sister-in-law Sue Gilbert and a smaller group of such letters to her friend Kate Scott Anthon. Hurston married twice but soon left each husband, scrambled her way from Florida to Harlem to Columbia University to Haiti and finally back to Florida, moved in and out of white patronage and poverty, professional success, and failure; her survival relationships were all with women, beginning with her mother. Both of these women in their vastly different circumstances were marriage resisters, committed to their own work and selfhood, and were later characterized as 'apolitical'. Both were drawn to men of intellectual quality; for both of them women provided the ongoing fascination and sustenance of life.

If we think of heterosexuality as *the* natural emotional and sensual inclination for women, lives such as these are seen as deviant, as pathological, or as emotionally and sensually deprived. Or, in more recent and permissive jargon, they are banalized as 'life styles'. And the work of such women, whether merely the daily work of individual or collective survival and resistance or the work of the writer, the activist, the reformer, the anthropologist, or the artist – the work of self-creation – is undervalued, or seen as the bitter fruit of 'penis envy' or the sublimation of repressed eroticism or the meaningless rant of a 'man-hater'. But when we turn the lens of vision and consider the degree to which and the methods whereby hetero-sexual 'preference' has actually been imposed on women, not only can we understand differ-ently the meaning of individual lives and work, but we can begin to recognize a central fact of women's history: that women have always resisted male tyranny. A feminism of action, often though not always without a theory, has constantly re-emerged in every culture and in every period. We can then begin to study women's struggle against powerlessness, women's radical rebellion, not just in male-defined 'concrete revolutionary situations' (Petchesky, 1979, p. 387) but in all the situations male ideologies have not perceived as revolutionary – for example, the refusal of some women to produce children, aided at great risk by other women;[17] the refusal to produce a higher standard of living and leisure for men (Leghorn and Parker show how both are part of women's unacknowledged, unpaid, and ununionized economic contribution). We can no longer have patience with Dinnerstein's view that women have simply collaborated with men in the 'sexual arrangements' of history. We begin to observe behaviour, both in history and in individual biography, that has hitherto been invis-ible or misnamed, behaviour which often constitutes, given the limits of the counterforce exerted in a given time and place, radical rebellion. And we can connect these rebellions and the necessity for them with the physical passion of woman for woman which is central to lesbian existence: the erotic sensuality which has been, precisely, the most violently erased fact of female experience.

Heterosexuality has been both forcibly and subliminally imposed on women. Yet everywhere women have resisted it, often at the cost of physical torture, imprisonment, psychosurgery, social ostracism, and extreme poverty. 'Compulsory heterosexuality' was named as one of the 'crimes against women' by the Brussels International Tribunal on Crimes against Women in 1976. Two pieces of testimony from two very different cultures reflect the degree to which persecution of lesbians is a global practice here and now. A report from Norway relates:

> A lesbian in Oslo was in heterosexual marriage that didn't work, so she started taking tranquillizers and ended up at the health sanatorium for treatment and rehabilitation … The moment she said in family group therapy that she believed she was a lesbian, the doctor told her she was not. He knew from 'looking into her eyes' he said. She had the eyes of a woman who wanted sexual intercourse with her husband. So she was subjected to so-called 'couch therapy'. She was put into a comfortably heated room, naked, on a bed, and for an hour her husband was to … try to excite her sexually … The idea was that

the touching was always to end with sexual intercourse. She felt stronger and stronger aversion. She threw up and sometimes ran out of the room to avoid this 'treatment'. The more strongly she asserted that she was a lesbian, the more violent the forced hetero-sexual intercourse became. This treatment went on for about six months. She escaped from the hospital, but she was brought back. Again she escaped. She has not been there since. In the end she realized that she had been subjected to forcible rape for six months.

(Russell and van der Ven, 1976, pp. 42–3)

And from Mozambique:

I am condemned to a life of exile because I will not deny that I am a lesbian, that my primary commitments are, and will always be to other women. In the new Mozambique, lesbianism is considered a left-over from colonialism and decadent Western civilization. Lesbians are sent to rehabilitation camps to learn through self-criticism the correct line about themselves ... If I am forced to denounce my own love for women, if I therefore denounce myself, I could go back to Mozambique and join forces in the exciting and hard struggle of rebuilding a nation, including the struggle for the emancipation of Mozambiquan women. As it is, I either risk the rehabilitation camps, or remain in exile.

(Russell and van der Ven, 1976, pp. 56–7)

Nor can it be assumed that women like those in Carroll Smith-Rosenberg's study, who married, stayed married, yet dwelt in a profoundly female emotional and passional world, 'preferred' or 'chose' heterosexuality. Women have married because it was necessary, in order to survive economically, in order to have children who would not suffer economic deprivation or social ostracism, in order to remain respectable, in order to do what was expected of women, because coming out of 'abnormal' childhoods they wanted to feel 'nor-mal' and because heterosexual romance has been represented as the great female adventure, duty, and fulfilment. We may faithfully or ambivalently have obeyed the institution, but our feelings – and our sensuality – have not been tamed or contained within it. There is no statis-tical documentation of the numbers of lesbians who have remained in heterosexual marriages for most of their lives. But in a letter to the early lesbian publication *The Ladder*, the play-wright Lorraine Hansberry had this to say:

I suspect that the problem of married woman who would prefer emotional-physical rela-tionships with other women is proportionally much higher than a similar statistic for men. (A statistic surely no one will ever really have.) This because the estate of woman being what it is, how could we ever begin to guess the numbers of women who are not prepared to risk a life alien to what they have been taught all their lives to believe was their 'natural' destiny – *and* – their only expectation for *economic* security. It seems to be that this is why the question has an immensity that it does not have for male homosexuals ... A woman of strength and honesty may, if she chooses, sever her marriage and marry a new male mate and society will be upset that the divorce rate is rising so – but there are few places in the United States, in any event, where she will be anything remotely akin to an 'outcast'. Obviously this is not true for a woman who would end her marriage to take up life with another woman.[18]

This *double life* – this apparent acquiescence to an institution founded on male interest and prerogative – has been characteristic of female experience: in motherhood and in many kinds of heterosexual behaviour, including the rituals of courtship; the pretence of asexuality by the nineteenth-century wife, the simulation of orgasm by the prostitute, the courtesan, the twentieth-century 'sexually liberated' woman.

Meridel LeSueur's documentary novel of the Depression, *The Girl* (1978), is arresting as a study of female double life. The protagonist, a waitress in a St Paul working-class speakeasy, feels herself passionately attracted to the young man Butch, but her survival relationships are with Clara, an older waitress and prostitute, with Belle, whose husband owns the bar, and with Amelia, a union activist. For Clara and Belle and the unnamed protagonist, sex with men is in one sense an escape from the bedrock misery of daily life, a flare of intensity in the grey, relentless, often brutal web of day-to-day existence:

> It was like he was a magnet pulling me. It was exciting and powerful and frightening. He was after me too and when he found me I would run, or be petrified, just standing in front of him like a zany. And he told me not to be wandering with Clara to the Marigold where we danced with strangers. He said he would knock the shit out of me. Which made me shake and tremble, but it was better than being a husk full of suffering and not knowing why.
>
> (LeSueur, 1978, pp. 10–11)[19]

Throughout the novel the theme of double life emerges; Belle reminisces about her marriage to the bootlegger Hoinck:

> You know, when I had that black eye and said I hit it on the cupboard, well he did it the bastard, and then he says don't tell anybody … He's nuts, that's what he is, nuts, and I don't see why I live with him, why I put up with him a minute on this earth. But listen kid, she said, I'm telling you something. She looked at me and her face was wonderful. She said, Jesus Christ, Goddam him I love him that's why I'm hooked like this all my life, Goddam him I love him.
>
> (1978, p. 20)

After the protagonist has her first sex with Butch, her women friends care for her bleeding, give her whiskey, and compare notes.

> My luck, the first time and I got into trouble. He gave me a little money and I come to St Paul where for ten bucks they'd stick a huge vet's needle into you and you start it and then you were on your own … I never had no child. I've just had Hoinck to mother, and a hell of a child he is.
>
> (1978, pp. 53–4)

> Later they made me go back to Clara's room to lie down … Clara lay down beside me and put her arms around me and wanted me to tell her about it but she wanted to tell about herself. She said she started it when she was twelve with a bunch of boys in an old shed. She said nobody had paid any attention to her before and she became very popular … They like it so much, she said, why shouldn't you give it to them and get presents and attention? I never cared anything for it and neither did my mama. But it's the only thing you got that's valuable,
>
> (1978, p. 55)

Sex is thus equated with attention from the male, who is charismatic though brutal, infantile, or unreliable. Yet it is the women who make life endurable for each other, give physical affection without causing pain, share, advise, and stick by each other. (*I am trying to find my strength through women – without my friends, I could not survive.*) LeSueur's *The Girl* parallels Toni Morrison's remarkable *Sula*, another revelation of female double life:

> Nel was the one person who had wanted nothing from her, who had accepted all aspects of her … Nel was one of the reasons Sula had drifted back to Medallion … The men … had merged into one large personality: the same language of love, the same entertainments of love, the same cooling of love. Whenever she introduced her private thoughts into their rubbings and goings, they hooded their eyes. They taught her nothing but love tricks, shared nothing but worry, gave nothing but money. She had been looking all along for a friend, and it took her a while to discover that a lover was not a comrade and could never be – for a woman.
>
> (Morrison, 1973, pp. 103–4)

But Sula's last thought at the second of her death is 'Wait'll I tell Nel'. And after Sula's death, Nel looks back on her own life:

> 'All that time all that time, I thought I was missing Jude.' And the loss pressed down on her chest and came up into her throat. 'We was girls together', she said as though explaining something. 'O Lord Sula', she cried, 'Girl, girl, girlgirlgirl!' It was a fine cry – loud and long – but it had no bottom and it had no top, just circles and circles of sorrow.[20]
>
> (1973, p. 149)

The Girl and *Sula* are both novels which examine what I am calling the lesbian continuum, in contrast to the shallow or sensational 'lesbians scenes' in recent commercial fiction (Brady and McDaniel, 1979). Each shows us woman identification untarnished (till the end of LeSueur's novel) by romanticism; each depicts the competition of heterosexual compulsion for women's attention, the diffusion and frustration of female bonding that might, in a more conscious form, reintegrate love and power.

IV

Woman identification is a source of energy, a potential springhead of female power, curtailed and contained under the institution of heterosexuality. The denial of reality and visibility to women's passion for women, women's choice of women as allies, life companions, and community, the forcing of such relationships into dissimulation and their disintegration under intense pressure have meant an incalculable loss to the power of all women *to change the social relations of the sexes, to liberate ourselves and each other*. The lie of compulsory female heterosexuality today afflicts not just feminist scholarship, but every profession, every reference work, every curriculum, every organizing attempt, every relationship or conversation over which it hovers. It creates, specifically, a profound falseness, hypocrisy, and hysteria in the heterosexual dialogue, for every heterosexual relationship is lived in the queasy strobe light of that lie. However we choose to identify ourselves, however we find ourselves labelled, it flickers across and distorts our lives.[21]

The lie keeps numberless women psychologically trapped, trying to fit mind, spirit, and sexuality into prescribed script because they cannot look beyond the parameters of the acceptable. It pulls on the energy of such women even as it drains the energy of 'closeted' lesbians – the energy exhausted in the double life. The lesbian trapped in the 'closet', the woman imprisoned in prescriptive ideas of the 'normal' share the pain of blocked options, broken connections, lost access to self-definition freely and powerfully assumed.

The lie is many-layered. In Western tradition, one layer – the romantic – asserts that women are inevitably, even if rashly and tragically, drawn to men; that even when that attraction is suicidal (e.g., *Tristan and Isolde*, Kate Chopin's *The Awakening*, 1978), it is still an organic imperative. In the tradition of the social sciences it asserts that primary love between the sexes is 'normal'; that women *need* men as social and economic protectors, for adult sexuality, and for psychological completion; that the heterosexually constituted family is the basic social unit; that women who do not attach their primary intensity to men must be, in functional terms, condemned to an even more devastating outsiderhood than their outsiderhood as women. Small wonder that lesbians are reported to be a more hidden population than male homosexuals. The Black lesbian-feminist critic Lorraine Bethel, writing on Zora Neale Hurston, remarks that for a Black woman – already twice an outsider – to choose to assume still another 'hated identity' is problematic indeed. Yet the lesbian continuum has been a life line for Black women both in Africa and the United States.

> Black women have a long tradition of bonding together ... in a Black/women's community that has been a source of vital survival information, psychic and emotional support for us. We have a distinct Black woman-identified folk culture based on our experiences as Black women in this society; symbols, language and modes of expression that are specific to the realities of our lives ... Because Black women were rarely among those Blacks and females who gained access to literary and other acknowledged forms of artistic expression, this Black female bonding and Black woman-identification has often been hidden and unrecorded except in the individual lives of Black women through our own memories of our particular Black female tradition.
>
> (Bethel, 1982)

Another layer of the lies is the frequently encountered implication that women turn to women out of hatred for men. Profound scepticism, caution, and righteous paranoia about men may indeed be part of any healthy woman's response to the misogyny of male-dominated culture, to the forms assumed by 'normal' male sexuality, and to *the failure even of 'sensitive' or 'political' men to perceive or find these troubling*. Lesbian existence is also represented as mere refuge from male abuses, rather than as an electric and empowering charge between women. One of the most frequently quoted literary passages on lesbian relationship is that in which Colette's Renée, in *The Vagabond* (1968), describes 'the melancholy and touching image of two weak creatures who have perhaps found shelter in each other's arms, there to sleep and weep, safe from man who is often cruel, and there to taste *better than any pleasure, the bitter happiness of feeling themselves akin, frail and forgotten* [emphasis added]'.[22] Colette is often considered a lesbian writer. Her popular reputation has, I think, much to do with the fact that she writes about lesbian existence as if for a male audience; her earliest 'lesbian' novels, the Claudine series, were written under compulsion for her husband and published under both their names. At all events, except for her writings on her mother, Colette is a less reliable source on the lesbian continuum than, I would think, Charlotte Brontë, who understood that while women may, indeed must, be one another's allies, mentors, and comforters in the female struggle for survival, there is quite extraneous delight in each other's company and attraction to each other's minds and character, which attend a recognition of each other's strengths.

By the same token, we can say that there is a *nascent* feminist political content in the act of choosing a woman lover or life partner in the face of institutionalized heterosexuality.[23] But for lesbian existence to realize this political content in an ultimately liberating form, the erotic choice must deepen and expand into conscious woman identification – into lesbian feminism.

The work that lies ahead, of unearthing and describing what I call here 'lesbian existence', is potentially liberating for all women. It is work that must assuredly move beyond the limits of white and middle-class Western Women's Studies to examine women's lives, work, and groupings within every racial, ethnic, and political structure. There are differences, moreover, between 'lesbian existence' and the 'lesbian continuum', differences we can discern even in the movement of our own lives. The lesbian continuum, I suggest, needs delineation in light of the 'double life' of women, not only women self-described as heterosexual but also of self-described lesbians. We need a far more exhaustive account of the forms the double life has assumed. Historians need to ask at every point how heterosexuality as institution has been organized and maintained through the female wage scale, the enforcement of middle-class women's 'leisure', the glamorization of so-called sexual liberation, the withholding of education from women, the imagery of 'high art' and popular culture, the mystification of the 'personal' sphere, and much else. We need an economics which comprehends the institution of heterosexuality, with its doubled workload for women and its sexual divisions of labour, as the most idealized of economic relations.

The question inevitably will arise: are we then to condemn all heterosexual relationships, including those which are least oppressive? I believe this question, though often heartfelt, is the wrong question here. We have been stalled in a maze of false dichotomies which prevents our apprehending the institution as a whole: 'good' versus 'bad' marriages; 'marriage for love' versus arranged marriage; 'liberated' sex versus prostitution; heterosexual intercourse versus rape; *Liebeschmerz* versus humiliation and dependency. Within the institution exist, of course, qualitative differences of experience; but the absence of choice remains the great unacknowledged reality, and in the absence of choice, women will remain dependent upon the chance or luck of particular relationships and will have no collective power to determine the meaning and place of sexuality in their lives. As we address the institution itself, moreover, we begin to perceive a history of female resistance which has never fully understood itself because it has been so fragmented, miscalled, erased. It will require a courageous grasp of the politics and economics, as well as the cultural propaganda, of heterosexuality to carry us beyond individual cases or diversified group situations into the complex kind of overview needed to undo the power men everywhere wield over women, power which has become a model for every other form of exploitation and illegitimate control.

Afterword [1986]

In 1980, Ann Snitow, Christine Stansell, and Sharon Thompson, three Marxist-feminist activists and scholars, sent out a call for papers for an anthology on the politics of sexuality. Having just finished writing 'Compulsory Heterosexuality' for *Signs*, I sent them that manuscript and asked them to consider it. Their anthology, *Powers of Desire*, was published by the Monthly Review Press New Feminist Library in 1983 and included my paper. During the intervening period, the four of us were in correspondence, but I was able to take only limited advantage of this dialogue due to ill health and resulting surgery. With their permission, I reprint here excerpts from that correspondence as a way of indicating that my essay should be read as one contribution to a long exploration in progress, not as my own 'last word' on sexual politics. I also refer interested readers to *Powers of Desire* itself.

Dear Adrienne,

... In one of our first letters, we told you that we were finding parameters of leftwing/ feminist sexual discourse to be far broader than we imagined. Since then, we have perceived what we believe to be a crisis in the feminist movement about sex, an intensifying debate (although not always an explicit one), and a questioning of assumptions once taken for granted. While we fear the link between sex and violence, as do Women Against Pornography, we wish we better understood its sources in ourselves as well as in men. In the Reagan era, we can hardly afford to romanticize any old norm of a virtuous and moral sexuality.

In your piece, you are asking the question, what would women choose in a world where patriarchy and capitalism did *not* rule? We agree with you that heterosexuality is an institution created between these grind stones, but we don't conclude, therefore, that it is entirely a male creation. You only allow for female historical agency insofar as women exist on the lesbian continuum while we would argue that women's history, like men's history, is created out of a dialectic of necessity and choice.

All three of us (hence one lesbian, two heterosexual women) had questions about your use of the term 'false consciousness' for women's heterosexuality. In general, we think the false consciousness model can blind us to the necessities and desires that comprise the lives of the oppressed. It can also lead to the too easy denial of others' experience when that experience is different from our own. We posit, rather, a complex social model in which all erotic life is a continuum, one which therefore includes relations with men.

Which brings us to this metaphor of the continuum. We know you are a poet, not an historian, and we look forward to reading your metaphors all our lives – and standing straighter as feminists, as women, for having read them. But the metaphor of the lesbian continuum is open to all kinds of misunderstandings, and these sometimes have odd political effects. For example, Sharon reports that at a recent meeting around the abortion-rights struggle, the notions of continuum arose in the discussion several times and underwent divisive transformation. Overall, the notion that two ways of being existed on the same continuum was interpreted to mean that those two ways were the same. The sense of range and gradation that your description evokes disappeared. Lesbianism and female friendship became exactly the same thing. Similarly, heterosexuality and rape became the same. In one of several versions of the continuum that evolved, a slope was added, like so:

Lesbianism
Sex with men, no penetration
Sex with men, penetration
Rape

This sloped continuum brought its proponents to the following conclusion: an appropriate, workable abortion-rights strategy is to inform all women that heterosexual penetration is rape, whatever their subjective experience to the contrary. All women will immediately recognize the truth of this and opt for the alternative of nonpenetration. The abortion-rights struggle will thus be simplified into a struggle against coercive sex and its consequences (since no enlightened woman would voluntarily undergo penetration unless her object was procreation – a peculiarly Catholic-sounding view).

The proponents of this strategy were young women who have worked hard in the abortion-rights movement for the past two or more years. They are inexperienced but they are dedicated. For this reason, we take their reading of your work seriously. We don't think, however, that it comes solely, or even at all, from the work itself. As likely a source is the tendency to dichotomize that has plagued the women's movement. The source of that tendency is harder to trace.

In that regard, the hints in 'Compulsory' about the double life of women intrigue us. You define the double life as 'the apparent acquiescence to an institution founded on male interest and prerogative'. But that definition doesn't really explain your other references to, for instance, the 'intense mixture' of love and anger in lesbian relationships – and to the peril of romanticizing what it means 'to love and act against the grain'. We think these comments raise extremely important issues for feminists right now; the problem of division and anger among us needs airing and analysis. Is this, by any chance, the theme of a piece you have in the works? … We would still love it if we could have a meeting with you in the next few months. Any chance? … Greetings and support from us – in all your undertakings.

We send love,
Sharon, Chris, and Ann
New York City
April 19, 1981

Dear Ann, Chris, and Sharon,

… It's good to be back in touch with you, you who have been so unfailingly patient, generous, and persistent. Above all, it's important to me that you know that ill health, not a withdrawal because of political differences, delayed my writing back to you …

'False consciousness' can, I agree, be used as a term of dismissal for any thinking we don't like or adhere to. But, as I tried to illustrate in some detail, there is a real, identifiable system of heterosexual propaganda, of defining women as existing for the sexual use of men, which goes beyond 'sex role' or 'gender' stereotyping or 'sexist imagery' to include a vast number of verbal and nonverbal messages. And this I call 'control of consciousness'. The possibility of a woman who does not exist sexually for men – the lesbian possibility – is buried, erased, occluded, distorted, misnamed, and driven underground. The feminist books – Chodorow, Dinnerstein, Ehrenreich and English, and others – which I discuss at the beginning of my essay contribute to this invalidation and erasure, and as such are part of the problem.

My essay is founded on the belief that we all think from within the limits of certain solipsisms – usually linked with privilege, racial, cultural, and economic as well as sexual – which present themselves as 'the universal', 'the way things are', 'all women', etc., etc. I wrote it equally out of the belief that in becoming conscious of our solipsisms we have certain kinds of choices, that we can and must re-educate ourselves. I never have maintained that heterosexual feminists are walking about in a state of 'brainwashed' false consciousness. Nor have such phrases as 'sleeping with the enemy' seemed to me either profound or useful. *Homophobia* is too diffuse a term and does not go very far in helping us identify and talk about the sexual solipsism of heterosexual feminism. In this paper I was trying to ask heterosexual feminists to examine their experience of heterosexuality critically and antagonistically, to critique the institution of which they are a part, to struggle with the norm and its implications for women's freedom, to become more open to the considerable resources offered by the lesbian-feminist perspective, to refuse to settle for the personal privilege and solution of the individual 'good relationship' within the institution of heterosexuality.

As regards 'female historical agency', I wanted, precisely, to suggest that the victim model is insufficient; that there *is* a history of female agency and choice which has actually challenged aspects of male supremacy; that, like male supremacy, these can be found in many different cultures … It's not that I think all female agency has been solely and avowedly lesbian. But by erasing lesbian existence from female history, from theory, from literary criticism … from feminist approaches to economic structure, ideas about 'the family', etc., an enormous amount of female agency is kept unavailable, hence unusable. I wanted to demonstrate that that kind of obliteration continues to be acceptable in seriously regarded feminist texts. What surprised me in the responses to my essay, including your notes, is how almost every aspect of it has been considered, except this – to me – central one. I was taking a position which was neither lesbian/separatist in the sense of dismissing heterosexual women nor a 'gay civil rights' plea for … openness to lesbianism as an 'option' or an 'alternate life style'. I was urging that lesbian existence has been an unrecognized and unaffirmed claiming by women of their sexuality, thus a pattern of resistance, thus also a kind of borderline position from which to analyse and challenge the relationship of heterosexuality to male supremacy. And that lesbian existence, when recognized, demands a conscious restructuring of feminist analysis and criticism, not just a token reference or two.

I certainly agree with you that the term *lesbian continuum* can be misused. It was, in the example you report of the abortion-rights meeting, though I would think anyone who had read my work from *Of Woman Born* onward would know that my position on abortion and sterilization abuse is more complicated than that. My own problem with the phrase is that it can be, is, used by women who have not yet begun to examine the privileges and solipsisms of heterosexuality, as a safe way to describe their felt connections with women, without having to share in the risks and threats of lesbian existence. What I had thought to delineate rather complexly as a continuum has begun to sound more like 'life-style shopping'. *Lesbian continuum* – the phrase – came from a desire to allow for the greatest possible variation of female-identified experience, while paying a different kind of respect to lesbian existence – the traces and knowledge of women who have made their primary erotic emotional choices for women. If I were writing the paper today, I would still want to make this distinction, but would put more caveats around *lesbian continuum*. I fully agree with you that Smith-Rosenberg's 'female world' is not a social ideal, enclosed as it is within prescriptive middle-class heterosexuality and marriage.

My own essay could have been stronger had it drawn on more of the literature by Black women toward which Toni Morrison's *Sula* inevitably pointed me. In reading a great deal more of Black women's fiction I began to perceive a different set of valences from those found in white women's fiction for the most part: a different quest for the woman hero, a different relationship both to sexuality with men and to female loyalty and bonding …

You comment briefly on your reactions to some of the radical-feminist works I cited [Barry, 1979; Brownmiller, 1975; Daly, 1978; Griffin, 1978; Russell and van der Ven, 1976; *Aegis: Magazine on Ending Violence Against Women*, (n.d.)]. I am myself critical of some of them even as I found them vitally useful. What most of them share is a taking seriously of misogyny – of organized, institutionalized, normalized hostility and violence against women. I feel no 'hierarchy of oppressions' is needed in order for us to take misogyny as seriously as we take racism, anti-Semitism, imperialism. To take misogyny seriously needn't mean that we perceive women merely as victims, without responsibilities or choices; it does mean recognizing the 'necessity' in that 'dialectic of necessity and choice' – identifying, describing, refusing to turn aside our eyes. I think that some of the apparent reductiveness, or even obsessiveness, of some white radical-feminist theory derives from racial and/or class solipsism, but also from the immense effort of trying to render woman hating visible amid so much denial ...

Finally, as to poetry and history: I want both in my life; I need to see through both. If metaphor can be misconstrued, history can also lead to misconstrual when it obliterates acts of resistance or rebellion, wipes out transformational models, or sentimentalizes power relationships. I know you know this. I believe we are all trying to think and write out of our best consciences, our most open consciousness. I expect that quality in this book which you are editing, and look forward with anticipation to the thinking – and the actions – toward which it may take us.

In sisterhood,
Adrienne
Montague, Massachusetts
November 1981

Notes

1 See, for example, Allen (1986); Brant (1984); Anzaldúa and Moraga (1981); Roberts (1981); Smith (1984). As Bethel and Smith pointed out in *Conditions 5: The Black Women's Issue* (1980), a great deal of fiction by Black women depicts primary relationships between women. I would like to cite here the work of Ama Ata Aidoo, Toni Cade Bambara, Buchi Emecheta, Bessie Head, Zora Neale Hurston, Alice Walker. Donna Allegra, Red Jordan Arobateau, Audre Lorde, Ann Allen Shockley, among others, write directly as Black lesbians. For fiction by other lesbians of colour, see Bulkin (1981). See also, for accounts of contemporary Jewish-lesbian existence, Beck (1982); Block (1982); and Kantrowitz and Klepfisz (1986). The earliest formulation that I know of heterosexuality as an institution was in the lesbian feminist paper *The Furies*, founded in 1971. For a collection of articles from that paper, see Myron and Bunch (1975).

2 I could have chosen many other serious and influential books, including anthologies, which would illustrate the same point: e.g., Boston Women's Health Book Collective, *Our Bodies, Ourselves* (1976), which devotes a separate (and inadequate) chapter to lesbians, but whose message is that heterosexuality is most women's life preference; Carroll (1976), which does not include even a token essay on the lesbian presence in history, though it cites an essay by Linda Gordon, Persis Hunt, *et al.* notes the use by male historians of 'sexual deviance' as a category to discredit and dismiss Anna Howard Shaw, Jane Addams, and other feminists ('Historical Phallacies: Sexism in American Historical Writing'); and Bridenthal and Koonz (1977), which contains three mentions of male homosexuality but no materials that I have been able to locate on lesbians. Lerner (1977) contains an abridgment of two lesbian-feminist-position papers from the contemporary movement but no other documentation of lesbian existence. Lerner does note in her preface, however, how the charge of deviance has been used to fragment women and discourage women's resistance. Linda Gordon (1976) notes accurately that 'it is not that feminism has produced more lesbians. There have always been many lesbians, despite the high levels of repression; and most lesbians experience their sexual preference as innate' (p. 410). [A.R., 1986: I am glad to update the first annotation in this footnote. 'The New' *Our Bodies, Ourselves* (1984) contains an expanded chapter on 'Loving Women: Lesbian Life and Relationships' and furthermore emphasizes choices for women throughout – in terms of sexuality, health care, family, politics, etc.]

3 This is a book which I have publicly endorsed. I would still do so, though with the above caveat. It is only since beginning to write this article that I fully appreciated how enormous is the unasked question in Ehrenreich and English's book.

4 [A.R., 1986: Work on both incest and on woman battering has appeared in the 1980s which I did not cite in the essay. See Rush (1980); Armstrong (1979); Butler (1978); Delacoste and Newman (1981); Freespirit (1982); Herman (1981); McNaron and Morgan (1982); and Betsy Warrior's richly informative, multipurpose compilation of essays, statistics, listings, and facts, the *Battered Women's Directory* (1982).]

5 [A.R., 1986: See especially 'Circumcision of Girls', in Nawal El Saadawi (1982, pp. 33–43).]

6 The issue of 'lesbian sadomasochism' needs to be examined in terms of dominant cultures' teachings about the relation of sex and violence. I believe this to be another example of the 'double life' of women.

7 Susan Schecter writes: 'The push for heterosexual union at whatever cost is so intense that ... it has become a cultural force of its own that creates battering. The ideology of romantic love and its jealous possession of the partner as property provide the masquerade for what can become severe abuse' (1979, pp. 50–1).

8 [A.R., 1986: See also Barry, Bunch, and Castley (1984).]

9 [A.R., 1986: This statement has been taken as claiming that 'all women are victims' purely and simply, or that 'all heterosexuality equals sexual slavery'. I would say, rather, that all women are affected, though differently, by dehumanizing attitudes and practices directed at women as a group.]

10 Elsewhere I have suggested that male identification has been a powerful source of white women's racism and that it has often been women already seen as 'disloyal' to male codes and systems who have actively battled against it (Rich, 1979b).

11 Cavin, 'Lesbian Origins' unpublished, ch. 6. [A.R., 1986: This dissertation was recently published as *Lesbian Origins* (San Francisco: Ism Press, 1986).]

12 For my perception of heterosexuality as an economic institution I am indebted to Lisa Leghorn and Katherine Parker, who allowed me to read the manuscript of their book *Woman's Worth: Sexual Economics and the World of Women* (1981).

13 I would suggest that lesbian existence has been most recognized and tolerated where it has resembled a 'deviant' version of heterosexuality – e.g., where lesbians have, like Stein and Toklas, played heterosexual roles (or seemed to in public) and have been chiefly identified with male culture. See also Claude E. Schaeffer (1965). (Berdache: 'an individual of a definite physiological sex [m. or f.] who assumes the role and status of the opposite sex and who is viewed by the community as being of one sex physiologically but as having assumed the role and status of the opposite sex' [Schaeffer, 1965, p. 231].) Lesbian existence has also been relegated to an upper-class phenomenon, an elite decadence (as in the fascination with Paris salon lesbians such as Renée Vivien and Natalie Clifford Barney), to the obscuring of such 'common women' as Judy Grahn depicts in her *The Work of a Common Woman* (1978a) and *True to Life Adventure Stories* (1978b).

14 'In a hostile world in which women are not supposed to survive except in relation with and in service to men, entire communities of women were simply erased. History tends to bury what it seeks to reject' (Cook, 1979). The Lesbian Herstory Archives in New York City is one attempt to preserve contemporary documents on lesbian existence – a project of enormous value and meaning, working against the continuing censorship and obliteration of relationships, networks, communities in other archives and elsewhere in the culture.

15 [A.R., 1986: The shared historical and spiritual 'crossover' functions of lesbians and gay men in cultures past and present are traced by Judy Grahn in *Another Mother Tongue: Gay Words, Gay Worlds* (1984). I now think we have much to learn both from the uniquely female aspects of lesbian existence and from the complex 'gay' identity we share with gay men.]

16 See Paulmé (1963, pp. 7, 266–7). Some of these sororities are described as 'a kind of defensive syndicate against the male element', their aims being 'to offer concerted resistance to an oppressive patriarchate', 'independence in relation to one's husband and with regard to motherhood, mutual aid, satisfaction of personal revenge'. See also Lorde (1984a); Topley (1978); Smedley (1976).

17 [A.R., 1986: See Davis (1981, p. 102); Patterson (1982, p. 133).]

18 I am indebted to Jonathan Katz's *Gay American History* (1976) for bringing to my attention Hansberry's letters to *The Ladder* and to Barbara Grier for supplying me with copies of relevant pages from *The Ladder*, quoted here by permission of Barbara Grier. See also the reprinted series of *The Ladder*, ed. Jonathan Katz *et al.* (1975), and Camody (1979).

19 LeSueur describes, in an afterword, how this book was drawn from the writings and oral narrations of women in the Workers Alliance who met as a writers' group during the Depression.

20 I am indebted to Lorraine Bethel's essay '"This Infinity of Conscious Pain": Zora Neale Hurston and the Black Female Literary Tradition' (1982).

21 See Russell and van der Ven: 'Few heterosexual women realize their lack of free choice about their sexuality, and few realize how and why compulsory heterosexuality is also a crime against them' (1976, p. 40).
22 Dinnerstein, the most recent writer to quote this passage, adds ominously: 'But what has to be added to her account is that these "women enlaced" are sheltering each other not just from what men want to do to them, but also from what they want to do to each other' (Dinnerstein, 1976, p. 103). The fact is, however, that woman-to-woman violence is a minute grain in the universe of maleagainst-female violence perpetuated and rationalized in every social institution.
23 Conversation with Blanche W. Cook, New York City, March 1979.

References

AEGIS: MAGAZINE ON ENDING VIOLENCE AGAINST WOMEN, [no publication details available].

ALLEN, P.G. (1986) *The Sacred Hoop: Recovering the Feminine American Indian Traditions*, Boston, MA: Beacon.

ANZALDÚA, G. and MORAGA, C. (eds) (1981) *This Bridge Called My Back: Writings by Radical Women of Color*, Watertown, MA: Persephone Press.

ARMSTRONG, L. (1979) *Kiss Daddy Goodnight: A Speakout on Incest*, New York: Pocket Books.

BARRY, K. (1979) *Female Sexual Slavery*, Englewood Cliffs, NJ: Prentice-Hall.

——, BUNCH, C., and CASTLEY, S. (eds) (1984) *International Feminism: Networking against Female Sexual Slavery*, New York: International Women's Tribune Centre.

BECK, E.T. (ed.) (1982) *Nice Jewish Girls: A Lesbian Anthology*, Watertown, MA: Persephone Press.

BETHEL, L. (1982) '"This infinity of conscious pain": Zora Neale Hurston and the black female literary tradition', in HALL, G.T., SCOTT, P.B. and SMITH, B. (eds) *All the Women Are White, All the Blacks Are Men, but Some of Us Are Brave: Black Women's Studies*, Old Westbury, NY: Feminist Press.

—— and SMITH, B. (1980) *Conditions*, 5, The Black Women's Issue, [n.p.n.].

BLOCK, A. (1982) *Lifetime Guarantee*, Watertown, MA: Persephone Press.

BOSTON WOMEN'S HEALTH BOOK COLLECTIVE (1976) *Our Bodies, Ourselves*, New York: Simon and Schuster.

BRADY, M., and MCDANIEL, J. (1979) 'Lesbians in the mainstream: the image of lesbians in recent commercial fiction', *Conditions*, 6, pp. 82–105.

BRANT, B. (ed.) (1984) *A Gathering of Spirit: A Collection of Writing by North American Indian Women*, Montpelier, VT: Sinister Wisdom Books.

BRIDENTHAL, R. and KOONZ, C. (eds) (1977) *Becoming Visible: Women in European History*, Boston, MA: Houghton Mifflin.

BROWNMILLER, S. (1975) *Against Our Will: Men, Women and Rape*, New York: Simon and Schuster.

BULKIN, E. (ed.) (1981) *Lesbian Fiction: An Anthology*, Watertown, MA: Persephone Press.

BUTLER, S. (1978) *Conspiracy of Silence: The Trauma of Incest*, San Francisco: New Glide.

CAMODY, D. (1979) 'Letters by Eleanor Roosevelt detail friendship with Lorena Hickok', *New York Times*, 21 October, [n.p.n.].

CARROLL, B. (ed.) (1976) *Liberating Women's History: Theoretical and Critical Essays*, Urbana: University of Illinois Press.

CAVIN, S. (1986) *Lesbian Origins*, San Francisco: Ism Press (original date 1978).

CHODOROW, N. (1978) *The Reproduction of Mothering*, Berkeley: University of California Press.

CHOPIN, K. (1978) *The Awakening*, London: Women's Press.

CLARK, G. (1975) 'The Beguines: a medieval women's community', *Quest: A Feminist Quarterly*, 1(4), pp. 73–80.

CLIFF, M. (1979) 'The resonance of interruption', *Chrysalis: A Magazine of Women's Culture*, 8, pp. 29–37.

COLETTE, S.G. (1968) *The Vagabond*, trans. Enid McLeod, Harmondsworth: Penguin.

COOK, B.W. (1979) '"Women alone stir my imagination": lesbianism and the cultural tradition', *Signs*, 4, pp. 719–20.

DALY, M. (1973) *Beyond God the Father*, Boston, MA: Beacon.

—— (1978) *Gyn/Ecology: The Metaethics of Radical Feminism*, Boston, MA: Beacon.

DAVIS, A. (1981) *Women, Race and Class*, New York: Random House.

DELACOSTE, F. and NEWMAN, F. (eds) (1981) *Fight Back! Feminist Resistance to Male Violence*, Minneapolis, MN: Cleis Press.

DEMETER, A. (1977) *Legal Kidnapping*, Boston, MA: Beacon.

DINNERSTEIN, D. (1976) *The Mermaid and the Minotaur: Sexual Arrangements and the Human Malaise*, New York: Harper & Row.

DWORKIN, A. (1974) *Woman Hating*, New York: Dutton.

EHRENREICH, B. and ENGLISH, D. (1973) *Witches, Midwives and Nurses: A History of Women Healers*, Old Westbury, NY: Feminist Press.

—— and ENGLISH, D. (1978) *For Her Own Good: 150 Years of the Experts' Advice to Women*, Garden City, NY: Doubleday, Anchor.

FREESPIRIT, J. (1982) *Daddy's Girl: An Incest Survivor's Story*, Langlois: Diaspora Distribution.

GORDON, L. (1976) *Woman's Body, Woman's Right: A Social History of Birth Control in America*, New York: Viking, Grosman.

GOUGH, K. (1975) 'The origin of the family', in REITER, R.R. (ed.) *Toward an Anthropology of Women*, New York: Monthly Review Press.

GRAHN, J. (1978a) *The Work of a Common Woman*, Oakland, CA: Diana Press.

—— (1978b) *True to Life Adventure Stories*, Oakland, CA: Diana Press.

—— (1984) *Another Mother Tongue: Gay Words, Gay Worlds*, Boston, MA: Beacon.

GRIFFIN, S. (1978) *Woman and Nature: The Roaring Inside Her*, New York: Harper & Row.

H.D. (1971) *Tribute to Freud*, Oxford: Carcanet.

HERMAN, J. (1981) *Father–Daughter Incest*, Cambridge, MA: Harvard University Press.

HOSKEN, F.P. (1979) 'The violence of power: genital mutilation of females', *Heresies: A Feminist Journal of Art and Politics*, 6, pp. 28–35.

KANTROWITZ, M.K. and KLEPFISZ, I. (eds) (1986) *The Tribe of Dina: A Jewish Women's Anthology*, Montpelier, VT: Sinister Wisdom Books.

KATZ, J. (ed.) (1976) *Gay American History: Lesbians and Gay Men in the USA*, New York: Thomas Y. Crowell.

—— et al. (eds) (1975) *The Ladder*, New York: Arno.

LEGHORN, L. and PARKER, K. (1981) *Woman's Worth: Sexual Economics and the World of Women*, London: Routledge and Kegan Paul.

LERNER, G. (ed.) (1977) *The Female Experience: An American Documentary*, Indianapolis, IN: Bobbs-Merrill.

LESSING, D. (1977) *The Golden Notebook*, New York: Bantam.

LESUEUR, M. (1978) *The Girl*, Cambridge, MA: West End Press.

LORDE, A. (1984a) 'Scratching the surface: some notes on barriers to women and loving', in *Sister Outsider*, Trumansburg, NY: Crossing Press.

—— (1984b) 'Use of the erotic: the erotic as power', in *Sister Outsider*, Trumansburg, NY: Crossing Press.

MACKINNON, C.A. (1979) *Sexual Harassment of Working Women: A Case of Sex Discrimination*, New Haven, CT: Yale University Press.

MCNARON, T. and MORGAN, Y. (eds) (1982) *Voices in the Night: Women Speaking about Incest*, Minneapolis, MN: Cleis Press.

MILLER, J.B. (1976) *Toward a New Psychology of Women*, Boston, MA: Beacon.

MORRISON, T. (1973) *Sula*, New York: Bantam.

MYRON, N. and BUNCH, C. (eds) (1975) *Lesbianism and the Women's Movement*, Oakland, CA: Diana Press.

OLSEN, T. (1978) *Silences*, Boston, MA: Delacorte.

PATTERSON, O. (1982) *Slavery and Social Death: A Comparative Study*, Cambridge, MA: Harvard University Press.

PAULME, D. (ed.) (1963) *Women of Tropical Africa*, Berkeley: University of California Press.

PETCHESKY, R. (1979) 'Dissolving the hyphen: a report on marxist-feminist groups 1–5', in EISENSTEIN, Z. (ed.) *Capitalist Patriarchy and the Case for Socialist Feminism*, New York: Monthly Review Press.

RICH, A. (1979a) 'Conditions for work: the common world of women', in *On Lies, Secrets, and Silence: Selected Prose, 1966–1978*, New York: W.W. Norton.

——(1979b) 'Disloyal to civilization: feminism, racism, gynephobia', in *On Lies, Secrets, and Silence: Selected Prose, 1966–1978*, New York: W.W. Norton.

ROBERTS, J.R. (1981) *Black Lesbians: An Annotated Bibliography*, Tallahassee, FL: Naiad.

ROSSI, A. (1976) 'Children and work in the lives of women', paper delivered at the University of Arizona, Tucson, February.

RUSH, F. (1980) *The Best-Kept Secret*, New York: McGraw-Hill.

RUSSELL, D. and VAN DER VEN, N. (eds) (1976) *Proceedings of the International Tribunal of Crimes against Women*, Millbrae, CA: Les Femmes.

SAADAWI, N. EL (1982) *The Hidden Face of Eve: Women in the Arab World*, Boston, MA: Beacon.

SAHLI, N. (1979) 'Smashing women's relationships before the fall', *Chrysalis: A Magazine of Women's Culture*, 8, pp. 817–27.

SCHAEFFER, C.E. (1965) 'The Kuterai female berdache: courier, guide, prophetess and warrior', *Ethnohistory*, 12, pp. 193–236.

SCHECTER, S. (1979) *Aegis: Magazine on Ending Violence against Women*, [no issue no.], July–August, [n.p.n.].

SMEDLEY, A. (1976) *Portraits of Chinese Women in Revolution*, MACKINNON, J. and MACKINNON, S. (eds), Old Westbury, NY: Feminist Press.

SMITH, B. (ed.) (1984) *Home Girls: A Black Feminist Anthology*, Albany, NY: Kitchen Table/Women of Color Press.

TOPLEY, M. (1978) 'Marriage resistance in rural Kwangtung', in WOLF, M. and WITKE, R. (eds) *Women in Chinese Society*, Stanford, CA: Stanford University Press.

WARRIOR, B. (1982) *Battered Women's Directory* (formerly entitled *Working on Wife Abuse*), 8th edition, [n.p.], Cambridge, MA: B. Warrior.

WOOLF, V. (1929) *A Room of One's Own*, London: Hogarth.

——(1966 [1938 orig.]) *Three Guineas*, New York: Harcourt Brace.

12 The *hijras* of India

Cultural and individual dimensions of an institutionalized third gender role

Serena Nanda [1985]

The *hijra*, an institutionalized third gender role in India, is 'neither male or female', containing elements of both. The *hijra* are commonly believed by the larger society to be intersexed, impotent men, who undergo emasculation in which all or part of the genitals are removed. They adopt female dress and some other aspects of female behaviour. *Hijras* traditionally earn their living by collecting alms and receiving payment for performances at weddings, births and festivals. The central feature of their culture is their devotion to Bahuchara Mata, one of the many Mother Goddesses worshipped all over India, for whom emasculation is carried out. This identification with the Mother Goddess is the source both of the *hijras*' claim for their special place in Indian society and the traditional belief in their power to curse or confer blessings on male infants.

The census of India does not enumerate *hijras* separately so their exact numbers are unknown. Estimates quoted in the press range from 50,000 (*India Today*, 1982) to 500,000 (*Tribune*, 1983). *Hijras* live predominantly in the cities of North India, where they find the greatest opportunity to perform their traditional roles, but small groups of *hijras* are found all over India, in the south as well as the north. Seven 'houses', or subgroups, comprise the *hijra* community; each of these has a guru or leader, all of whom live in Bombay. The houses have equal status, but one, Laskarwallah, has the special function of mediating disputes which arise among the others. Each house has its own history, as well as rules particular to it. For example, members of a particular house are not allowed to wear certain colours. *Hijra* houses appear to be patterned after the *gharanas* (literally, houses), or family lineages among classical musicians, each of which is identified with its own particular musical style. Though the culturally distinct features of the *hijra* houses have almost vanished, the structural feature remains.[1]

The most significant relationship in the *hijra* community is that of the *guru* (master, teacher) and *chela* (disciple). When an individual decides to (formally) join the *hijra* community, he is taken to Bombay to visit one of the seven major *gurus*, usually the *guru* of the person who has brought him there. At the initiation ritual, the *guru* gives the novice a new, female name. The novice vows to obey the *guru* and the rules of the community. The *guru* then presents the new *chela* with some gifts.

The *chela*, or more likely, someone on her behalf, pays an initiation fee and the *guru* writes the *chela*'s name in her record book. This *guru–chela* relationship is a lifelong bond of reciprocity in which the *guru* is obligated to help the *chela* and the *chela* is obligated to be loyal and obedient to the *guru*.[2] *Hijras* live together in communes generally of about 5 to 15 members, and the heads of these local groups are also called *guru*. *Hijras* make no distinctions within their community based on caste origin or religion, although in some parts of India, Gujerat, for example, Muslim and Hindu *hijras* reportedly live apart (Salunkhe, 1976).

In Bombay, Delhi, Chandigarh and Bangalore, *hijras* of Muslim, Christian, and Hindu origin live in the same houses.

In addition to the hierarchical *guru–chela* relationship, there is fictive kinship by which *hijras* relate to each other. Rituals exists for 'taking a daughter' and the 'daughters' of one 'mother' consider themselves 'sisters' and relate on a reciprocal, affectionate basis. Other fictive kinship relations, such as 'grandmother' or 'mother's sister' (aunt) are the basis of warm and reciprocal regard. Fictive kin exchange small amounts of money, clothing, jewellery and sweets to formalize their relationship. Such relationships connect *hijras* all over India, and there is a constant movement of individuals who visit their *gurus* and fictive kin in different cities. Various annual gatherings, both religious and secular, attract thousands of *hijras* from all over India.[3]

The extant literature on the *hijras* is scant, confusing, misleading, contradictory, and judgemental. With few exceptions (Salunkhe, 1976; Sinha, 1967) it lacks a basis in fieldwork or intensive interviewing. A major dispute in that literature has been whether or not the *hijra* role encompasses homosexuality.

In my view, the essential cultural aspect of the *hijra* role is its asexual nature. Yet, empirical evidence also indicates that many *hijras* do engage in homosexual activity. This difference between the cultural ideal and the real behaviour causes a certain amount of conflict within the community. The present paper, based on a year's fieldwork among *hijra* communes in various parts of India, examines both the cultural ideal of asexuality and the behavioural dimension of homosexuality, and how the conflict is experienced and handled within the community.

Cultural dimensions of the *hijra* role

Hijras *as neither man nor woman*

A commonly told story among *hijras*, which conceptualizes them as a separate, third gender, connects them to the Hindu epic, the *Ramayana*:

> In the time of the Ramayana, Ram … had to leave Ayodhya (his native city) and go into the forest for 14 years. As he was going, the whole city followed him because they loved him so. As Ram came to … the edge of the forest, he turned to the people and said, 'Ladies and gents, please wipe your tears and go away.' But these people who were not men and not women did not know what to do. So they stayed there because Ram did not ask them to go. They remained there 14 years and snake hills grew around them. When Ram returned from Lanka, he found many snake hills. Not knowing why they were there he removed them and found so many people with long beards and long nails, all meditating. And so they were blessed by Ram. And that is why we *hijras* are so respected in Ayodhya.

Individual *hijras* also speak of themselves as being 'separate', being 'neither man nor woman', being 'born as men, but not men', or being 'not perfect men'. *Hijras* are most clearly 'not men' in relation to their claimed inability and lack of desire to engage in the sexual act as men with women, a consequence of their claimed biological intersexuality and their subsequent castration. Thus, *hijras* are unable to reproduce children, especially sons, an essential element in the Hindu concept of the normal, masculine role for males.

But if *hijras* are 'not men', neither are they women, in spite of several aspects of feminine behaviour associated with the role. These behaviours include dressing as women, wearing their hair long, plucking (rather than shaving) their facial hair, adopting feminine mannerisms, taking on women's names, and using female kinship terms, and a special, feminized vocabulary. *Hijras* also identify with a female goddess or as wives of certain male deities in ritual contexts. They claim seating reserved for 'ladies only' in public conveyances. On one occasion, they demanded to be counted as women in the census.[4]

Although their role requires *hijras* to dress like women, few make any real attempt to imitate or to 'pass' as women. Their female dress and mannerisms are exaggerated to the point of caricature, expressing sexual overtones that would be considered inappropriate for ordinary women in their roles as daughters, wives, and mothers. *Hijra* performances are burlesques of female behaviour. Much of the comedy of their behaviour derives from the incongruities between their behaviour and that of traditional women. They use coarse and abusive speech and gestures in opposition to the Hindu ideal of demure and restrained femininity. Further, it is not at all uncommon to see *hijras* in female clothing sporting several days' growth of beard, or exposing hairy, muscular arms. The ultimate sanction of *hijras* to an abusive or unresponsive public is to lift their skirts and expose the mutilated genitals. The implicit threat of this shameless, and thoroughly unfeminine, behaviour is enough to make most people give them a few cents so they will go away. Most centrally, as *hijras* themselves acknowledge, they are not born as women, and cannot reproduce. Their impotence and barrenness, due to a deficient or absent male organ, ultimately precludes their being considered fully male; yet their lack of female reproductive organs or female sexual organs precludes their being considered fully female.

Indian belief and the *hijra*'s own claims commonly attribute the impotence of the *hijra* as male to a hermaphroditic morphology and psychology. Many informants insisted 'I was born this way', implying hermaphroditism; such a condition is the standard reason given for joining the community. Only one of 30 informants, however, was probably born intersexed. Her words clearly indicate how central this status is to the *hijra* role, and make explicit that *hijras* are not males because they have no male reproductive organ:

> From my childhood I am like this. From birth my organ was very small. My brother tried taking me to doctors and all but the doctors said, 'No, it won't grow, your child is not a man and not a woman, this is God's gift and all … ' From that time my mother would dress me in girl's clothes. But then she saw it was no use, so she sent me to live with the *hijras*. I am a real *hijra*, not like those others who are converts; they are men and can have children, so they have the (emasculation) operation, but I was born this way.

> (Field notes, 1981–82)

Hijra *impotence and creative asceticism*

If, in Indian reality, the impotent male is considered useless as a man because he is unable to procreate, in Indian mythology, impotence can be transformed into generativity through the ideal of *tapasya*, or the practice of asceticism. *Tapas*, the power that results from ascetic practices and sexual abstinence, becomes an essential feature in the process of creation. Ascetics appear throughout Hindu mythology in procreative roles. In one version of the Hindu creation myth, Siva carries out an extreme, but legitimate form of *tapasya*, that of self-castration. Because the act of creation he was about to undertake had already been accomplished by Brahma, Siva breaks off his *linga* (phallus), saying, 'there is no use for this *linga* … ' and throws it into the earth. His act results in the fertility cult of *linga*-worship, which expresses the paradoxical theme of creative asceticism (O'Flaherty, 1973). This theme provides one explanation of the positive role given the *hijras* in Indian society. Born intersexed and impotent, unable themselves to reproduce, *hijras* can, through the emasculation operation, transform their liability into a source of creative power which enables them to confer blessings of fertility on others.

The link between the Hindu theme of creative asceticism and the role and power of the *hijras* is explicitly articulated in the myths connecting them to their major point of religious identification – their worship of Bahuchara Mata, and her requirement that they undergo emasculation. Bahuchara was a pretty, young maiden in a party of travellers passing through the forest in Gujerat. The party was attacked by thieves, and, fearing they would outrage her modesty, Bahuchara drew her dagger and cut off her breast, offering it to the outlaws in place of her body. This act, and her ensuing death, led to Bahuchara's deification and the practice of self-mutilation and sexual abstinence by her devotees to secure her favour.

Bahuchara has a special connection to the *hijras* because they are impotent men who undergo emasculation. This connection derives special significance from the story of King Baria of Gujerat. Baria was a devout follower of Bahucharaji, but was unhappy because he had no son. Through the goddess' favour a son, Jetho, was born to him. The son, however, was impotent. The King, out of respect to the goddess, set him apart for her service. Bahucharaji appeared to Jetho in a dream and told him to cut off his genitalia and dress himself as a woman, which he did. This practice has been followed by all who join the *hijra* cult (Metha, 1945–46).

Emasculation is the *dharm* (caste duty) of the *hijras*, and the chief source of their uniqueness. The *hijras* carry it out in a ritual context, in which the client sits in front of a picture of the goddess Bahuchara and repeats her name while the operation is being performed. A person who survives the operation becomes one of Bahuchara Mata's favourites, serving as a vehicle of her power through their symbolic rebirth. While the most popular image of Bahuchara is that of the goddess riding on a cock, Shah (1961) suggests that her original form of worship was the *yantra*, a conventional symbol for the vulva. A relation between this representation of the goddess and emasculation may exist: emasculation certainly brings the *hijra* devotee in to a closer identification with the female object of devotion.

Identification of the *hijras* with Bahuchara specifically and through her, with the creative powers of the Mother Goddess worshipped in many different forms in India, is clearly related to their major cultural function, that of performing at homes where a male child has been born. During these performances the *hijras*, using sexual innuendos, inspect the genitals of the infant whom they hold in their arms as they dance. The *hijras* confer fertility, prosperity, and health on the infant and family.

At both weddings and births, *hijras* hold the power to bless and to curse, and families regard them ambivalently. They have both auspicious functions and inauspicious potential. In regard to the latter, charms are used during pregnancy against eunuchs, both to protect against stillbirth, and a transformation of the embryo from male to female. Hiltebeitel (1980) suggests that the presence of eunuchs at births and weddings:

> … marks the ambiguity of those moments when the nondifferentiation of male and female is most filled with uncertainty and promise – in the mystery that surrounds the sexual identity of the still unborn child and on that [occasion] which anticipates the re-union of male and female in marital sex.
>
> (Hiltebeitel, 1980, p. 168)

Thus, it is fitting that the eunuch-transvestites, themselves characterized by sexual ambiguity, have ritual functions at moments that involve sexual ambiguity.

The eunuch-transvestite role of the *hijras* links them not only to the Mother Goddess, but also to Siva, through their identification with Arjuna, the hero of the Mahabharata. One origin myth of the *hijras* is the story of Arjuna's exile. He lives incognito for one year as part of the price he must pay for losing a game of dice, and also for rejecting the advances of one of the celestial nymphs. Arjuna decides to hide himself in the guise of a eunuch-transvestite, wearing bangles made of white conch, braiding his hair like a woman, clothing himself in female attire, and serving the ladies of the King's court (Rajagopalachari, 1980). Some *hijras* say that whoever is born on Arjuna's day, no matter where in the world, will become a *hijra*. Hiltebeitel (1980) makes a persuasive case for the identification of Arjuna with Siva, especially in his singer/dancer/eunuch/transvestite role.

The theme of the eunuch state is elaborated in a number of ways in the Mahabharata, and it is Arjuna who is the theme's central character. Arjuna, in the disguise of eunuch-transvestite, participates in weddings and births, and thus provides a further legitimization for the ritual contexts in which the *hijras* perform. At one point, for example, Arjuna in this disguise helps prepare the King's daughter for her marriage and her future role as mother-to-be. In doing this, he refuses to marry the princess himself, thus renouncing not only his sovereignty, but also the issue of an heir. His feigned impotence paves the way for the birth of the princess' child, just as the presence of the impotent *hijras* at the home of a male child paves the way for the child's fertility and the continuation of the family line.

This evidence suggests that intersexuality, impotence, emasculation and transvestism are all variously believed to be part of the *hijra* role, accounting for their inability to reproduce and the lack of desire (or the renunciation of the desire) to do so. In any event, sexual abstinence, which Hindu mythology associates with the powers of the ascetic, is in fact, the very source of the *hijras*' powers. The *hijras* themselves recognize this connection: they frequently refer to themselves as *sannyasin*, the person who renounces his role in society for the life of a holy wanderer and beggar. This vocation requires renunciation of material possessions, the duties of caste, the life of the householder and family man, and, most particularly, the renunciation of sexual desire (*kama*). In claiming this vocation, *hijras* point out how they have abandoned their families, live in material poverty, live off the charity of the others, and 'do not have sexual desires as other men do'.

Hijras understand that their 'other-worldliness' brings them respect in society, and that if they do not live up to these ideals, they will damage that respect. But just as Hindu mythology contains many stories of ascetics who renounce desire but nevertheless are moved by desire to engage in sexual acts, so, too, the *hijra* community experiences the tension between their religious, ascetic ideal community and the reality of the individual human's desire and sensuality.

Individual dimensions of the *hijra* role

Hijras *as homosexuals*

The remainder of this paper focuses on the sexual activities of *hijras*, and the ways in which the community experiences the conflict between the real and the ideal.

A widespread belief in India is that *hijras* are intersexed persons claimed or kidnapped by the *hijra* community as infants. No investigator has found evidence to support this belief. Given the large and complex society of India, the *hijra* community attracts different kinds of persons, most of whom join voluntarily as teenagers or adults. It appears to be a magnet for persons with a wide range of cross-gender characteristics arising from either a psychological or organic condition (Money and Wiedeking, 1980). The *hijra* role accommodates different personalities, sexual needs, and gender identities without completely losing its cultural meaning.

While the core of the positive meaning attached to the *hijra* role is linked to the negation of sexual desire, the reality is that many *hijras* do, in fact, engage in sexual activities. Because sexual behaviour is contrary to the definition of the role such activity causes conflict for both the individuals and the community. Individual *hijras* deal with the conflict in different ways, while the community as a whole resorts to various mechanisms of social control.

Though it is clear from the literature that some *hijras* engage in homosexual activity, there has been controversy over the centrality of this activity in the institutionalization of the role in India.[5] In his psychoanalytical study of high castes in a village in Rajasthan, Carstairs (1957) asserted that the *hijra* role is primarily a form of institutionalized homosexuality that developed in response to tendencies toward latent homosexuality in Indian national character. Morris Opler (1960) contested both Carstairs' evaluation of Indian character and his assertion that *hijras* are primarily conceptualized as homosexuals or that they engaged in any sexual activity.

Opler argued that the cultural definition of their role in Indian society was only one of performers. Sinha (1967), who worked in Lucknow in North India, acknowledged their performing role, but treated *hijras* primarily as homosexuals who join the community specifically to satisfy their sexual desires. Lynton and Rajan (1974), who interviewed *hijras* in Hyderabad, indicate that a period of homosexual activity, involving solicitation in public, sometimes precedes a decision to join the *hijras*. Their informants led them to believe, however, that sexual activity is prohibited by *hijra* rules and that these are strictly enforced by the community elders. Freeman (1979), who did fieldwork in Orissa at the southern edge of North Indian culture, discusses *hijras* as transvestite prostitutes and hardly mentions their ritual roles.

My own data (Nanda, 1984), gathered through fieldwork in Bangalore and Bombay, and in several North Indian cities, confirm beyond doubt that, however deviant it may be regarded within the *hijra* community, *hijras* in contemporary India extensively engage in sexual relations with men. This phenomenon is not entirely modern; nineteenth-century accounts (Bhimbhai, 1901; Faridi, 1899) claim that *hijras* were known to kidnap small boys for the purpose of sodomy or prostitution. Such allegations still find their way into the contemporary popular press (*India Today*, 1982).

Although *hijras* attribute their increased prostitution to declining opportunities to earn a living in their traditional manner, eunuch-transvestites in Hindu classical literature also had the reputation of engaging in homosexual activity. The classic Hindu manual of love, the *Kama Sutra* (Burton, 1986), specifically outlines sexual practices that were considered appropriate for eunuch-transvestites to perform with male partners.[6] Classical Hinduism taught that there was a 'third sex', divided into various categories, two of which were castrated men, eunuchs, and hermaphrodites, who wore false breasts, and imitated the voice, gestures, dress and temperaments of women. These types shared the major function of providing alternative techniques of sexual gratification (Bullough, 1976). In contemporary India, concepts of eunuch, transvestite and male homosexual are not distinct, and the *hijras* are considered all of these at once (O'Flaherty, 1980).

The term *hijra*, however, which is of Urdu origin and the masculine gender, has the primary meaning of hermaphrodite. It is usually translated as eunuch, never as homosexual. Even Carstairs' informants, among whom the homosexuality of the *hijras* was well known, defined them as either drum players at the birth of male children, or eunuchs, whose duty was to undergo castration. In parts of North India, the term for effeminate males who play the passive role in homosexual relations is *zenanas* (women); by becoming a *hijra*, one removes oneself from this category (see also Lynton and Rajan, 1974). Furthermore, a covert homosexual subculture exists in some of the larger cities in North India (Anderson, 1977), but persons who participate in it are not called *hijras*. In fact, as in other cultures (Carrier, 1980; Wikan, 1977) men who play the inserter role in sexual activities between men have no linguistically or sociologically distinguished role. Unlike western cultures, in India sexual object choice alone does not define gender. In some South Indian regional languages, the names by which *hijras* are called, such as *kojja*, in Telegu (Anderson, 1977) or *potee* in Tamil, are, unlike the term *hijra*, epithets used derogatorily to mean a cowardly or feminine male or homosexual. This linguistic difference, however, is consistent with the fact that in South India the *hijras* do not have the cultural role which they do in North India.

According to my research, homosexual activity is widespread among *hijras*, and teenage homosexual activity figures significantly in the lives of many individuals who join the community. As Sinha's interviews also indicate (1967), those *hijras* who engage in homosexual activity share particular life patterns before joining the community. Typically, such individuals liked during childhood to dress in feminine clothes, play with girls, do traditionally female work, and avoid the company of boys in rough play. In lower-class families, the boy's effeminacy is both ridiculed and encouraged by his peers, who may persuade him to play the insertee role for them, possibly with some slight monetary consideration. At this stage the boy lives with his family, though in an increasingly tense atmosphere. He thinks of himself as a male and wears male clothing, at least in public. As his interest in homosexual activity increases, and his relations with his family become more strained, he may leave home. In most cases their families make serious attempts to inhibit their feminine activity with scoldings, surveillance, restrictions, and beatings, so that the boy finally has no choice but to leave.[7]

There are two modes of sexual relations among *hijras*. One is casual prostitution, the exchange of sexual favours with different men for a fixed sum of money, and the other is 'having a husband'. *Hijras* do not characterize their male sexual partners as homosexual; they quite explicitly distinguish them as being different from homosexuals. One *hijra*, Shakuntala, characterizes the customers in the following way:

> ... these men ... are married or unmarried, they may be the father of many children. Those who come to us, they have no desire to go to a man ... they come to us for the sake of going to a girl. They prefer us to their wives ... each one's tastes differ among people ... It is God's way; because we have to make a living, he made people like this so we can earn.

> (Field notes, 1981–82)

Shakuntala clearly expressed a feminine gender identity and was, in fact, the person who came closest to what would be called in the west a transsexual, that is, experiencing himself as a 'female trapped in a male body'. She remembered having felt that she was a female since childhood, liking to dress in female clothing, doing woman's work inside the house and playing with girls rather than boys. She was introduced to homosexual activity in her teens, which she claims 'spoiled' her for the normal, heterosexual male role. She has a very maternal, nurturing temperament, and emphasizes the maternal aspect of the *guru* role to her young *chelas*.[8] She is currently involved in a long-term, monogamous relationship with a young man who lives in her neighbourhood and whom she hopes will 'marry' her. She underwent the emasculation operation because she wanted 'to become more beautiful, like woman'. She was the only *hijra* interviewed who was taking hormones 'to develop a more feminine figure'. She always dressed as a woman and was very convincing in a feminine role, not exhibiting the more flamboyant mannerisms and gestures of the typical *hijra*. Because of her strong attachment to her present boyfriend, she is sometimes criticized by her *hijra* friends as having 'husband fever'. As one of her friends says:

> Those people, like Shakuntala, with husband fever, they are mad over their husbands, even to the point of suicide. If that fellow even talks to a[nother] girl, immediately they'll fight with him. If he is out at night, even if it is three o'clock in the morning, they'll go in search of him. They won't even sleep till he returns.
>
> (Field notes, 1981–82)

This devotion to one man is seen as typical of Shakuntala's extremely feminine identification.

Not all *hijras* who engage in sexual relation with other men express such complete feminine identification. One *hijra*, for example, explained the attraction of men to *hijras* on different grounds:

> See, there is a proverb, 'For a normal lady [prostitute] it is four annas and for a *hijra* it is twelve annas'. These men, they come to us to have pleasure on their own terms. They may want to kiss us or do so many things. For instance, the customer will ask us to lift the legs (from a position lying on her back) so that they can do it through the anus. We allow them to do it by the back [anal intercourse], but not very often.
>
> (Field notes, 1981–82)

This statement suggests that the attraction of the *hijras* is that they will engage in forms of sexual behaviour in which Indian women will normally not engage. Several of my non-*hijra* male informants confirmed this view.

Having a husband is the preferred alternative for those *hijras* who engage in sexual relations. Many of my informants have, or recently had, a relatively permanent attachment to one man whom they referred to as their husband. They maintain warm and affectionate, as well as sexually satisfying and economically reciprocal, relationships with these men, with whom they live, sometimes alone, or sometimes with several other *hijras*. Lalitha, a very feminine-looking *hijra* in her middle thirties, has had the same husband for nine years. He used to come for prostitution to the *hijra* commune in which Lalitha lived and then they lived together in a small house until he got married. Now Lalitha has moved back with the *hijras*, where she cooks their meals in return for free food and lodging. But she still maintains her relationship with her 'husband':

> My husband is a Christian. He works in a cigarette factory and earns 1000 rupees a month. He is married to [another] woman and has got four children. I encouraged him to get married and even his wife and children are nice to me. His children call me *chitti* [mother's sister] and even his wife's parents know about me and don't say anything. He gives me saris and flowers and whenever I ask for money he never says no. When he needs money, I would give him also.
>
> (Field notes, 1981–82)

Hijras who have husbands do not break their ties with the *hijra* community, although sometimes their husbands urge them to do so. Sushila, an attractive, assertive, and ambitious *hijra* in her early thirties has a husband who is a driver for a national corporation headquarters and earns 600 rupees a month. She continues to be very active in the local *hijra* community, however, and even refuses to give up practising prostitution in spite of her husband's objections:

> My husband tells me, 'I earn enough money. Why do you go for prostitution?' I tell him, 'You are here with me today. What surety is there you will be with me forever? I came to you from prostitution, and if you leave me, I'll have to go back to it. Then all those other *hijras* will say, "Oh, she lived as a wife and now look at her fate, she has come back to prostitution."' So I tell him, 'Don't put any restrictions on me; now they all think of me as someone nice, but when I go back to prostitution, they will put me to shame.' If he gives me too much back talk, I give him good whacks.
>
> (Field notes, 1981–82)

Sushila is saving the money she makes from prostitution and from that her husband gives to her so that she can buy a business, probably a bathhouse for working-class men. In Bangalore, bathhouses are commonly run by *hijras*.

Although many *hijras* complain that it is hard for them to save money, some have a good business sense and have invested in jewellery and property so that they can be relatively independent financially in their old age. For *hijras* who are not particularly talented singers and dancers, or who live in cities where their ritual performances are not in demand prostitution provides an adequate way of earning a living. It is a demanding and even occasionally dangerous profession, however, because some customers turn out to be 'rowdies'. Although a *hijra* living in a commune has to pay 50 per cent of her fees from prostitution to her household head, few of the younger *hijra* prostitutes can afford their own place; and living with others provides a certain amount of protection from rough customers and the police. In spite of the resentment and constant complaints by younger *hijra* prostitutes that they are exploited by their elders, they are extremely reluctant to live on their own.

Hijra sexuality as a source of conflict

The attraction that the *hijra* role holds for some individuals is the opportunity to engage in sexual relations with men, while enjoying the sociability and relative security of an organized community; these advantages are apparent in contrast to the insecurity and harassment experienced by the effeminate homosexual living on his own. But, whether with husbands or customers, sexual relations run counter to the cultural definitions of the *hijra* role, and are a source of conflict within the community. *Hijra* elders attempt to maintain control over those who would 'spoil' the *hijras*' reputation by engaging in sexual activity.

Hijras are well aware that they have only a tenuous hold on respectability in Indian society, and that this respectability is compromised by even covertly engaging in sexual relations. Ascetics have always been regarded with scepticism and ambivalence in Indian society. While paying lip service to the ascetic, conventional Hinduism maintained a very real hostility to it. It classed the non-Vedic ascetic with the dregs of society, 'such as incendiaries, poisoners, pimps, spies, adulterers, abortionists, atheists and drunkards'; these fringe members of society found their most respectable status among the Siva sects (O'Flaherty, 1973, p. 67). This ambivalence toward ascetics accurately describes the response of Indian society to the *hijra* as well, who are also, not coincidentally, worshippers of Siva. In addition, the notion of the false ascetic (those who pretend to be ascetics in order to satisfy their lust) abounds in Hindu mythology. This contradictory attitude, a high regard for asceticism coupled with disdain for those who practise it, characterizes contemporary as well as classical India. Even those families who allow the *hijras* to perform at births and weddings ridicule the notion that they have any real power.

Indian audiences express their ambivalence toward the *hijras* by challenging the authenticity of *hijra* performers. The *hijras*' emasculation distinguishes them from *zenanas*, or practising effeminate homosexuals, who do not have the religious powers ascribed to the *hijras*, but who sometimes impersonate them in order to earn a living. Thus, *hijras* state that emasculation is necessary because, when they are performing or asking for alms, people may challenge them. If their genitals have not been removed, they will be reviled and driven away as imposters. *Hijra* elders themselves constantly deride those 'men who are men and can have children' and join their community only to make a living from it, or to enjoy sexual relations with men. The parallel between such 'fake' *hijras* and the false ascetics is clear.

Hijras consider sexual activity offensive to the *hijra* goddess, Bahuchara Mata. Upon initiation into the community, the novice vows to abstain from sexual relations or to marry. *Hijra* elders claim that all *hijra* houses lock their doors by nine o'clock at night, implying that no sexual activities occur there. In the cities where *hijra* culture is strongest, *hijras* who practise prostitution are not permitted to live with *hijras* who earn their living by traditional ritual performances. Those who live in these respectable or 'family' houses are carefully watched to see that they do not have contact with men. In areas more peripheral to the core of *hijra* culture, including most of South India, prostitutes do live in houses with traditional *hijra* performers, and may, in fact, engage in such performances themselves whenever they have an opportunity to do so.

Sexually active *hijras* usually assert that all *hijras* join the community so that they can engage in sexual relations with men. As Sita, a particularly candid informant, said:

> Why else would we wear saris? Those who you see who are aged now, when they were young they were just like me. Now they say they haven't got the sexual feeling and they talk only for God and all, but I tell you, that is all nonsense. In their younger days, they also did this prostitution and it is only for the sexual feeling that we join.
>
> (Field notes, 1981–82)

The *hijras* who most vehemently denied having sexual relations with men were almost always over 40. It appears that as they get older, *hijras* give up sexual activity. Such change over the life cycle parallels that in India generally; in the Hindu cultural ideal, women whose sons are married are expected to give up sexual activity. In fact, not all women do so, but there is social pressure to do so. People ridicule and gossip about middle-aged women who act in ways that suggest active sexual interest (Vatuk, 1985). The presentation of self as a non-sexual person that occurs with age also appears among the *hijras*. The elderly ones may wear male clothing in public, dress more conservatively, wearing white rather than boldly coloured saris, act in a less sexually suggestive manner, and take on household domestic roles that keep them indoors.

Although *hijra* elders are most vocal in expressing disapproval of *hijra* sexual relations, even younger *hijras* who have husbands or practise prostitution admit that such behaviour runs counter to *hijra* norms and lowers their status in the larger society. *Hijra* prostitutes say that prostitution is a necessary evil for them, the only way for them to earn a living. They attribute the frequency of *hijra* prostitution to the declining economic status of the *hijras* in India since the time of Independence. At that time the rajas and nawobs in the princely states, who were important patrons of *hijra* ritual performances, lost their offices. *Hijras* also argue that in modern India, declining family size and the spread of Western values, which undermine belief in their powers, also contributes to their lowered economic position, making prostitution necessary.

India as an accommodating society

India is characteristically described as a sexually tolerant society (Bullough, 1976; Carrier, 1980). Indeed, the *hijra* role appears to be elastic enough to accommodate a wide variety of individual temperaments, identities, behaviours, and levels of commitment, and still function in a culturally accepted manner. This elasticity derives from the genius of Hinduism: although not every *hijra* lives up to the role at the highest level, the role nonetheless gives religious meaning to cross-gender behaviour, that is despised, punished and pushed beyond the pale of the cultural system in other societies.

Several different aspects of Hindu thought explain both the ability of Indian society to absorb an institutionalized third gender role, as well as to provide several contexts within which to handle the tension between the ideal and real aspects of the role. Indian mythology contains numerous examples of androgynes (see O'Flaherty, 1980), impersonators of the opposite sex, and among both deities and humans individuals with sex changes. Myths are an important part of popular culture. Sivabhaktis (worshippers of Siva) give *hijras* special respect because one of the forms of Siva is Ardhanarisvara ('the lord who is half woman'). *Hijras* also associate themselves with Vishnu, who transforms himself into Mohini, the most beautiful woman in the world, in order to take back the sacred nectar from the demons who have stolen it. Further, in the worship of Krishna, male devotees may imagine themselves to be female, and even dress in female clothing; direct identification with Krishna is forbidden, but the devotee may identify with him indirectly by identifying with Radha, that is, by taking a female form. Thousands of *hijras* identify themselves as Krishna's wives in a ritual performed in South India. These are only a few of the contexts within which the *hijras* link themselves to the Great Tradition of Hinduism and develop a positive definition for their feminine behaviour.

In handling the conflict between the real and the ideal, *hijras* and other groups in the Indian population are confronted with the seemingly conflicting value which Hinduism places on both eroticism and procreation, on the one hand, and non-attachment and asceticism, on the other. Both Hinduism and Islam are what Bullough calls 'sex-positive' religions (1976). Both allow for the tolerance of a wider range of sexual expression than exists in Western culture with its restrictive Judeo-Christian, religious heritage. Hinduism explicitly recognizes that humans achieve their ultimate goals – salvation, bliss, knowledge and (sexual) pleasure – by following many different paths because humans differ in their special abilities and competencies. Thus, Hinduism allows a different ethic according to one's own nature and affords the individual temperament the widest latitude, from highly idealistic morality, through genial toleration, and, finally, to compulsive extremes (Lannoy, 1975).

Hindu thought attempts to reconcile the value conflict between sexuality and chastity through the concept of a life cycle with four stages. Each stage has its appropriate sexual behaviour: in the first stage one should be a chaste student, in the second a married householder, in the third a forest dweller preparing for withdrawal from society, and in the final stage, a *sannyasin*, the ascetic who has renounced everything. Thus, the Hindu ideal is a fully integrated life in which each aspect of human nature, including sexuality, has its time. *Hijras* implicity recognize these stages in their social organization through a hierarchy in which one begins as a *chela* and moves into the position of *guru* as one gets older, taking on *chelas* and becoming less sexually active.

Hindu mythology also provides some contexts within which the contradictions between the ascetic ideal and the sexual activity are legitimate: Siva himself is both the great erotic and the great ascetic. In myths he alternates between the two forms. In some mythic episodes Siva is unable to reconcile his two roles as ascetic and householder, and in others he is a hypocritical ascetic because of his sexual involvement with Parvati, his consort (O'Flaherty, 1973). Indian goddesses as sexual figures also exist in abundance and in some stories a god will take on a female form specifically to have sexual relations with a male deity.

Where Western culture feels uncomfortable with contradictions and makes strenuous attempts to resolve them, Hinduism allows opposites to confront each other without a resolution, 'celebrating the idea that the universe is boundlessly various, and ... that all possibilities may exist without excluding each other' (O'Flaherty, 1973, p. 318). It is this characteristically Indian ability to tolerate, and even embrace, contradictions at social, cultural and personality levels, that provides a context for *hijras*. *Hijras* express in their very bodies the confrontation of femaleness and maleness as polar opposites. In Indian society they are not only tolerated but also valued.

Acknowledgements

For their assistance in developing the ideas in this paper, grateful acknowledgement is made to Joseph Carrier, David Greenberg, A.M. Shah, Rajni Chopra, Evelyn Blackwood, John Money, the participants of the Columbia University Seminar on the Indian Self, and most especially, Owen Lynch and Alan Roland. I am also grateful to Mr Banu Vasudevan, Bharati Gowda, and Shiv Ram Apte, as well as my friends among the *hijras*, without whom this paper could not have been written.

Notes

1 I would like to thank Veena Oldenburg for calling this to my attention. A similar pattern exists among the courtesans in North India (Oldenburg, 1984).
2 Alan Roland (1982) has insightfully examined some of the emotional and psychological aspects of hierarchy within the Hindu joint family, and many of his conclusions could well be applied to the *hijra* hierarchy.
3 Some of these religious occasions are participated in by non-*hijras* as well, while others celebrate events specific to the *hijra* community, such as the anniversary of the deaths of important gurus.
4 More recently, *hijras* have been issued ration cards for food in New Delhi, but must apply only under the male names.
5 A more detailed description of this literature is found in Nanda (1984).
6 'Mouth Congress' is considered the appropriate sexual activity for eunuchs disguised as women, in the *Kama Sutra*. An Editor's note (Burton, 1986, p. 124) suggests that this practice is no longer common in India, and is perhaps being replaced by sodomy, which has been introduced since the Muslim period.
7 Social class factors are relevant here. Boys who are born with indeterminate sex organs (I came across three such cases by hearsay) to upper-middle-class families would not be likely to join the *hijras*. In two of these cases the men in question were adults; one had been sent abroad to develop his career in science with the expectation that he would not marry, but at least would have the satisfaction of a successful and prestigious career. The other was married by his parents to a girl who, it was known, could not have children. The third is still a toddler and is being brought up as a boy. I also had the opportunity to interview a middle-aged, middle-class man who was desperately trying to find a doctor to perform the transsexual operation on him in a hospital. He chose not to join the *hijras* because of their 'reputation' but envied them their group life and their ability to live openly as women.

8 *Gurus* are sometimes considered like mothers, sometimes like fathers, and sometimes like husbands. Their female aspect is related to the nurturing and care and concern they have for their *chelas*; the male aspect refers more to the authority they have over their *chelas* and the obedience and loyalty that is due them.

References

ANDERSON, C. (1977) 'Gay men in India', unpublished manuscript, University of Wisconsin.

BHIMBHAI, K.P. (1901) 'Gujarat population, Hindus', in CAMPBELL, J.M. (Compiler) *Gazetteer of the Bombay Presidency*, 4(1), Bombay: Government Central Press.

BULLOUGH, V.L. (1976) *Sexual Variance in Society and History*, Chicago: University of Chicago Press.

BURTON, R.F. (trans. and ed.) *The Kama Sutra of Vatsyayana: The Classic Hindu Treatise on Love and Social Conduct*, New York: Dorset Press.

CARRIER, J. (1980) 'Homosexual behaviour in cross-cultural perspective', in MARMOR, J. (ed.) *Homosexual Behaviour: A Modern Reappraisal*, New York: Basic Books.

CARSTAIRS, G.M. (1957) *The Twice Born*, London: Hogarth Press.

FARIDI, F.L. (1899) '*Hijras*', in CAMPBELL, J.M. (Compiler) *Gazetteer of the Bombay Presidency*, 9(2), Bombay: Government Central Press.

FREEMAN, J.M. (1979) *Untouchable: An Indian Life History*, Stanford, CA: Stanford University Press.

HILTEBEITEL, A. (1980) 'Siva, the goddess, and the disguises of the Pandavas and Draupadi', *History of Religions*, 20, pp. 147–74.

INDIA TODAY (1982) 'Fear is the key', 15 September, pp. 84–5.

LANNOY, R. (1975) *The Speaking Tree*, New York: Oxford University Press.

LYNTON, H.S. and RAJAN, M. (1974) *Days of the Beloved*, Berkeley: University of California Press.

METHA, S. (1945–46) 'Eunuchs, Pavaiyas and Hijadas', *Gufarat ahitya Sabja*, Amdavad, Karyavahi, 2, Ahmedabad.

MONEY, J. and WIEDEKING, C. (1980) *Handbook of Human Sexuality*, WOLMAN, B. and MONEY, J. (cds) Englewood Cliffs, NJ: Prentice-Hall.

NANDA, S. (1984) 'The *Hijras* of India: a preliminary report', *Medicine and Law*, 3, pp. 59–75.

O'FLAHERTY, W. (1973) *Asceticism and Eroticism in the Mythology of Siva*, Oxford: Oxford University Press.

—— (1980) *Women, Androgynes, and Other Mythical Beasts*, Chicago: University of Chicago Press.

OLDENBURG, V. (1984) *The Making of Colonial Lucknow*, Princeton: Princeton University Press.

OPLER, M. (1960) 'The Hijaras (hermaphrodities) of India and Indian national character: a rejoinder', *American Anthropologist*, 62, pp. 505–11.

RAJAGOPALACHARI, C. (1980) *Mahabharata*, Bombay: Bharatiya Vidya Bhavan.

ROLAND, A. (1982) 'Toward a psychoanalytical psychology of hierarchical relationships in Hindu India', *Ethos*, 10, pp. 232–53.

SALUNKHE, G. (1976) 'The cult of the Hijaras', *Illustrated Weekly*, 8 August, pp. 16–21.

SHAH, A.M. (1961) 'A note on the Hijaras of Gujerat', *American Anthropologist*, 61, pp. 1325–30.

SINHA, A.P. (1967) 'Procreation among the eunuchs', *Eastern Anthropologist*, 20, pp. 168–76.

THE TRIBUNE (1983) '500,000 eunuchs in India, Pak.', 26 August, p. 2.

VATUK, S. (1985) 'South Asian cultural conceptions of sexuality', in BROWN, J.K. and KERNS, V. (eds) *In Her Prime: A New View of Middle-Aged Women*, S. Hadley, MA: Bergin and Harvey.

WIKAN, U. (1977) 'Man becomes woman: transsexualism in Oman as a key to gender roles', *Man*, 12, pp. 304–19.

13 Capitalism and gay identity

John D'Emilio [1983]

For gay men and lesbians, the 1970s were years of significant achievement. Gay liberation and women's liberation changed the sexual landscape of the nation. Hundreds of thousands of gay women and men came out and openly affirmed same-sex eroticism. We won repeal of sodomy laws in half the states, a partial lifting of the exclusion of lesbian and gay men from federal employment, civil rights protection in a few dozen cities, the inclusion of gay rights in the platform of the Democratic Party, and the elimination of homosexuality from the psychiatric profession's list of mental illnesses. The gay male subculture expanded and became increasingly visible in large cities, and lesbian feminists pioneered in building alternative institutions and an alternative culture that attempted to embody a liberating vision of the future.

In the 1980s, however, with the resurgence of an active right wing, gay men and lesbians face the future warily. Our victories appear tenuous and fragile; the relative freedom of the past few years seems too recent to be permanent. In some parts of the lesbian and gay male community, a feeling of doom is growing: analogies with McCarthy's America, when 'sexual perverts' were a special target of the right, and with Nazi Germany, where gays were shipped to concentration camps, surface with increasing frequency. Everywhere there is a sense that new strategies are in order if we want to preserve our gains and move ahead.

I believe that a new, more accurate theory of gay history must be part of this political enterprise. When the gay liberation movement began at the end of the 1960s, gay men and lesbians had no history that we could use to fashion our goals and strategy. In the ensuing years, in building a movement without a knowledge of our history, we instead invented a mythology. This mythical history drew on personal experience, which we read backward in time. For instance, most lesbians and gay men in the 1960s first discovered their homosexual desires in isolation, unaware of others, and without resources for naming and understanding what they felt. From this experience, we constructed a myth of silence, invisibility, and isolation as the essential characteristics of gay life in the past as well as the present. Moreover, because we faced so many oppressive laws, public policies, and cultural beliefs, we projected this into an image of the abysmal past: until gay liberation, lesbians and gay men were always the victims of systematic, undifferentiated, terrible oppression.

These myths have limited our political perspectives. They have contributed, for instance, to an overreliance on a strategy of coming out – if every gay man and lesbian in America came out, gay oppression would end – and have allowed us to ignore the institutionalized ways in which homophobia and heterosexism are reproduced. They have encouraged, at times, an incapacitating despair, especially at moments like the present: how can we unravel a gay oppression so pervasive and unchanging?

There is another historical myth that enjoys nearly universal acceptance in the gay movement, the myth of the 'eternal homosexual'. The argument runs something like this: gay men and lesbians always were and always will be. We are everywhere; not just now, but throughout history, in all societies and all periods. This myth served a positive political function in the first years of gay liberation. In the early 1970s, when we battled an ideology that either denied our existence or defined us as psychopathic individuals or freaks of nature, it was empowering to assert that 'we are everywhere'. But in recent years it has confined us as surely as the most homophobic medical theories, and locked our movement in place.

Here I wish to challenge this myth. I want to argue that gay men and lesbians have not always existed. Instead, they are a product of history, and have come into existence in a specific historical era. Their emergence is associated with the relations of capitalism; it has been the historical development of capitalism – more specifically, its free-labour system – that has allowed large numbers of men and women in the late twentieth century to call themselves gay, to see themselves as part of a community of similar men and women, and to organize politically on the basis of that identity.[1] Finally, I want to suggest some political lessons we can draw from this view of history.

What, then, are the relationships between the free-labour system of capitalism and homosexuality? First, let me review some features of capitalism. Under capitalism workers are 'free' labourers in two ways. We have the freedom to look for a job. We own our ability to work and have the freedom to sell our labour power for wages to anyone willing to buy it. We are also freed from the ownership of anything except our labour power. Most of us do not own the land or the tools that produce what we need, but rather have to work for a living in order to survive. So, if we are free to sell our labour power in the positive sense, we are also freed, in the negative sense, from any other alternative. This dialectic – the constant interplay between exploitation and some measure of autonomy – informs all of the history of those who have lived under capitalism.

As capital – money used to make more money – expands so does this system of free labour. Capital expands in several ways. Usually it expands in the same place, transforming small firms into larger ones, but it also expands by taking over new areas of production: the weaving of cloth, for instance, or the baking of bread. Finally, capital expands geographically. In the United States, capitalism initially took root in the Northeast, at a time when slavery was the dominant system in the South and when noncapitalist Native American societies occupied the western half of the continent. During the nineteenth century, capital spread from the Atlantic to the Pacific, and in the twentieth, US capital has penetrated almost every part of the world.

The expansion of capital and the spread of wage labour have effected a profound transformation in the structure and functions of the nuclear family, the ideology of family life, and the meaning of heterosexual relations. It is these changes in the family that are most directly linked to the appearance of a collective gay life.

The white colonists in seventeenth-century New England established villages structured around a household economy, composed of family units that were basically self-sufficient, independent, and patriarchal. Men, women, and children farmed land owned by the male head of the household. Although there was a division of labour between men and women, the family was truly an interdependent unit of production: the survival of each member depended on all. The home was a workplace where women processed raw farm products into food for daily consumption, where they made clothing, soap, and candles, and where husbands, wives, and children worked together to produce the goods they consumed.

By the nineteenth century, this system of household production was in decline. In the Northeast, as merchant capitalists invested the money accumulated through trade in the production of goods, wage labour became more common. Men and women were drawn out of the largely self-sufficient household economy of the colonial era into a capitalist system of free labour. For women in the nineteenth century, working for wages rarely lasted beyond marriage; for men, it became a permanent condition.

The family was thus no longer an independent unit of production. But although no longer independent, the family was still interdependent. Because capitalism had not expanded very far, because it had not yet taken over – or socialized – the production of consumer goods, women still performed necessary productive labour in the home. Many families no longer produced grain, but wives still baked into bread the flour they bought with their husbands' wages; or, when they purchased yarn or cloth, they still made clothing for their families. By the mid-nineteenth century, capitalism had destroyed the economic self-sufficiency of many families, but not the mutual dependence of the members.

This transition away from the household family-based economy to a fully developed capitalist free-labour economy occurred very slowly, over almost two centuries. As late as 1920, 50 per cent of the US population lived in communities of fewer than 2,500 people. The vast majority of blacks in the early twentieth century lived outside the free-labour economy, in a system of sharecropping and tenancy that rested on the family. Not only did independent farming as a way of life still exist for millions of Americans, but even in towns and small cities women continued to grow and process food, make clothing, and engage in other kinds of domestic production.

But for those people who felt the brunt of these changes, the family took on new significance as an affective unit, an institution that provided not goods but emotional satisfaction and happiness. By the 1920s among the white middle class, the ideology surrounding the family described it as the means through which men and women formed satisfying, mutually enhancing relationships and created an environment that nurtured children. The family became the setting for a 'personal life', sharply distinguished and disconnected from the public world of work and production (see Zaretsky, 1976; Fass, 1977).

The meaning of heterosexual relations also changed. In colonial New England the birth rate averaged over seven children per woman of childbearing age. Men and women needed the labour of children. Producing offspring was as necessary for survival as producing grain. Sex was harnessed to procreation. The Puritans did not celebrate heterosexuality but rather marriage; they condemned all sexual expression outside the marriage bond and did not differentiate sharply between sodomy and heterosexual fornication.

By the 1970s, however, the birth rate had dropped to under two. With the exception of the post-World-War-Two baby boom, the decline has been continuous for two centuries, paralleling the spread of capitalist relations of production. It occurred when access to contraceptive devices and abortion was systematically curtailed. The decline has included every segment of the population – urban and rural families, blacks and whites, ethnics and WASPS, the middle class and the working class.

As wage labour spread and production became socialized, then, it became possible to release sexuality from the 'imperative' to procreate. Ideologically, heterosexual expression came to be a means of establishing intimacy, promoting happiness, and experiencing pleasure. In divesting the household of its economic independence and fostering the separation of sexuality from procreation, capitalism has created conditions that allow some men and women to organize a personal life around their erotic/emotional attraction to their own sex. It has made possible the formation of urban communities of lesbians and gay men and, more recently, of a politics based on sexual identity.

Evidence from colonial New England court records and church sermons indicates that male and female homosexual behaviour existed in the seventeenth century. Homosexual behaviour, however, is different from homosexual identity. There was, quite simply, no 'social space' in the colonial system of production that allowed men and women to be gay. Survival was structured around participation in a nuclear family. There were certain homosexual acts – sodomy among men, 'lewdness' among women – in which individuals engaged, but family was so pervasive that colonial society lacked even the category of homosexual or lesbian to describe a person. It is quite possible that some men and women experienced a stronger attraction to their own sex than to the opposite sex – in fact, some colonial court cases refer to men who persisted in their 'unnatural' attractions – but one could not fashion out of that preference a way of life. Colonial Massachusetts even had laws prohibiting unmarried adults from living outside family units (see Katz, 1976, pp. 16–24, 568–71; Oaks, 1978; Roberts, 1980).

By the second half of the nineteenth century, this situation was noticeably changing as the capitalist system of free labour took hold. Only when individuals began to make their living through wage labour, instead of as parts of an interdependent family unit, was it possible for homosexual desire to coalesce into a personal identity – an identity based on the ability to remain outside the heterosexual family and to construct a personal life based on attraction to one's own sex. By the end of the century, a class of men and women existed who recognized their erotic interest in their own sex, saw it as a trait that set them apart from the majority, and sought others like themselves. These early gay lives came from a wide social spectrum: civil servants and business executives, department store clerks and college professors, factory operatives, ministers, lawyers, cooks, domestics, hoboes, and the idle rich; men and women, black and white, immigrant and native-born.

In this period, gay men and lesbians began to invent ways of meeting each other and sustaining a group life. Already, in the early twentieth century, large cities contained male homosexual bars. Gay men stalked out cruising areas, such as Riverside Drive in New York City and Lafayette Park in Washington. In St Louis and the nation's capital, annual drag balls brought together large numbers of black gay men. Public bath houses and YMCAs became gathering spots for male homosexuals. Lesbians formed literary societies and private social clubs. Some working-class women 'passed' as men to obtain better-paying jobs and lived with other women – forming lesbian couples who appeared to the world as husband and wife. Among the faculties of women's colleges, in the settlement houses, and in the professional associations and clubs that women formed, one could find lifelong intimate relationships supported by a web of lesbian friends. By the 1920s and 1930s, large cities such as New York and Chicago contained lesbian bars. These patterns of living could evolve because capitalism allowed individuals to survive beyond the confines of the family.[2]

Simultaneously, ideological definitions of homosexual behaviour changed. Doctors developed theories about homosexuality, describing it as a condition, something that was inherent in a person, a part of his or her 'nature'. These theories did not represent scientific breakthroughs, elucidations of previously undiscovered areas of knowledge; rather, they were an ideological response to a new way of organizing one's personal life. The popularization of the medical model, in turn, affected the consciousness of the women and men who experienced homosexual desire, so that they came to define themselves through their erotic life.[3]

These new forms of gay identity and patterns of group life also reflected the differentiation of people according to gender, race, and class that is so pervasive in capitalist societies. Among whites, for instance, gay men have traditionally been more visible than lesbians. This partly stems from the division between the public male sphere and the private female sphere. Streets, parks, and bars, especially at night, were 'male space'. Yet the greater visibility of white men also reflected their larger numbers. The Kinsey studies of the 1940s and 1950s found significantly more men than women with predominantly homosexual histories, a situation caused, I would argue, by the fact that capitalism had drawn far more men than women into the labour force, and higher wages. Men could more easily construct a personal life independent of attachments to the opposite sex, whereas women were more likely to remain economically dependent on men. Kinsey *et al.* (1948, 1953) also found a strong positive correlation between years of schooling and lesbian activity. College-educated white women, far more able than their working-class sisters to support themselves, could survive more easily without intimate relationships with men.

Among working-class immigrants in the early twentieth century, closely knit kin networks and an ethic of family solidarity placed constraints on individual autonomy that made gayness a difficult option to pursue. In contrast, for reasons not altogether clear, urban black communities appeared relatively tolerant of homosexuality. The popularity in the 1920s and 1930s of songs with lesbian and gay male themes – 'B.D. Woman', 'Prove It On Me', 'Sissy Man', 'Fairey Blues' – suggests an openness about homosexual expression at odds with the mores of whites. Among men in the rural West in the 1940s, Kinsey found extensive incidence of homosexual behaviour, but, in contrast with the men in large cities, little consciousness of gay identity. Thus even as capitalism exerted a homogenizing influence by gradually transforming more individuals into wage labourers and separating them from traditional communities, different groups of people were affected in different ways.[4]

The decisions of particular men and women to act on their erotic/emotional preference for the same sex, along with the new consciousness that this preference made them different, led to the formation of an urban subculture of gay men and lesbians. Yet at least through the 1930s this subculture remained rudimentary, unstable, and difficult to find. How, then, did the complex, well-developed gay community emerge that existed by the time the gay liberation movement exploded? The answer is to be found in the dislocations of World War Two, a time when the cumulative changes of several decades coalesced into a qualitatively new shape.

The war severely disrupted traditional patterns of gender relations and sexuality, and temporarily created a new erotic situation conducive to homosexual expression. It plucked millions of young men and women, whose sexual identities were just forming, out of their homes, out of towns and small cities, out of the heterosexual environment of the family, and dropped them into sex-segregated situations – as GIs, as WACs and WAVES, in same-sex rooming houses for women workers who relocated to seek employment. The war freed millions of men and women from the settings where heterosexuality was normally imposed. For men and women already gay, it provided an opportunity to meet people like themselves. Others could become gay because of the temporary freedom to explore sexuality that the war provided.[5]

The gay men and women of the 1940s were pioneers. Their decisions to act on their desires formed the underpinnings of an urban subculture of gay men and lesbians. Throughout the 1950s and 1960s the gay subculture grew and stabilized, so that people coming out then could more easily find other gay women and men than in the past. Newspapers and magazines published articles describing gay male life. Literally hundreds of novels with lesbian themes were published.[6] Psychoanalysts complained about the new ease with which their gay male patients found sexual partners. And the gay subculture was not to be found just in the largest cities. Lesbians and gay male bars existed in places like Worcester, Massachusetts, and Buffalo, New York; in Columbia, South Carolina, and Des Moines, Iowa. Gay life in the 1950s and 1960s became a nationwide phenomenon. By the time of the Stonewall Riot in New York City in 1969 – the event that ignited the gay liberation movement – our situation was hardly one of silence, invisibility, and isolation. A massive, grass-roots liberation movement could form almost overnight precisely because communities of lesbians and gay men existed.

Although gay community was a precondition for a mass movement, the oppression of lesbians and gay men was the force that propelled the movement into existence. As the subculture expanded and grew more visible in the post-World-War-Two era, oppression by the state intensified, becoming more systematic and inclusive. The Right scapegoated 'sexual perverts' during the McCarthy era. Eisenhower imposed a total ban on the employment of gay women and men by the federal government and government contractors. Purges of lesbians and homosexuals from the military rose sharply. The FBI instituted widespread surveillance of gay meeting places and of lesbians and gay organizations, such as the Daughters of Bilitis and the Mattachine Society. The Post Office placed tracers on the correspondence of gay men and passed evidence of homosexual activity on to employers. Urban vice squads invaded private homes, made sweeps of lesbians and gay male bars, entrapped gay men in public places, and fomented local witchhunts. The danger involved in being gay rose even as the possibilities of being gay were enhanced. Gay liberation was a response to this contradiction.

Although lesbians and gay men won significant victories in the 1970s and opened up some safe social space in which to exist, we can hardly claim to have dealt a fatal blow to heterosexism and homophobia. One could even argue that the enforcement of gay oppression has merely changed locales, shifting somewhat from the state to the arena of extralegal violence in the form of increasingly open physical attacks on lesbians and gay men. And, as our movements have grown, they have generated a backlash that threatens to wipe out our gains. Significantly, this New Right opposition has taken shape as a 'pro-family' movement. How is it that capitalism, whose structure made possible the emergence of a gay identity and the creation of urban gay communities, appears unable to accept gay men and lesbians in its midst? Why do heterosexism and homophobia appear so resistant to assault?

The answers, I think, can be found in the contradictory relationship of capitalism to the family. On the one hand, as I argued earlier, capitalism has gradually undermined the material basis of the nuclear family by taking away the economic functions that cemented the ties between family members. As more adults have been drawn into the free-labour system, and as capital has expanded its sphere until it produces as commodities most goods and services we need for our survival, the forces that propelled men and women into families and kept them there have weakened. On the other hand, the ideology of capitalist society has enshrined the family as the source of love, affection, and emotional security, the place where our need for stable, intimate human relationships is satisfied.

This evaluation of the nuclear family to preeminence in the sphere of personal life is not accidental. Every society needs structures for reproduction and childrearing, but the possibilities are not limited to the nuclear family. Yet the privatized family fits well with capitalist relations of production. Capitalism has socialized production while maintaining that the products of socialized labour belong to the owners of private property. In many ways, childrearing has also been progressively socialized over the last two centuries, with schools, the media, peer groups, and employers taking over functions that once belonged to parents. Nevertheless, capitalist society maintains that reproduction and childrearing are private tasks, that children 'belong' to parents, who exercise the rights of ownership. Ideologically, capitalism drives people into heterosexual families: each generation comes of age having internalized a heterosexist model of intimacy and personal relationships. Materially, capitalism weakens the bonds that once kept families together so that their members experience a growing instability in the place they have come to expect happiness and emotional security. Thus, while capitalism has knocked the material foundation away from family life, lesbians, gay men, and heterosexual feminists have become the scapegoats for the social instability of the system.

This analysis, if persuasive, has implications for us today. It can affect our perception of our identity, our formulation of political goals, and our decisions about strategy.

I have argued that lesbian and gay identity and communities are historically created, the result of a process of capitalist development that has spanned many generations. A corollary of this argument is that we are not a fixed social minority composed for all time of a certain percentage of the population. There are more of us than one hundred years ago, more of us than forty years ago. And there may very well be more gay men and lesbians in the future. Claims made by gays and nongays that sexual orientation is fixed at an early age, that large numbers of visible gay men and lesbians in society, the media, and the schools will have no influence on the sexual identities of the young, are wrong. Capitalism has created the material condition for homosexual desire to express itself as a central component of some individuals' lives; now, our political movements are changing consciousness, creating the ideological conditions that make it easier for people to make that choice.

To be sure, this argument confirms the worst fears and most rabid rhetoric of our political opponents. But our response must be to challenge the underlying belief that homosexual relations are bad, a poor second choice. We must not slip into the opportunistic defence that society need not worry about tolerating us, since only homosexuals become homosexual. At best, a minority group analysis and a civil rights strategy pertain to those of us who already are gay. It leaves today's youth – tomorrow's lesbians and gay men – to internalize heterosexist models that it can take a lifetime to expunge.

I have also argued that capitalism has led to the separation of sexuality from procreation. Human sexual desire need no longer be harnessed to reproductive imperatives, to procreation; its expression has increasingly entered the realm of choice. Lesbians and homosexuals most clearly embody the potential of this spirit, since our gay relationships stand entirely outside a procreative framework. The acceptance of our erotic choices ultimately depends on the degree to which society is willing to affirm sexual expression as a form of play, positive and life-enhancing. Our movement may have begun as the struggle of a 'minority', but what we should now be trying to 'liberate' is an aspect of the personal lives of all people – sexual expression.[7]

Finally, I have suggested that the relationship between capitalism and the family is fundamentally contradictory. On the one hand, capitalism continually weakens the material foundation of family life, making it possible for individuals to live outside the family, and for a lesbian and gay male identity to develop. On the other, it needs to push men and women into families, at least long enough to reproduce the next generation of workers. The elevation of the family to ideological preeminence guarantees that a capitalist society will reproduce not just children, but heterosexism and homophobia. In the most profound sense, capitalism is the problem.[8]

How do we avoid remaining the scapegoats, the political victims of the social instability that capitalism generates? How can we take this contradictory relationship and use it to move toward liberation?

Gay men and lesbians exist on social terrain beyond the boundaries of the heterosexual nuclear family. Our communities have formed in that social space. Our survival and liberation depend on our ability to defend and expand that terrain, not just for ourselves but for everyone. That means, in part, support for issues that broaden the opportunities for living outside traditional heterosexual family units: issues like the availability of abortion and the ratification of the Equal Rights Amendment, affirmative action for people of colour and for women, publicly funded daycare and other essential social services, decent welfare payments, full employment, the rights of young people – in other words, programmes and issues that provide a material basis for personal autonomy.

The rights of young people are especially critical. The acceptance of children as dependents, as belonging to parents, is so deeply ingrained that we can scarcely imagine what it would mean to treat them as autonomous human beings, particularly in the realm of sexual expression and choice. Yet until that happens, gay liberation will remain out of our reach.

But personal autonomy is only half the story. The instability of families and the sense of impermanence and insecurity that people are now experiencing in their personal relationships are real social problems that need to be addressed. We need political solutions for these difficulties of personal life. These solutions should not come in the form of a radical version of the pro-family position, of some left-wing proposals to strengthen the family. Socialists do not generally respond to the exploitation and economic inequality of industrial capitalism by calling for a return to the family farm and handicraft production. We recognize that the vastly increased productivity that capitalism has made possible by socializing production is one of its progressive features. Similarly, we should not be trying to turn back the clock to some mythic age of the happy family.

We do need, however, structures and programmes that will help to dissolve the boundaries that isolate the family, particularly those that privatize childrearing. We need community – or worker-controlled day care, housing where privacy and community coexist, neighbourhood institutions – from medical clinics to performance centres – that enlarge the social unit where each of us has a secure place. As we create structures beyond the nuclear family that provide a sense of belonging, the family will wane in significance. Less and less will it seem to make or break our emotional security.

In this respect gay men and lesbians are well situated to play a special role. Already excluded from families as most of us are, we had to create, for our survival, networks of support that do not depend on the bonds of blood or the licence of the state, but that are freely chosen and nurtured. The building of an 'affectional community' must be as much a part of our political movement as are campaigns for civil rights. In this way we may prefigure the shape of personal relationships in a society grounded in equality and justice rather than exploitation and oppression, a society where autonomy and security do not preclude each other but coexist.

Notes

1 I do not mean to suggest that no one has ever proposed that gay identity is a product of historical change. See, for instance, McIntosh, 1968 and Weeks, 1977. It is also implied in Foucault, 1978. However, this does represent a minority viewpoint and the works cited above have not specified how it is that capitalism as a system of production has allowed for the emergence of a gay male and lesbian identity. As an example of the 'eternal homosexual' thesis, see Boswell, 1980, where 'gay people' remains an unchanged social category through fifteen centuries of Mediterranean and Western Europe history.

2 For the period from 1870 to 1940 see the documents in Katz, 1976 and 1983. Other sources include Bérubé, 1979; Bullough and Bullough, 1977.

3 On the medical model see Weeks, 1977, pp. 23–32. The impact of the medical model on the consciousness of men and women can be seen in Hyde, 1978, p. 47, and in the story of Lucille Hart in Katz, 1976, pp. 258–79. Radclyffe Hall's classic novel about lesbianism, *The Well of Loneliness*, published in 1928, was perhaps one of the most important vehicles for the popularization of the medical model.

4 On black music, see Various Artists, 1977, and Albertson, 1974; on the persistence of kin network in white ethnic communities see Smith, 1979; on differences between rural and urban male homoerotism see Kinsey *et al.*, 1948, pp. 455–7 and pp. 630–1.

5 The argument and the information in this and the following paragraphs come from my book *Sexual Politics, Sexual Communities: The Making of a Homosexual Minority in the United States, 1940–1970* (D'Emilio, 1983). I have also developed it with reference to San Francisco in 'Gay politics, gay community: San Francisco's experience' (D'Emilio, 1981).

6 On lesbian novels see the *Ladder*, March 1958, p. 18; February 1960, pp. 14–15; April 1961, pp. 12–13; February 1962, pp. 6–11; January 1963, pp. 6–13. The *Ladder* was the magazine published by the Daughters of Bilitis.

7 This especially needs to be emphasized today. The 1980 annual conference of the National Organization for Women, for instance, passed a lesbian rights resolution that defined the issue as one of 'discrimination based on affectional/sexual preference/orientation', and explicitly disassociated the issue from other questions of sexuality such as pornography, sadomasochism, public sex, and pederasty.

8 I do not mean to suggest that homophobia is 'caused' by capitalism, or is to be found only in capitalist societies. Severe sanctions against homoeroticism can be found in European feudal society and in contemporary socialist countries. But my focus in this essay has been the emergence of a gay identity under capitalism, and the mechanisms specific to capitalism that made this possible and that reproduce homophobia as well.

References

ALBERTSON, C. (1974) *Bessie*, New York: Stein and Day.

BERUBE, A. (1979) 'Lesbians and gay men in early San Francisco: notes toward a social history of lesbians and gay men in America', unpublished paper.

BOSWELL, J. (1980) *Christianity, Social Tolerance, and Homosexuality*, Chicago: University of Chicago Press.

BULLOUGH, V. and BULLOUGH, B. (1977) 'Lesbianism in the 1920s and 1930s: a newfound study', *Signs*, 2, summer, pp. 895–904.

D'EMILIO, J. (1981) 'Gay politics, gay community: San Francisco's experience', *Socialist Review*, 55, January–February, pp. 77–104.

—— (1983) *Sexual Politics, Sexual Communities: The Making of a Homosexual Minority in the United States, 1940–1970*, Chicago: University of Chicago Press.

FASS, P. (1977) *The Damned and the Beautiful: American Youth in the 1920s*, New York: Oxford University Press.

FOUCAULT, M. (1978) *The History of Sexuality, vol. 1: An Introduction*, New York: Pantheon.

HALL, R. (1928) *The Well of Loneliness*, London: Jonathan Cape.

HYDE, L. (Ed.) (1978) *Rat and the Devil: The Journal Letters of F. Matthiessen and Russel Cheney*, Hamden, CT: Archon.

KATZ, J. (1976) *Gay American History*, New York: Crowell.

—— (1983) *Gay/Lesbian Almanac*, New York: Crowell.

KINSEY, A. *et al.* (1948) *Sexual Behavior in the Human Male*, Philadelphia, PA: W.B. Saunders.

—— *et al.* (1953) *Sexual Behavior in the Human Female*, Philadelphia, PA: W.B. Saunders.

LADDER, March 1958, p. 18; February 1960, pp. 14–15; April 1961, pp. 12–13; February 1962, pp. 6–11; January 1963, pp. 6–13; published by the Daughters of Bilitis.

MCINTOSH, M. (1968) 'The homosexual role', *Social Problems*, 16, pp. 182–92.

OAKS, R.F. (1978) 'Things fearful to name: sodomy and buggery in seventeenth century New England', *Journal of Social History*, 12, pp. 268–81.

ROBERTS, J.R. (1980) 'The case of Sarah Norman and Mary Hammond', *Sinister Wisdom*, 24, pp. 57–62.

SMITH, J. (1979) 'Our own kind: family and community networks in Providence', in COTT, N.F. and PLECK, E.H. (eds) *A Heritage of Her Own*, New York: Simon and Schuster.

VARIOUS ARTISTS (1977) *AC/DC Blues: Gay Jazz Reissues*, Stash Records, ST–106.

WEEKS, J. (1977) *Coming Out: Homosexual Politics in Britain*, New York: Quartet Books.

ZARETSKY, E. (1976) *Capitalism, the Family, and Personal Life*, New York: Harper & Row.

Section II

Sexual meanings, health and rights

Part 5

Gender, power and rights

14 Masculinities and globalization

The men and the boys

R.W. Connell [2000]

Connell (2000a) outlines some major findings of the new social research on the construction of masculinities. If we compare this picture with earlier accounts of the 'male sex role', it is clear that the ethnographic moment in research has already had important intellectual fruits.

Nevertheless, it has always been recognized that some issues go beyond the local. For instance, any study of the mythopoetic movement must recognize it is only part of a spectrum of masculinity politics (Messner, 1997; Schwalbe, 1996). Historical studies such as Phillips (1987) on New Zealand and Kimmel (1996) on the United States have traced the changing public constructions of masculinity for whole countries over long periods. Ultimately, the large historical context, the big picture, is essential for understanding the small picture, the ethnographic detail.

This logic must now be taken a step further. What happens in localities is affected by the history of whole countries, but what happens in countries is affected by the history of the world. Locally situated lives are now (indeed have long been) powerfully influenced by geopolitical struggles, global markets, multinational corporations, labour migration, and transnational media.

To understand local masculinities, then, we must think in global terms. But how? That is the problem pursued in this chapter. I will offer a framework for thinking about masculinities as a feature of world society, and for thinking about men's gender practices in terms of the global structure and dynamics of gender.

The world gender order

Masculinities do not first exist and then come into contact with femininities; they are produced together, in the process that makes a gender order. Accordingly, to understand the masculinities on a world scale we must first have a concept of the globalization of gender.

This is one of the most difficult points in current gender analysis because the very conception is counterintuitive. We are so accustomed to thinking of gender as the attribute of an individual, even as a particularly intimate matter, that it requires a considerable wrench to think of gender on the vast scale of global society, currently numbering about 6000 million people.

Some relevant discussions, such as the literature on 'women and development', blur the issue of gender. They treat the institutions or processes that cross national boundaries (markets, corporations, intergovernmental programmes, etc.) as being gender neutral in principle, but impacting on men and women unequally because of bad attitudes or bad policies. Such conceptions reproduce the familiar liberal-feminist view of the state as being in principle gender-neutral even though it is empirically dominated by men.

But the picture changes if we recognize that very large-scale institutions such as the state are themselves gendered, in quite precise ways (Connell, 1990). The picture changes if we recognize that international relations, international trade and global markets are inherently, not accidentally, arenas of gender formation and gender politics (Enloe, 1990). Then we can recognize the existence of a world gender order. This can be defined as the structure of relationships that connect the gender regimes of institutions, and the gender orders of local society, on a world scale.

A definition, however, is only a beginning. The substantial questions remain: what is the shape of that structure, how tightly are its elements linked, how has it arisen in history, what is its trajectory into the future?

Current business and media talk about 'globalization' pictures a tide sweeping across the world, driven by new technologies, producing vast unfettered global markets in which all participate on equal terms. This is certainly a misleading image. As Hirst and Thompson (1996) show, the global economy in fact is highly unequal and the degree to which it has become homogenized is wildly overestimated in business rhetoric. Multinational corporations based in the three great economic powers (the United States, the European Union, and Japan) are the major economic actors worldwide.

The structure bears the marks of its history. Modern global society was historically produced, as Wallerstein (1974) argued, by the economic and political expansion of European states from the fifteenth century on, leading to the creation of colonial empires. It is in this process that we find the roots of the modern world gender order.

Imperialism was, from the start, a gendered process. Its first phase, colonial conquest and settlement, was carried out by gender-segregated forces and resulted in massive disruption of indigenous gender orders. In its second phase, the stabilization of colonial societies, new gender divisions of labour were produced in plantation economies and colonial cities, while gender ideologies were linked with racial hierarchies and the cultural defence of empire. The third phase, marked by political decolonization, economic neo-colonialism, and the current growth of world markets and systems of financial control, has seen gender divisions of labour remade on a massive scale in the 'global factory' (Fuentes and Ehrenreich, 1983), as well as the spread of gendered violence alongside Western military technology.

The result of this history is a partially integrated, highly unequal, and turbulent world society, in which gender relations are unevenly linked on a global scale. The unevenness becomes clear when the different substructures of gender defined in Connell (2000b) are examined separately.

Power relations

The colonial and post-colonial world has tended to break down purdah systems of patriarchy in the name of modernization, if not of women's emancipation (Kandiyoti, 1994). At the same time, large-scale organizations have appeared, notably the state and corporations, which, with few exceptions, are culturally masculinized and controlled by men. As Enloe (1990) has vividly shown, the world of international politics is heavily gendered, with women marginalized in diplomacy, military aid, and trade negotiations. In post-colonial capitalism the power of local elites depends on their relations with the metropolitan powers. So the hegemonic masculinities of neo-colonial societies are uneasily poised between local and global cultures.

Production relations (division of labour)

A characteristic feature of colonial and neo-colonial economies was the restructuring of local production systems to produce a male wage-worker/female domestic-worker couple (Mies, 1986). This need not produce a 'housewife' in the Western suburban sense. For instance where the wage work required male migration to plantations or mines (Moodie, 1994) the result might be more economic responsibility for women, not less. But it has generally produced the same identification of masculinity with the public realm and the money economy, and femininity with the domestic realm, which is a core feature of the modern European gender system (Holter, 1997).

Cathexis (emotional relations)

Missionary activity, both religious and cultural, has attacked indigenous homosexual and cross-gender practices, such as the Native American 'berdache' and the Chinese 'passion of the cut sleeve' (Hinsch, 1990). Recently created Western models of romantic heterosexual love as the basis for marriage, and of gay identity as the main alternative, have now circulated globally. Yet as Altman (1996) observed, they do not simply displace indigenous models, but interact with them in extremely complex ways.

Symbolism

Mass media, especially electronic media, in most parts of the world follow North American and European models and relay a great deal of metropolitan content, including its gender imagery. A striking example is the reproduction of a North American imagery of femininity by Xuxa, the blonde television superstar in Brazil (Simpson, 1993). In counterpoint, 'exotic' gender imagery has been used in the marketing strategies of newly industrializing countries (e.g. airline advertising from South-East Asia) – a tactic based on the longstanding combination of the exotic and the erotic in the colonial imagination (Jolly, 1997). Major powers also may use gender symbolism to renegotiate their position in the world system. Jeffords (1989) shows this in the 'remasculinization of America' after defeat in the Vietnam War, through the symbolic media of films and novels.

Clearly the world gender order is not simply a blown-up copy of a European-American gender order. The European-American gender order was changed by colonialism; and elements from other cultures now circulate globally. Yet in no sense do they mix on equal terms to produce a United Colors of Benetton gender order. The culture and institutions of the North Atlantic countries are hegemonic within the emergent world system. This is crucial for understanding the kinds of masculinities produced in globalization.

The repositioning of men and the remaking of masculinities

The positioning of men and the making of masculinities may be analysed at any of the levels at which gender practice is configured, including the body, personal life or collective social practice. At each level we need to consider how globalization influences configurations of gender. Here I will discuss the process at the levels of personal life and collective practice. Issues about bodies are discussed in greater detail in Connell (2000c).

The impact of global forces on personal life can be seen in individual life histories. Sometimes the link is indirect. An example is young working-class men on the fringe of the regular labour market (Connell, 1995; Connell, 2000c). The fact of chronic unemployment, which makes it impossible for them to construct a masculinity organized around being a 'breadwinner', arises from the local economy's changing position in the global economy.

In other cases, such as executives of multinational corporations and the financial sector servicing international trade, the link is obvious. The requirements of a career in international business set up strong pressures on domestic life. Almost all multinational executives are men, and the assumption in their trade magazines and advertising is that they will have dependent wives running their homes and bringing up their children.

At the level of collective practice, masculinities are involved in the cultural remaking of gender meanings under globalization; they are also affected by a rather different process, the reshaping of the institutional contexts of practice.

The growth of global mass media, especially electronic media, is an obvious vector for the globalization of gender. Popular entertainment circulates stereotyped gender images, deliberately made attractive for marketing purposes. The example of Xuxa in Brazil has already been mentioned. International news media are also controlled or strongly influenced from the metropole, and circulate Western definitions of authoritative masculinity, criminality, desirable femininity, etc. At places and times where local cultures are in flux, such as Eastern Europe after the collapse of communism, these imported definitions can have tremendous impact.

But there are limits to the power of global mass communications. Some local centres of mass entertainment differ from the Hollywood model; for example, the Indian popular film industry centred in Mumbai. Further, media research shows that audiences are highly selective in their reception of media messages. Audiences do know there is an element of fantasy in mass entertainment. Just as economic globalization can be exaggerated, so can cultural homogenization. The creation of a 'global culture' is a more turbulent and uneven process than is often assumed (Featherstone, 1995).

More important than cultural standardization, I would argue, is a process that began long before electronic media existed – the export of institutions. Gendered institutions not only circulate definitions of masculinity and femininity. Gendered institutions, creating specific conditions for social practice, call into existence specific patterns of practice.

Thus, certain patterns of collective violence are embedded in the organization and culture of a Western-style army, and these are different from the patterns of pre-colonial violence. Certain patterns of calculative egocentrism are embedded in the working of a stock market; certain patterns of rule-following and domination are embedded in a bureaucracy.

The colonial and post-colonial world saw the installation, on a very large scale, of institutions on the North Atlantic model: armies, states, bureaucracies, corporations, capital markets, labour markets, schools, law courts, transport systems. These are gendered institutions, and their functioning has directly reconstituted masculinities in the periphery. This is not necessarily by direct modelling or copying of the gender patterns themselves; it can also occur indirectly, as a result of pressures for change that are inherent in the institutional form.

To the extent particular institutions become dominant in world society, the patterns of masculinity embedded in them may become global standards. Masculine dress is an interesting indicator. Almost every political leader in the world now wears the uniform of the Western business executive.

The more common pattern, however, is not the complete displacement of local patterns but an articulation between the local gender order and the gender regime of the new institutions. Case studies such as Hollway's (1994) account of bureaucracy in Tanzania illustrate the point. There, domestic patriarchy linked up with masculine authority in the state, in ways that subverted the government's formal commitment to equal opportunity for women.

The world gender order is patriarchal, in the sense that it privileges men over women. There is a 'patriarchal dividend' for men arising from unequal wages, unequal labour-force participation, and a highly unequal structure of ownership, as well as cultural and sexual privileging. This has been extensively documented by feminist work on women's situation globally (e.g. Taylor, 1985), though its implications for masculinity have mostly been ignored.

The conditions thus exist for the production of a hegemonic masculinity on a world scale, that is to say, a dominant form of masculinity which embodies, organizes and legitimates men's domination in the gender order as a whole.

The conditions of globalization, which involve the interaction of many local gender orders, multiply the forms of masculinity in the global gender order. At the same time, the specific shape of globalization, concentrating economic and cultural power on an unprecedented scale, provides new resources for dominance by particular groups of men.

This dominance may become institutionalized in a pattern of masculinity which becomes, to some degree, standardized across localities. I will call such patterns 'globalizing masculinities'. It is among globalizing masculinities, rather than narrowly within the metropole, that we are likely to find candidates for hegemony in the world gender order.

Globalizing masculinities

In this section I will offer a sketch of major forms of globalizing masculinity, in three historical phases of the making of a world gender order.

Masculinities of conquest and settlement

The creation of the world-spanning empires and their social order involved peculiar conditions for the gender practices of men. Colonial conquest itself was mainly carried out by groups of men – soldiers, sailors, traders, administrators, and a good many who were all these by turn (such as the 'Rum Corps' in the early days of the colony of New South Wales).

These men were drawn from the more segregated occupations and milieux in the metropole, and it is likely that the men drawn into colonization tended to be the more rootless. Certainly the process of conquest could produce frontier masculinities that combined the occupational culture of these groups with an unusual level of violence and egocentric individualism. The vehement debate among their contemporaries about the genocidal violence of the Spanish conquistadors – who in 50 years completely exterminated the population of Hispaniola in the West Indies – suggests that the pattern was recognized at the time (Las Casas, 1971).

The political history of empire is full of evidence of the tenuous control over the frontier exercised by the state. The Spanish monarchs were unable to rein in the conquistadors, the governors in Sydney were unable to hold back the squatters and the governors in Capetown were unable to hold back the Boers. Gold rushes broke boundaries everywhere. At one stage what was virtually an independent republic was set up by escaped slaves in Brazil.

This lack of control probably extended to other forms of social control too, such as customary controls on men's sexuality. Extensive sexual exploitation of indigenous women was a common feature of conquest. In certain circumstances frontier masculinities might be reproduced as a local cultural tradition long after the frontier had passed, such as the gauchos of southern South America and the cowboys of the western United States.

In other circumstances, however, the frontier of conquest and exploitation was replaced by a frontier of settlement. Sex ratios in the colonizing population changed, as women arrived and locally born generations succeeded. A shift back towards the family patterns of the metropole was likely.

As Cain and Hopkins (1993) have shown for the British Empire, the ruling group in the colonial world as a whole was an extension of the dominant class in the metropole – the landed gentry – and tended to reproduce its social customs and ideology. The creation of a certain pattern of masculinity among settlers might be the goal of state policy, as it seems to have been in late nineteenth-century New Zealand, part of a general process of pacification and the creation of an agricultural social order (Phillips, 1987). Or it might be undertaken through institutions created by settler groups, such as the elite schools in Natal studied by Morrell (1994).

The impact of colonialism on the construction of masculinity among the colonized is much less documented, but there is every reason to think it was severe. Conquest and settlement disrupted all the structures of indigenous society, whether or not this was intended by the colonizing powers (Bitterli, 1989). Indigenous gender orders were no exception. Their disruption could result from the pulverization of indigenous communities (as in the seizure of land in eastern North America and Southeastern Australia), gendered labour migration (as in gold mining with black labour in South Africa: Moodie, 1994), or ideological attacks on local gender arrangements (as in the missionary assault on the transgender 'berdarche' tradition in North America: Williams, 1986).

The varied course of resistance to colonization is also likely to have affected the making of masculinities. This is clear in the region of Natal in South Africa, where sustained resistance to colonization by the Zulu kingdom was a key to the mobilization of ethnic-national masculine identities in the twentieth century (Morrell 1996).

Masculinities of empire

The imperial social order created a hierarchy of masculinities, as it created a hierarchy of communities and races. The colonizers distinguished 'more manly' from 'less manly' groups among their subjects. In British India, for instance, Bengali men were supposed effeminate while Pathans and Sikhs were regarded as strong and warlike. Similar distinctions were made in South Africa between 'Hottentots' and Zulus, in North America between Iroquois, Sioux and Cheyenne on one side and southern and southwestern tribes on the other.

At the same time, the growing emphasis on gender difference in European culture in the eighteenth and nineteenth centuries provided symbols of overall superiority and inferiority. Within the imperial 'poetics of war' (MacDonald, 1994), the conqueror was virile, while the colonized were dirty, sexualized and effeminate or childlike. In many colonial situations indigenous men were called 'boys' by the colonizers (e.g. Zimbabwe: Shire, 1994).

Sinha's (1995) interesting study of the language of political controversy in India in the 1880s and 1890s shows how the images of 'manly Englishman' and 'effeminate Bengali' were deployed to uphold colonial privilege and restrain movements for change. In the late nineteenth century, it was generally true that racial barriers in colonial societies were hardening rather than weakening. Gender ideology began to fuse with racism in forms that the twentieth century never untangled.

The power relations of empire meant that indigenous gender orders were generally under pressure from the colonizers, rather than the other way around. But the colonizers too might change. The barriers of late colonial racism were not only to prevent pollution from below. They were also to forestall 'going native', a well-recognized possibility – the starting-point, for instance, of Kipling's famous novel *Kim* (1901).

The pressures and profits of empire might also work changes in gender arrangements among the colonizers. In the colonies, a large supply of indigenous domestic servants made wives more leisured and managerial, as shown in Bulbeck's (1992) study of Australian women in Papua New Guinea, and entrenched a division of spheres between men and women. In the metropole, empire also had effects on the gender order, most spectacularly in symbolic definitions of masculinity. Frontier heroes such as Lawrence of Arabia (Dawson, 1991) became exemplars of masculinity. A whole social movement, the Boy Scouts, drew imagery and rituals from empire for its programme for the training of boys.

The world of empire created two very different settings for the modernization of masculinities. In the periphery, the forcible restructuring of economies and workforces tended to individualize on the one hand and rationalize on the other. A widespread result was masculinities in which the rational calculation of self-interest was the key to action, emphasizing the European gender contrast of rational man/irrational woman. The specific form might be local – for instance the Japanese 'salaryman', a type first named in the 1910s, was specific to the Japanese context of large, stable industrial conglomerates (Kinmonth, 1981). But the result generally was masculinities defined around economic action, with both workers and entrepreneurs increasingly adapted to emerging market economies.

In the metropole, the accumulation of wealth made possible a specialization of leadership in the dominant classes. Struggles for hegemony occurred in which masculinities organized around domination or violence were split from masculinities organized around expertise. The class compromises that allowed the development of the welfare state in Europe and North America were paralleled by gender compromises. Gender reform movements, most notably the women's suffrage movement, contested the legal privileges of men and forced concessions from the state.

In this context, agendas of reform in masculinity emerged in the metropole from the late nineteenth century: the temperance movement, companionate marriage, homosexual rights movements. Eventually this led to the pursuit of androgyny in 'men's liberation' in the 1970s (Kimmel and Mosmiller, 1992).

Not all reconstructions of masculinity, however, emphasized tolerance or moved towards androgyny. The vehement masculinity politics of fascism, for instance, emphasized dominance and difference, and glorified violence, a pattern still found in contemporary racist movements (Tillner, 1997).

Masculinities of post-colonialism and neo-liberalism

The process of decolonization naturally disrupted the gender hierarchies of the colonial order. Where armed struggle was involved, there might be a deliberate cultivation of masculine hardness and violence (as in South Africa: Xaba, 1997). Some activists and theorists of liberation struggles celebrated this as a necessary response to colonial violence and emasculation. Women in liberation struggles were perhaps less impressed. However one evaluates the process, one of the consequences of decolonization was another round of disruptions of community-based gender orders, and another step in the reorientation of masculinities towards national and international contexts.

Nearly half a century after the main wave of decolonization, gender hierarchies persist in new shapes. With the collapse of Soviet communism, the decline of post-colonial socialism, and the ascendancy of the new right in Europe and North America, world politics is more and more organized around the needs of transnational capital and the creation of global markets.

Neo-liberal politics has little to say, explicitly, about gender. It speaks a gender-neutral language of 'markets', 'individuals' and 'choice'. New-right politicians and journalists denounce 'political correctness' and 'feminazis', and new-right governments have abolished or downgraded equal opportunity programmes and women's policy units.

But the world in which neo-lialism rules is still a gendered world, and neo-liberalism has an implicit gender politics. The 'individual' of neo-liberal theory has the attributes and interests of a male entrepreneur. The attack on the welfare state generally weakens the position of women, while the increasingly unregulated power of transnational corporations places strategic power in the hands of particular groups of men.

It is not surprising that the installation of market capitalism in Eastern Europe and the former Soviet Union has been accompanied by a reassertion of dominating masculinities and, in some situations, a sharp worsening in the social position of women (Novikova, 2000).

In these circumstances it is reasonable to conclude that the hegemonic form of masculinity in the current world gender order is the masculinity associated with those who control its dominant institutions: the business executives who operate in global markets, and the political executives who interact (and in many contexts merge) with them. I will call this pattern 'transnational business masculinity'.

This form of masculinity is not readily available for ethnographic study, but we can get some clues to its character from its reflections in management literature, business journalism, corporate self-promotion, and from studies of local business elites (e.g. Donaldson, 1998).

Transnational business masculinity appears to be marked by increasing egocentrism, very conditional loyalties (even to the corporation), and a declining sense of responsibility for others (except for purposes of image-making). Gee *et al.* (1996), studying recent management textbooks, noted the peculiar construction of the executive in 'fast capitalism' as a person with no permanent commitments, except to the idea of accumulation itself. The occupational world here is characterized by a limited technical rationality ('management theory'), which is increasingly separate from science.

Transnational business masculinity differs from traditional bourgeois masculinity by its increasingly libertarian sexuality, with a growing tendency to commodify relations with women. Hotels catering for businessmen in most parts of the world now routinely offer pornographic videos. In many parts of the world there is a well-developed prostitution industry catering for international businessmen.

Businessmen themselves do not require bodily force, since the patriarchal dividend they benefit from is accumulated by impersonal, institutional means. But corporations increasingly use the exemplary bodies of elite sportsmen as a marketing tool (note the phenomenal growth of corporate 'sponsorship' of sport in the last generation), and indirectly as a means of legitimation for the whole gender order.

Masculinity politics on a world scale

Recognizing global society as an arena where masculinities are formed allows us to pose new questions about the politics of masculinity. What social dynamics in the global arena give rise to masculinity politics, and what shape does global masculinity politics take?

As I have noted, the gradual creation of a world gender order has meant many local instabilities of gender. These range from the disruption of men's local cultural dominance as women move into the public realm and higher education, through the disruption of sexual identities that produced 'queer' politics in the metropole, to the shifts in the urban intelligentsia that produced 'the new sensitive man' and other images of gender change.

One response to such instabilities, on the part of groups whose power is challenged but still dominant, is to reaffirm local gender hierarchies. A masculine fundamentalism is, accordingly, a common response in gender politics at present.

A soft version, searching for an essential masculinity among myths and symbols, is offered by the 'mythopoetic' men's movement in the United States, and by the religious revivalists of the Promise Keepers (Messner, 1997). A much harder version is found, in the United States, in the right-wing militia movement (Gibson, 1994). An equally hard version is found in contemporary Afghanistan, if we can trust Western media reports, in the militant misogyny of the Taliban. It is no coincidence that in these two cases, hardline masculine fundamentalism goes together with a marked anti-internationalism. The world system – rightly enough – is seen as the source of pollution and disruption.

Not that the emerging global order is a hotbed of gender progressivism. Indeed, the neo-liberal agenda for the reform of national and international economies involves closing down historic possibilities for gender reform. I have noted how neo-liberalism subverts the gender compromise embodied in the metropolitan welfare state. It has also undermined the progressive liberal agendas of sex-role reform represented by affirmative action programmes, anti-discrimination provisions, child-care services, and the like. Right-wing governments have persistently cut such programmes in the name either of individual liberties or global competitiveness. Through these means the patriarchal dividend to men is defended or restored, without an explicit masculinity politics in the form of a mobilization of men.

In the arenas of international relations, the international state, multinational corporations and global markets, masculinities are deployed and a reasonably clear hegemony exists. The transnational business masculinity described above has had only one major competitor for hegemony in recent decades: the rigid, control-oriented masculinity of military command, a variant of which is the military-style bureaucratic dictatorships of Stalinism. With the collapse of Stalinism and the end of the cold war, Big Brother (Orwell's famous parody of this form of masculinity) is a fading threat. The more flexible, calculative, egocentric masculinity of the 'fast capitalist' entrepreneur holds the world stage.

We must, however, recall two important conclusions of the ethnographic moment in masculinity research described in Connell (2000a). Different forms of masculinity exist together, and the hegemony of any given form is constantly subject to challenge. These are possibilities in the global arena too.

Transnational business masculinity is not completely homogeneous. Variations are embedded in different parts of the world system, which may not be completely compatible. We may distinguish a Confucian variant, based in East Asia, with stronger commitment to hierarchy and social consensus, from a secularized Christian variant, based in North America, which shows more hedonism and individualism, and greater tolerance to social conflict. In certain arenas there is already conflict between the business and political leaderships embodying these forms of masculinity. Such conflict is found in debates over 'human rights' versus 'Asian values', and over the extent of trade and investment liberalization.

If these are contenders for hegemony, there is also opposition to hegemony. The global circulation of 'gay' identity (Altman, 1996) is an important indication that non-hegemonic masculinities may operate in global arenas, and may even find certain political articulation, in the case of gay masculinities, around human rights and AIDS prevention.

Critiques of dominant forms of masculinity have also been circulating internationally, among heterosexual men or among groups that are predominantly heterosexual. Three examples in the English-speaking world are the 'anti-sexist' or 'profeminist' men's groups in the United States, with their umbrella group NOMAS (National Organization of Men Against Sexism), which has been running since the early 1980s (Cohen, 1991); the British new left men's groups, which produced the remarkable magazine *Achilles Heel* (Seidler, 1991); and the Canadian White Ribbon campaign, the most successful mass mobilization of men opposing men's violence against women (Kaufman, 1999).

There are parallel developments in other language communities. In Germany, for instance, feminists launched a discussion of the gender of men in the 1980s (Hagemann-White and

Rerrich, 1988; Metz-Göckel and Müller, 1985). This has been followed by an educational (Kindler, 1993), a popular psychology (Hollstein, 1992), a critical (*Widersprüche*, 1995; BauSteineMänner, 1996), and a religious (Zulehner and Volz, 1998) debate about masculinities and how to change them.

In Scandinavia, gender reform has led to the 'father's quota' of parental leave in Norway (Gender Equality Ombudsman, 1997) and to a particularly active network of masculinity researchers. In Japan, a media debate about 'men's liberation' and some pioneering books about changing masculinities (Ito, 1993; Nakamura, 1994) have been followed by the foundation of a men's centre and diversifying debates on change.

These developments at national or regional level have, very recently, begun to link internationally. An International Association for Studies of Men has begun to link men involved in critical studies of masculinity. Certain international agencies, including UNESCO, have sponsored conferences to discuss the policy implications of new perspectives on masculinity (Breines *et al.*, 2000).

Compared with the concentration of institutional power in multinational businesses, these initiatives remain small-scale and dispersed. They are, nevertheless, important in potential. The global gender order contains, necessarily, a greater diversity of forms than any local gender order. This must reinforce the consciousness that masculinity is not one fixed form. The plurality of masculinities at least symbolically prefigures the variety and creativity of a democratic gender order.

References

ALTMAN, D. (1996) 'Rupture or continuity? The internationalization of gay indentities', *Social Text 48*, 14(3), pp. 77–94.

BAUSTEINEMÄNNER (1996) *Kritische Männerforschung*, Berlin: Argument.

BITTERLI, U. (1989) *Cultures in Conflict: Encounters between European and non-European Cultures, 1492–1800*, Stanford, CA: Stanford University Press.

BREINES, I., CONNELL, R. and EIDE, I. (2000) *Male Roles and Masculinities: A Culture of Peace Perspective*, Paris: UNESCO.

BULBECK, C. (1992) *Australian Women in Papua New Guinea: Colonial Passages 1920–1960*, Cambridge: Cambridge University Press.

CAIN, P.J. and HOPKINS, A.G. (1993) *British Imperialism: Innovation and Expansion, 1688–1914*, New York: Longman.

COHEN, J. (1991) 'NOMAS: challenging male supremacy', *Changing Men*, winter/spring, pp. 45–46.

CONNELL, R.W. (1990) 'The state, gender and sexual politics: theory and appraisal', *Theory and Society*, 19, pp. 507–44.

—— (1995) *Masculinities*, Cambridge: Polity.

—— (2000a) 'Debates about men, new research on masculinities', in *The Men and The Boys*, Berkeley and Los Angeles: University of California Press.

—— (2000b) 'New directions in theory and research', in *The Men and The Boys*, Berkeley and Los Angeles: University of California Press.

—— (2000c) 'Globalization and men's bodies', in *The Men and The Boys*, Berkeley and Los Angeles: University of California Press.

DAWSON, G. (1991) 'The bond bedouin: Lawrence of Arabia, imperial adventure and the imagining of English-British masculinity', in ROPER, M. and TOSH, J. (eds) *Manful Assertions: Masculinities in Britain since 1800*, London: Routledge.

DONALDSON, M. (1998) 'Growing up very rich: the masculinity of the hegemonic', *Journal of Interdisciplinary Gender Studies*, 3(2), pp. 95–112.

ENLOE, C. (1990) *Bananas, Beaches and Bases: Making Feminist Sense of International Politics*, Berkeley and Los Angeles: University of California Press.

FEATHERSTONE, M. (1995) *Undoing Culture: Globalization, Postmodernism and Identity*, London: Sage.

FUENTES, A. and EHRENREICH, B. (1983) *Women in the Global Factory*, Boston, MA: South End.

GEE, J.P., HULL, G. and LANKSHEAR, C. (1996) *The New Work Order: Behind the Language of the New Capitalism*, Sydney: Allen & Unwin.

GENDER EQUALITY OMBUDSMAN (1997) 'The father's quota, information sheet on parental leave entitlements', Ohio.

GIBSON, J.W. (1994) *Warrior Dreams: Paramilitary Culture in Post-Vietnam America*, New York: Hill & Wang.

HAGEMANN-WHITE, C. and RERRICH, M.S. (1988) *FrauenMännerBilder*, Bielefeld: AJZ-Verlag.

HINSCH, B. (1990) *Passions of the Cut Sleeve: The Male Homosexual Tradition in China*, Berkeley and Los Angeles: University of California Press.

HIRST, P. and THOMPSON, G. (1996) *Globalization in Question: The International Economy and the Possibilities of Governance*, Cambridge: Polity.

HOLLSTEIN, W. (1992) *Machen Sie Platz, mein Herr! Teilen statt Herrschen*, Hamburg: Rowohlt.

HOLLWAY, W. (1994) 'Gender difference and the production of subjectivity' in HENRIQUES, J., HOLLWAY, W., URWIN, C., VENN, C. and WALKERDINE, V. (eds) *Changing the Subject*, London: Methuen.

HOLTER, O.G. (1997) 'Gender, patriarchy and capitalism: a social forms analysis', doctoral dissertation, Faculty of Social Science, University of Oslo.

ITO, K. (1993) *Otokorashisa-no-yukue*, Tokyo: Shinyo-sha.

JEFFORDS, S. (1989) *The Remasculization of America: Gender and the Vietnam War*, Bloomington: Indiana University Press.

JOLLY, M. (1997) 'From point Venus to Bali Ha'i: eroticism and exoticism in representations of the Pacific' in MANDERSON, L. and JOLLY, M. (eds) *Sites of Desire, Economies of Pleasure: Sexualities in Asia and the Pacific*, Chicago: The University of Chicago Press.

KANDIYOTI, D. (1994) 'The paradoxes of masculinity: some thoughts on segregated societies' in CORNWALL, A. and LINDISFARNE, N. (eds) *Dislocating Masculinity: Comparative Ethnographies*, London: Routledge.

KAUFMAN, M. (1999) 'Men and violence', *International Association for Studies of Men Newsletter*, special issue, 6, [n.p.n.].

KIMMEL, M.S. (1996) *Manhood in America: A Cultural History*, New York: Free Press.

—— and MOSMILLER, T.E. (1992) *Against the Tide: Profeminist Men in the United States, 1776–1990, A Documentary History*, Boston, MA: Beacon Press.

KINDLER, H. (1993) *Maske(r)ade: Jungen- und Männerarbeit für die Praxis*, Neuling: Schwäbisch Gmünd und Tübingen.

KINMONTH, E.H. (1981) *The Self-made Man in Meiji Japanese Thought: From Samurai to Salary Man*, Berkeley: University of California Press.

KIPLING, R. (1987 [orig. 1901]) *Kim*, London: Penguin.

LAS CASAS, B. (1971) *History of the Indies*, trans. A. Collard, New York: Harper & Row.

MACDONALD, R.H. (1994) *The Language of Empire: Myths and Metaphors of Popular Imperialism 1880–1918*, Manchester: Manchester University Press.

MESSNER, M.A. (1997) *The Politics of Masculinities: Men in Movements*, Thousand Oaks, CA: Sage.

METZ-GÖCKEL, S. and MÜLLER, U. (1985) *Der Mann: Die Brigitte-Studie*, Hamburg: Beltz.

MIES, M. (1986) *Patriarchy and Accumulation on a World Scale: Women in the International Division of Labour*, London: Zed.

MOODIE, T.D. (1994) *Going for Gold: Men, Mines, and Migration*, Johannesburg: Witwatersrand University Press.

MORRELL, R. (1994) 'Boys, gangs, and the making of masculinity in the white secondary schools of Natal, 1880–1930', *Masculinities*, 2(2), pp. 56–82.

——— (1996) *Political Economy and Identities in KwaZulu-Natal: Historical and Social Perspectives*, Durban: Indicator Press.

NAKAMURA, A. (1994) *Watashi-no Danseigaku, Kindaibugei-sha*, Tokyo, National Men's Health Conference: 10–11 August 1995, Canberra: Australian Government Publishing Service.

NOVIKOVA, J. (2000) 'Soviet and post-Soviet masculinities: after men's wars in women's memories' in BREINES, I., CONNELL, R.W., and EIDE, I. (eds) *Male Roles and Masculinities: A Culture of Peace Perspective*, Paris: UNESCO.

PHILLIPS, J. (1987) *A Man's Country? The Image of the Pakeha Male: A History*, Auckland: Penguin.

SCHWALBE, M. (1996) *Unlocking the Iron Cage: The Men's Movement, Gender Politics, and the American Culture*, New York: Oxford University Press.

SEIDLER, V.J. (1991) *Achilles Heel Reader: Men, Sexual Politics, and Socialism*, London: Routledge.

SHIRE, C. (1994) 'Men don't go to the moon: language, space and masculinities in Zimbabwe' in CORNWALL, A. and LINDISFARNE, N. (eds) *Dislocating Masculinity: Comparative Ethnographies*, London: Routledge.

SIMPSON, A. (1993) *Xuxa: The Mega-Marketing of Gender, Race and Modernity*, Philadelphia: Temple University Press.

SINHA, M. (1995) *Colonial Masculinity: The Manly Englishman and the Effeminate Bengali in the Late Nineteenth Century*, Manchester: Manchester University Press.

TAYLOR, D. (1985) 'Women: an analysis' in *Women: A World Report*, London: Methuen.

TILLNER, G. (1997) 'Masculinity and xenophobia', paper presented at UNESCO meeting on Male Roles and Masculinities in the Perspective of a Culture of Peace, Oslo.

WALLERSTEIN, I. (1974) *The Modern World-System: Capitalist Agriculture and the Origins of the European World-Economy in the Sixteenth Century*, New York: Academic Press.

WIDERSPRÜCHE (1995) *Männlichkeiten*, special issue, 56/57, [n.p.n.].

WILLIAMS, W.L. (1986) *The Spirit and the Flesh: Sexual Diversity in American Indian Culture*, Boston, MA: Beacon.

XABA, T. (1997) 'Masculinity in a transitional society: the rise and fall of the "young lions"', paper presented at the conference on Masculinities in Southern Africa, University of Natal, Durban.

ZULEHNER, P.M. and VOLZ, R. (1998) *Männer im Aufbruch: Wie Deutschlands Männer sich selbst und wie Frauen sie sehen*, Ostfildern: Schwabenverlag.

15 Violence, sexuality, and women's lives

Lori L. Heise [1995]

My feminist project over the last three years has been to interject the reality of violence against women into the dominant discourse on AIDS, women's health, and international family planning. My overall aim has been two-fold: to improve public health policy by making it more reflective of the reality of women's lives, and to marshal some of the resources and technical know-how of the international health community to assist women's organizations fighting gender violence in the developing world.[1]

To date, the failure of the global health community to recognize gender-based abuse has put both important public health objectives and individual women at risk. By ignoring the pervasiveness of violence within relationships, for example, the current global AIDS strategy (which is based heavily on condom promotion) dooms itself to failure. The research shows that many women are afraid to even broach the subject of condom use for fear of male reprisal (Elias and Heise, 1993; Gupta and Weiss, 1995). As Anke Ehrhardt, co-director of the HIV Center for Clinical and Behavioral Studies [in New York], observes, 'We have not only ignored the fact that women do not control condom use, but we have rushed headlong into prevention efforts aimed at getting women to insist on condom use without taking into account that they may risk severe repercussions, such as violence and other serious threats to their economic and social support' (Ehrhardt, 1991).

This is but one example of the potential costs of failing to explore the intersection of violence, sexuality, gender, and public health. In this chapter, I lay out what is known about violence and sexuality, especially with respect to its implications for women's sexual and reproductive lives. More importantly, I discuss several risks I see present in the feminist project of introducing ideas about violence and sexuality into the professional world of public health. Focusing the 'biomedical gaze' on violence risks reinforcing negative images of woman as 'victim', an impression that can undermine women's own sense of self-efficacy and can justify continued inattention to women's needs. (For example, when faced with women's initial difficulty in 'negotiating' condom use, some AIDS experts recommended shifting the entire focus of condom promotion and training to men, instead of exploring ways to strengthen women's ability to protect themselves.) Increased attention to the pervasiveness of violence, especially sexual violence, also risks fuelling popular notions of sexuality as biologically driven and of male sexuality as 'inherently predatory' – both notions experiencing a resurgence in popular culture. As I will show, however, the cross-cultural record does not support a vision of male sexuality as inherently aggressive. To the extent that male sexual behaviour is aggressive in certain cultures, it is because sexuality expresses power relations based on gender.

A multiplicity of discourses

Sexuality and gender have become the subjects of sociological and biomedical inquiry only within the last century or so. Within this short history, several distinct discourses have laid claim to the domain of human sexual experience. The first, 'sexology', emerged as a discipline in the late nineteenth century. Typified by Havelock Ellis, Alfred Kinsey, and Masters and Johnson, sexology has been most concerned with sexual function, dysfunction, and the physiology of the sexual response. To its credit, sexology views women as agents of their own sexual lives, and takes as given women's right to sexual pleasure (see Table 15.1).

Many feminists have criticized sexology, however, for neglecting the 'dangerous' side of sex for women: abuse, unwanted pregnancy, STDs, humiliation, rape. As feminist Lenore Tiefer points out, 'Sexology's nomenclature of sexual disorders does not describe what makes women unhappy about sex in the real world, but narrows and limits the vision of sexual problems to failures of genital performance' (Tiefer, 1992). According to Tiefer, sexology looks at sexuality from the position of male privilege, where the sexual narrative has to do with erotics: intercourse, arousal, pleasure, erection, orgasm, 'All well and good', she notes, 'but hardly the stuff at the centre of many women's sexual experience' (Tiefer, 1992, p. 4).

Feminists also fault sexology for failing to confront and work against gender-based power differentials. Significantly, none of the breakthrough studies that first documented the pervasiveness of non-consensual sex, illegal abortion, and STDs in women came from mainstream sex research. Sexology has resisted challenging male power over female sexuality – in the form of coercive sex, male-defined religious doctrine, or lack of contraceptive research –

Table 15.1 Sex research paradigms

Sexology	Population control/ public health	Anti-violence feminism	Integrated feminist approach
Acknowledges PLEASURE but focuses on genital performance.	Focuses on DANGER (STDs; unwanted pregnancy; 'high-risk sex')	Focuses on DANGER (rape, child sexual abuse; pornography)	Acknowledges DANGER but claims women's right to sexual PLEASURE
Ignores gender power imbalances	Attempts to override imbalances through technology	Fights against gender-based power inequities	Fights against gender-based power inequities
Focuses on behaviour and physiology	Focuses on behaviour and technology	Focuses on context and meaning (although tends toward negative)	Focuses on context and meaning but recognizes pragmatic realities
Women seen as agents	Women seen as a means to an end (e.g. to achieve demographic targets)	Women seen as victims (or potential victims)	Women seen as agents operating within restricted options
Adherents see themselves as scientists	Adherents see themselves as practitioners	Adherents see themselves as activists	Adherents see themselves as activists and practitioners
Risks trivializing women's reality by ignoring 'danger' part of sex for women	Ignores gender-based power relations to the detriment of programme success	Fuels essentialist notions of male sexuality as inherently 'predatory'. Reinforces image of women as victims	Seeks strategies that empower women and promote long-term social change while meeting women's immediate needs

because it fears 'politicizing' what it sees as a basically neutral, 'scientific' subject. According to feminists, however, sexologists – like all professionals – can either support institutional norms that ignore women's reality, or they can subvert those norms. As Tiefer maintains: 'Any attempt to be neutral, to be "objective" is to support the status quo' (Tiefer, 1992, p. 5).

A second, more recent discourse on sexuality emerges from the 'population control' and international health establishment. International health's interest in sex focuses almost exclusively on behaviours that have implications for demographics and/or for disease. A review of over 2,100 articles from five of the top family planning and health journals, for example, reveals that between 1980 and 1992 sexuality and male–female power dynamics are mentioned only within three narrow contexts: how women's attitudes about sexuality influence contraception use and effectiveness (41 articles); how adolescent sexual activity and contraception use are related to teen pregnancy (24 articles); and how 'high-risk' sexual behaviours are related to the spread of sexually transmitted diseases, including AIDS (11 articles) (Dixon-Mueller 1992). The preoccupation in public health has been with sexual danger and with counting disembodied acts (e.g., the number of instances of unprotected penetrative intercourse in the last month) not with meaning, context, or pleasure. In this discourse, women are frequently seen as means to an end – as 'targets' for demographic initiatives or as reproductive vessels – rather than as individuals with independent needs and a right to sexual self-determination and pleasure (Dixon-Mueller, 1993).

A third prominent discourse, which I shall call 'anti-pornography feminism', is best represented by women such as Andrea Dworkin, Catherine MacKinnon, Kathleen Barry, and Evelina Giobbe. These women have dominated one side of what has come to be known in feminist circles as the 'sex wars' – basically an internal debate over the 'appropriate' boundaries (from a feminist perspective) of human sexual behaviour. At issue are such themes as pornography, sadomasochism, prostitution, and how society should respond to these phenomena (Valverde, 1987; Cole, 1989). The anti-pornography feminists argue for intervention and insist that women will never achieve equality as long as their sexuality is commercialized, and as long as domination and economic exploitation are conflated with sexual pleasure. The 'sex radical' critique on the other hand sees long-term danger in any effort to censor sexual behaviour between consenting adults, arguing that such efforts can too easily be used against sexual minorities and women (Vance, 1984).

While my work shares a common motivation with the anti-pornography feminists, there are strains in their thought that I find troubling. I commend this paradigm for its focus on gender-based power inequities and for its activist stance, but it tends to be profoundly pessimistic, and easily degenerates into portraying women solely as victims. In their zeal to highlight the dangers of sex, anti-pornography feminists have also tended to overlook sex's pleasures. In a radically 'sex-negative' culture, overcompensation – even in the face of a culture largely indifferent to women's victimization – carries certain dangers. It also contributes to the popular 'demonization' of men and of male sexuality. It is the importation of these pitfalls that I fear in my effort to introduce the reality of violence into the family planning and international health field. To the uninitiated, the very pervasiveness of violence can be so overwhelming as to justify dismissing the situation as impossible to change.

Understanding, such concerns have been used to question efforts to integrate violence into the public-health mainstream. Rather than tolerate naïveté and gender-blindness in the health and development field, however, I think anti-violence activism must seek to transform public health discourse and research, encouraging a greater emphasis on social context, meaning, power differentials, and gender. It is with this vision that I offer a new paradigm for sex research and practice within public health, combining the strengths of the three other models.

Table 15.1 includes a brief summary of the existing sex paradigms as well as a suggested model for a new approach. This new option – which I call the 'integrated feminist approach' – is most closely approximated today by the feminist women's health movement (for example, groups such as the Boston Women's Health Book Collective, authors of *Our Bodies, Ourselves*, and the Coletivo Feminista Sexualidade e Saúde in São Paulo, Brazil).

While this chart admittedly oversimplifies three complex and pluralistic fields of inquiry, it nonetheless allows a quick (and I hope useful) comparison of some of the existing stakeholders in women's sexuality. It also summarizes the integrated approach to sexuality that I strive for in my own work. The following section explores what we currently know about violence and coercion as it relates to women's sexual and reproductive health. In the last section of this chapter, I offer an interpretation of this data and explore my concerns about the anti-pornography discourse in greater detail.

The impact of violence on women's sexual and reproductive lives

Regrettably, we know very little in social science about how violence or fear of violence operates in women's lives. Only recently have researchers begun to document the pervasiveness of gender-based abuse and virtually no attempt has been made to investigate how violence affects women's sexuality. There are important questions in need of exploration: what is the role of coercion in sexual initiation? How do force and fear affect women's experience of sexual pleasure? How does violence affect women's reproductive health? The following section summarizes the information available on each of these questions. Of necessity, much of the analysis remains speculative.

The prevalence of violence against women

The most endemic form of violence against women is wife abuse, or more accurately, abuse of women by intimate male partners. Table 15.2 summarizes twenty studies from a wide variety of countries that document that one-quarter to over half of women in many countries of the world report having been physically abused by a person or former partner. Although some of these studies are based on convenience sample, the majority are based on probability samples with a large number of respondents (e.g., Mexico, United States, Colombia, Kenya).[2]

Statistics around the world also suggest that rape is a common reality in the lives of women and girls. Six population-based surveys from the United States, for example, suggest that between one in five and one in seven US women will be the victim of a completed rape in her lifetime (Kilpatrick, Edmund and Seymor, 1992).[3] Moreover, there are well-designed studies of rape among college-aged women from New Zealand (Gavey, 1991), Canada (Dekeseredy and Kelly, 1992), the United States (Koss, Gidycz and Wisniewski, 1987), and the United Kingdom (Beattie, 1992) that reveal remarkably similar rates of completed rape across countries, when using similar survey instruments (based on Koss and Oros, 1982).[4] A study among adult women (many of them college students) in Seoul, Korea, yielded slightly lower rates of completed rape, but an equally high rate of attempts (Shim, 1992) (see Table 15.3).

Not surprisingly, given the extremely sensitive nature of the subject, reliable data on child sexual abuse are even scarcer. Nonetheless, the few studies that do exist – along with ample indirect evidence – suggest that sexual abuse of children and adolescents is a widespread phenomenon. In the United States, for example, population-based studies indicate that 27 to 62 per cent of women recall at least one incident of sexual abuse before the age of eighteen

Table 15.2 Prevalence of wife abuse, selected countries

Country	Sample size	Sample type	Findings	Comments
Barbados (Handwerker 1991)	264 women and 243 men aged 20–45	Island-wide national probability sample	30% of women battered as adults	Women and men report 50% of their mothers were beaten
Antigua (Handwerker 1993)	97 women aged 20–45	Random subset of national probability sample	30% of women battered as adults	Women and men report that 50% of mothers were beaten
Kenya (Raikes 1990)	733 women from Kissi District	District-wide cluster sample	42% 'beaten regularly'	Taken from survey of contraceptive prevalence
Papua New Guinea (Toft, 1987)	Rural 736 men, 715 women; urban low income 368 men, 298 women; urban elite 178 men, 99 women	Rural survey in 19 villages in all regions and provinces; urban survey with oversample of elites	67% of rural women beaten; 56% of urban low-income women beaten; 62% of urban elite women beaten	Almost perfect agreement between percentage of women who claim to have been beaten and percentage of men who admit to abuse
Sri Lanka (Sonali, 1990)	200 mixed ethnic, low-income women from Colombo	Convenience sample from low-income neighbourhood	60% have been beaten	51% said husbands used weapons
India (Mahajan, 1990)	109 men and 109 women from village in Jullundur District Punjab	50% sample of all scheduled (low) caste households and 50% of non-scheduled (higher) caste houses	75% of lower caste men admit to beating their wives; 22% of higher caste men admit to beatings	75% of scheduled caste wives report being beaten 'frequently'
Malaysia (WAO, 1992)	713 women and 508 males over 15 years old	National random probability sample of peninsular Malaysia	39% of women have been 'physically beaten' by a partner in the last year	Note: This is an annual figure. 15% of adults consider wife beating acceptable (22% of Malays)
Colombia (Profamilia, 1992)	3,272 urban women; 2,118 rural women	National probability sample	20% physically abused; 33% psychologically abused; 10% raped by husband	Part of Colombia's DHS survey
Costa Rica (Chacon *et al.*, 1990)	1,388 women	Convenience sample of women attending child-welfare clinic	50% report being physically abused	Sponsored by UNICEF/PAHO
Costa Rica (Chacon *et al.*, 1990)	1,312 women aged 15 to 49 years	Random probability sample of urban women	51% report being beaten up to several times per year; 35% report being hit regularly	—
Mexico (Jalisco) (Ramirez and Vazquez, 1993)	1,163 rural women; 427 urban women in the state of Jalisco	Random household survey of women on DIF register	56.7% of urban women and 44.2% of rural women	Experienced some form of 'interpersonal violence'

continued on next page

Table 15.2
Cont.

Country	Sample size	Sample type	Findings	Comments
Mexico (Valdez and Cox, 1990)	342 women from Nezahualcoyotl	Random probability sample of women from city adjacent to Mexico City	33% had lived in a 'violent relationship'	—
Ecuador (CEPLAES, 1992)	200 low-income women	Convenience sample of Quito barrio	60% had been 'beaten' by a partner	Of those beaten, 37% were assaulted with frequency between once a month and every day
Chile (Larrain, 1993)	1,000 women in Santiago aged 22 to 55 years involved in a relationship of 2 years or more	Stratified random probability sample with a maximum sampling error of 3%	60% abused by a male intimate; 26.2% physically abused (more severe than pushes, slaps, or having an object thrown at you)	70% of those abused are abused more than once a year
Norway (Schei and Bakkesteig, 1989)	150 women aged 20 to 49 years in Trondheim	Random sample selected from census data	25% had been physically or sexually abused by a male partner	Definition does not include less severe forms of violence like pushing, slapping, or shoving
New Zealand (Mullen *et al.*, 1988)	2,000 women sent questionnaire; stratified random sample of 349 women selected for interview	Random probability sample selected from electoral rolls of five contiguous parliamentary constituencies	20.1% report being 'hit and physically abused' by a male partner; 58% of these women (>10% of sample) were battered more than 3 times	—
USA (Straus and Gelles, 1986)	2,143 married or co-habitating couples	National random probability sample	28% report at least one episode of physical violence	—
USA (Grant, Preda and Martin, 1991)	6,000 women state-wide from Texas	State-wide random probability sample	39% have been abused by male partner after age 18; 31% have been physically abused	>12% have been sexually abused by male partner after age 18
USA (Teske and Parker, 1983)	3,000 rural women in Texas	Random probability sample of communities with 50,000 people or less	40.2% have been abused after age 18; 31% have been physically abused	22% abused within the last 12 months

(Peters, Wyatt and Finkelhor, 1986).[5] An anonymous, island-wide, probability survey of Barbados revealed that one woman in three and one to two men per one hundred reported behaviour constituting childhood or adolescent sexual abuse (Handwerker, 1991). And in Canada, a government commission estimated that one in four female children and one in ten male children are sexually assaulted prior to the age of seventeen years (Canadian Government, 1984).

Table 15.3 Prevalence of rape among college-aged women

Country	Authors	Sample	Definition of rape[a]	Completed rape	Completed and attempts
Canada	Dekeseredy and Kelly, 1992	National probability sample of 1,835 women at 95 colleges and universities	Anal, oral or vaginal intercourse by force or threat of force SES # 9, 10	8.1% (by dating partners since high school)	23.3% (rape or sexual assault by anyone ever)
New Zealand	Gavey, 1991	347 women psychology students	Anal, vaginal intercourse by force or threat; or because a man gave alcohol or drugs SES # 8, 9, 10	14.1%	25.3%
UK	Beattie, 1992	1,574 women at six universities	Vaginal intercourse by force or because a man gave alcohol or drugs SES # 8, 9	11.3%	19.3%
USA	Koss *et al.*, 1987	3,187 women at 32 colleges and universities	SES # 8, 9, 10	15.4%	27.5%
USA	Moore, Nord and Peterson, 1989	Nationally representative sample of 18 to 22 years old	Forced to have sex against your will, or were raped?	12.7% of whites; 8% of blacks (before age 21)	—
Seoul Korea	Shim, 1992	2,270 adult women (quota sample)	SES # 9, 10	7.7%	21.8%

[a] Estimates of rape and attempted rape are based on the legal definition of rape in the country concerned and are derived from different combinations of the following questions taken from the Sexual Experiences Survey (Koss and Oros, 1984): 4) Has a man attempted sexual intercourse (getting on top of you, attempting to insert his penis) when you didn't want to by threatening or using some degree of physical force (twisting your arm, holding you down, etc.) but intercourse did not occur? 8) Have you had sexual intercourse when you didn't want to because a man gave you alcohol or drugs? 9) Have you had sexual intercourse when you didn't want to because a man threatened or used some degree of physical force (twisting your arm, holding you down, etc.) to make you? 10) Have you engaged in sex acts (anal or oral intercourse or penetration by objects other than a penis) when you didn't want to because a man threatened or used some degree of phyiscal force (twisting your arm, holding you down, etc.) to make you?

Elsewhere, indirect evidence suggests cause for concern. Two studies from Nigeria, for example, document that a large percentage of female patients at STD clinics are young children. A 1988 study in Zaria, Nigeria found that 16 per cent of female patients seeking treatment for STDs were children under the age of five and another 6 per cent were children between the ages of six and fifteen (Kisekka and Otesanya, 1988). An older study in Ibadan found that 22 per cent of female patients attending one STD clinic were children under the age of ten (Sogbetun *et al.*, 1977). Likewise, a study conducted in the Maternity Hospital of Lima, Peru revealed that 90 per cent of the young mothers aged twelve to sixteen had been raped by their father, stepfather or another close relative.[6]

A final indication of the prevalence of sexual abuse comes from the observations of children themselves. In 1991, when the Nicaraguan NGO, CISAS held a national conference for the children involved in their 'Child to Child' programme (a project that trains youngsters aged eight to fifteen to be better child-care providers for their siblings), participants identified 'sexual abuse' as the number one health priority facing young people in their country.

Experience of sexual pleasure

When coercion enters the sexual arena, it invariably affects women's experience of sex. While we know something about the impact of rape or sexual abuse on women's sexual functioning, little is known about how subtle or overt coercion within consensual unions affects women's sexual lives. Research indicates that from 50 to 60 per cent of women who are raped experience severe sexual problems, including fear of sex, problems with arousal, and decreased sexual functioning (Becker *et al.*, 1982; Burnam, 1988). But what about forced sex within relationships, or about the role of coercion in women's sexual initiation? Both are topics deserving much greater exploration.

Little information is available, for example, on the degree to which young women feel coerced into their first sexual experience. In one study, 40 per cent of girls aged eleven to fifteen in Jamaica reported the reason for their first intercourse as 'forced' (Allen, 1982). A qualitative study of sexual initiation among adolescent girls in the United States – aptly entitled 'Putting a Big Thing into a Little Hole' – indicates that many girls recall their first intercourse negatively (Thompson, 1990).[7] Many girls mention pain, fear, disappointment, and a sense of not being in control of the situation. While most do not frame their experiences as 'coercive', few in this group were prepared for or actively wanted the sex to happen. As author Sharon Thompson observes; 'Often they did not agree to sex. They gave in, they gave up, they gave out' (Thompson, 1990, p. 358).

Also at issue is how young girls experience first intercourse when forced into arranged marriages at a very young age. While the rate of child marriage is declining, a significant portion of girls are still married off at a very young age, often to unknown men many years their senior (see Table 15.4). Evidence from a qualitative study of sexual initiation among child brides in Iran confirms that early intercourse, even when culturally supported, can be very traumatic for young girls, anthropologist Mary Hegland interviewed exiled Iranian women living in

Table 15.4 Percentage of women aged 20 to 24 today who were married before the age of fifteen, selected countries

Country	per cent	Year of Report
Nigeria	26.7	1990
Mali	26.7	1987
Cameroon	21.3	1991
Uganda	17.8	1989/90
Liberia	16.6	1986
Egypt*	15.0	1988
Guatemala	12.6	1987
Pakistan	11.4	1990/91
Indonesia	10.0	1991
Dominican Republic	9.0	1991
Mexico	6.2	1987
Trinidad/Tobago	6.0	1987

* Before the age of sixteen

Source: Selected Demographic and Health Surveys

the United States about sexual initiation in Iran (Hegland, n.d.). Many gave graphic details of forced defloration of young girls, most of whom were totally ignorant of sex (often a young girl was held down by relatives while the man forced himself on her). While the women said the term 'rape' would never be applied to this experience in Iran, they freely used terms like 'rape' and 'torture' to describe the experience, after being exposed to this language in the United States. This new language merely gave voice to feelings they already had.

Given the prevalence of violence in women's lives, there is a remarkable lack of information on how it affects women's sexuality. Only one study, published recently in the *Journal of Family Violence*, explicitly looks at the effects of violence on women's experience of sex (Apt and Hurlbert, 1993). Compared to non-abused women in distressed marriages, women living in violent relationships had significantly lower (i.e., more negative) responses on nine scales designed to measure sexual satisfaction, intimacy, arousal, and attitudes toward sex. Nonetheless, they had significantly more intercourse. *Why? pressure? Rape? etc.*

This high rate of intercourse is not surprising given the frequency of coerced sex within physically abusive relationships. Whereas 14 per cent of all US wives report being physically forced to have sex against their will, the prevalence of coercive intercourse among battered women is at least 40 per cent (Campbell and Alford, 1989). In Bolivia and Puerto Rico, 58 per cent of battered wives report being sexually assaulted by their partner, and in Colombia the reported rate is 46 per cent (Isis International 1988; Profamilia, 1992). Given the percentage of women around the world who live with physically abusive partners, it is likely that sexual coercion within consensual unions is quite common.

There is also a remarkable gap in our knowledge about the meaning and experience of sex among women who live in non-violent relationships. Even here, the experience of sex for women is often humiliating and degrading – one that they tolerate rather than enjoy. Commenting on how their husbands treated them sexually, the Iranian women interviewed above used such phrases as 'I'm not a toilet', 'I'm not just a hole', 'It's like swallowing nasty medicine' (Hegland, n.d.). In focus group discussions with Mexican women about men, sex, and marriage, many women likewise expressed deep resentment about how men treated them in sexual relationships (Folch-Lyon, Macorra and Schearer, 1981). Women in particular mentioned:

- physical abuse by husbands to coerce the wife's sexual compliance;
- widespread male infidelity;
- men's authoritarian attitude toward their wives;
- threats of abandonment if a wife failed to meet her husband's sexual demands or his demand for more children; and
- an abiding sense of depersonalization, humiliation, and physical dissatisfaction during sex.

Perhaps more than anything, the Spanish phrase women commonly use for sex captures their sentiment: 'el me usa' (he uses me). Such comments raise the question of the nature of 'consent' within the patriarchal institution of marriage. Would women consent to such treatment if they had the economic resources to survive independently and the social permission to seek sexual gratification elsewhere?

Ability to control fertility

The family planning literature documents that, for many women, fear of male reprisal greatly limits their ability to use contraception (Dixon-Mueller, 1992). Men in many cultures react negatively to birth control because they think it signals a woman's intentions to be unfaithful (their logic being that protection against pregnancy allows women to be promiscuous). Where children are a sign of male virility, a woman's attempts to use birth control may also be interpreted as an affront to her partner's masculinity. While male approval is not always the deciding factor, studies from countries as diverse as Mexico, South Africa, and Bangladesh have found that partner approval is the single greatest predictor of women's contraceptive use.[8] When partners disapprove, women either forgo contraception or they resort to family planning methods they can use without their partner's knowledge.

The unspoken reality behind this subterfuge is that women can be beaten or otherwise abused if they do not comply with men's sexual and childbearing demands. In a recent interview, Hope Mwesigye of FIDA-Uganda, a non-profit legal aid organization for women in Kampala, recounted the story of a young married mother who was running from a husband who regularly beat her. Despite earning a decent wage, the woman's husband refused to maintain her and their two children. To avoid bringing more children into the world whom she could not feed, the woman began using birth control without her husband's consent. The beatings began when she failed to bring forth more children; they became more brutal when he learned of her contraceptive use (Banwell, 1990).

In other countries, legal provisions requiring spousal permission before dispensing birth control can actually put women at increased risk of violence. According to Pamela Onyango of Family Planning International Assistance, women in Kenya have been known to forge their partner's signature rather than open themselves to violence or abandonment by requesting permission to use family planning services (Banwell, 1990). Nor are Kenyan women alone in their fear of such consequences. Researchers conducting focus groups on sexuality in Mexico and Peru found that women held similar concerns – fear of violence, desertion, or accusations of infidelity – if they brought up birth control (Folch-Lyon, Macorra, and Schearer, 1981; Fort, 1989). Not surprisingly, when family planning clinics in Ethiopia removed their requirement for spousal consent, clinic use rose 26 per cent in just a few months (Cook and Maine, 1987).

Not all women who fear violence in this context are necessarily at risk of actual abuse. In fact, some recent studies suggest that many men may be more open to family planning than most women suspect (Gallen, 1986). Communication in marriage can be so limited, however, that spouses often do not know their partner's views on family planning. Women thus assume that their husband's attitude will mirror the cultural norm, which frequently says that men want large families and distrust women who use birth control. The discrepancy between women's perceptions and reality also speaks to the ability of violence to induce fear by example.

Risk of acquiring STDs

Not surprisingly, male violence also impedes women's ability to protect themselves from HIV and other STDs. Violence can increase a woman's risk either through non-consensual sex or by limiting her willingness and/or ability to enforce condom use. In many cultures, suggesting condom use is even more threatening than raising birth control in general, because condoms are widely associated with promiscuity, prostitution, and disease. By bringing up condom use, women either insinuate their own infidelity or implicitly challenge a male part-ner's right to conduct outside relationships. Either way, a request for condoms may trigger a violent response (Elias and Heise, 1993; Worth, 1991).

Indeed, an AIDS prevention strategy based solely on 'negotiating' condom use assumes equity of power between men and women that simply does not exist in many relationships. Even within consensual unions, women often lack control over the dynamics of their sexual lives. A study of home-based industrial workers in Mexico, for example, found that wives' bargaining power in marriage was lowest with regard to decisions about if and when to have sexual intercourse (Beneria and Roldan, 1987). Studies of natural family planning in the Phil-ippines, Peru, and Sri Lanka (Liskin, 1981) and sexual attitudes among women in Guatemala (DataPro and Asociación Guatemalteco para la Prevención y Control de SIDA, 1991) also mention forced sex in marriage, especially when the men arrive at home drunk.

Childhood sexual abuse also appears to generate responses that put individuals at increased risk of STDs, including AIDS. Several studies, for example, link a history of sexual abuse with a high risk of entering prostitution (Finkelhor, 1987; James and Meyerding, 1977). Researchers from Brown University found that men and women who had been raped or forced to have sex in either childhood or adolescence were four times more likely than non-abused individuals to have worked in prostitution (Zierler, 1991). They were also twice as likely to have multiple partners in any single year and to engage in casual sex with partners they did not know. Women survivors of childhood sexual assault were twice as likely to be heavy consumers of alcohol and nearly three times more likely to become pregnant before the age of eighteen. These behaviours did not translate directly into higher rates of HIV among women, but men who experienced childhood sexual abuse were twice as likely to be HIV positive as men who did not.

Impacts of sexual abuse on sexual risk-taking have also been documented in a developing country – on the island of Barbados. Based on a probability survey of 407 men and women, anthropologist Penn Handwerker has shown that sexual abuse is the single most important determinant of high-risk sexual activity during adolescence for both Barbadian men and women (Handwerker, 1991). After controlling for a wide range of socio-economic and home-environment variables (e.g., absent father), sexual abuse remains strongly linked to both the number of partners adolescents have and to their age at first intercourse. Further analysis shows that direct effects of childhood sexual abuse on partner change remain significant into the respondent's mid-thirties. For men, physical, emotional, and/or sexual abuse in childhood is also highly correlated with lack of condom use in adulthood, after controlling for many other variables.[9]

Pregnancy complication and birth outcomes

While pregnancy should be a time when the health and well-being of women is specially protected, surveys suggest that pregnant women are prime targets for abuse. Results from a large, prospective study of battery during pregnancy among low-income women in Houston and Baltimore in the United States, for example, indicate that one out of every six pregnant women was battered during her present pregnancy (MacFarlane *et al.*, 1992). The study, sponsored by the Centers for Diseases Control, followed a stratified cohort of 691 White, African-American and Hispanic women for three years in Houston and Baltimore. Of the abused women in this study, 60 per cent reported two or more episodes of violence, and they were three times as likely as non-abused women to begin prenatal care in the third trimester. Other studies indicate that women battered during pregnancy run twice the risk of miscarriage and four times the risk of having a low-birth-weight baby compared with women who are not beaten (Stark *et al.*, 1981; Bullock and MacFarlane, 1989). Birth weight is a powerful predictor of a child's survival prospects in the first year of life. Battering during pregnancy is likely to have an even greater impact on Third World mothers who are already malnourished and overworked. A survey of 342 randomly sampled women in Mexico City revealed that 20 per cent of those battered reported blows to the stomach during pregnancy (Valdez and Cox, 1990). In another study of 80 battered women who sought judicial intervention against their partner in San José, Costa Rica, 49 per cent report being beaten during pregnancy. Of these, 7.5 per cent reported miscarriages due to the abuse (Ugalde, 1988).

A prospective study of 161 women living is Santiago, Chile, likewise revealed that those women living in areas of high social and political violence had a significantly increased risk of pregnancy complications compared to women living in lower-violence neighbourhoods. After adjusting for potential confounders (income, education, marital status, underweight, cigarette smoking, dissatisfaction with neighbourhood, life events, alienation, uncertainty and depression), researchers found that high levels of socio-political violence were associated with an approximately fivefold increase in risk of pregnancy complications (such as pre-eclampsia, premature labour, threat of miscarriages, gestational hypertension, etc.) (Zapata *et al.*, 1992). If the stress and trauma of living in a violent neighbourhood can induce complications, it is reasonable to assume that living in the private hell of an abusive relationship could as well.

Some thoughts on the implications of these findings

After reading the above review, it is hard not to share the profound pessimism about men and about male sexuality that runs throughout much of the anti-pornography literature. It is important to consider, however, the appropriate message to be taken from these data. Unfortunately, the conclusion some have drawn is that women are essentially powerless and that men must be aggressive by nature. Generally there is indignation at male abuse, but it is often accompanied by a sense that the problem runs too deep to be addressed. Whether justified by biological arguments (evolution has endowed men with an aggressive sexual nature) or socio-cultural determinism (patriarchy is everywhere and not easily changed), these beliefs can rationalize inaction.

Ironically, the very research and ideas that can be used to justify inaction often come from individuals who probably would not support the use of their data in this way. I, for example, oppose the view that male sexuality is inherently aggressive or that women are essentially victims. Most of my anti-violence colleagues would likely agree, although few have made a point of arguing against the interpretation of their work in this way. Given the appeal of 'essentialist' notions of sex and gender in popular culture (and the political implications of such arguments), it is my belief, however, that anyone who promotes new ideas in mainstream discourse has a responsibility not only for what they meant to say, but for how their words can be construed and used. It is out of this sense of responsibility that I offer the following interpretation of the data on sexuality and violence that I present above.

First, despite the powerful ability of violence to exact obedience and exert control, women are not powerless. In fact, women have proven incredibly capable of exerting agency even within the most constrained social conditions. Extremely poor women in India, for example, have been known to exert control over their sexual lives by declaring extended religious fasts, a socially sanctioned activity (imbued with taboos against sexual relations) that even violent men are reluctant to violate (Savara, personal communication). Likewise, research has shown that far from being passive, battered women often adopt complex coping and management strategies that serve to lessen the impact of the violence on themselves and their children (Bowker, 1983; Browne, 1987; Okun, 1986). Even some prostitutes interpret their decision to turn tricks as an empowered choice – a way to make money for sexual services exacted from other women through marriage (Delacoste and Alexander, 1987). This is not to say that women do not deserve broader choices than these examples imply. Such acts do represent, however, creativity and resourcefulness in the face of powerful social forces, and it is important to acknowledge and affirm these at all times. Failure to recognize the possibility of agency within patriarchal structures fuels fatalism and can undermine women's sense of self, with disempowering results.

In her speech 'Does Sexuality Have a History?', for example, feminist attorney, Catherine MacKinnon advances a very deterministic and fatalistic picture of women and sexuality. Taking issue with the prevailing view of academic historians that sexuality is basically socially constructed and highly plastic, MacKinnon (1991) writes:

> I would hypothesize that while ideologies about sex and sexuality may ebb and flow … the actual practices of sex may look relatively flat … underneath all of these hills and valleys, these ebbs and flows, there is this bedrock, this tide that has not changed much, namely male supremacy and the subordination of women … For this feminists have been called ahistorical. Oh, dear. We have disrespected the profundity and fascination of all the different ways in which men fuck us in order to emphasize that however they do it, they do it. And they do it to us.

> (MacKinnon, 1991, p. 6)

In a later edition of the *Michigan Quarterly*, the same journal which reprinted the original speech, author Suzanne Rhodenbaugh (1991) accuses MacKinnon of committing a 'new violence' by denying women the agency to define their own sexuality. In her reply essay, 'MacKinnon, May I Speak?' Rhodenbaugh writes:

> MacKinnon, with probably good intention to empower women, seems to me in her essay another voice reducing us, one saying we are creatures mainly acted upon. This feels greatly over-simplified, and finally untrue. It feels further, like new injustice. For if my 'history of sexuality' includes such facts as my having been raped, having been beaten by a husband, having gone through a pregnancy against my will, and all that has happened to my body and my sexual attention that I did not seek but was subjected to … then presumably as a sexual creature I'm little more than victim, and am predominantly passive.

> (Rhodenbaugh, 1991, p. 442)

MacKinnon likewise implies that male sexual behaviour is hegemonically abusive ('however they do it, they do it. And they do it to us'). But Rhodenbaugh refuses to cede her agency, saying. 'I'm just one individual woman, but I'm not of a mind to exchange the name "invisible" for the name "victim". Neither name will hold me' (Rhodenbaugh, 1991, p. 422).

Indeed, Rhodenbaugh's comments capture the essence of the dilemma faced by anti-violence activists: in exposing the reality of violence, we risk gaining visibility at the price of promoting the image of woman as victim and the notion of sex as all danger and no pleasure. One way to avoid this pitfall is to always counterbalance the pessimism engendered by the tenacity of patriarchy with examples of women's creative attempts at resistance within existing constraints. Another is to constantly imbue the anti-violence discourse with reminders of why feminists fight sexual violence in the first place. As author Naomi Wolf points out, 'Feminists agitate against rape not just because it is a form of violence – but because it is a form of violence that uniquely steals from the survivor her sexual spontaneity and delight ... The right to say no must exist for the right to say yes to have any meaning' (Wolf, 1992). Regrettably, this recognition is all too often lost in feminist discussions of sexual violence.

A second pitfall of anti-violence work is the danger of fuelling popular notions of sexual essentialism by drawing attention to the pervasiveness of gender violence. Essentialist explanations for social phenomenon are generally dangerous because they provide a powerful justification for the *status quo*. If what exists is biologically based, then it is 'natural' and by extension, 'good' (or at least not open to change). Essentialist interpretations have a long history, beginning with scientists such as Freud and Konrad Lorenz who saw aggression and sexuality as 'drives' or 'instincts' that needed periodic release or they were likely to 'discharge' in destructive ways. This 'hydraulic' image of sexuality is one that still holds much popular appeal. Indeed, the notion that men 'need' frequent sex with many partners is a myth used in many cultures (including my own) to justify and condone sexual behaviour by men that can be exploitive and hurtful to women.

While most psychologists now reject the drive theory it still captures the imagination of many in the general public. The meteoric rise of author/academic Camille Paglia attests to the enduring appeal that such essentialist notions command. Although Paglia, a latter-day Freudian, would likely object to being characterized as a biological determinist, her writings and public statements smack of determinism and her analysis of sexual violence draws exclusively from biology, psychology, and ethics rather than from an analysis of power or gender-role socialization. In *Sex, Art and American Culture*, for example, Paglia writes:

> Aggression and eroticism are deeply intertwined. Hunt, pursuit, and capture are biologically programmed into male sexuality ... I see in the simple, swaggering masculinity of the jock and in the noisy posturing of the heavy-metal guitarist certain fundamental, unchangeable truths about sex ... We must remedy social injustice wherever we can. But there are some things we cannot change. There are sexual differences based in biology. Academic feminism is lost in a fog of social constructionism.
>
> (Paglia, 1992, pp. 50–3)

A careful reading of Paglia's text reveals that she does believe that the male 'tendency toward brutishness' can be overridden through socialization (in some cases, at least), but it is easy to see how her purposefully provocative statements about male sexuality could be constructed to support popular notions that 'boys will be boys'. Given the potential of such rationalizations to promote behaviour harmful to women, Paglia has a responsibility not only for her beliefs but for how her words are likely to be heard. Once she steps out of academia and onto the TV talk-show circuit, Paglia has an increased duty to guard against the misuse of her ideas by paying careful attention to language and by countering likely misinterpretations of her ideas.

Likewise, feminists who uncover the pervasiveness of violence should not leave the impression that aggression is an immutable part of male sexuality. With understandable frustration, some in the health and development field have reacted to the violence data with the question: What is it about male sexuality that makes men that way? I think, however, that this is the wrong question. Rather we should be asking: what is it about the construction of masculinity in different cultures that promotes aggressive sexual behaviour by men? And what is it about the construction of femininity and the structure of economic and social power relations in societies that permits this behaviour to continue?

The reason it is wrong to frame the question in terms of 'maleness' (which is normally interpreted to have biological roots) is because the cross-cultural record does not support the view that male violence against women is universal. Three separate cross-cultural studies confirm that there are at least a handful of societies where rape and/or wife abuse does not exist (or did not exist in the recent past). In her study of 156 tribal societies, for example, feminist anthropologist Peggy Reeves Sanday classified 47 per cent of the cultures she studied as essentially 'rape free' (i.e., rape was totally absent or extremely rare) (Sanday, 1981). Even if one cedes that some of the societies designated 'rape free' probably represent inadequacies in the ethnographic record rather than truly non-violent societies, the number of examples cited (and the descriptions of life in these societies) suggest that there are (or have been) at least some cultures not plagued by gender-based abuse.

Likewise, two other studies of wife abuse cross-culturally (Levinson, 1989; Counts, Brown, and Campbell, 1992) unearth additional examples of cultures where gender-based violence is absent or exceedingly rare. In his ethnographic review of ninety peasant and small-scale societies, Levinson (1989) identified sixteen that could be described as 'essentially free or untroubled by family violence'. Among the Central Thai, for example, domestic violence was extremely rare according to detailed ethnographies collected in the 1960s. Central Thai families were remarkable for the absence of any meaningful division of labour by sex: men were as likely as women to carry out household duties including child care, and women as likely as men to plough or manage the family business. Divorce was common, people preferring to separate rather than live with discord. Community norms disdained aggression; other non-violent means of conflict resolution were plentiful and preferred (Phillips, 1966).

The existence of such cultures – even if few in number – stands as proof that violence against women is not an inevitable outgrowth of male biology, male sexuality, or male hormones. It is 'male conditioning', not the 'condition of being male', that appears to be the problem. Although what it means to be 'male' varies among different cultures and within different segments of the same culture, the importance of the masculine mystique appears to be a common element in many, but not all, societies. In his book *Manhood in the Making: Cultural Concepts of Masculinity*, anthropologist David Gilmore notes that across many cultures 'there is a constantly recurring notion that real manhood is different from simple anatomical maleness, that it is not a neutral condition that comes about spontaneously through biological maturation but rather is a precarious or artificial state that boys must win against powerful odds' (Gilmore, 1990, p. 11). Gilmore observes that this notion exists among both peasants and sophisticated urban people, and among both warrior people and those who have never killed in anger. He argues further that 'manhood' represents an 'achieved status' different from parallel notions of womanhood. 'As a social icon', he writes, 'femininity ... usually involves questions of body ornament or sexual allure, or other essentially cosmetic behaviours that enhance, rather than create, an inherent quality of character. An authentic femininity rarely involves tests or proofs of action ... ' (Gilmore, 1990, p. 11).

Although I would disagree with Gilmore's last statement (in many cultures a woman must bear a child before she is considered fully human, much less a mature, adult woman), his observations about the elusive quality of manhood are nonetheless important for our analysis of sexually aggressive behaviour in men. It is my belief, shared by other theorists (such as Lancaster, 1992; Olsson, 1984; and Stolenberg, 1989) that it is partly men's insecurity about their masculinity that promotes abusive behaviour toward women. The fear that accompanies this insecurity derives in part from a gendered system that assigns power and status to that which is male and denigrates or subordinates that which is female. Men in many cultures wage daily battle to prove to themselves and others that they qualify for inclusion in the esteemed category 'male'. To be 'not male', is to be reduced to the status of woman, or worse, to be 'queer' (see below).

Since gender is socially constructed, it must be actualized through action and sensation – by doing things that repeatedly affirm that one is really male or really female while avoiding things that leave room for doubt. As social theorist John Stoltenberg observes:

> Most people born with a penis between their legs grow up aspiring to feel and act unambigu-ously male, longing to belong to the sex that is male and daring not to belong to the sex that is not, and feeling this urgency for a visceral and constant verification of their male sexual (read: gender) identity – for a fleshy connection to manhood – as the driving force of their life. The drive does not originate in the anatomy. The sensations derive from the idea. The idea gives the feelings social meaning; the idea determines which sensations shall be sought.
>
> (Stolenberg, 1989, p. 31)

Many societies have evolved elaborate rituals and rites of passage to help induct young men into manhood. Some involve brutal hazing and tests of courage while others require endur-ance, aptitude, and skill. They all share the underlying premise that real men are made, not born. This feeds into men's gender insecurity.

One way to feel unambiguously male in many cultures is to dominate women, to behave aggressively, and to take risks. A 'real man' in the Balkans, for example, is one who drinks heavily, fights bravely, and shows 'indomitable virility' by fathering many children (Denich, 1974, p. 250). In eastern Morocco, 'true men' are distinguished based on their physical prowess and heroic acts of both feuding and sexual potency (Marcus, 1987, p. 50). On the South Pacific island of Truk, fighting, drinking, defying the sea, and sexually conquering women are the true measures of manhood (Caughey 1970; Gilmore, 1990; Marshall, 1979).

Significantly, sexual conquest and potency appear as repeated themes in many cultural definitions of manhood, placing women at increased risk of coercive sex. This is as true in the United States as it is elsewhere. Recently, nine teenage boys from an upper-working-class suburb of Long Beach were arrested for allegedly molesting and raping a number of girls, some as young as ten. The boys, members of a group called the Spur Posse, acknowledge having sex with scores, or underage girls, as part of a sexual competition. In tabulating their sexual exploits, the boys make reference to the uniform number of the sports stars who are their heroes – 'I'm 44 now – Reggie Jackson. I'm 50 – David Robinson'. Tellingly, some of the boys' fathers appear boastful of their son's conquest. In a *New York Times* article, one father praised his son as 'all man' and insisted that the girls his son had had sex with were 'giving it away' (Gross, 1993).

The salience of sex to some versions of masculine identity is likewise recognized in a Swedish government report on prostitution, published in 1981:

> The male confirms and proves his maleness, his virility, through his sexuality. It becomes the core, the very essence around which he consciously and unconsciously forms his ideas about himself as a man. The female sexual identity has not been formed in relationship to sexuality, but in the need to be chosen by a man … By being chosen the woman receives the necessary proof of her value as a woman – both in her own eyes and in others.
>
> (Olsson, 1984, p. 73)

Indeed, some theorists go so far as to assert that notions of masculinity help construct the experience of sex itself. Speaking from an Anglo-American perspective, John Stolenberg argues that 'so much of most men's sexuality is tied up with gender-actualizing – with feeling like a real man – that they can scarcely recall an erotic sensation that had no gender-specific cultural meaning. As most men age, they learn to cancel out and deny erotic sensations that are not specifically linked to what they think a real man is supposed to feel' (Stolenberg, 1989, p. 33).

To the extent that masculine ideals are associated with violence, virility, and power, it is easy to see how male sexual behaviour might emerge as predatory and aggressive. Indeed, the more I work on violence against women, the more I become convinced that the real way forward is to redefine what it means to be male. When masculinity is associated with aggression and sexual conquest, domineering sexual behaviour and violence become not only a means of structuring power relations between men and women, but a way of establishing power relations among men. As Roger Lancaster observes in his ethnographic study of gender relations in Nicaragua, within many gendered systems sexual exploits are part of a system of posturing among men where women are merely the medium of competition (see Lancaster, 1992, 1995, this volume, chapter 7).

Since men have a collective interest in the perpetuation of gender hierarchies, individual male behaviour is closely monitored by the male community (and sometimes by mothers acting on behalf of their sons). When the behaviour of men or boys does not live up to the masculine ideal, they are frequently rebuked by invoking another gendered symbol: the male homosexual, however culturally defined. 'Real men' are almost always defined in opposition to the queer, the *hueco*, the *cochón*, the sissy. Homosexual stigma is invoked to enforce the masculine ideal; it becomes part of the glue that holds male dominance together.

As Lancaster points out in his Nicaraguan example, homosexual stigma helps structure and perpetuate male sexual and gender norms. Lancaster maintains that by adolescence, boys are in open competition for the status of manhood. 'The signs of masculinity', he argues, 'are actively struggled for, and can only be won by wresting them away from other boys around them' (Lancaster, 1992, 1995).

Fortunately, the ethnographic record provides us with examples to prove that the world need not be constructed this way. After exhaustively reviewing existing information on masculinity cross-culturally, Gilmore notes that while 'ideas and anxieties about masculinity as a special-status category of achievement are widespread in societies around the world, being expressed to varying degrees ... they do not seem to be absolutely universal' (Gilmore, 1990). He cites several exceptions; cultures where manhood is of minimal interest to men and where there is little or no social pressure to act 'manly'.

Among Gilmore's examples are the Semai people of Malaysia and inhabitants of Tahiti. In Tahiti, for example, there are no strict gender roles, no concept of male honour to defend, and no social expectations to 'get even'. Men share a cultural value of 'timidity' that forbids retaliation, and even when provoked, men rarely become violent. According to Gilmore, the concept of 'manliness' as separate from femininity is simply foreign to them (Gilmore, 1990). An extensive ethnographic record reveals that a similar description would be appropriate for the Semai of Malaysia as well (Dentan, 1979).

What is intriguing about these two examples is that they conform well to the picture of other societies known to have low or non-existent levels of violence against women. Indeed, both Peggy Sanday's cross-cultural study of rape and the anthology *Sanctions and Sanctuary*, a cross-cultural look at wife beating, found that one of the strongest predictors/correlates of societies with high violence against women was the presence of a masculine ideal that emphasized dominance, toughness, or male honour (Counts, Brown, and Campbell, 1992).[10] While these types of studies cannot prove causality, they do begin to suggest which factors appear

Table 15.5 Correlates of gender violence based on cross-cultural studies

Predictive of high violence	Predictive of low violence
1. Violent interpersonal conflict resolution[1, 3]	1. Female power outside of the home[1, 2, 3]
2. Economic inequality between men and women[3]	2. Active community interference in violence[2, 3]
3. Masculine ideal of male dominance/toughness/honour[1, 2]	3. Presence of exclusively female groups (work or solidarity)[2, 3]
4. Male economic and decision-making authority in the family[3]	4. Sanctuary (shelters/friends/family)[2]

[1]   Sanday, 1981
[2]   Counts, Brown and Campbell, 1992
[3]   Levinson, 1989

especially predictive of high rates of violence against women versus those that predict low rates of gender violence. Table 15.5 presents a simplified account of the major findings of the Levinson, Sanday, and *Sanctions and Sanctuary* studies.

Interestingly, the findings strongly support the feminist contention that hierarchical gender relations – perpetuated through gender socialization and the socio-economic inequalities of society – are integrally related to violence against women. Male decision-making in the home and economic inequality between men and women are strongly correlated with high rates of violence against women, while women having power outside of the home (whether political, economic, or magical) seems to offer some protection against abuse. Another particularly strong factor seems to be the social acceptance of violence as a way to resolve conflict: where interpersonal violence is tolerated in the society at large, women are at higher risk. Given that much behaviour is learned by children through modelling, this finding is hardly surprising.

This generic picture conforms well to actual ethnographic descriptions of societies with little or no violence against women. Sanday uses the Mbuti Pygmies, a forest-dwelling people, to illustrate her point. Violence between the sexes, or between anybody, is virtually absent among the Mbuti Pygmies when they are in their forest environment. There is little division of labour by sex. A man is not ashamed to pick mushrooms and nuts if he finds them, or to wash and clean a baby. Decision-making is by common consent; men and women have equal say because hunting and gathering are both important to the economy (Turnbull, 1965). This description sounds remarkably similar to that offered for the Cental Thai, the Semai of Malaysia, and the Tahitians, described earlier.

The factors that emerge as predictive of low violence are also enlightening. In addition to female power, the presence of all-female coalitions or work groups appears to be significant. Whether this operates by increasing women's economic power or through female solidarity and consciousness-raising remains unclear. Especially significant appears to be the presence of strong sanctions against violence and access to sanctuary (hence the name of the anthology, *Sanctions and Sanctuary*). Sanctions can take the form of swift legal response, or they can involve informal community sanctions, like public humiliation. Likewise, 'sanctuary' can be formal shelters or merely the cultural understanding that neighbours and/or family members will take in a woman whose partner is threatening her. Violence appears especially common in cultures where women leave their natal village to get married; not only are family members not present to intervene in disputes, but it is more difficult for the woman to seek refuge when relatives are distant (Counts, Brown and Campbell, 1992). In fact, active community or family interference in violent events emerged as important predictors of low violence in both of the wife-beating studies.

Conclusion

These cross-cultural titbits suggest that the possibility of a world without violence against women is not a hopeless fantasy. Societies have existed, and may still exist, that are essentially free of gender-based abuse. But social movements must have both vision and a sense of responsibility to those who must live within today's reality. The overwhelming presence of violence in many women's lives demands that we work on two fronts; to challenge the gender-based inequities and beliefs that perpetuate male violence and to provide services and support to those attempting to survive, despite the social forces allied against them. A range of professions – public health, family planning, sexuality research – have important roles to play. They can marshal their resources to help untangle the complex web of social forces that encourage violent behaviour; they can design programmes to empower women and enlighten men; and they can identify and refer women to helpful services. Given the health and social consequences of abuse, this is not only their prerogative, but their obligation.

Notes

1　As it stands, most international development funders see violence as outside of their area of responsibility. International funding tends to be very sectoral, with aid streams targeted specifically to education, agriculture, population control, or health. Since anti-violence initiatives – such as crisis centres, law-reform efforts, and public education – do not fall easily within any of these categories, they frequently cannot get outside funding or support. The *Violence, Health and Development* project helps articulate the links between violence and women's health with an eye towards recruiting more health dollars for violence-related programming.

2　Although individually valid, these studies are not directly comparable because each uses a different set of questions to probe for abuse. The vast majority of studies ask the respondents whether they have been 'abused', 'beaten', or 'involved in a violent relationship'. A subset (e.g., the studies from Barbados and United States) make this determination based on a list of 'acts' that a woman may or may not have been subjected to during her lifetime (e.g., hitting with fist, biting, being hit with an object, etc). Clinical and research experience suggests that allowing women to self-define abuse, if anything, underestimates the level of physical and psychological violence in intimate relationships. In many cultures, women are socialized to accept physical and emotional chastisement as part of a husband's marital prerogative, thereby limiting the range of behaviour women consider 'abuse'. Moreover, women are sometimes reluctant to report abuse out of shame or fear of incriminating other family members. Both factors suggest that the prevalence rates in Table 15.2 are likely to be underestimates of actual abuse.

3　All of the studies use legally grounded definitions of rape; thus, forms of penetration other than penile-vaginal are included and women were not instructed to exclude rape by husbands. Questions were typically framed to define explicitly the behaviours that should be included in the definition. For example: 'Has a man made you have sex by using force or threatening to harm you? When we use the word "sex" we mean a man putting his penis in your vagina even if he didn't ejaculate (come)?' This is followed by: 'If he did not try to put his penis in your vagina, has a man made you do other sexual things like oral sex, or put fingers or objects inside you by using force or threatening to harm you?'

4　The estimates in Table 15.3 are based on existing legal definitions of rape in the United States, which recognize penetration of any orifice by physical force or threat of force, or because a woman is incapacitated due to drugs or alcohol.

5　In evaluating the sources of variability in prevalence of sexual abuse, Peters, Wyatt and Finkelhor (1986) suggest that differences in definitions and the various methods used in these studies probably account for most of the variations reported.

6　This figure is quoted in 'Rape: Can I have this Child?' a photonovela produced by Movimiento Manuela Ramos, Lima, Peru, as part of their campaign to decriminalize abortion in cases of rape.

7　Another significant subset reported positive initiations. While recalling some lack of pleasure due to inexperience, these girls actively agreed to intercourse and considered it part of an on-going process of sexual discovery that began earlier in life with sex play, petting, and masturbation

8   By no means is male approval always the greatest determinant of contraceptive use. For examples of cases where it is, see Gallen (1986) and Kincaid (1992).
9   Variables controlled for include: years in legal or common-law union during previous five years; raised in lower-class home; education of mother; education of father; raised in stable nuclear family; raised solely by mother; raised with a step-father; degree of affection mother's partner showed her; degree of physical and emotional abuse to mother; degree of affection mother showed son; degree of affection mother's partner showed son; degree to which mother's partner physically and emotionally abused son; man's education status; man's occupational status.
10 There are examples of peaceful societies that do have a notion of 'achieved manhood', but generally this manhood is not linked to dominance, male honour, or aggression but to skill, often in the realm of hunting. In these societies – such as the Mbuti Pygmies and the !Kung Bushmen – hunting is not an 'outlet for aggression', but is seen as 'a contribution to society of both indispensable economic and spiritual value ... truly a kind of indirect nourishment or nurturing' (Gilmore, 1990, p. 116).

References

ALLEN, S.M. (1982) 'Adolescent pregnancy among 11–15 year old girls in the parish of Manchester', dissertation for diploma in community health, Kingston, University of the West Indies, cited in MACCORMACK, C.P. and DRAPER, A., 'Social and cognitive aspects of female sexuality in Jamaica', in P. CAPLAN (ed.) (1987), *The Cultural Construction of Sexuality*, London: Tavistock Publications.

APT, C. and HURLBERT, D. (1993) 'The sexuality of women in physically abusive marriage: a comparative study', *Journal of Family Violence*, 8(1), pp. 57–69.

BANWELL, S.S. (1990) *Law, Status of Women and Family Planning in Sub-Saharan Africa: A Suggestion for Action*, Nairobi: The Pathfinder Fund.

BEATTIE, V. (1992) 'Analysis of the Results of a Survey on Sexual Violence in the UK', Cambridge: Women's Forum, unpublished manuscript.

BECKER, J.V., SKINNER, L.J., ABEL, G.G. and TREACY, E.C. (1982) 'Incidence and types of sexual dysfunctions in rape and incest victims', *Journal of Sex and Marital Therapy*, 8, pp. 65–74.

BENERIA, L. and ROLDAN, M. (1987) *The Crossroads of Class and Gender*, Chicago: University of Chicago Press.

BOWKER, L.H. (1983) *Beating Wife Beating*, Lexington, KY: Lexington Books.

BROWNE, A. (1987) *When Battered Women Kill*, New York: The Free Press.

BULLOCK, L.F. and MACFARLANE, J. (1989) 'The birthweight/battering connection', *American Journal of Nursing*, 89, pp. 1153–5.

BURNAM, M.A. (1988) 'Sexual assault and mental disorders in a community population', *Journal of Consulting and Clinical Psychology*, 56(6), pp. 843–50.

CAMPBELL, J. and ALFORD, P. (1989) 'The dark consequences of marital rape', *American Journal of Nursing*, July, pp. 946–8.

CANADIAN GOVERNMENT (1984) *Sexual Offenses Against Children*, Vol. 1, Ottawa: Canadian Publishing Centre.

CAUGHEY, J.L. (1970) 'Cultural values in Micronesian society', unpublished PhD dissertation, University of Pennsylvania.

CHACON, K. *et al.* (1990) 'Caracteristicas de la mujer agredida atendida en el Patronato Nacional de la Infancia (PANI)', San José, Costa Rica, cited in BATRES, G. and CLARAMUT, C., *La violencia contra la mujer en la familia costarricense: un problema de salud publica*, San Jose: Costa Rica: ILANUD.

COLE, S. (1989) *Pornography and the Sex Crisis*, Toronto: Amanita Enterprises.

COOK, R. and MAINE, D. (1987) 'Spousal veto over family planning services', *American Journal of Public Health*, 77(3), pp. 339–44.

COUNTS, D., BROWN, J. and CAMPBELL, J. (eds) (1992) *Sanctions and Sanctuary*, Boulder, CO: Westview Press.

DATAPRO AND ASOCIACION GUATEMALTECO PARA LA PREVENCION Y CONTROL DE SIDA (1991) *Guatemala City Women: Empowering a Vulnerable Group for HIV Prevention*, Guatemala City: DataPro.

DEKESEREDY, W. and KELLY, K. (1992) Private Communication. 'Preliminary data from first national study on dating violence in Canada', Ottawa: Family Violence Prevention Division, Department of Health and Welfare.

DELACOSTE, F. and ALEXANDER, P. (1987) *Sex Work: Writings by Women in the Sex Industry*, Pittsburgh, PA: Cleis Press.

DENICH, B. (1974) 'Sex and power in the Balkans', in ROSALDO, M. and LAMPHERE, L. (eds), *Women, Culture and Society*, Palo Alto, CA: Stanford University Press.

DENTAN, R. (1979) *The Semai: A Nonviolent People of Malaya*, New York: Holt, Rinehart and Winston.

DIXON-MUELLER, R. (1992) 'Sexuality, gender and reproductive health', working paper prepared for International Women's Health Coalition, New York.

—— (1993) *Population Policy and Women's Rights: Transforming Reproductive Choice*, Westport, CT: Praeger.

EHRHARDT, A.A. (1991) 'Speech delivered at the first National Conference on Women and HIV Infection', sponsored by the National Institutes of Health and Centers for Disease Control, Washington, DC.

ELIAS, C. and HEISE, L. (1993) 'The development of microbicides: a new method of HIV prevention for women', *Programs Division Working Paper 6*, New York: The Population Council, Routledge.

FINKELHOR, D. (1987) 'The sexual abuse of children: current research reviewed', *Psychiatric Annals*, 17, pp. 233–41.

FOLCH-LYON, E., MACORRA, L., and SCHEARER, S.B. (1981) 'Focus group and survey research on family planning in Mexico', *Studies in Family Planning*, 12(12), pp. 409–32.

FORT, A.L. (1989) 'Investigation of the social context of fertility and family planning: a qualitative study in Peru', *International Family Planning Perspectives*, 15(3), pp. 88–94.

GALLEN, M.A. (1986) 'Men – new focus for family planning programs', *Population Reports*, Series J., pp. 33.

GAVEY, N. (1991) 'Sexual victimization prevalence among New Zealand University students', *Journal of Consulting and Clinical Psychology*, 59, pp. 464–6.

GILMORE, D.D. (1990) *Manhood in the Making: Cultural Concepts of Masculinity*, New Haven, CT: Yale University Press.

GRANT, R., PREDA, M. and MARTIN, J.D. (1991) *Domestic Violence in Texas: A Study of State-wide and Rural Spouse Abuse*, Midwestern State University: Bureau of Business and Government Research.

GROSS, J. (1993) 'Where "boys will be boys" and adults are befuddled', *New York Times*, 29 March.

GUPTA, G.R. and WEISS, E. (1995) 'Women's lives and sex: implications for AIDS prevention' in PARKER, R.G. and GAGNON, J.H. (eds) *Conceiving Sexuality: Approaches to Sex Research in a Postmodern World*, New York and London: Routledge.

HANDWERKER, P. (1991) 'Gender power difference may be STD risk factor for the next generation', paper presented at the 90th Annual Meeting of the American Anthropological Association, Chicago.

—— (1993) 'Power, gender violence, and high risk sexual behavior: AIDS/STD risk factors need to be defined more broadly', private communication, Department of Anthropology, Humboldt State University, 10 February.

HEGLAND, M.E. (n.d.) Personal Communication.

ISIS INTERNATIONAL (1988) 'Campaña sobre la violencia en contra de la mujer', Boletin 16–17, Red de Salud de las Mujeres Latinoamericanas y del Caribe, Santiago, Chile: Isis International.

JAMES, J. and MEYERDING, J. (1977) 'Early sexual experience and prostitution', *American Journal of Psychiatry*, 134, pp. 1381–5.

KILPATRICK, D.G., EDMUND, C.N. and SEYMOR, A.K. (1992) *Rape in America: A Report to the Nation*, Arlington, VN: The National Victims Center.

KINCAID, D.L. (1992) 'Family planning and the empowerment of women in Bangledesh', paper presented at the 119th Annual Meeting of the American Public Health Association, Atlanta, GA, 13 November.

KISEKKA, M. and OTESANYA, B. (1988) 'Sexually transmitted disease as a gender issue: example from Nigeria and Uganda', paper presented at the AFARD/AAWORD Third General Assembly on 'The African crisis and the women's vision of the way out', Dakar, August.

KOSS, M.P., GIDYCZ, C.A. and WISNIEWSKI, N. (1987) 'The scope of rape: incidence and prevalence of sexual aggression and victimization in a national sample of higher education students', *Journal of Consulting and Clinical Psychology*, 55, pp. 162–70.

—— and OROS, C.J. (1982) 'Sexual experiences survey: a research instrument investigating sexual aggression and victimization', *Journal of Consulting and Clinical Psychology*, 50, pp. 455–7.

LANCASTER, R.N. (1992) *Life is Hard: Machismo, Danger, and the Intimacy of Power in Nicaragua*, Berkeley and Los Angeles: University of California Press.

—— (1995) 'That we should all turn queer?' homosexual stigma in the making of manhood and the breaking of a revolution in Nicaragua', in PARKER, R.G. and GAGNON, J.H. (eds) *Conceiving Sexuality: Approaches to Sex Research in a Postmodern World*, New York and London: Routledge.

LARRAIN, S. (1993) *Estudio de frecuencia de la violencia intrafamiliar y la condición de la mujer en Chile*, Santiago, Chile: Pan American Health Organization.

LEVINSON, D. (1989) *Violence in Cross-Cultural Perspective*, Newbury Park, CA: Sage Publishers.

LISKIN, L.S. (1981) 'Periodic abstinence: how well do new approaches work?', *Population Reports*, Baltimore, MD: Population Information Program, Johns Hopkins Schools of Hygiene and Public Health.

MACKINNON, C. (1991) 'Does sexuality have a history?', *Michigan Quarterly Review*, 30(1), pp. 1–11.

MACFARLANE, J., *et al.* (1992) 'Assessing for abuse during pregnancy: severity and frequency of inquiries and associated entry into prenatal care', *Journal of the American Medical Society*, 267(23), pp. 3176–8.

MAHAJAN, A. (1990) 'Instigators of wife battering', in SOOD, S. (ed.) *Violence Against Women*, Jaipur, India: Arihant Publishers.

MARCUS, M. (1987) 'Horsemen are the fence of the land: honor and history among the Ghiyata of Eastern Morocco', in GILMORE, D.D. (ed.), *Honor and Shame and the Unity of the Mediterranean*, Washington DC: American Anthropological Association, special publication, No. 22.

MARSHALL, M. (1979) *Weekend Warriors*, Palo Alto, CA: Mayfield.

MOORE, K.A., NORD, C.W. and PETERSON, J. (1989) 'Nonvoluntary sexual activity among adolescents', *Family Planning Perspectives*, 21(3), p. 110–14.

MULLEN, P.E. *et al.* (1988) 'Impact of sexual and physical abuse on women's mental health', *Lancet*, 1, pp. 841.

OKUN, L.E. (1986) *Woman Abuse: Facts Replacing Myths*, Albany: State University of New York Press.

OLSSON, H. (1984) 'The woman, the love, and the power', in BARRY, K., BUNCH, C. and CASTLEY, S. (eds) *International Feminism: Networking Against Female Sexual Slavery*, New York: International Tribune Center.

PAGLIA, C. (1992) *Sex, Art and American Culture*, New York: Vintage Books.

PETERS, S.D., WYATT, G.E. and FINKELHOR, D.P. (1986) 'Prevalence', in FINKELHOR, D. (ed.), *A Source Book on Child Sexual Abuse*, Beverly Hills, CA: Sage.

PHILLIPS, H.P. (1966) *Thai Peasant Personality: The Patterning of Interpersonal Behavior in the Village of Bang Chan*, Berkeley: University of California Pres.

PROFAMILIA (1992) 'Estudio sobre la violencia contra la mujer en la familia basado en la encuesta realizada a las mujeres maltratadas que acudieron al servicio jurídico de ProFamilia entre el 15 de Marzo de 1989 y el 30 de Marzo de 1990', in *La violencia e los derechos humanos de la mujer*, Bogota: ProFamilia.

RAIKES, A. (1990) *Pregnancy, Birthing and Family Planning in Kenya: Changing Patterns of Behavior: A Health Utilization Study in Kissi District*, Copenhagen: Centre for Development Research.

RAMIREZ, J.C.R. and VAZQUEZ, G.U. (1993) 'Mujer y violencia: un hecho cotidiano', in *Salud publica de Mexico*, Cuernavaca: Instituto Nacional de Salud Publica.

RHODENBAUGH, S. (1991) 'Catherine MacKinnon: may I speak?', *Michigan Quarterly Review*, 30, 3, pp. 415–22.

SANDAY, P. (1981) 'The socio-cultural context of rape: a cross cultural study', *Journal of Social Issues*, 37(4), pp. 5–27.

SCHEI, B. and BAKKESTEIG, L.S. (1989) 'Gynaecological impact of sexual and physical abuse by spouse: a study of a random sample of Norwegian women', *British Journal of Obstetrics and Gynaecology*, 96, pp. 1379–83.

SHIM, Y.H. (1992) 'Sexual violence against women in Korea: a victimization survey of Seoul women', paper presented at the conference on 'International perspectives: crime, justice, and public order', St Petersburg, Russia, 21–27 June.

SOGBETUN, A.O., ALAUSA, K.O., and OSOBA, A.O. (1977) 'Sexually transmitted disease in Ibadan, Nigeria', *British Journal of Venereal Disease*, 53, pp. 158.

SONALI, D. (1990) *Brave New Families: Stories of Domestic Upheavel in Late Twentieth Century America*, New York: Basic.

STARK, E., FLITCRAFT, A., ZUCKERMAN, B., GREY, A., ROBINSON, J. and FRAZIER, W. (1981) 'Wife abuse in the medical setting: an introduction for health personnel', monograph 7, Washington, DC: Office of Domestic Violence.

STOLENBERG, J. (1989) *Refusing to Be a Man: Essays on Sex and Justice*, Portland, OR: Breiten Bush Books.

STRAUS, M.A. and GELLES, R.J. (1986) 'Societal change and change in family violence from 1975 to 1985 as revealed by two national surveys', *Journal of Marriage and the Family*, 48, pp. 465–79.

THOMPSON, S. (1990) 'Putting a big thing into a little hole: teenage girls' accounts of sexual initiation', *The Journal of Sex Research*, 27(3), pp. 341–61.

TESKE, R. Jr. and PARKER, M. (1983) 'Spouse abuse in Texas: a study of women's attitudes and experiences', Austin: Texas Department of Human Resources.

TIEFER, L. (1992) 'Feminism matters in sexology', in BEZEMER, W. *et al.* (eds), *Sex Matters*, Amsterdam: Elsevier Science Publishers.

TURNBULL, C. (1965) 'The Mbuti Pygmies: an ethnographic survey', *Anthropological Papers of the American Museum of Natural History*, 50, pp. 137–282.

TOFT, S. (ed.) (1987) *Domestic Violence in Papua New Guinea*, Law Reform Commission Occasional Paper No. 19, Port Morseby, Papua New Guinea.

UGALDE, J.G. (1988) 'Sindrome de la mujer agredida', *Mujer*, No. 5, San Jose, Costa Rica: Cefemina.

VALDEZ, R.S. and COX, E.S. (1990) *La violencia hacia la mujer Mexicana como problema de salud pública: la incidencia de la violencia domestica en una microregión de Ciudad Nexahualcoyotl*, Mexico City: CECOVID.

VALVERDE, M. (1987) *Sex, Power, and Pleasure*, Philadelphia, PA: New Society Publishers.

VANCE, C.S. (1984) *Pleasure and Danger: Exploring Women's Sexuality*, New York: Routledge and Kegan Paul.

WAO (Woman's Action Organization) (1992) *Draft Report of the National Study on Domestic Violence*, Kuala Lampur: Malaysia.

WOLF, N. (1992) 'Feminist fatale', *New Republic*, 16 March.

WORTH, D. (1991) 'Sexual violence against women and substance abuse', paper presented to The Domestic Violence Task Force, New York, January.

ZAPATA, C. *et al.* (1992) 'The influence of social and political violence on the risk of pregnancy complications', *American Journal of Public Health*, 82(5), pp. 685–90.

ZIERLER, S. (1991) 'Adult survivors of childhood sexual abuse and subsequent risk of HIV infection', *American Journal of Public Health*, 81(5), pp. 572–5.

16 Reproductive and sexual rights

A feminist perspective

Sonia Corrêa and Rosalind Petchesky [1994]

In current debates about the impact of population policies on women, the concept of reproductive and sexual rights is both stronger and more contested than ever before. Those who take issue with this concept include religious fundamentalists, as well as opponents of human rights in general, who associate human rights with individualist traditions deriving from Western capitalism. Some feminists, too, are sceptical about the readiness with which advocates of fertility reduction programmes, whose primary concern is neither women's health nor their empowerment, have adopted the language of reproductive rights to serve their own agendas.

As a Southern and a Northern feminist who have written about and organized for women's reproductive health for many years, we are conscious of the tensions and multiple perspectives surrounding this conceptual territory. Our purpose in this chapter is not to impose a concept, but to explore a different way of thinking about it in order to advance the debate. We define the terrain of reproductive and sexual rights in terms of power and resources: power to make informed decisions about one's own fertility, childbearing, child rearing, gynaecologic health, and sexual activity; and resources to carry out such decisions safely and effectively. This terrain necessarily involves some core notion of 'bodily integrity', or 'control over one's body'. However, it also involves one's relationships to one's children, sexual partners, family members, community, caregivers, and society at large; in other words, the body exists in a socially mediated universe.

Following a review of the epistemological and historical underpinnings of this concept, we address several fundamental problems that critics have raised about rights discourse: its indeterminate language, its individualist bias, its presumption of universality, and its dichotomization of 'public' and 'private' spheres. We argue that rather than abandoning rights discourse, we should reconstruct it so that it both specifies gender, class, cultural, and other differences and recognizes social needs. Our principal point is that sexual and reproductive (or any other) rights, understood as private 'liberties' or 'choices', are meaningless, especially for the poorest and most disenfranchised, without *enabling conditions* through which they can be realized. These conditions constitute *social rights* and involve social welfare, personal security, and political freedom. Their provision is essential to the democratic transformation of societies to abolish gender, class, racial, and ethnic injustice.

We then analyse the ethical bases of reproductive and sexual rights, and propose four component principles: bodily integrity, personhood, equality, and respect for diversity. In examining each of these principles, we emphasize the broader social implications that ethicists, legal scholars, and demographers often ignore. All four principles, as we interpret them, both derive from and further society's interest in empowered and politically responsible citizens, including all women. By thus linking reproductive and sexual rights to development, we challenge legalistic notions of civil and political rights that still dominate the human rights field.

Throughout this discussion, we raise a number of policy-related issues. When are reproductive and sexual decisions freely made and when coerced? What is the relationship between women's reproductive and sexual rights and responsibilities and men's, and should women's social and biological positioning in reproduction give us a privileged voice in the construction of rights? Is there a 'right to procreate' or a 'socially responsible' way to make procreative decisions? What conditions predicate 'socially responsible' decision-making? What are the obligations of state governments and international organizations to provide the necessary conditions for 'free and responsible choices'?

We are suggesting not that reproductive and sexual rights are absolute or that women have the right to reproduce under any circumstances, but that policies to enforce those rights must address existing social conditions and begin to change them. We conclude by proposing a feminist social rights approach to population and development policies.

Epistemological and historical premises

Contrary to many social critics, we are not convinced that reproductive and sexual rights (or human rights) are simply a 'Western' concept. As Kamla Bhasin and Nighat Khan (1986) have argued with regard to feminism in South Asia, 'an idea cannot be confined within national or geographic boundaries'. Postcolonial writers and Southern governments have readily adopted, and adapted, the theories of Marx, Malthus, or Milton Friedman to suit their own purposes. Democracy movements in postcolonial societies easily invoke rights when it comes to voting, or forming political parties or trade unions. Why should concepts such as 'reproductive rights', 'bodily integrity', and women's right to sexual self-determination be any less adaptable?

Second, we assume that ethical norms and language itself are always subject to historical variation and political contestation. Feminist engagement in the debate over the meanings of rights, including reproductive and sexual rights, is a necessary part of our efforts to transform women's situation as citizens, nationally, and internationally. Changing the rhetoric of legal instruments or official policies can be one strategic step toward transforming the conditions of people's lives.

The term 'reproductive rights' is of recent – and probably North American[1] – origin, but its roots in ideas of bodily integrity and sexual self-determination have a much older and culturally broader genealogy. The idea that women in particular must be able 'to decide whether, when, and how to have children' originated in the feminist birth-control movements that developed at least as early as the 1830s among the Owenite socialists in England and spread to many parts of the world over the course of a century (Chesler, 1992; Gordon, 1976; Huston, 1992; Jayawardena, 1993; Ramusack, 1989; Weeks 1981). Leaders of these movements in Western countries, such as Margaret Sanger in North America and Stella Browne in England, linked 'the problem of birth control' not only with women's struggle for social and political emancipation, but also with their need to 'own and control' their bodies and to obtain sexual knowledge and satisfaction (Sanger, 1920). Their counterparts among women's rights advocates in nineteenth-century Europe and America and among the early birth-control pioneers in twentieth-century Asia, North Africa, and Latin America were more reticent about women's sexuality, emphasizing instead a negative right: that of women (married or single) to refuse unwanted sex or childbearing.

Underlying both the defensive and the affirmative versions of these early feminist prototypes of reproductive rights language were the same basic principles of *equality, personhood,* and *bodily integrity*. They held a common premise: in order for women to achieve equal status with men in society, they must be respected as full moral agents with projects and ends of their own; hence they alone must determine the uses – sexual, reproductive, or other – to which their bodies (and minds) are put.[2]

In the late 1970s and early 1980s, women's health movements emerged throughout Asia, Latin America, Europe and North America (DAWN, 1993; García-Moreno and Claro, 1994). These movements aimed at achieving the ability of women, *both* as individuals *and* in their collective organizational forms and community identities, to determine their own reproductive and sexual lives in conditions of optimum health and economic and social well-being. They did not imagine women as atoms completely separate from larger social contexts; rather, they consciously linked the principle of 'women's right to decide' about fertility and childbearing to 'the social, economic and political conditions that make such decisions possible' (Women's Global Network for Reproductive Rights, 1991).

Increasingly, as women of colour in Northern societies and women from Southern countries have taken leadership in developing the meanings of sexual and reproductive rights for women, these meanings have expanded. They have come to encompass both a broader range of issues than fertility regulation (including, for example, maternal and infant mortality, infertility, unwanted sterilization, malnutrition of girls and women, female genital mutilation, sexual violence, and sexually transmitted diseases); and a better understanding of the structural conditions that constrain reproductive and sexual decisions (such as reductions in social-sector expenditures resulting from structural adjustment programmes; lack of transportation, water, sanitation, and child care; illiteracy; and poverty). In other words, the concept of sexual and reproductive *rights* is being enlarged to address the *social needs* that erode reproductive and sexual choice for the majority of the world's women, who are poor (Desai, 1994; Petchesky and Weiner, 1990).

In the past decade, the integral tie between reproductive rights and women's sexual self-determination, including the right to sexual pleasure, has gained recognition not only in the North, but in Latin America, Africa and Asia.[3] As the Women's Resource and Research Center (WRRC) in the Philippines states in its *Institutional Framework and Strategies on Reproductive Rights* (Fabros, 1991), 'self-determination and pleasure in sexuality is one of the primary meanings of the idea of "control over one's body" and a principal reason for access to safe abortion and birth control'. Anchoring the possibility of women's *individual* right to health, well-being, and 'self-determined sexual lives' to the *social* changes necessary to eliminate poverty and empower women, this framework dissolves the boundary between sexuality, human rights, and development. It thus opens a wider lens not only on reproductive and sexual rights, but on rights in general.

Rights discourse: rethinking rights as individual and social

The discourse of (human) rights has come under heavy assault in recent years, from, among others, feminist, Marxist, and postmodernist sources (Olsen, 1984; Tushnet, 1984; Unger, 1983). Critics point out, first, that the value and meaning of rights are always contingent upon the political and social context; even the most traditional, authoritarian, patriarchal regimes will have some notion of correlative rights and duties that may be turned to the advantage of the state or corporate powers and made to perpetuate the burdens of citizens or the powerless. Second, rights language is indeterminate; if women demand their sexual and reproductive rights, male partners can demand theirs, foetuses (or foetal advocates) can demand theirs, clinicians and pharmaceutical companies theirs, and so forth. Finally there is the problem of abstract individualism and universality typically ascribed to rights language. In the classical liberal model of supposedly equal individuals choosing and bargaining to get satisfaction of their rights, differences of economic condition, race, gender, or other social circumstance that structure real people's lack of choice are rendered invisible (Rosenfeld, 1992).

While these criticisms are theoretically compelling, they offer no alternative discourse for social movements to make collective political claims. Whatever its theoretical weaknesses, the polemical power of rights language as an expression of aspirations for justice across widely different cultures and political-economic conditions cannot easily be dismissed (Heller, 1992). In practice, then, the language of rights remains indispensable but needs radical redefinition.

Feminist theorists and activists have figured prominently in efforts to shed the abstract universality, formalism, individualism and antagonism encumbering rights language (Bunch, 1990; Crenshaw, 1991; Friedman, 1992; Nedelsky, 1989; Petchesky, 1994; Schneider, 1991; Williams, 1991). Allying themselves with worldwide struggles for democratization among indigenous peoples, ethnic minorities, sexual minorities, immigrant groups, and oppressed majorities – all of whom invoke the language of 'human rights' – they seek to recast rights discourse in a more inclusive 'referential universe' (Williams, 1991). The purpose is to transform the classical liberal rights model in order: (1) to emphasize the *social*, not just individual, nature of rights, thus shifting the major burden of correlative duties from individuals to public agencies; (2) to acknowledge the *communal* (relational) *contexts* in which individuals act to exercise or pursue their rights; (3) to foreground the *substantive* basis of rights in human needs and a redistribution of resources; and (4) to recognize the bearers of rights in their self-defined, multiple identities, including their gender, class, sexual orientation, race, and ethnicity.

Classical liberal rights discourse has traditionally assumed a sharp division between 'public' and 'private' spheres and a tendency of individuals to act only with reference to narrow self-interests rather than any concept of public good. According to this dualistic vision of society, rights exist in a 'private' domain where 'individuals' ought to be pretty much left alone by the state to maximize their self-interests according to market demands. Feminist political theorists have amply criticized this presumed public–private division, pointing out that both domains in most societies tend to be dominated by men and that male dominance in one sphere reinforces it in the other (Eisenstein, 1983; Elshtain, 1981; Kelly, 1984; Okin, 1979). Thus the construction of a legal and normative boundary between 'public' and 'private' insulates the daily, routine practices of gender subordination – in the home, the workplace, the streets, and religious institutions. It masks the ways in which women's labour and services as caretakers and reproducers provide the material and emotional basis for 'publics' to survive:

> For many girls and women, the most severe violations of their human rights are rooted deeply within the family system, bolstered by community norms of male privilege and frequently justified by religious doctrines or appeals to custom or tradition. These hidden injuries of gender are rarely addressed in public policies and international assemblies because they threaten collective beliefs in the 'sanctity, harmony, and stability' of the family unit.
>
> (Dixon-Mueller, 1993)

Feminist writings and actions in defence of women's human rights build on these critiques to challenge the customary reluctance of states and international agencies to intervene in traditionally defined 'family matters'. Through vigorous international campaigns leading up to and beyond the United Nations Human Rights Conference in Vienna in 1993, they have called for national and international sanctions against gender-based violations of human rights, and they have shown how such violations occur most frequently in the supposedly private realms of family, reproduction, and sexuality (for example, through endemic violence against women). Inaction by public authorities in response to such violations – whether at the hand of state officials, nongovernmental organizations (NGOs), or spouses – constitutes, they argue, a form of acquiescence (Bunch, 1990; Cook, 1993b; Copelon, 1994; Freedman and Isaacs, 1993; Heise, 1992).

By prying open the 'citadel of privacy', feminist legal and political theory offers a wedge with which to challenge the claims of 'tradition' and 'local culture' used to defeat domestic application of international human rights norms (see Boland, Rao and Zeidenstein, 1994). Feminist deconstructions of the public–private division also point to a model of reproductive and sexual behaviour that is socially contextualized, contrasting sharply with the assumption of the classical liberal model and of many family planners and demographers (echoing Malthus) that women's reproductive decisions reflect only narrow self-interest. Supported by sociological and anthropological data, they show, on the contrary, that such decisions are usually made under enormous pressures from family, community, and society to comply with prevailing gender and reproductive norms, as well as internalized commitments to act responsibly toward others.

A social model of human behaviour does not assume that individuals make decisions in a vacuum or that 'choices' are equally 'free' for everyone. Group identities that are complex and 'intersectional' (across gender, class, ethnicity, religion, age, nationality) pull women's decisions in multiple directions. Moreover, because of existing social inequalities, the resources and range of options women have at their disposal differ greatly, affecting their ability to exercise their rights (Crenshaw, 1991; Eisenstein, 1994; Williams, 1991).

How does this interactive, socially embedded model of personal decision-making apply to the realm of sexual and reproductive rights? Qualitative data across a variety of cultural and historical settings suggest that the extent to which reproductive and sexual decisions are 'freely' made eludes easy classification; but 'free' or 'voluntary', whatever its meaning, is not the same as isolated or individualistic. In each concrete case we must weigh the multiple social, economic, and cultural factors that come to bear on a woman's decision and constitute its local meaning. Women's decisions about whether or not to bring a pregnancy to term are most frequently made in consultation with, under the constraint of, and sometimes in resistance against networks of significant others – mothers, mothers-in-law, sisters, other kin, neighbours; sometimes husbands or male partners, sometimes not (Adams and Castle, 1994; Ezeh, 1993; Gilligan, 1982; Jeffery, Jeffery and Lyon, 1989; Khattab, 1992; Petchesky, 1990). While some communities or female kin networks may function as sites of support for women's reproductive freedom – for example, facilitating clandestine abortion or contraception, or refusal of unwanted sex – others may present direct barriers or antagonisms. Jealous or violent husbands or vigilant in-laws may prevent women from visiting clinics, using condoms, getting abortions, or attending workshops on women's health, thus not only constricting their 'choices' but increasing their risks of unwanted pregnancy, maternal mortality, sexually transmitted diseases (STDs), and AIDS (Heise, 1992; Protacio, 1990; Ramasubban, 1990). Indeed, rightwing religious movements to restore 'family values' and 'community traditions' may harbour some men's distrust of the communities women make and their aim to refortify the conjugal dyad, where women are isolated from natal and friendship bonds.

Here we confront the nagging problem, always a dilemma for feminist advocates, of how to critique the kinds and range of choices available to women without denigrating the decisions women do make for themselves, even under severe social and economic constraints.[4] The debate concerning sterilization prevalence rates in Brazil provides a striking illustration. In a context of rapid fertility decline, female sterilization has become a 'preferred' method in Brazil, used by 44 per cent of current contraceptors. In some regions, the sterilization rate reaches more than 64 per cent, as in the case of the Northeast, and the average age of sterilization has rapidly declined since the early 1980s (15 per cent of sterilized women in the Northeast are under 25 years of age). A complex mix of factors explains this trend: concerns about the side effects or effectiveness of reversible contraception, failure of the public health system to provide adequate information about and access to other methods, severe economic conditions, women's employment patterns, and cultural and religious norms making sterilization less 'sinful' than abortion (Corrêa, 1993; Lopez, 1993; Petchesky, 1979).

In their analysis of the sterilization trends, Brazilian feminists are caught between the urgent need to denounce the inequities in sterilization rates – particularly among black women – and the evidence of research findings that many women have consciously chosen and paid for the procedure and are satisfied with their decision. On the one hand, this is a clear example of the 'constrained choices' that result from circumstances of gender, poverty, and racism; the very notion that women in such conditions are exercising their 'reproductive rights' strains the meaning of the term (Lopez, 1993). On the other hand, the call for criminal sanctions against sterilization by some groups in Brazil seems a denial of women's moral agency in their search for reproductive self-determination.

We need to develop analytical frameworks that respect the integrity of women's reproductive and sexual decisions, however constrained, while also condemning social, economic, and cultural conditions that may force women to 'choose' one course over another. Such conditions prevail in a range of situations, curtailing reproductive choices and creating dilemmas for women's health activists. Women desperate for employment may knowingly expose themselves to reproductively hazardous chemicals or other toxins in the workplace. Women hedged in by economic dependence and the cultural preference for sons may 'choose' abortion as a means of sex selection. Where female genital mutilation is a traditional practice, women must 'choose' for their young daughters between severe health risk and sexual loss on the one hand, and unmarriageable pariah status on the other.

For reproductive decisions to be in any real sense 'free', rather than compelled by circumstance or desperation, requires the presence of certain *enabling conditions*. These conditions constitute the foundation of reproductive and sexual rights and are what feminists mean when they speak of women's 'empowerment'. They include material and infrastructural factors, such as reliable transportation, child care, financial subsidies, or income supports, as well as comprehensive health services that are accessible, humane, and well staffed. The absence of adequate transportation alone can be a significant contributor to higher maternal mortality and failure to use contraceptives (see Asian and Pacific Women's Resource Collection Network, 1990; and McCarthy and Maine, 1992). They also include cultural and political factors, such as access to education, earnings, self-esteem, and the channels of decision-making. Where women have no education, training, or status outside that which comes from bearing sons, childbearing may remain their best option (Morsy, 1994; Pearce, 1994; Ravindran, 1993).

Such enabling conditions, or social rights, are integral to reproductive and sexual rights. And directly entail the responsibility of states and mediating institutions (for example, population and development agencies) for their implementation. Rights involve not only *personal liberties* (domains where governments should leave people alone), but also *social entitlements* (domains where affirmative public action is required to ensure that rights are attainable by everyone). They thus necessarily imply public responsibilities and a renewed emphasis on the linkages between personal well-being and social good, including the good of public support for gender equality in all domains of life.

This is not meant to suggest a mystical 'harmony of interests' between individual women and public authorities, nor to deny that conflicts between 'private' and 'public' interests will continue to exist. In societies governed by competitive market values, for example, middle-class couples and entrepreneurs may raise serious ethical questions by exploiting reproductive technologies to produce the 'right sex' or the 'perfect child'. Meanwhile, under repressive or dictatorial regimes, the reproductive desires of individuals may be sacrificed altogether to an ethics of public expediency: witness the harsh anti-natalist campaign in China. These realities prompt us to rethink the relationship between the state and civil society, and to map out an ethical framework for reproductive and sexual rights in the space where the social and the individual intersect.

The ethical content of reproductive and sexual rights

We propose that the grounds of reproductive and sexual rights for women consist of our ethical principles: *bodily integrity*, *personhood*, *equality*, and *diversity*. Each of these principles can be violated through acts of invasion or abuse – by government officials, clinicians and other providers, male partners, family members, and so on – or through acts of omission, neglect, or discrimination by public (national or international) authorities. Each also raises dilemmas and contradictions that can be resolved only under radically different social arrangements from those now prevailing in most of the world.

Bodily integrity

Perhaps more than the other three principles, the principle of bodily integrity, or the right to security in and control over one's body, lies at the core of reproductive and sexual freedom. As suggested in our introduction, this principle is embedded in the historical development of ideas of the self and citizenship in Western political culture. Yet it also transcends any one culture or region, insofar as some version of it informs all opposition to slavery and other involuntary servitude, torture, rape, and every form of illegitimate assault and violence. As the Declaration of the International Women's Year Conference in Mexico City put it in 1975, 'the human body, whether that of women or men, is inviolable and respect for it is a fundamental element of human dignity and freedom' (quoted in Freedman and Isaacs, 1993).

To affirm the right of women to 'control over' or 'ownership of' their bodies does not mean that women's bodies are mere things, separate from themselves or isolated from social networks and communities. Rather, it connotes the body as an integral part of one's self, whose health and wellness (including sexual pleasure) are a necessary basis for active participation in social life. Bodily integrity, then, is not just an individual but a social right, since without it women cannot function as responsible community members (Freedman and Isaacs, 1993; Petchesky, 1990, 1994). Yet in its specific applications, the bodily integrity principle reminds us that while reproductive and sexual rights are necessarily social, they are also ir-reducibly personal. While they can never be realized without attention to economic development, political empowerment, and cultural diversity, ultimately their site is individual women's bodies (DAWN, 1993; Petchesky, 1990).

Bodily integrity includes both 'a woman's right *not to be alienated from her sexual and reproductive capacity* (e.g., through coerced sex or marriage, … [genital mutilation], denial of access to birth control, sterilization without informed consent, prohibitions on homosexuality) and … her right to the *integrity of her physical person* (e.g., freedom from sexual violence, from false imprisonment in the home, from unsafe contraceptive methods, from unwanted pregnancies or coerced childbearing, from unwanted medical interventions)' (Dixon-Mueller, 1993). Such negative abuses occur at multiple levels or sites, including not only relations with sexual partners and kin, clinicians and other providers, but also state or military campaigns (for example, coercive fertility reduction programmes or the rape of women as a tool of 'ethnic cleansing').

But bodily integrity also implies *affirmative* rights to enjoy the full potential of one's body for health, procreation, and sexuality. Each of these raises a host of complex questions we can only touch upon here. In regard to health, the very term 'integrity' connotes *wholeness* – treating the body and its present needs as a unity, not as piecemeal mechanical functions or fragments. Dr Rani Bang in India found that in one district in Maharashtra State, 92 per cent of the women who used local family planning clinics suffered from untreated gynaecologic infections or diseases (Bang, 1989, cited in Bruce, 1990). How can this happen if clinicians are treating women's bodies and reproductive health as a whole? Similarly, family planning programmes that emphasize so-called medically efficacious methods of contraception at the cost or even to the exclusion of barrier methods fail to offer women protection against STD and Human Immunodeficiency Virus (HIV) infection, thus exposing them to morbidity, infertility, or death.

The question of whether there is a 'fundamental right to procreate' based in one's biological reproductive capacity is clearly more complicated than whether one has a right, as a matter of bodily integrity, to prevent or terminate a pregnancy. Yet we can recognize that childbearing has consequences for others besides an individual woman, man, or lineage without subscribing to the claim that women have a duty to society (or the planet!) to abstain from reproducing. Such a duty could begin to exist only when all women are provided sufficient resources for their well-being, viable work alternatives, and a cultural climate of affirmation outside of childbearing so that they no longer depend on children for survival and dignity (Berer, 1990; Freedman and Isaacs, 1993). And even then, anti-natalist policies that depend on coercion or discriminate against or target particular groups would be unacceptable.

Our hesitancy about a 'right to procreate' is not based on any simple correlation between population growth, environmental degradation, and women's fertility, persuasively refuted elsewhere (see Sen, Germain and Chen, 1994). Rather, it comes from apprehensions about how patriarchal kinship systems throughout history have used such claims to confine and subordinate women, who alone have bodies that can be impregnated. Procreative rights are, however, an important part of reproductive and sexual rights. They include the right to participate in the basic human practice of raising and nurturing children; the right to bring wanted pregnancies to term in conditions of safety, decency, and good health, and to raise one's children in such conditions; and the right of gay and lesbian families to bear, foster, or adopt children in the same dignity as other families. They also include a transformation in the prevailing gender division of labour so that men are assigned as much responsibility for children's care as women.

Finally, what shall we say of the body's capacity for sexual pleasure and the right to express it in diverse and non-stigmatized ways? If the bodily integrity principle implies such a right, as we believe, its expression surely becomes more complicated and fraught with dangers for women and men in the context of rising prevalence of HIV and STD infection

(Berer, 1993a; DAWN, 1993). In addition to these immediate dangers – compounded by the now well-documented fact that many STDs increase women's susceptibility to HIV – there is the 'vicious cycle' in which 'women suffering the consequences of sexually transmitted disease find themselves in a social circumstance that further increases their risk of exposure to sexually transmitted infections and their complications' (Elias, 1991). This cycle currently affects sub-Saharan African women most drastically, but is rapidly becoming a worldwide phenomenon. It includes women's lack of sexual self-determination; the high risk they incur of infertility and ectopic pregnancy from STD infection; their dependence on men and in-laws for survival; the threat of ostracism or rejection by the family or male partner following infection or infertility; then the threat of unemployment, impoverishment, and prostitution, followed by still greater exposure to STD and HIV infection (Elias, 1991; Wasserheit, 1993).

The global crisis of HIV and AIDS complicates but does not diminish the right of all people to responsible sexual pleasure in a supportive social and cultural environment. For women and men of diverse sexual orientations to be able to express their sexuality without fear or risk of exclusion, illness, or death requires sex education and male and female re-socialization on a hitherto unprecedented scale. This is why bodily integrity has a necessary social rights dimension that, now more than ever, is a matter of life and death.

Personhood

Listening to women is the key to honouring their moral and legal personhood – that is, their right to self-determination. This means treating them as principal actors and decision-makers in matters of reproduction and sexuality – as subjects, not merely objects, and as ends, not only means, of population and family planning policies. As should be clear from our earlier discussion emphasizing a relational-interactive model of women's reproductive decisions, our concept of decision-making autonomy implies respect for how women make decisions, the values they bring to bear, and the networks of others they choose to consult; it does not imply a notion of solitude or isolation in 'individual choices'. Nor does it preclude full coun-selling about risks and options regarding contraception, prenatal care, childbearing, STDs and HIV, and other aspects of gynaecologic health.

At the clinical level, for providers to respect women's personhood requires that they trust and take seriously women's desires and experiences, for example, concerning contraceptive side effects. When clinicians trivialize women's complaints about such symptoms as head-aches, weight gain, or menstrual irregularity, they violate this principle. Qualitative studies of clinical practices regarding the use of Norplant® in the Dominican Republic, Egypt, Indo-nesia, and Thailand found that women's concerns about irregular bleeding were often dismissed, and their requests for removal of the implant not honoured (Zimmerman *et al.*, 1990).

Respect for personhood also requires that clients be offered a complete range of safe options, fully explained, without major discrepancies in cost or government subsidization. When some contraceptive methods are *de facto* singled out for promotion (for instance, long-acting implants or sterilization), or clinical practices manifest strong pro-natalist or anti-natalist biases (as in programmes governed by demographic targets), or safe legal abortion is denied, respect for women's personhood is systematically abused. 'Quality of care' guide-lines, which originated in women's health activism and were codified by Judith Bruce, reflect not only good medical practice but an ethic of respect for personhood (Bruce, 1990; DAWN, 1993; Jain, Bruce and Mensch, 1992; Mintzes, 1992).

At the level of national and international policies and programmes, treating women as persons in sexual and reproductive decision-making means assuring that women's organizations are represented and heard in the processes where population and health policies are made and that effective mechanisms of public accountability, in which women participate, are established to guard against abuses. It also means abandoning demographic targets in the service of economic growth, cost containment, or ethnic or nationalist rivalries and replacing them with reproductive health and women's empowerment goals (see Jain and Bruce, 1994). Demographic targeting policies that encourage the use of material incentives or disincentives often work to manipulate or coerce women, particularly those who are poor, into accepting fertility control methods they might otherwise reject, thus violating their decision-making autonomy.

The question of 'incentives' is clearly a complicated one, since in some circumstances they may expand women's options and freedom (Dixon-Mueller, 1993). Feminists and human-rights activists have justly criticized programmes that promote particular fertility control methods or anti-natalist campaigns through monetary inducements or clothing to 'acceptors', fines or denials of child care or health benefits to 'offenders', or quotas reinforced with 'bonuses' for village officials or clinic personnel (Freedman and Isaacs, 1993; Ravindran, 1993). What would be our reaction, however, to a system of women-managed comprehensive care clinics that provided child care or free transportation to facilitate clinic visits? A distinct difference exists between these two cases, since the former deploys the targeting and promotional strategies that undermine women's personhood, whereas the latter incorporates the kinds of enabling conditions we earlier found necessary for equalizing women's ability to exercise their reproductive rights. To distinguish *supportive* or *empowering* conditions from *coercive* incentives or disincentives, we need to assure that they respect all four ethical principles of reproductive rights (bodily integrity, personhood, equality, and diversity). When poor or incarcerated women are expected to purchase other rights 'for the price of their womb' (for example, a job for sterilization or release from prison for Norplant®), 'incentives' become corrupted into bribes (Williams, 1991). Women's social location determines whether they are able to make sexual and reproductive decisions with dignity.

Equality

The principle of equality applies to sexual and reproductive rights in two main areas: relations between men and women (gender divisions), and relations among women (conditions such as class, age, nationality, or ethnicity that divide women as a group). With respect to the former, the impetus behind the idea of reproductive rights as it emerged historically was to remedy the social bias against women inherent in their lack of control over their fertility and their assignment to primarily reproductive roles in the gender division of labour. 'Reproductive rights' (or 'birth control') was one strategy within a much larger agenda for making women's position in society equal to men's. At the same time, this notion contains the seeds of a contradiction, since women alone are the ones who get pregnant, and in that sense, their situation – and degree of risk – can never be reducible to men's.

This tension, which feminists have conceptualized in the debate over equality versus 'difference', becomes problematic in the gender-neutral language of most United Nations documents pertaining to reproductive rights and health. For example, article 16(e) of the Convention on the Elimination of All Forms of Discrimination against Women (CEDAW) gives men and women 'the same rights to decide freely and responsibly on the number and spacing of their children and to have access to the information, education and means to enable *them* to exercise these rights [emphasis added]'. Might this article be used to mandate husbands' consent to abortion or contraception? Why should men and women have 'the same' rights with regard to reproduction when, as not only childbearers but those who in most societies have responsibility for children's care, women have so much greater stake in the matter – when, indeed, growing numbers of women raise children without benefit of male partners? (The language of 'couples' in family planning literature raises the same kinds of questions.)

If we take the issue of contraception as an illustration, the principle of equality would seem to require that, where contraceptive methods carry risks or provide benefits, those risks and benefits must be distributed on a fair basis between women and men, as well as among women. This would suggest a population policy that puts greater emphasis on encouraging male responsibility for fertility control and scientific research into effective 'male' contraceptives. In fact, many women express a sense of unfairness that they are expected to bear nearly all the medical risks and social responsibility for avoiding unwanted pregnancies (Pies, n.d.). But such a policy might also conflict with the basic right of women to control their own fertility and the need many women feel to preserve that control, sometimes in conditions of secrecy and without 'equal sharing' of risks.

On the surface, this dilemma seems to be a contradiction within feminist goals, between the opposing principles of equality and personhood. The feminist agenda that privileges women's control in reproductive rights would seem to reinforce a gender division of labour that confines women to the domain of reproduction. Yet exploring the problem more deeply reveals that women's distrust of men's taking responsibility for fertility control and reluctance to relinquish methods women control are rooted in other kinds of gendered power imbalances that work against a 'gender equality' approach to reproductive health policies. These include social systems that provide no educational or economic incentives toward men's involvement in child care and cultural norms that stigmatize women's sexuality outside the bounds of heterosexual monogamy. Thus, while a reproductive health policy that encourages the development and use of 'male methods' of contraception may increase the total range of 'choices', in the long run it will not help to realize women's social rights nor gender equality until these larger issues are also addressed.

Applying the equality principle in the implementation of sexual and reproductive rights also requires attention to potential inequalities *among* women. This means, at the least, that risks and benefits must be distributed on a fair basis and that providers and policy-makers must respect women's decision-making authority without regard to differences of class, race, ethnic origin, age, marital, status, sexual orientation, nationality, or region (North–South). Returning to our example of contraception, there is certainly ample evidence that access to safe methods of fertility control can play a major role in improving women's health, but some contraceptive methods can have negative consequences for some women's health (National Research Council, 1989). Issues of equal treatment may arise when certain methods – particularly those that carry medical risks or whose long-term effects are not well known – are tested, targeted, or promoted primarily among poor women in Southern or Northern countries. Indeed, when clinical trials are conducted among poor urban women, who tend to move frequently or lack transportation, the necessary conditions for adequate medical follow-up may not exist, and thus the trials themselves may be in violation of the equality principle. Meanwhile, issues of discrimination arise when safe, beneficial methods such as condoms or diaphragms, low-dose hormonal pills, or hygienic abortion facilities are available only to women with the financial resources to pay for them.

For governments and international organizations to promote sexual and reproductive rights in ways that respect equality among women requires addressing at least the most blatant differences in power and resources that divide women within countries and internationally. In the case of safe, effective methods of contraception, laws that guarantee the 'freedom' of all women to use whatever methods they 'choose' are gratuitous without geographic access, high-quality services and supplies, and financing for all women who need them. We are saying that the economic and political changes necessary to create such conditions are a matter not just of development, but of (social) *rights*; indeed, they are a good example of why development *is* a human right and why women's reproductive rights are inseparable from this equation (Sen, 1992).

Diversity

While the equality principle requires the mitigation of inequities among women in their access to services or their treatment by health providers and policy-makers, the diversity principle requires respect for differences among women – in values, culture, religion, sexual orientation, family or medical condition, and so on. The universalizing language of international human rights instruments, reflecting a Western liberal tradition, needs to be reshaped to encompass such differences (see Freedman and Isaacs, 1993; Cook, 1993a, 1993b). While defending the universal applicability of sexual and reproductive rights, we must also acknowledge that such rights often have different meanings, or different points of priority, in different social and cultural contexts. Differences in cultural or religious values, for example, affect attitudes toward children and childbearing, influencing how diverse groups of women think about their entitlements in reproduction. In her study of market women in Ile-Ife, Nigeria, anthropologist Tola Olu Pearce (1994) found that the high value placed on women's fertility and the subordination of individual desires to group welfare in Yoruba tradition made the notion of a woman's individual right to choose alien. Yet Yoruba women in Ile-Ife have also used methods of fertility control to space their children and 'avoid embarrassment' for untold generations and no doubt consider it part of their collective 'right' as women to do so. A similar communal ethic governing women's reproductive decisions emerges in a study of Latina single mothers in East Harlem (New York City), who consider their 'reproductive rights' to include the right to receive public assistance in order to stay home and care for their children (Benmayor, Torruellas and Juarbe, 1992).

Local religious and cultural values may also shape women's attitudes toward medical technologies or their effects, such as irregular menstrual bleeding. Clinic personnel involved in disseminating Norplant® have not always understood the meanings menstrual blood may have in local cultures and the extent to which frequent bleeding – a common side effect of Norplant® – may result in the exclusion of women from sex, rituals, or community life (Zimmerman *et al.*, 1990). Imposing standards of what is 'normal' or 'routine' bleeding (for example, to justify refusal to remove the implant upon request) could constitute a violation of the diversity principle, as well as the bodily integrity and personhood principles.[5]

It is important to distinguish between the feminist principle of respect for difference and the tendency of male-dominated governments and fundamentalist religious groups of all kinds to use 'diversity' and 'autonomy of local cultures' as reasons to deny the universal validity of women's human rights.[6] In all the cases cited above, women's assertion of their particular needs and values, rather than denying the universal application of rights, clarifies what those rights mean in specific settings. Women's multiple identities – whether as members of cultural, ethnic, and kinship groups, or as people with particular religious and sexual orientations, and so forth – challenge human-rights discourse to develop a language and methodology that are pluralistic yet faithful to the core principles of equality, personhood, and bodily integrity. This means that the diversity principle is never absolute, but always conditioned upon a conception of human rights that promotes women's development and respects their self-determination.

Traditional patriarchal practices that subordinate women – however local or time-worn, or enacted by women themselves (for example, genital mutilation) – can never supersede the social responsibility of governments and intergovernmental organizations to enforce women's equality, personhood, and bodily integrity, through means that respect the needs and desires of the women most directly involved.

Bringing a feminist social rights approach to population and development policies

The above analysis has attempted to show that the individual (liberty) and the social (justice) dimensions of rights can never be separated, as long as resources and power remain unequally distributed in most societies. Thus the affirmative obligations of states and international organizations become paramount, since the ability of individuals to exercise reproductive and sexual rights depends on a range of conditions not yet available to many people and impossible to access without public support. In this respect, the language of 'entitlement' seems to us overly narrow, insofar as it implies claims made by individuals on the state without expressing the idea of a mutual public interest in developing empowered, educated, and politically responsible citizens, including all women. Likewise, the language of 'choosing freely and responsibly' still contained in most international instruments that address family planning and reproductive rights is at best ambiguous and at worst evasive (see Boland, Rao and Zeidensteinin, 1994). What does it mean to choose 'responsibly'? Who, in fact, is responsible, and what are the necessary conditions – social, economic, cultural – for individuals to act, in socially responsible ways? The correlative duties associated with sexual and reproductive rights belong not only to the bearers of those rights, but to the governmental and intergovernmental agencies charged with their enforcement.

Health policies and programmes that treat reproduction and women holistically, across the lifecycle and through means appropriate to women's social situations, require comprehensive services with well-trained staff and adequate facilities for all women. If women are to be empowered to speak out in clinical settings and to make claims about their sexual and reproductive health needs – particularly where the quality of care is inadequate – they must have 'a culture of health awareness', which may in turn rest on their having opportunities for economic independence and political self-determination (Basu, 1990). Ultimately such ends are a question not so much of economic transformations as of political priorities and values. As the participants in the Expert Group Meeting on Population and Women, held in Botswana in 1992, stated: 'Equality for women depends not on the level of development or the economic resources available but on the political will of Governments and on the cultural setting in which women have to live' (1992).

The necessary conclusion is that governments and population agencies professing to uphold women's reproductive and sexual rights must do a lot more than avoid abuses. They must do more even than enforce 'quality of care' guidelines, which reach only to conditions in the clinic and not to local communities and the larger society. Beyond this, they must seek a reordering of international economic policies (including so-called structural adjustment programmes), national budgetary priorities, and national health and population policies to de-emphasize debt servicing and militarism in favour of social welfare and primary healthcare. And they need to adopt affirmative programmes that promote 'a culture of health awareness' and empowerment among women, and an attitude of respect, non-violence, and responsibility toward women and children among men.

Documents developed in preparation for the 1994 International Conference on Population and Development (ICPD), in Cairo, have begun to reflect the vision of reproductive and sexual rights as social rights that we have presented here. This is true not only of documents produced by women's NGOs, but also of official conference preparatory meetings and summaries, where for the first time in international population discourse, issues of gender equality and women's empowerment overshadow demographic targets and economic growth and are recognized as part of 'sustainable development'. In both the topical outline adopted for the new World Population Plan of Action and the Second Preparatory Committee chairman's summary, issues of gender equality, women's rights, and reproductive rights cut across all sections, rather than being limited to the customary one or two token references. In sharp contrast to the previous World Population Plan of Action, the Preparatory Committee chairman's summary emphasizes the importance, in relation to family planning and reproductive health, of sexuality, sexual health, and STD and HIV/AIDS prevention. Unlike most UN documents, moreover, it includes 'sexual orientation' in listing conditions that 'many delegations' recognized should not be discriminated against in women's 'access to information, education and services to exercise their reproductive and sexual rights'.

We need to see this marked shift from the emphases of the plans of action adopted in 1974 and 1984 as a direct consequence of the strength and global impact of the women's health and rights movements during the last decade (see García-Moreno and Claro, 1994). Years of organizing and advocacy by women's health groups throughout the world have clearly had an important effect *at the level of official rhetoric* on intergovernmental forums concerned with 'population' issues. To what extent are we likely to see governments, UN agencies, and international population organizations move from awareness to action to translate this rhetoric into concrete policies and programmes that truly benefit women?

Many women's health groups, in both the South and the North, are concerned that feminist-sounding rhetoric is being used by international population agencies to legitimate and gloss over what remain instrumentalist and narrowly quantitative ends. Perceiving the history of population control policies and programmes as all too frequently oblivious to women's needs and the ethical principles outlined above, they fear the language of reproductive rights and health may simply be co-opted by the Cairo process to support business as usual.

Our position is slightly more optimistic but nonetheless cautious. Feminists are putting pressure on population and family planning agencies to acknowledge women's self-defined needs and our conceptions of reproductive and sexual rights. This should move us closer to social and policy changes that empower women, but whether it does will depend on even more concerted action by women's NGOs, including alliances with many other groups concerned with health, development, and human rights. One such action should be to insist on full participation by women's rights and health groups in all relevant decision-making bodies and accountability mechanisms. In the long run, however, it is not enough that we call population agencies to account. To bridge the gap between rhetoric about reproductive and sexual rights and the harsh realities most women face demands a much larger vision. We must integrate, but not subordinate, those rights with health and development agendas that will radically transform the distribution of resources, power, and wellness within and among all the countries of the world (DAWN, 1993; Sen, 1992). These are the enabling conditions to transform rights into lived capacities. For women, Cairo is just a stop along the way.

Notes

1   The term seems to have originated with the founding of the Reproductive Rights National Network (R2N2) in the United States in 1979. R2N2 activists brought it to the European-based International Campaign for Abortion Rights in the early 1980s; at the International Women and Health Meeting in Amsterdam in 1984, the Campaign officially changed its name to the Women's Global Network for Reproductive Rights (Berer, 1993b). Thereafter, the concept rapidly spread throughout women's movements in the South (for example, in 1985, under the influence of feminist members who had attended the Amsterdam meeting, the Brazilian Health Ministry established the Commission on the Rights of Human Reproduction). See also García-Moreno and Claro, 1994.

2   In fact, the principle of 'ownership of one's body and person' has much deeper roots in the history of radical libertarian and democratic thought in Western Europe. Historian Natalie Zemon Davis traced this idea to sixteenth-century Geneva, when a young Lyonnaise girl, brought before the Protestant elders for sleeping with her fiancé before marriage, invoked what may have been a popular slogan: 'Paris est au roi, et mon corps est à moi' (Paris is the king's, and my body is mine). The radical Levellers in seventeenth-century England developed the notion of a 'property in one's person', which they used to defend their members against arbitrary arrest and imprisonment (Petchesky, 1994). But the principle is not only of European derivation. Gandhi's concept of *Brahmacharya*, or 'control over the body', was rooted in Hindu ascetic traditions and the Vedas' admonition to preserve the body's vital fluids. Like that of nineteenth-century feminists and the Catholic Church, Gandhi's concept was rhetorically gender-neutral, requiring both men and women to engage in sexual restraint except for purposes of procreation (Fischer, 1962; O'Flaherty, 1980). Islamic law goes further toward a sexually affirmative concept of self-ownership. Quranic provisions not only entitle women to sexual satisfaction in marriage, as well as condoning abortion and contraception; they also allow that, upon divorce – which wives as well as husbands may initiate – a woman regains her body (Ahmed, 1992; Musallam, 1983; Ruthven, 1984).

3   In Latin America, a new resolution of the Colombian Ministry of Public Health 'orders all health institutions to ensure women the right to decide on all issues that affect their health, their life, and their sexuality, and guarantees rights to information and orientation to allow the exercise of free, gratifying, responsible sexuality which cannot be tied to maternity' (quoted in Cook, 1993a). In North Africa, Dr Hind Khattab's field research among rural Egyptian women has revealed strong sentiments of their sexual entitlement to pleasure and gratification from husbands (Khattab, 1993).

4   Feminist theory and practice have witnessed a long history of division over this question. Whether with regard to protective labour legislation, prosecution, pornography, or providing contraceptive implants to teenagers or poor women, conflicts between 'liberals' (advocates of 'freedom to choose') and 'radicals' (advocates of social protection or legal prohibition) have been bitter and protracted.

5   Not only clinicians but feminist activists may be guilty of imposing their own values and failing to respect diversity. Feminist groups that condemn all reproductive technologies (for example, technologies that artificially assist fertility) as instruments of medical control over women and against 'nature' ignore the ways that such technologies may expand the rights of particular women (for example, lesbians seeking pregnancy through artificial insemination or *in vitro* fertilization).

6   It seems crucial to us to recognize that religious fundamentalist movements are on the upswing in all the world's regions and major religions – Catholicism, Protestantism, Judaism, and Hinduism as well as Islam. Despite vast cultural and theological differences, these fundamentalisms share a view of women as reproductive vessels that is antipathetic to any notion of women's reproductive rights. In an otherwise excellent discussion of the clash between religious and customary law and human rights, Lynn Freedman and Stephen Isaacs (1993) place undue emphasis on Muslim countries and Islamic law.

References

ADAMS, A. and CASTLE, S. (1994) 'Gender Relations and Household Dynamics', in SEN, G., GERMAIN, A., and CHEN, L.C. (eds) *Population Policies Reconsidered: Health, Empowerment, and Rights*, Cambridge, MA: Harvard University Press.

AHMED, L. (1992) *Women and Gender in Islam*, New Haven, CT: Yale University Press.

ASIAN AND PACIFIC WOMEN'S RESOURCE COLLECTION NETWORK (1990) *Asia and Pacific Women's Resource and Action Series*: Health, Kuala Lumpur: Asia and Pacific Development Centre.

BANG, R. (1989) 'High prevalence of gynaecological diseases in rural Indian women', *Lancet*, 337, pp. 85–8.

BASU, A.M. (1990) 'Cultural influences on health care use: two regional groups in India', *Studies in Family Planning*, 21, pp. 275–86.

BENMAYOR, R., TORRUELLAS, R.M., and JUARBE, A.L. (1992) *Responses to Poverty among Puerto Rican Women: Identity, Community, and Cultural Citizenship*, New York: Centro de Estudios Puertorriqueños, Hunter College.

BERER, M. (1990) 'What would a feminist population policy be like?', *Women's Health Journal*, 18, pp. 4–7.

—— (1993a) 'Population and family planning policies: women-centered perspectives', *Reproductive Health Matters*, 1, pp. 4–12.

—— (1993b) Personal communication.

BHASIN, K., and KHAN, N. (1986) *Some Questions on Feminism for Women in South Asia*, New Delhi: Kali.

BOLAND, R., RAO, S. and ZEIDENSTEN, G. (1994) 'Honoring human rights in population policies: from declaration to action', in SEN, G., GERMAIN, A. and CHEN, L.C. (eds) *Population Policies Reconsidered: Health, Empowerment, and Rights*, Cambridge, MA: Harvard University Press.

BRUCE, J. (1990) 'Fundamental elements of the quality of care: a simple framework', *Studies in Family Planning*, 21, pp. 61–91.

BUNCH, C. (1990) 'Women's rights as human rights: towards a re-vision of human rights', *Human Rights Quarterly*, 12, pp. 486–98.

CHESLER, E. (1992) *Woman of Valor: Margaret Sanger and the Birth Control Movement in America*, New York: Simon & Schuster.

COOK, R.J. (1993a) 'International human rights and women's reproductive health', *Studies in Family Planning*, 24, pp. 73–86.

—— (1993b) 'Women's international human rights law: the way forward', *Human Rights Quarterly*, 15, pp. 230–61.

COPELON, R. (1994) 'Intimate terror: understanding domestic violence as torture', in COOK, R.J. (ed.), *International Women's Human Rights*, Philadelphia: University of Pennsylvania.

CORREA, S. (1993) 'Sterilization in Brazil: reviewing the analysis', unpublished paper.

CRENSHAW, K. (1991) 'Demarginalizing the intersection of race and sex: a black feminist critique of antidiscrimination doctrine, feminist theory, and anti-racist politics', in BARRLERR, K.T. and KENNEDY, R. (eds), *Feminist Legal Theory*, Boulder, CO: Westview Press.

DEVELOPMENT ALTERNATIVES WITH WOMEN FOR A NEW ERA (DAWN) (1993) 'Population and reproductive rights component: platform document/preliminary ideas', unpublished paper.

DESAI, S. (1994) 'Women's burdens: easing the structural constraints' in SEN, G., GERMAIN, A. and CHEN, L. (eds) *Population Policies Reconsidered: Health, Empowerment and Rights*, Cambridge, MA: Harvard University Press.

DIXON-MUELLER, R. (1993) *Population Policy and Women's Rights: Transforming Reproductive Choice*, Westport, CT: Praeger.

EISENSTEIN, Z. (1983) *The Radical Future of Liberal Feminism*, Boston, MA: Northeastern University Press.

—— (1994) *The Color of Gender*, Berkeley and Los Angeles: University of California Press.

ELIAS, C. (1991) *Sexually Transmitted Diseases and the Reproductive Health of Women in Developing Countries*, New York: Population Council.

ELSHTAIN, J.B. (1981) *Public Man, Private Woman*, Princeton: Princeton University Press.

EXPERT GROUP MEETING ON POPULATION AND WOMEN (1992) *Substantive Preparations for the Conference Recommendations*, New York: United Nations Economic and Social Council.

EZEH, A.C. (1993) 'The influence of spouses over each other's contraceptive attitudes in Ghana', *Studies in Family Planning*, 24, pp. 163–74.

FABROS, M.L. (1991) *The WRRC's institutional framework and strategies on reproductive rights. Flights 4.* Official publication of the Women's Resource & Research Center, Quezon City, Philippines.

FISCHER, L. (1962) *The Essential Gandhi*, New York: Vintage.

FREEDMAN, L.P., and ISAACS, S. L. (1993) 'Human rights and reproductive choice', *Studies in Family Planning*, 24, pp. 18–30.

FRIEDMAN, M. (1992) 'Feminism and modern friendship: dislocating the community', in AVINERI, S. and DE-SHALIT, A. (eds), *Communitarianism and Individualism*, New York: Oxford University Press.

GARCIA-MORENO, C. and CLARO, A. (1994) 'Challenges from the women's health movement: women's rights versus population control', in SEN, G., GERMAIN, A. and CHEN, L.C. (eds) *Population Policies Reconsidered: Health, Empowerment, and Rights*, Cambridge, MA: Harvard University Press.

GILLIGAN, C. (1982) *In a Different Voice: Psychological Theory and Women's Development*, Cambridge, MA: Harvard University Press.

GORDON, L. (1976) *Woman's Body, Woman's Right: A Social History of Birth Control in America*, New York: Penguin.

HEISE, L. (1992) 'Violence against women: the missing agenda', in KOBLINSKY, M.A., TIMYAN, J. and GAY, J. (eds), *Women's Health: A Global Perspective*, Boulder, CO: Westview Press.

HELLER, A. (1992) 'Rights, modernity, democracy', in CORNELL, D., ROSENFELD, M. and CARLSON, D.G. (eds), *Deconstruction and the Possibility of Justice*, New York: Routledge.

HUSTON, P. (1992) *Motherhood by Choice: Pioneers in Women's Health and Family Planning*, New York: Feminist Press.

JAIN, A. and BRUCE, J. (1994) 'A reproductive health approach to the objectives and assessment of family planning programs' in SEN, G., GERMAIN, A. and CHEN, L. (eds) *Population Policies Reconsidered: Health, Empowerment and Rights*, Cambridge, MA: Harvard University Press.

——, BRUCE, J. and MENSCH, B. (1992) 'Setting standards of quality in family planning programs', *Studies in Family Planning*, 23, pp. 392–5.

JAYAWARDENA, K. (1993) *With a Different Voice: White Women and Colonialism in South Asia*, London: Zed.

JEFFERY, P., JEFFERY, R. and LYON, A. (1989) *Labour Pains and Labour Power: Women and Childbearing in India*, London: Zed.

KELLY, J. (1984) *Women, History, and Theory*, Chicago: The University of Chicago Press.

KHATTAB, H. (1992) *The Silent Endurance: Social Conditions of Women's Reproductive Health in Rural Egypt*, Amman: UNICEF.

—— (1993) Personal communication.

LOPEZ, I. (1993) 'Constrained Choices: An Ethnography of Sterilization and Puerto Rican Women in New York City', unpublished manuscript.

MCCARTHY, J. and MAINE, D. (1992) 'A framework for analyzing the determinants of maternal mortality', *Studies in Family Planning*, 23, pp. 23–33.

MINTZES, B. (ed.) (1992) *A Question of Control: Women's Perspectives on the Development and Use of Contraceptives*, Amsterdam, WEMOS: Women & Pharmaceuticals Project.

MORSY, S. (1994) 'Maternal morality in Egypt: selective health strategy and the medicalization of population control', in GINSBURG, F.D. and RAPP, R. (eds), *Conceiving the New World Order: The Global Stratification of Reproduction*, Berkeley and Los Angeles: University of California Press.

MUSALLAM, B.F. (1983) *Sex and Society in Islam: Birth Control Before the Nineteenth Century*, Cambridge: Cambridge University Press.

NATIONAL RESEARCH COUNCIL (1989) *Contraception and Reproduction: Health Consequences for Women and Children in the Developing World*, Washington, DC: National Academy Press.

NEDELSKY, J. (1989) 'Reconceiving autonomy', *Yale Journal of Law and Feminism*, 1, pp. 7–36.

O'FLAHERTY, W.D. (1980) *Women, Androgynes, and Other Mythical Beasts*, Chicago: The University of Chicago.

OKIN, S.M. (1979) *Women in Western Political Thought*, Princeton: Princeton University.

OLSEN, F. (1984) 'Statutory rape: a feminist critique of rights analysis', *Texas Law Review*, 63, pp. 387–432.

PEARCE, T.O. (1994) 'Women's reproductive practices and biomedicine: cultural conflicts and trans-formations', in GINSBURG, F.D. and RAPP, R. (eds), *Conceiving the New World Order: The Global Stratification of Reproduction*, Berkeley and Los Angeles: University of California Press.

PETCHESKY, R.P. (1979) 'Reproductive choice in the contemporary United States: a social analysis of female sterilization', in MICHAELSON, K. (ed.), *And the Poor Get Children*, New York: Monthly Review.

—— (ed.) (1990) *Abortion and Woman's Choice: The State, Sexuality and Reproductive Freedom*, revised, Boston, MA: Northeastern University Press.

—— (1994) 'The body as property: A feminist revision', in GINSBURG, F.D. and RAPP, R. (eds), *Conceiving the New World Order: The Global Stratification of Reproduction*, Berkeley: University of California.

—— and WEINER, J. (1990) 'Global feminist perspectives on reproductive rights and reproductive health', New York: Reproductive Rights Education Project, Hunter College.

PIES, C. (n.d.) *Creating Ethical Reproductive Health Care Policy*, San Francisco: Education Programs Associates.

PROTACIO, N. (1990) 'From womb to tomb: the Filipino women's struggle for good health and justice', paper presented at the Fourth International Interdisciplinary Congress on Women, 12 June, at Hunter College, New York.

RAMASUBBAN, R. (1990) 'Sexual behaviour and conditions of health care: potential risks for HIV transmission in India', paper prepared for the International Union for the Scientific Study of Population Seminar on Anthropological Studies Relevant on the Sexual Transmission of HIV, in Sonderborg, Denmark.

RAMUSACK, B.N. (1989) 'Embattled advocates: the debate over birth control in India, 1920–40', *Journal of Women's History*, 1, pp. 34–64.

RAVINDRAN, T.K.S. (1993) 'Women and the politics of population and development in India', *Reproductive Health Matters*, 1, pp. 26–38.

ROSENFELD, M. (1992) 'Deconstruction and legal interpretation: conflict, indeterminacy and the temptations of the new legal formalism', in CORNELL, D., ROSENFELD, M. and CARLSON, D.G. (eds), *Deconstruction and the Possibility of Justice*, New York: Routledge.

RUTHVEN, M. (1984) *Islam in the World*, New York: Oxford University Press.

SANGER, M. (1920) *Woman and the New Race*, New York: Truth.

SCHNEIDER, E.M. (1991) 'The dialectic of rights and politics: perspectives from the women's move-ment', in BARDEN, K.T. and KENNEDY, R. (eds), *Feminist Legal Theory*, Boulder, CO: Westview Press.

SEN, G. (1992) *Women, Poverty and Population: Issues for the Concerned Environmentalist*, Cambridge, MA: Center for Population and Development Studies, Harvard University.

——, GERMAIN, A., and CHEN, L. (eds) (1994) *Population Policies Reconsidered: Health, Empow-erment, and Rights*, Cambridge, MA: Harvard University Press.

TUSHNET, M. (1984) 'An essay on rights', *Texas Law Review*, 62, pp. 1363–403.

UNGER, R. (1983) 'The critical legal studies movement', *Harvard Law Review*, 96(3), pp. 561–675.

WASSERHEIT, J. (1993) 'The costs of reproductive tract infections in women', in BERER, M. and RAY, S. (eds), *Women and HIV/AIDS: An International Resource Book*, London: Pandora.

WEEKS, J. (1981) *Sex, Politics and Society: The Regulation of Sexuality Since 1800*, New York: Longman.

WILLIAMS, P.J. (1991) *The Alchemy of Race and Rights*, Cambridge, MA: Harvard University Press.

WOMEN'S GLOBAL NETWORK FOR REPRODUCTIVE RIGHTS (1991) *Statement of Purpose*, general leaflet.

ZIMMERMAN, M., *et al.* (1990) 'Assessing the acceptability of Norplant® implants in four countries: findings from focus group research', *Studies in Family Planning*, 21, pp. 92–103.

Part 6

Sexual categories and classifications

17 HIV, heroin and heterosexual relations

Stephanie Kane [1991]

In urban areas dominated by the illegal drug trade, re-use of needles, drug injection, unsafe sex, and the human immunodeficiency virus (HIV) are a dangerous combination of social practice and biology. It is here that epidemiologists, ethnographers and the media are tracking the fastest progression of HIV infection in the United States (Turner, Miller and Moses, 1989; Des Jarlais, Friedman and Stoneburner, 1988). But HIV moves insidiously through bodily fluids. Behind the attention-getting drug scene, the virus may tap more and more deeply into the roots of our minority communities, constituting the gradual, rather than explosive spread into the heterosexual population predicted by the chief epidemiologist for the Centers for Disease Control (Altman, 1987). As intravenous (IV) drug users become exposed and infected to HIV through used needles and have unprotected, penetrative sex with their part- ners, HIV continues to spread. A 'general public' immune to HIV infection is a fiction that undermines public health efforts to prevent AIDS among individuals who do not necessarily identify themselves or their partners with high-risk groups even though epidemiologically they may fit in such categories. Ethnographic analysis of individual experience and social practice reveals the weakness of the opposition between 'general public' and 'high-risk groups' when used for research or education.

This research documents the personal experience of sex partners of intravenous drug users – their girlfriends and wives, boyfriends and husbands – in relation to the risk of HIV infec- tion. Analysis focuses on how sex partners negotiate the risk of HIV infection in the context of sexual relationships that are shaped by drug-use practices. The study is part of a larger street outreach project sponsored by the National Institute on Drug Abuse (NIDA Grant No. 5R18 DAO 5285). Analysis is based on epidemiological and ethnographic interviews with 35 African American male and female sex partners from Chicago's southside in 1988–89. It is supported by additional ethnographic interviews with 22 other sex partners and 10 intrave- nous (IV) drug-using partners of both genders and white, Latino, as well as African American ethnicities from north-, west- and southsides of the city.

As defined by the study, sex partners are individuals who had vaginal intercourse with an active IV drug user of the opposite sex within six months preceding interview. This is not a self-defined group; until they become study participants, sex partners do not identify them- selves as such. Participants qualified for the sex partner study only if they did not shoot drugs, although many used drugs by other routes of administration. Indeed, 80 per cent of the sample reportedly used a variety of drugs bought on the street at least occasionally. Most of the sex partners who used drugs preferred a synthetic form of heroin called 'karachi' that is used intranasally – that is, 'tooted'. While injected heroin may bring infected blood with it through a used needle, intranasal heroin use does not present a direct AIDS-related risk. Yet it produces the same problems of addiction. Sex partners who are habitual heroin users are closer to being in 'the life', the subculture dominated by illegal drug and sex trades. Thus the habit of tooting heroin affects the level and kind of risk of HIV infection that people take, as well as their potential for creating risk-reducing change (Mondanaro, 1987).

Thus, for the defined group of sex partners in this sample, it is not drug use that presents the most immediate risk of HIV infection. Nor is it casual sex with numerous partners of prostitution – the factors that are the focus of most previous research on heterosexual transmission of HIV. This study focuses on a different aspect of risk, one which is more embedded in core mainstream values: the risk that accompanies primary relationships of some years and some stability. Unprotected sex with long-term heterosexual partners who shoot drugs presents the most immediate risk of HIV infection in this group.

Sex partners whose most stable relationship presents them with the highest risk in regard to HIV infection have a different set of concerns from those generally considered appropriate to 'high-risk groups' in the limelight of street action. By documenting the situations and concerns of sex partners, and analysing these from their perspectives and in their language, it becomes possible to understand how and why people do or do not respond to public health information about HIV infection as currently presented by the scientific community. This research begins to identify the dimensions of everyday experience that are relevant to the AIDS epidemic in urban minority communities where heroin use is prevalent, but which are as yet unaddressed by epidemiological studies.

If the strategic aspect of discursive representations of experience is taken into account (Clifford, 1986), and if discursive representations are interpreted within appropriate social and historical contexts, they can provide a rich source of material for understanding the social impact of the AIDS epidemic. Without this discursive dimension, analytic power to interpret seroprevalence data cross-culturally would be lacking. In addition, and independently of the problem of interpreting seroprevalence data, ethnographic analysis of discourse recorded in interviews provides a way to link the experience of sexual intimacies implicated in HIV transmission with broader patterns of social relations and the historical conditions that structure these patterns. For instance, the interviews documented here examine the relation between the risk of HIV infection through the intimate sexual practices of intravenous drug users and their sex partners, the social organization of experience in an urban African American community, and the way that experience of sexual relations and sexual risk is shaped by drug-related practices. Ethnographic analysis of discourse thus links local, culturally specific meanings through which AIDS is interpreted to our understanding of AIDS as a global phenomenon.

Method

Background on the epidemiology of heterosexual transmission

Bidirectional heterosexual intercourse is an established route of transmission globally, but its efficiency and related risk factors remain unclear (Padian, 1987). In the United States, there is an urgent need to understand the epidemiology of HIV transmission: in our minority communities where IV drugs use is prevalent, increasing numbers of AIDS cases are attributed to heterosexual transmission (Guinan and Hardy, 1987; Wofsy, 1987). Between 1988 and 1989, twice as many women as men were infected via heterosexual transmission, and over twice as many black women as compared to white women were infected via sex with a partner who used drugs intravenously (Centers for Disease Control, 1989a).

In Central Africa, where heterosexual transmission is the dominant mode and there is little or no reported IV drug use, studies of female prostitutes have identified numerous sex partners as an important factor in heterosexual HIV transmission. For example, in Kinshasa, Zaire, HIV seroprevalence rates were shown to increase steadily among female prostitutes who had a range of lifetime sex partners numbering between less than 200 and more than 1000 (Mann, Quinn and Francis, 1986). As Padian (1987, p. 947) points out, reporting bias, incidence of other sexually transmitted diseases, cultural differences in sexual practices and the role of prostitutes, make it difficult to interpret data such as this. While statistical probabilities suggest that there are increased risks inherent in the sexual behaviour of individuals such as the prostitutes sampled in Zaire, they are a questionable basis for public health messages that warn against 'promiscuity' and emphasize a reduction in the number of partners as a primary AIDS prevention strategy in the United States.

In a recent study evaluating the impact of public health messages in the US, a mathematical probability analysis of HIV infection patterns indicates that in both high and low seroprevalence groups, consistent and careful condom use is a far more effective method of reducing risk of HIV infection than is reducing the number of partners (Reiss and Leik, 1989). Although the latter lowers the risk of selecting an infected partner, repeated exposure to a single infected partner raises the risk of HIV infection from that individual. Hearst and Hulley (1988) point out that having one partner in a 'high-risk group' is more dangerous than having safe sex with many partners who are not. There is also evidence from Italy that the risk of being infected with HIV from steady partners is greater than from occasional partners (Centers for Disease Control, 1989b). Padian (1988) does point out, however, that HIV transmission displays a tremendous heterogeneity in infectivity: some women experience transmission after only a few contacts with an infected man, whereas other women remain uninfected despite thousands of repeated unprotected contacts.

The identification of 'promiscuity' as a causal factor in the epidemiology of AIDS has been the subject of a number of critiques (see Watney, 1987; Oppenheimer, 1988, p. 267; Treichler, 1988; Bolton, 1989; Murray and Payne, 1989) to which this research lends further support. While the risk of even single, casual encounters cannot be ignored, this research indicates that to reach individuals who may be at risk of HIV infection from long-term partners, public health education must emphasize the safeness of sex, not the diversity of partners or casualness. Sex plays a different kind of role, and sexual risk has different meanings in the lives of people with only one or two partners (as in 71 per cent of this study sample of $n = 35$) than in those individuals who engage in sex with numerous partners. Among most of the sex partners of intravenous drug users in this sample, it is not a high number of casual partners, but unsafe sex with a monogamous or primary partner that represents the greatest risk of exposure to HIV.

Research context of the sex partner study

Research with sex partners of intravenous drug users on the predominantly black southside of Chicago was carried out as part of a street outreach project focusing on IV drug users in three sites with contrasting ethnic composition in that city. Research included a standard interview administered nationally and designed for quantitative assessments, open-ended ethnographic interviews, and testing for HIV antibodies. All data is strictly confidential; the staff in direct contact with participants did not know their HIV status and participants chose whether or not they wanted to find out the results of the HIV test. Preliminary calculations (from August 1990) of HIV seropositivity rates in all three sites of the Chicago study are 22 per cent ($n = 224$ out of 1014) for IV drug users and 6 per cent ($n = 10$ out of 171) for sex partners. For the southside site alone, HIV seropositivity is 16 per cent ($n = 51$ out of 311) for IV drug users and 3 per cent ($n = 1$ out of 40) for sex partners. Note that for the most part, IV drug user and sex partners' samples had to be recruited independently, so that individuals in the sex partner sample are not necessarily partners with individuals in the IV-drug-user sample. Although on the increase, seropositivity rates associated with IV drug use in Chicago are generally much lower than New York City, reflecting the epidemic lag time between urban areas of the east coast and midwest (Des Jarlais *et al.*, 1987). It is this lag time that provides the opportunity for effective intervention.

The research purpose of the larger Chicago project is the testing of a social network model of AIDS intervention that employs indigenous ex-addicts as outreach workers (Wiebel, 1988). In order to carry out AIDS intervention, ex-addicts re-enter social networks within which they once engaged in shooting behaviour. The model conceptualizes intervention as the institution of risk-reduction behaviours as group norms. A step-wise approach to risk reduction encourages intravenous drug users to actively use the AIDS prevention method that they are best able to achieve – in other words, if people cannot stop shooting drugs, and cannot avoid shooting with used needles, then perhaps they can incorporate a regular practice of disinfecting needles with bleach and rinsing with clean water. If a person must engage in penetrative sex with a partner whose HIV status is unknown, then careful condom use should become routine. At the same time outreach workers work the streets, distributing bleach, condoms and AIDS information, they assess risk behaviours with individuals. Outreach workers also establish and maintain relations of trust between IV-drug-using networks and field-station staffs, which include ethnographers, medical personnel and interviewers.

The southside field station is located in a storefront on the street that marks the area's largest centre of the drug shooting subculture, an area that also includes a major prostitution 'stroll'. The field station is identified as a place where intravenous drug users come to participate in formal, paid, research tasks. It is also a place where intravenous drug users ('hypes' or 'shooters') come to pass the time. In large part due to the magetism of one senior outreach worker who has shared much experience with local intravenous drug users, first in the street and in prison as an addict, then later as counsellor and administrator in drug-treatment programmes, the station has become incorporated into street life. He is a well-known figure in the network of intravenous drug users who come in on a daily basis and play dominos and bridge in the front room. Their lively presence forms the ongoing ambiance of the station, contextualizing the scheduled research tasks of interviewing and blood-drawing within a friendly and protective social environment. Working at the station provides a way for ethnographers to engage in participant observation without continually exposing themselves to the stress, unpredictability, and potential violence of illegal activities on city streets.

Recruitment and interviewing for the sex partner study

As awareness of the mounting risk of HIV infection from male intravenous drug users to their female sexual partners grew in the United States, the sexual partner component of the Chicago project was added to outreach and research efforts. The social network model was adapted to accommodate sex partner recruitment on the southside. But the outreach team found that intravenous drug users in the networks already targeted were reluctant to share information about their partners with staff, or information about AIDS and IV drug use with their non-shooting partners, as discussion of these issues could prejudice their relationships. At the same time, as Sterk *et al.* (1989) also describe, even after contact with outreach workers, many sex partners are reluctant to participate in a project associated with intravenous drug users. In December of 1988, a woman was hired and trained to do outreach specifically to sex partners of intravenous drug users. By the end of April 1989 she recruited the sample of 35 men and women upon which this study is based.

The relatively small size of the sample is a result of our difficulties in discovering and verifying sex partner status. In contrast to the verification of IV-drug-user status, often as simple as rolling up the sleeves and demonstrating 'fresh tracks' where drugs had been recently injected, there is no physical sign of past sexual behaviour with an IV drug user. Because we paid project participants (sex partners received a total of $30 for two interviews and a blood test), motivation to fabricate sex partner relations existed. For the most part, we assured sex partner status by limiting recruitment to individuals of whom the outreach worker had some prior knowledge. In the case of 24 of the 35 sex partners (69 per cent), the outreach worker either knew the sex partner or IV drug user personally or had seen them around enough to know relevant facts about them. Five (14 per cent) sex partners were recruited through their IV-drug-using partners who were already known to station staff. Four (11 per cent) sex partners reached the station through friends who had already been recruited as sex partners; and two (6 per cent) sex partners unknown to staff were contacted directly through street outreach. When prior information was not available, the outreach worker and the ethnographer for sex partner component (the author), recruited the senior outreach worker to engage the person in conversation. We questioned candidates on criteria for participation, and tested their knowledge of minor details regarding IV drug use, which they would know if they had intimate contact. We also checked their arms to make sure there were no track marks from IV drug use. The aim of this screening procedure was to eliminate individuals who might be 'conning' us for the money. If we had no reason to suspect a person of being insincere, we accepted them into the sample. At the time of contact, all participants already knew that their partners did shoot drugs.

The resulting sample extends out of the outreach worker's personal network – that is, people whom she knows through her kin, friends, and acquaintances; past careers as student, addict, and person in treatment; and general familiarity of the areas of the southside where she grew up. In contrast to the IV-drug-user networks the main project focused on, which have an existence independent of the AIDS epidemic, sex partners have not identified themselves as a group prior to AIDS intervention, and are at some distance from the IV-drug-user network. Thus the sample most closely reflects a strategic use of the web of lifetime social interactions created by one dynamic individual in a complex, yet circumscribed, urban environment.

The dynamic nature of the outreach worker's personality and history, and her commitment to the project, cannot be underestimated in understanding the success of her efforts. Another difficulty that she had to overcome was that several members of the sample made a regular practice of avoiding sites of social interaction frequented by intravenous drug users. Our field station, created for intravenous drug users, was one such site that sex partners tended to avoid. In these cases, the money we offered was little inducement. The outreach worker had to overcome the resistance of sex partners who did not want to frequent the station, allay the anxiety provoked by discussion of personal and difficult matters with a stranger, and convince them of the importance of AIDS education and research.

To minimize anxieties sex partners might have in coming into the station and maximize the depth of acquaintance, after introduction and screening, the ethnographer administered the standard epidemiological interview as well as the ethnographic interview. Each took about an hour. The standard form was designed by NIDA for use on all National AIDS Demonstration research projects with intravenous drug users. It elicits quantifiable data on demographics, history of drug use, needle use and sexual behaviour, drug treatment, prison experience, travel, health, current knowledge of AIDS transmission and prevention, and HIV antibody testing. The form was designed primarily for use with intravenous drug users. When administered to sex partners, many of whom had little direct connection with drugs and crime, the subject matter, explicit style, and level of specificity in regard to illegal behaviour, posed problems of appropriateness which had to be overcome in the ethnographic interview that followed.

Recording life histories is a form of qualitative, ethnographic interviewing that can be adapted to the dual purpose of AIDS research and intervention (Rosenbaum, 1981, p. 139; Geiger, 1986). The topic of AIDS and related risk behaviours reviewed in the initial standard interview served as a frame of reference for the ethnographic interview that followed. With AIDS as a frame of reference, each person's history and present approach towards sexual relationships were discussed and reinterpreted. The social context of sexual relationships and the everyday, practical aspects of how sexual relationships are formed and experienced were discussed. Topics include: a reconstruction of everyday routines with details of how, when and why individual routines intersect; points of argument and decision-making that have affected a couple's course through time and space; interacting characteristics of multiple sexual relationships, also changing with time.

Description of sample

This summary is based on data reported by 35 African Americans (17 men and 18 women) between the ages 23 to 59 (mean age for men = 40; for women = 36) who had sexual relations with an IV drug user in the six months prior to interview. Although habitual drug use had levelled economic differences among them, the sample represents a diversity of interests, attitudes, and lifestyles that draw from past and present differences in class, education, profession, responsibility to children, and involvement in the sex and drug trades (see Table 17.1).

Non-intravenous use of street drugs is a common but not universal practice in this sample (see Table 17.2). A pattern of multiple drug use – in other words, different drugs used simultaneously or sequentially depending on cost availability, and purity – predominates among the users in this sample.

Nevertheless, there is a strong preference for opiate-related compounds. More specifically, most of the drug-using sex partners preferred a synthetic form of heroin called 'karachi' that is used intranasally.

At the time this research took place, karachi, a mix that laboratory analysis indicates may also contain phenobarbitol and methaqualone, was commonly sold on the southside. Its production and use may be unique to Chicago.

As reported, sexual practices show great homogeneity; the frequency and diversity of sexual practice in this sample is not remarkably high. Most adhere to a conventional pattern of vaginal intercourse. There are three different approaches to using condoms evident in the sample: using condoms never, sometimes, or always. Over half (54 per cent) of the sample reported never using condoms; 37 per cent reported using condoms sometimes. Only three sex partners, women of ages 23, 38, and 51 (9 per cent), reported always using condoms for vaginal sex (see Table 17.3). The low level of condom use is not consistent with the level of knowledge in regard to AIDS risk as measured by a True/False test on the standard interview: 100 per cent knew that they could be exposed to HIV through unprotected vaginal sex; 97 per cent knew that it is possible for intravenous drug users to be exposed through sharing dirty needles; 89 per cent knew that condoms could protect one from exposure to HIV during sex.

This is demonstrated by thirteen individuals who reported using condoms some of the time and not using them others. For eight of those individuals, the partial use of condoms does not

Table 17.1 Demographics of heterosexual sex partner sample. Medical history, education, income and residence as reported by sex partners (SPs). (IVDU = intravenous drug user)

	# Female SPs (n = 18)	# Male SPs (n = 17)	% Total sample
MEDICAL HISTORY (most common problem)			
gonorrhea	4	10	40%
pneumonia	4	4	23%
EDUCATION			
some college	4	8	34%
high-school degree	7	3	29%
no high-school degree	7	6	37%
literacy	18	17	100%
INCOME (six months prior to interview)			
part- or full-time legal employment			
(all but two in service occupations)	5	4	26%
government aid only	9	3	34%
government aid supplemented by illegal sources (theft,	2	7	26%
prostitution/pimping, and/or drug dealing)			
illegal sources only	0	3	9%
supported by kin	1	0	3%
indigent	1	0	3%
RESIDENCE (six months prior to the interview)			
SP supports own residence	15	4	54%
SP fully or partially supports residence shared with IVDU	1	6	20%
SP lives with own kin	1	4	14%
SP lives in residence supported by IVDU	1	1	6%
or kin of IVDU			
SP has no stable residence	0	2	6%

reflect an inconsistent approach. Rather, these individuals have adapted public health information to fit their own situation, using personalized rules to guide sexual risk behaviour that they then reported following in a consistent manner. For example, four women and two men reported always using condoms with partners other than their IV-drug-using partner(s). By following this rule, they leave themselves and their IV-drug-using partners open to the possibility of HIV infection or reinfection, but protect all other partners. In contrast, one man and one woman followed the reverse rule, always using condoms with IV-drug-using partner(s), but never with others. The transformation of public health messages into personalized rules of condom use tailored to conform to the constraints and complications of sexual relationships shape the direction of possible HIV transmission.

The number and stability of sexual relationships affects the probability that HIV will be transmitted to and from a sex partner. In this sample, there is not a characteristically high number of 'casual' partners. For 94 per cent of the women and 65 per cent of the men, their primary relationship is the factor most implicated in AIDS-related risk – that is, the one they have with an IV drug user (see Table 17.4). As defined here, primary relationships, like monogamous ones, involve sharing, fidelity, exchange and emotional commitment; in contrast to monogamy, primary relationships allow for the possibility of secondary relationships with 'outside' individuals. While there may be additional partners with whom sex is practised, these relationships tended to be more occasional and less emotionally significant.

Table 17.2   Non-intravenous drug use in a small heterosexual sample. Reported use of street drugs and alcohol by partners (SPs) of IV drug users in 6 months preceding interview

	# Female SPs (n = 17)	# Male SPs (n = 18)	% Total sample
HABITUAL USERS			46%
Heroin/karachi	6	6	34%
cocaine*	0	2	(6%)
heroin/karachi and cocaine	0	2	(6%)
OCCASIONAL USERS			
(miscellaneous drugs)	6	6	34%
Non-users			
(abstinence includes alcohol)	6	1	20%

* Cocaine was sold in hydrochloride form and tooted or smoked as freebase; crack was not commonly sold in southside Chicago during this research period

Nevertheless, when sex partners have unprotected sex, they put all their partners as well as themselves at risk for HIV infection.

Both men and women reported receiving money in exchange for sexual relations, or in the case of men, 'pimping' for women who did so. But for the most part, the distinction between prostitution, on the one hand, and on the other hand social/sexual relationships in which monetary exchange constituted a form of gift-giving, is quite blurry. Only one woman, the youngest in the sample, explicitly said that she engaged in street prostitution. All together, the 18 women in the sample reported having sex with an average of 2.3 men in the six months prior to interview; men reported the same average number of 2.3 women. The woman who did work sex on the street had the highest number of partners ($n = 13$). If she is not included in this calculation, the average number of men with whom women practised sex is 1.6, a number more representative of this mostly middle-aged, child-rearing, 'low profile' sample.

Table 17.3   Sex practices in a small heterosexual sample. Reported frequency of sexual practices and condom use by sex partners (SPs) in 6 months preceding interview, including, but not limited to sex with IV-drug-using partner. (+c = used condoms always; ±c = used condoms sometimes; -c = never used condoms)

	#Female SPs (n = 18)			#Male SPs (n = 17)			% Total sample
	+c	+/–c	–c	+c	+/–c	–c	
VAGINAL SEX							100%
once/week or less	2	2	4	0	2	3	(37%)
once/day or less	1	3	4	0	5	6	(54%)
more than once/day	0	1	1	0	1	0	(9%)
ORAL/PENILE SEX							46%
once/week	0	1	4	1	0	3	(26%)
once/day or less	1	0	0	0	0	6	(20%)
ANAL SEX							9%
once/week or less	0	1	0	0	0	2	(9%)

Table 17.4 Age and sexual relationships of a small heterosexual sample. Age and sexual relationships with intravenous-drug-using partners (IVDUs) and others reported as active in 6 months prior to interview by male and female sex partners (SPs)

	n	*Mean years of age (range)*	*Mean # SPs (range)*	*Mean duration (years) SP–IVDU relation (range)*	*% SP–IVDU relations that are primary*
female SP	18	36 (23–54)	2.3 (1–13)	4.9 (1–15)	94.4%
male SP	17	40 (29–59)	2.3 (1–6)	8.1* (2–17)	64.7%

* Calculation based on *n* = 14 (incomplete data)

For the sex partners in this sample, relationships with intravenous drug users tend to be long term. The estimated duration of these relationships averages 4.9 years (*n* = 18) for female sex partners with male IV drug users, and 8.1 years (*n* = 14) for male sex partners with female IV drug users. Despite the relative stability of relationships over time, however, sex partners do not tend to develop relationships of economic inter-dependence with IV-drug-using partners. Given the destructive economics of drug addiction, this comes as no surprise. Only two women and two men interviewed reported being dependent on their IV-drug-using partners for financial support in the six months preceding interview. Fourteen (78 per cent) of the women and eleven (65 per cent) of the men reported that they were financially independent of their male IV-drug-using partners. Over half (54 per cent) of all sex partners maintain a residence different from their IV-drug-using partners (see Table 17.1).

There are gender differences apparent in residence patterns, which may be due in part to governmental conditions for receiving economic aid (Stack, 1974). Women were more likely to rely solely on government aid, have a stable residence, and bear the burden of child care and support. Female sex partners more often supported households that included children and excluded male IV-drug-using partners. Ten (56 per cent) of the women supported children under 18 years of age in their households, but only one (6 per cent) reported sharing her household with a male IV-drug-using partner. In contrast, male sex partners were more likely to support households which included female IV-drug-using partners (*n* = 6; 35 per cent) than ones that included children (*n* = 2; 12 per cent).

In sum, although the patterns represented cannot be over-generalized because of the small sample number, some tendencies can be noted. The lives of most sex partners interviewed are circumscribed by poverty, lack of rewarding employment, and use of addictive drugs. Sex partners are involved in long-term, primary relationships with IV drug users. The stability of these relationships does not depend on the establishment of joint households, indeed, sex partners show a marked tendency toward financial and residential independence. Vaginal intercourse without condoms or with partial use of condoms are the predominant forms of sexual practice in the sample. The multiple strategies of risk-reduction represented, dependent as they are on variable interpretation and application of public health information, indicate the need to understand the effect of social context in the design and implementation of AIDS intervention and education programmes.

Results: one take on a complex scene

Pressures impinging on the process of risk-reduction

Decisions to adopt sexual risk-reduction methods take place in a social and economic context that is shaped by a constellation of interacting conditions and events. Relationships are dynamic; the dynamics of the relationships between sex partner and IV drug user are complicated by single or double drug addiction. Severe heroin addiction has the power to push everything else in a person's life to the side, sapping the ability and concern to deal with everyday life. AIDS awareness as a motivator for risk reduction may fade in and out of importance as addictions cycle and attitudes toward relationships change. Other factors influence the ability to incorporate new information and active changes in behaviour. For sex partners who have a number of sexual relationships in addition to their steady one, the integration of risk-reduction methods is more complicated, and life is generally more chaotic. Public health information may need to be integrated in different ways at different times.

The significance accorded AIDS as a risk factor in everyday life is also determined by pressures external to sexual relationships. It's hard to deal with possible futures in an overwhelming present. In ghetto life, the possibility of AIDS is just one of many threats to well-being. Women are trying to raise kids alone in a crime-ridden environment with barely enough money to live. People get sick and, not infrequently, someone close to them dies. Many are unemployed and on the street when they're not in jail. Low-level jobs are stressful. Those who make it out to work in downtown Chicago or the suburbs strain to resolve the irresolvable pressures of getting paid in the white world and living in the black ghetto. There's never enough money, not much to do, and violence an everpresent possibility. When life is rough, survival day to day, it's hard to think about the possibility of HIV infection too.

The social context of relationships between sex partner and IV drug user

Identity and participation with the drug subculture is different for sex partners and their IV-drug-using partners. This difference shapes the way negotiations regarding AIDS risk-reduction are carried out. Most sex partners reported that they did not find out that their IV-drug-using partner actually shot drugs till well after the relationship was established. In part, this is because the two do not participate together in group activities that would make differences in drug use apparent. They form relationships that cross group boundaries (see Figure 17.1). The 'square' sex partners in this sample orient their lives toward mainstream black culture, organizing activities around family, work, and church. They may never use drugs, or may use them as alcohol is commonly used – for example, to celebrate special occasions. In any case, they do not identify with the drug subculture (from whence their classification as 'square' derives), and are connected to it only through their partners. 'Mrs Jones', one such 50-year-old woman who has been married for 12 years to her second husband, an IV drug user, explains how they are part of different social groups:

> We [she and her husband] grew up together, and you know you keep those friendships. And now I speak and I socialize with people and everything. But I don't go out of my way to try and make no whole lot of friends, you know. So the ones that I know, my friends don't use no drugs. … I don't know his street friends.

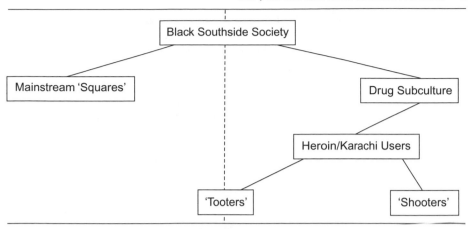

Figure 17.1 Social categories of heterosexual sample in respect to drug use

Her husband is a member of the IV-drug-using network that 'hangs out' in and around the field station. When I asked how she manages to distance herself from a drug scene that occupies the same few blocks that she lives and shops on, she sketches these typical social interactions:

> Now like, by me coming through, by them hanging on the corner, I don't speak to them, you know. We'll look at one another. Now if I see him hanging up there and they're all grouped up there together, well I'll walk up and I'll say, 'Hi. How is everybody?' or something like that. But I don't think they really hang nowhere; I think they just hanging on these corners, you know. I don't know their wives or their old ladies or nothing like that. And he don't take me to, say like me and you are friends and I would say, 'Well, why don't you guys come over this week end and we watch the VCR or some tapes'. His friends don't do that. … So that's just what makes me think that it's too much secretive, you know. I don't know where he go. I don't know where he be. And I'm wondering if he have got another friend, a girlfriend, that's friends with these people, you know, and they doing the thing this way. But it doesn't bother me.

In contrast to the squares, some sex partners use heroin occasionally or addictively, tooting instead of shooting it. Most of the sex partners who use heroin habitually are addicted to karachi, a synthetic form of heroin that is nearly always tooted (it is insoluble in water). Although they are part of the wider heroin-oriented drug subculture, they no more identify with social networks of intravenous drug users than squares do; heroin tooters and shooters form socially distinct groups (Kane, 1989b). A 23-year-old woman who had been dating an IV drug user for about three years puts it simply: 'He has his friends that like to shoot up and I have my friends that like to toot'. A 41-year-old man, married to an IV drug user for eleven years, looks down on the shooting lifestyle. He tells me:

> Matter of fact, most of the guys that I'm around have homes, families, and they indulge just to a point and after that, that's it. They set a limit and they live by it. They been at that for 15 or 20 years and so it's not nothing that they just started, it's always been that way. … Whether you believe this or not, it's a thing with us whether you might call us snobs. Because to a point, we look down on the other group and even though we may use, we

call them 'dope fiends'. I know that it's a snobbish attitude, but we always try to keep ourselves away from the depth of it. We don't want to get down to that point of where the corner is our main environment. … When I do get high, I get high at home, OK? I never ever get high on the street. Once I am high, I am never on a corner standing for the world to see me. … Generally it's two or three of us getting together on payday or something and spend $15 or $20 bucks apiece, then that's the way, and we all go home. Or we'll go to one person's house and when the [TV football or basketball] game is over then we're done with it.

Clear-cut distinctions between tooting and shooting may be self-deluding, at least from a drug treatment standpoint, as addiction can result from either practice (C. Rhoades, personal communication). But from the perspective of a demanding addiction, heroin tooters have practical reasons to form their own social networks. Heroin for tooting may vary in chemical form from heroin for shooting. 'Hot dope' for shooting often has quinine in it, in order, they say, to 'boost the rush', but this makes it burn when snorted up the nose. On the other hand, heroin in the form of karachi is hard to inject. Tooters therefore buy heroin at 'copping' sites that are often different from shooter's copping sites. The sites move around the city, and dealers may change face and supply unpredictably. Connections with reliable dealers are learned of through other tooters. Tooters may share information about good 'connect[ion]s', split the cost of a 'bag', and 'do it up' together.

When a sex partner is involved with an IV drug user, even when both are using heroin, drug administration is rarely a joint activity. A 27-year-old woman, who snorts karachi on occasion, has been dating an IV drug user three or four times a week for about three years. She explains:

OK, I've got some friends that shoot drugs and I socialize with them. I might go over and we might smoke a joint [of marijuana] or something together, you know, and that's it. I don't really hang out with them. I don't go with them to cop their drugs and they don't go with me to cop mine because most intravenous drug users think that karachi is a waste of money – because it's a synthetic drug – for one thing. And they just get pissed off with you because you tooting it, you know. And they feel like they could have been buying something else with that money that you wasted, [they could have been] firing up their arms. So, you know, y'all don't really socialize with another. Not on the get high tip. Cause they feel like it's a waste. But you feel like you really getting high, but they feel you just fucking up money. You just wasting time and money.

A 38-year-old man, now in methadone treatment, discusses how social relations are reorganized on the basis of drug use. In his case, differences in how they administered heroin has been forcing a separation between himself and a woman with whom he has been living for the preceding seven years, and intimate with for the preceding nine:

By her using, the people she dealt with, that she used to deal with, she don't deal with. She started hanging around the shooting crowd. I just couldn't really, how could I say it? They don't relate to me, because I don't do what they do. If you got a bag [of heroin], a person that is snorting, he wants to snort it; a person that shoot it he wants to put it in water. So now me and him, or me and her, we can't communicate no more. They gravitating more towards shooting; she is pulling more towards their way. Even though me and her – she will say, 'Everything is cool with me and you, and I still love you'. When she had to go take care of business, she had to go with them. Then I didn't like that because I figured sooner or later it ain't going to be me and her. I thought that maybe I could keep her here, that maybe some kind of way me and her could get some kind of treatment and so forth and so on. But it didn't work that way. I just accepted her like she was.

As this quote describes, tooters and shooter don't fit in the same social circles. It also indicates that it is possible for some people to live with a shooter without also starting to shoot, even if they are addicted to heroin. Tooting sex partners are excluded from IV-drug-user networks in which social relations are characteristically organized intensively around repeating cycles of obtaining money, copping, and injecting. Because tooting requires higher doses to produce the same effect, tooting heroin on a regular basis is not an economically acceptable practice among shooters. Recruitment into 'hard core' scenes is not an inevitable consequence of heroin use. Thus, in the relationships between sex partners and IV drug users, identities in respect to the drug subculture do not necessarily shift. Differential identities and participation in the drug scene lend these relationships their particular character and govern the enactment of joint behaviour in space and time. Differential identities of tooters and shooters in personal relationships are in some sense mutually beneficial: a tooter may be committed to a person who shoots but fears shooting because it represents getting in deeper into the life; a shooter who has a partner who is not caught up in the street scene can periodically share a measure of stability, or at least find a comfortable and warm place to rest. But how does commitment between a square or tooter and a shooter develop and how is it affected when a sex partner realizes that their partner's shooting behaviour has put them at risk from AIDS?

The formation and management of relationships between sex partners and IV drug users

Southside Chicago is a densely populated urban ghetto, but it can seem like a small town. Most people find their social lives within a fifty-block range, visiting regularly with neighbours and kin, taking the same paths to work and shop. Repetitive sightings make strange faces familiar. When opportunities arise, introductions are made. Sex partners meet intravenous drug users in neighbourhood bars, grocery and liquor stores, at parties, at work, in rooming houses, in school. When sex partners first get to know an IV drug user with whom a long-term relationship will develop, the IV drug user is often in a healthy phase of addiction. It is when they lose control over their habit that they are discovered. By the time the sex partner learns of the other's condition, they may already feel committed to them, and thus try and go ahead, live with it, and help. They've already 'gotten in too deep'.

The drug scene brings sex partners and intravenous drug users together. Dealers may sell cocaine to both. Cocaine is commonly used by tooters and shooters to either boost the heroin high or as a cheaper alternative to heroin. Besides selling drugs, 'connects' (dealers) provide an opportunity for customers to meet. Customers may toot up a bag of heroin or cocaine together for fun, developing a friendship that leads to sex. But meeting an IV drug user through a connect may be misleading. Intravenous drug users rarely mention a preference for injection in their initial presentations of self. And non-injected drug use is common, so there is no reason to presume that someone with whom one happens to toot or smoke drugs is more likely to shoot drugs at other times.

A 33-year-old man from a middle-class Chicago suburb tells how he came to have a girlfriend who shot heroin:

I was using drugs and that's simply because my sister and her old man was using drugs, cause they was like peddling drugs, OK? And I would hang around them. Upstairs they had like a little place for a den that they all got around and socialized with, you know [laugh]. I wanted to do what they were doing, you know, 'cause they were older than I was. So I sat in with them and I started using drugs with them. Sniffing heroin, OK? And it's a girl that I liked, a young lady that I liked, one of my sister's friends. She used to come up there ever so often, you know, to purchase a little drugs, you understand? So we got to know each other. We started going with each other off and on. We started dating regularly, on a regular basis, OK? Just so happened, and then months to months went on, I didn't notice anything until I started noticing red spots on her legs. Little red spots, you understand. So one night me and her was gonna have sex, OK? And she said she had to use the washroom. And she went in the washroom and stayed almost an hour. So I went and found out what the hell was going on. I just bust open the door and there she was. Had the needle in her. She was like in a daze, you understand? A daze.

Some sex partners are not so innocent. A pimp spoke about the mother of two of his children, a woman he recruited as a prostitute when she was 14 years old and who later started to shoot drugs:

I turned her out to drugs and the whole game. The game, period. ... But the intention wasn't for her to use drugs. 'Cause that kind of takes money out of my pocket. Just be straight up and down and square and go to work and get my money. Like that. But it didn't turn out like that. Cause she'd meet other people in the streets and other influences, pressures and stress dealing with going to get my money. And so, it wasn't about love and happiness.

On the other hand, for square partners, it's hard to believe anyone would want to do drugs, much less shoot drugs. Intravenous drug users may offer plausible origins for their problem to make it more acceptable. Mrs Jones, the woman married for 12 years to an IV drug user (quoted above) tells what her husband told her about slipping back into his heroin habit:

... He said, you know, he was in Vietnam. And he said that's really where he got hooked at. He said because it was so much shooting and fighting going on over there until you really did have to have something. And he was very young. He was like nineteen years old. And he said it was so much shooting and killing and carrying on before, he said that he had to have something to keep his self together. He said that's where he started getting hold of those drugs at. ... I didn't even know that he had been messing with drugs until he told me. ... after we got married. He just started using drugs about two years ago. Got back on it.

Sex partners may delay discovery as long as possible. In some ways, it is easier not to acknowledge their partner's shooting behaviour. Chances are if they have difficulty acknowledging shooting behaviour, they also have trouble acknowledging the risk of AIDS.

The social management of relationships between sex partners and IV drug users

Sex partners and IV drug users manage their relationships with each other by managing their differences. They do so by maintaining everyday routines that are independent of one another and by establishing specific rules that minimize the visibility of the injection ritual. While the masking contradictions inherent in their different involvements in the drug subculture provide the conditions for relationships to persist over the long term, this process may block attempts to effectively acknowledge the risk of HIV transmission.

Independent routines

For the most part, sex partners and intravenous drug users reportedly pursue their responsibilities and obsessions independently. Time spent together tends to be fixed in space but unpredictable in time. There is an agreed meeting place, but meeting time is more spontaneous, depending on the tempo of street action. The most common pattern reported is a female sex partner who is home with regularity. Her male IV-drug-using partner will show up there in a characteristically erratic pattern – for example, most evenings at some unspecified time, or every two or three days for a couple of days, or, in less steady relationships, just 'once in a blue moon'. While unpredictability may make it impossible to depend on a man, a woman burdened with child-care responsibilities may appreciate having a relationship that does not become full-time. If a male sex partner has his own household or shares a household with a female IV drug user, he would probably be subject to the same street-governed schedule of unpredictability. Depending on the situation and the drug(s), strong addictions may level some gender differences (Kane, 1989a). Younger couples with few responsibilities usually have their own rooms or apartments. They arrange to meet on occasion for outings, having sex in one of their rooms if privacy permits, or in hotels that can be rented by the hour. And there are married partners with children who manage to hold steady jobs, raise kids, and maintain addictions.

Hence, for most couples, even those maintaining long-term relationships, sex partners and intravenous drug users live their lives independently. They have their own routines, and they are not dependent upon one another to accomplish these routines. They come together for company, sex, and accompanying economic benefits, each getting as much as they can from the relationship. Maybe they get what they need, or maybe they know that asking too much would not work anyway under the circumstances. Some do not have many options. The question of why individuals choose each other to bond with cannot be answered from the interviews, although it is clear that AIDS awareness may directly affect this kind of choice.

Rules limit drug use and displays of drug injection

The way sex partners described it to me, when they are apart from their IV-drug-using partners, they travel different geographies and engage in different activities. When they are together, they tend to be together alone, without others. Unless specifically provoked, disturbing differences in habits are not spoken of or acted on. In this way, relative peace is managed. It takes the efforts of both partners to make this work. For intravenous drug users, this means keeping an addiction from escalating, from devouring more and more of their lives. Nobody wants to get 'caught in the whirlpool'. For this reason, intravenous drug users gravitate toward moderating influences, like sex partners, to keep themselves at a level of addiction they can handle. By setting limits for themselves, there are intravenous drug users who have sustained heroin addictions from youth to old age without destroying their bodies and their relationships with other people. The poor quality of street heroin contributes to these techniques of addiction management.

For example, in an interview I did with an IV drug user, a college-educated woman who was intimately involved with one of the male sex partners in the study described her adherence to self-imposed limits. She had begun to snort heroin while working a high-pressure job in a state prison, and had begun shooting not long before the interview:

> I never take my stuff out the house and sell it, you know. Some place you have to have a line that you draw, you know. And when you've gotten up to that line, then it's no more that you can do, even if you do want it. And I've wanted it too. But you just have to, there's no more money, and there's nothing else you can do. It's over. Take your ass to bed. It's like living a double life, you know. You get high or whatever, and you hang out. And then you come home and you go to bed. You take a bath. You get up in the morning. You put your clean clothes on. You get your briefcase and go to your job and play that role.

This person had to temporarily drop out of the career track she was on and is now in treatment. When limits are observed and beneficial conditions exist, a person addicted to heroin may pull themselves up out of the whirlpool temporarily or, less often, for good. Methadone treatment can be useful in this way, helping the addict to lower the dose to which he or she is addicted. This reduces the intensity of addiction, and thus the economic and physiological burden it presents. Indeed, it may be more useful to consider addiction as cyclic, rather than a phenomenon that is either present or absent. The status of relationships between sex partners and IV drug users can then be interpreted in relation to the phase of addiction being dealt with at any one time.

When both sex partner and IV drug user are habitual heroin users, their addictions interact. There is a tendency to pull one another in. One 32-year-old woman addicted to karachi says of her relationship with an IV drug user:

> … Every time that I wanted to straighten out my life and pull myself together I would start on this uphill climb and I would do OK. He would say, 'Well baby, now come on, let's go back together. Let's go do this and let's go to do and let's get high'. I listen at that and he would pull me right back into the circle of where we were before. Or either he would try to straighten out his life and try to straighten out things on his job and what have you, and then I would come along and then I would pull him back. It was like we went through this for almost four years. We were pulling up and down, up and down, up and down. One day I just got tired. I couldn't take it any more. I just got depressed. I was depressed for two months. I didn't get out of bed and I didn't call nobody. I shut the door in my bedroom where nobody else was. I made sure all the drapes were pulled. I didn't care if my rent was paid or my phone was paid, didn't care about nothing. I just laid in my bed and lost, what … forty pounds.

The sex partner just quoted passes through phases when she wants to overcome her addiction but can't because these phases are not synchronous with her partner's. Motivated by a desire to 'stay clean', sex partners will try to break off relations with IV drug users at such times. But breaking up is usually a slip and slide process of small-scale negotiated steps towards separation. A 28-year-old female sex partner, with one child and a once-a-day intranasal heroin habit, comments on her IV-drug-using boyfriend:

> … he's on the street. But our relationship is on and off, on and off. Two people doing bad ain't going to make it, you know, like that. We don't live together. We did once upon a time, but we don't live together.

Many of the sex partners interviewed said that they continued relationships with IV drug users that tended to hover between being happy and breaking up. In the meantime, they persist in their routines, and adapt systems of rules that make daily life supportable. Shooting drugs, the behaviour directly involved in high risk of HIV transmission, is the focus of the most specific set of rules. Rules vary according to levels of strictness and tolerance, but they all function to minimize visibility of the injection ritual for the benefit of both partners. Most partners agree that shooting will not take place in the home of a sex partner, whether or not the sex partner does drugs by other means, and whether or not the IV drug user contributes to the economic support of the household. As one 34-year-old supported by his IV-drug-using girlfriend says: 'Nothing goes on in her place. Not there and not them [her shooting friends]'. Fifty-year-old Mrs Jones explains her preference for the rule about not letting her husband shoot up in the apartment they share together. Despite the fact that she uses neither drink nor drugs, she says:

> … you know what I imagine? If I had it. If they were coming to my house and I was looking at this stuff and watching them do it, maybe one time they would catch me at a vulnerable time when I was depressed and feeling sorry for myself, and I would say, 'What the heck. Give me some too'. But by him not, like I say, I don't know where they doing this stuff at.

A 37-year-old woman, whose life for the past couple of years has been focused on caring for a disabled mother and sister, has also been dating an IV-drug-using man. They meet and have sex about once a week. She says:

> When he is getting high I'm not with him. I can't stand the sight of blood. I can't stand the little episode that they go through. It's sickening to me. I've seen it before, that's why I know that I can't stand to see it.

Some will allow their partners to shoot behind the closed door of a bathroom, but not in their immediate presence. Shooters reportedly prefer the privacy and convenience that bathroom sinks afford when in the home of their sex partners. For example, a 40-year-old man who owns real estate and a small business near the field station lives with a partner who shoots Ritalin (the stimulant methylphenidate). He is strict about not letting her friends in their apartment, but takes a pragmatic approach toward shooting:

> Rather than to have her go to one of these so-called shooting galleries where they share needles, I would rather see her in the room somewhere shooting it, you know. And incidentally, she'll hide in the closet or something just because she knows what my attitude towards shooting drugs is, you know. She'll never let me see her doing it.

Even where both partners enjoy being high on the same drug together, administration may take place separately. For example, a 23 year-old woman with a partner who shoots heroin and a karachi habit of her own says:

> We do them [drugs] together but, as he is an IV drug user, it sort of, I don't know, I hate to say this, it sort of turns me off to see him shoot up or anything. So, when he has his little thing and I have my little thing, we seem to turn our backs or go in other rooms, you know. We're just not looking at one another when we're getting high. But afterwards, after we finish whatever we're doing, we always come back and, you know, kiss and pet and whatever.

Extenuating circumstances do arise. A 27-year-old woman who usually meets her boyfriend in hotels finds herself in this situation:

> I told him, 'Don't shoot it in front of me'. If he had to shoot it, 'Go to another room, you
> know. Don't do that in front of me.' But one time he did, you know. And that's because
> we was at his parent's house and they knowed if he was in that room by himself, they
> knew he had been shooting drugs. So he called me in there for a front. Like me and him
> was talking. And he shot the shit and I didn't care for it, you know. And I told him. Ever
> since then he didn't do it.

As these quotes suggest, the level of tolerance for shooting activities varies among sex
partners and is expressed in the house rules that couples negotiate. The institution of rules
regarding time and place of drug injection excludes the act of shooting and its attendant practices and companionships from the domestic sphere and from the consciousness of sex partners. By masking the contradictions inherent in their different involvements in the drug
subculture, sex partners normalize their relationships with intravenous drug users. This is the
social management of relationships. It allows long-term bonds to develop. But being blind to
shooting behaviour when one has a partner with a shooting habit has direct implications for
AIDS prevention. As one sex partner aptly points out:

> We talked about these things. Drug addicts will argue the point about this AIDS thing.
> They are not as safe with it as the person that don't shoot up. I think most drug addicts
> prefer to use their own needles, but you know they get into them types. For instance, if I
> say, 'Don't bring no drugs home'. He would go some place else and use them. You know
> what I'm saying? All the time he might not have his outfit [injection equipment] with
> him. The spot that they be in, they might not have bleach there. So if he wanted to get
> high, they're going to get high. Probably if most people could bring it home, it might cut
> down AIDS. You know, if you could just lay your stuff out and just have it out in the
> open, they might be a little more careful. It's two sides to every story. Because I don't
> use, I don't want to see it. And I might have been helping him to see it. He might have
> been a little safer in using. I hope he don't get AIDS or that he don't have it you know.
> I'm just saying that if a person can have their own spot and have everything that they
> need right there, it's a little safer than going out in the streets doing it. But I'm sure that
> most everybody that is with somebody that don't use don't want it around. You know
> what I'm saying?

That was a twice-widowed 54-year-old woman, speaking her mind. She and her IV-drug-using
partner had been 'on the up and down' for some time and he'd left town a couple of months
before the interview. She never does drugs herself: 'I got nephews and nieces. They are teenagers and there is a certain profile I carry for them'. Nor is she lax about shooting practices in
others. However, she doesn't believe in rules: 'You can't make a man do like you can a child'.
But even if she could, her comments suggest that her rules about IV drug-using would be
governed more by therapeutic concern than fear, disgust, or social convention. Therapeutic
concern, together with a realistic evaluation of one's own vulnerabilities, is what sex partners
may need to activate AIDS intervention efforts within their own personal spheres.

Acknowledging sexual risk

In general, when sex partners first meet IV-drug-using partners they are unaware of the
latters' habits of drug administration. Upon discovery of these habits, the couple experiences
a crisis in their relationship that is negotiated in various ways. Everyday routines and rules are

established to mitigate the sex partners' awareness of their partners' continued shooting behaviour (for example, by hiding the injection ritual) and to mitigate the potentially negative effects that a partner's shooting behaviour may actually have on a relationship (for example, by maintaining independent households). This process of social management normalizes the relationship, allowing it to persist in time.

Unfortunately, sexual transmission of HIV is independent of this process of social management. Whether or not partners create a situation in which shooting behaviour is specifically excluded from experience shared intentionally, viral exposure may be a present, invisible, and deadly possibility. The virus picked up 'in the street' may unintentionally be brought into the protected domestic sphere. It is the personal consequences of this fact that are brought to bear in an intervention interview. Conflicts over shooting behaviour and contradictions resulting from differences in identity and participation in the drug subculture, masked by strategies of social management, are brought to the surface. Thus intervention may trigger another crisis in the relationship between sex partner and IV drug user. Like the crisis that typically occurs when a sex partner discovers that the person they are involved with shoots drugs, a crisis triggered by acknowledging the risk of AIDS is a distressing event that may either end a relationship or open the way for change.

Proposed change is threatening, especially in the case of sex partners who want to be protected from their lovers because of IV drug use: IV drug use is already a bone of contention. Sex is just one aspect of a relationship, but it is an important channel through which an emotional bond is expressed and balance between partners and between partners and the wider society is achieved (Rubin, 1984). Couples cannot easily make risk-reducing changes such as having less sex, or putting a condom between them, or touching each other outside more than inside. Before making such proposals, a sex partner needs to make it clear that proposing change is not an act of judgement motivated by bad faith, that physical distancing does not necessarily signify a desire to withdraw from intimacy. Otherwise such proposals lead to misinterpretation, whatever the habitual sexual patterns (everyone has heard of AIDS, why bring it up now?). The possibility of successfully proposing change also depends on the phase of addiction the partners are experiencing at the time. If both partners could participate in AIDS intervention and/or drug treatment programmes, there is all the more chance that risk-reducing can be reasonably discussed (Wermuth, Ham and Gibson, 1988). This is often not the case. But through private interviews as well as group exchanges, sex partners can become prepared to take a strong yet sensitive stance when they present these issues to their IV-drug-using partners (NIDA, 1989). With persistence and creativity, the ideal of healthy, caring change can displace negative feelings.

Being able to acknowledge risk also depends on personal character and history, the financial situation, and the kind of relationships in which a sex partner is involved (Kane, 1990). Some sex partners don't want to struggle with the strong and negative emotions that may be evoked by the mere mention of a condom. Partners who are already on the verge of breaking up might choose to be done with the relationship altogether. Those more committed to a relationship may decide to stop having sex until their partners have their blood tested for HIV. Sex partners might choose to continue ignoring their risk or choose to transform their understanding of risk so that they feel more comfortable with it, personalizing public health information so that it fits their situation, protecting themselves in some ways, but not adhering to any absolutes. There may be as many ways to deal with AIDS information as there are sex partners. But if partners do decide to keep a relationship and do try to incorporate risk-reducing sexual behaviour, they must jointly initiate a negotiated, on-going, inventive process that begins with acknowledging the problem.

Conclusion

This ethnographic research adds a dimension of human experience to epidemiological representations of 'IV drug users' and 'sex partners'. In so doing, it reveals a certain lack of correspondence between these risk group categories and the social reality to which these categories are meant to refer. This lack of correspondence has wider implications for the use of risk group classifications in AIDS research and prevention more generally.

The social organization of everyday life in minority communities such as the southside of Chicago has been transformed by the escalation of drug trade in the recent past. Holding out (false) promise of relief to people whose lives are constrained by poverty and lack of opportunity, taking drugs may sometimes have appeal. The drug subculture is active and heterogeneous, producing its own categories by which individuals may be organized. In the social context described by the sex partners recruited into this study, people were divided into groups differentiated by the technologies and sensations of different drugs effects ('highs') and by the methods and moralities of different modes of economic survival ('hustles'). Differential identity and participation in these groups lend the relationships between sex partners and IV drug users their particular character and govern the enactment of joint behaviour, including sexual risk, in space and time.

To recapitulate, in the context of long-term, sexually active relationships in which only one partner shoots drugs, the possible conjuncture of risks is determined in part by the particular ways that this kind of relationship is socially managed. Most sex partners live independently of IV-drug-using partners. They come together socially, but tend to keep the economies of household and heroin apart. When couples do come together, problematic differences tend to be suppressed in deed and discourse. However, the acknowledgement and renegotiation of the double risks of unsafe sex and needle re-use requires explicit discussion of that which has been left unsaid. The persistence of risk-taking, especially in sex, must be understood within this particular context.

On the classification of high-risk groups

The problem of AIDS can be approached epidemiologically, using the language of risk based on statistical calculations of HIV seroprevalence and AIDS cases in large-numbered samples. And it can be approached ethnographically, using the language of any number of people who may be experiencing the complex reality that is indexed by statistics. This research uses an epidemiological category as a starting-point – heterosexual sex partners of IV drug users – and constructs an ethnographic version of one aspect of the problem of HIV transmission in minority neighbourhoods dominated by the drug trade in the United States. Once discursive representations of sex partners' social identities and practices are analysed, however, the conceptual and pragmatic weakness of public health models that rely on distinguishing 'high-risk groups' from a 'general population' somehow not at risk of HIV infection becomes more apparent. This sample of individuals who fit in the category of sex partners identify with the so-called general public and they are at risk of HIV infection. In other words, sex partners do not necessarily identify with any high-risk group, their own or their IV-drug-using partners. This problem of non-identification associated with the sex partner category is similar to, and provides further support for, critiques of risk group classification schemes based on cross-cultural analyses of the use of 'homosexual' as a category in AIDS discourse (Treichler, 1988, p. 122; Alonso and Koreck, 1989; Parker, 1987; Treichler 1989).

Epidemiologically, mainstream and heroin-addicted sex partners who toot the drug are in the same AIDS-related risk group, but ethnographically, the behaviour of sex partners who habitually toot heroin must be understood from the perspective of a heroin subculture that includes IV drug users. The categories of 'sex partners', 'IV drug users', and 'general public' cannot be clearly separated in practice. Description and analysis of this particular social context of HIV transmission reveals the level at which risk group typologies become incompatible with social practice, suggesting that there are limits to the usefulness of elaborating risk group typologies as a long-term strategy and goal of AIDS research and prevention.

Acknowledgements

This research was part of a larger National AIDS Demonstration Research project supported in part by the National Institute on Drug Abuse Grant No. 5R18 DAO 5285. My thanks for research assistance and discussion to Wayne Wiebel, Wendel Johnson, Sinia Harper, Claude Rhoades, Dana Nicholas, Lessie Jean Williams. Discussions with Theresa Mason were especially helpful in clarifying the issues involved. Thanks also to Pauline Greenhill for her editorial comments.

References

ALONSO, A.M. and KORECK, M.T. (1989) 'Silences: "Hispanics", AIDS, and sexual practices', *Differences: Journal of Feminist Cultural Studies*, 1, pp. 101–24.

ALTMAN, L.K. (1987) 'Anxiety allayed on heterosexual AIDS', *New York Times*, 5 June, p. 11.

BOLTON, R. (1989) 'AIDS and promiscuity: what's the connection, if any?' presented at the Annual Meetings of the Society for Applied Anthropology, Santa Fe.

CENTERS FOR DISEASE CONTROL (1989a) 'HIV/AIDS surveillance', 10 June, p. 8.

—— (1989b) 'AIDS and human immunodeficiency virus infection in the US: 1988 update' [from abstract 4025, in Program and Abstracts of the 4th International Conference on AIDS, Stockholm, 1988], *Morbidity and Mortality Weekly Reports*, supplement, 38, p. 8.

CLIFFORD, J. (1986) 'Introduction: partial truths', in CLIFFORD, J. and MARCUS, G. (eds) *Writing Culture: The Poetics and Politics of Ethnography*, Berkeley: University of California Press.

DES JARLAIS, D., FRIEDMAN, S. and STONEBURNER, R. (1988) 'HIV infection and intravenous drug use: critical issues in transmission dynamics, infection outcomes, and prevention', *Reviews of Infectious Diseases*, 10, pp. 151–8.

——, WISH, E., FRIEDMAN, S. *et al.* (1987) 'Intravenous drug use and heterosexual transmission of human immunodeficiency virus: current trends in New York', *New York State Journal of Medicine*, 87, pp. 283–7.

GEIGER, S. (1986) 'Women's life histories: method and content', *Signs: Journal of Women, Culture and Society*, 11(2), pp. 334–51.

GUINAN, M.E. and HARDY, A. (1987) 'Epidemiology of AIDS in women in the US: 1981–86', *Journal of the American Medical Association*, 257, pp. 2039–42.

HEARST, N. and HULLEY, S. (1988) 'Preventing the heterosexual spread of AIDS: are we giving our patients the best advice?', *Journal of the American Medical Association*, 259, pp. 2428–32.

KANE, S.C. (1989a) 'The control of bodily fluids in the time of AIDS: Chicago 1989', presented at the Annual Meeting of the Society for Applied Anthropology, Santa Fe.

—— (1989b) 'Under the influence: street drugs, HIV, and the organization of experience', presented at the Annual Meeting of the American Anthropological Association, Washington, DC.

—— (1990) 'AIDS, addiction, and condom use: sources of sexual risk in heterosexual women', *Journal of Sex Research*, 27, pp. 427–49.

MANN, J.M., QUINN, T.C. and FRANCIS, H. (1986) 'Sexual practices associated with LAV/HTLV-III seropositivity among female prostitutes in Kinshasa, Zaire', 2nd International Conference on AIDS, Paris.

MONDANARO, J. (1987) 'Strategies for AIDS prevention: motivating health behaviour in drug dependent women', *Journal of Psychoactive Drugs*, 19, pp. 143–9.

MURRAY, S. and PAYNE, K. (1989) 'The social classification of AIDS in American epidemiology', *Medical Anthropology*, 10, pp. 115–28.

NIDA (NATIONAL INSTITUTE ON DRUG ABUSE) (1989) 'Conference on AIDS Intervention Strategies for Female Sexual Partners (National AIDS Demonstration Research and AIDS Targeted Outreach Model Contract Programs)', report prepared by NOVA Research Company, Bethesda.

OPPENHEIMER, G. (1988) 'In the eye of the storm: the epidemiological construction of AIDS', in FEE, E. and FOX, D. (eds) *AIDS: The Burdens of History*, Berkeley: University of California Press.

PADIAN, N.S. (1987) 'Heterosexual transmission of AIDS: international and national projections', *Review of Infectious Diseases*, 9, pp. 947–60.

—— (1988) 'Preventing the heterosexual spread of AIDS [letter]', *JAMA*, 260, p. 1879.

PARKER, R. (1987) 'Acquired immunodeficiency syndrome in Brazil', *Medical Anthropology Quarterly*, new series, 1, pp. 155–75.

REISS, I. and LEIK, R. (1989) 'Evaluating strategies to avoid AIDS', *Journal of Sex Research*, 26, pp. 411–33.

ROSENBAUM, M. (1981) *Women on Heroin*, New Brunswick, NJ: Rutgers University Press.

RUBIN, G. (1984) 'Thinking sex', in VANCE, C. (ed.) *Pleasure and Danger: Exploring Female Sexuality*, Boston, MA: Routledge and Kegan Paul.

STACK, C. (1974) *All Our Kin: Strategies for Survival in a Black Community*, New York: Harper and Row.

STERK, C., FRIEDMAN, S., SUFIAN, M., STEPHERSON, B. and DES JARLAIS, D. (1989) 'Barriers to AIDS: interventions among sexual partners of IV drug users', presented at the 5th International Conference on AIDS, Montreal.

TREICHLER, P. (1988) 'AIDS, gender, and biomedical discourse: current contests for meaning', in FEE, E. and FOX, D. (eds) *AIDS: The Burdens of History*, Berkeley: University of California Press.

—— (1989) 'AIDS and HIV infection in the third world: a first world perspective', in KRUGER, B. and MARIANI, P. (eds) *Remaking History*, Seattle, WA: Bay Press.

TURNER, C., MILLER, H. and MOSES, L. (1989) *AIDS: Sexual Behaviour and Intravenous Drug Use*, Washington, DC: National Academy Press.

WATNEY, S. (1987) *Policing Desire: Pornography, AIDS and the Media*, Minneapolis: University of Minnesota Press.

WERMUTH, L., HAM, J. and GIBSON, D. (1988) 'AIDS prevention outreach to female partners of IV drug users', paper presented to the Annual Meeting of the American Public Health Association, Boston.

WIEBEL, W.W. (1988) 'Combining ethnographic and epidemiologic methods in targeted AIDS interventions: the Chicago model', *National Institute on Drug Abuse Monograph No 80, Needle Sharing among Intravenous Drug Abusers: National and International Perspectives*, DHHS Publication No. (ADM) 88–1567, Rockville, MD.

WOFSY, C. (1987) 'Human immunodeficiency virus infection in women', *Journal of the American Medical Association*, 257, pp. 2074–6.

18 An explosion of Thai identities

Global queering and re-imagining queer theory

Peter A. Jackson [2000]

A growing number of authors (for example, Miller, 1992; Altman, 1995; Sullivan and Leong, 1995) have observed that the proliferation of gay, lesbian, bisexual and transgender/transsexual (g/l/b/t) identities is increasingly a global phenomenon. In particular, Altman's (1996) discussion of 'global queering' has provoked considerable debate, with Halperin (1996), Morton (1997), Connors (1997) and Stivens (1997) having presented critiques, to which Altman (1997) has responded.[1]

How are we to understand the global proliferation of gender and sexual diversity and, more particularly, the apparent similarities of new categories and identities in non-Western societies to Western-styled gay and lesbian forms? A number of explanatory models have been put forward. The global queering model, propounded by Altman, argues that globalizing economic and technological forces have facilitated cross-cultural borrowing from the West. For Altman, the emergence of 'the global gay' is best understood as 'the expansion of an existing Western category' and as being 'part of the rapid globalization of lifestyle and identity politics' (1996, p. 33). Another model, argued for by Morris (1994, 1997) in the case of Thailand, draws on Foucault's (1980) work to maintain that new gay and lesbian identities have emerged as a consequence of the institution of a new discursive regime based on sexuality. According to Morris, this contrasts with an older not yet fully superseded discursive regime based on gender. Morris's model also assumes processes of cross-cultural exchange and imposition within the broader context of globalization (Morris, 1994, p. 17).

Both Altman and Morris have referred to my research on historical shifts in Thai discourses in their respective accounts of the proliferation of gender/sex[2] diversity. Moreover, in the context of debates on global queering, Altman (1996) and Martin and Berry (1998) have correctly observed that I have emphasized cultural difference and local discursive continuities, and critiqued universalizing analyses that suggest we are witnessing a trend towards global gender/sex uniformity. I have located the emergence of new gender/sex identities in Thailand within micro-historical analyses of concrete events (see Jackson, 1999a) and, while not denying that globalizing processes have transformed and increasingly integrated diverse societies, my work has revealed how these processes impact in highly specific ways in different localities. As Appadurai (1996, p. 17) has suggested:

> globalization is ... a deeply historical, uneven and even *localizing* process. Globalization does not necessarily or even frequently imply homogenization or Americanization. [emphasis in original]

Foucault's ambiguous legacy

In her account of the emergence of new forms of male and female homosexual identity in Thailand, Morris (1994) criticizes critical theorists who, while ostensibly committed to championing sexual diversity and celebrating difference, remain committed to a homogenizing and Eurocentric framework. Elsewhere, it has been argued that while Foucauldian-modelled queer theory is open to the analysis of complexity and difference *within* Western societies, it is typically closed to acknowledging difference between Western and non-Western cultures (Jackson, 2000). Much of what passes for queer analysis of non-Western homosexualities, such as Bravman's (1997) study of accounts of Chinese homosexualities, takes the experience of immigrant ethnic diasporas within Western societies as the model for understanding the situation in homeland societies – a phenomenon that might be described as 'reducing China to Chinatown'(Jackson, 2000).

Failure to take cultural difference seriously means that within much critical theory the non-West often exists only as a site for the projection of Western expectations and fantasies, which are then misconstrued as 'data' to 'prove' the 'general validity' of Western theory. The American philosopher Alphonso Lingis, whose erotic travelogues (Lingis, 1983, 1995) are much cited by critical theorists (see for example Grosz, 1994), uses Thailand in just such a way (Jackson 1999b). Lingis (1995, pp. 105–28) offers a fantastic parody of Thai masculinity when he claims that all Thai men are potentially drag queens or *kathoey* in order to demonstrate the 'reality' of psychoanalytic notions of the polymorphous character of desire.

Morris has expressed ambivalence about the capacity of Western theories of sexuality to capture the specificity of Thai eroticisms:

> In the end, it might be simpler if one could carry out an investigation of Thai sexualities by simply forgetting Foucault. But, Baudrillard's witty polemic aside, no one writing about sexuality can forget Foucault. At best we can wilfully ignore him. And we are left with a burden of profound ethnocentrism.
>
> (1994, p. 38)

However, in a more recent study of Thai homosexualities Morris (1997) abandons these reservations about the cross-cultural applicability of Foucauldian history of sexuality, arguing that Thai forms are now on a trajectory of convergence with Western sexual identities. In this paper, I take up the concerns of Morris's earlier (1994) study, analysing Thai discourses in order to suggest how we may begin to cut through the ethnocentrism of current Foucauldian accounts of the history of sexuality. In doing this, it is not a question of forgetting Foucault, but rather of understanding the broader parameters of his *oeuvre*. While we do need to avoid using Foucault's texts as templates for a global sexual historiography, his methodology and his insights on discourses as regimes of power/knowledge remain highly productive analytical tools.

In many respects, this study develops a similar argument to that of Halperin (1998), who has critiqued the slavish invocation of Foucault's texts in much contemporary gay and queer historiography and called for reflective engagement with the broader parameters of Foucault's genealogical methodology. As will become clear, while I critique Morris's attachment to Foucault's (1980) text, her studies of Thai eroticisms remain repositories of considerable insight.

Structure of this study

I begin by summarizing the results of research on the emergence of new gender/sex categories in Thailand since the 1960s in order to document the stunning transformations that have taken place in the past four decades. From this base I consider, first, how we should describe the new categories and, second, how we are to account for the proliferation of gender/sex differences. Underlying such a quest is the task of understanding what exactly the new Thai categories are. In the global queering discussion the question of what is being 'seen' or 'described' in Asia and elsewhere has tended to be assumed as part of the explanatory theories that have been adduced. To adduce Foucauldian history of sexuality in explaining shifts in Thai discourses is to assume that the new categories and identities *are* sexualities. However, if identity is constituted within discourse, and if Asian gender/sex discourses are distinct from Western discourses, then Asian subjectivities are not reducible to Western forms of sexual identity. If this is true, then in Thailand the 'objects' of this inquiry are not sexual identities, but rather varieties of what in Thai discourses are called *phet* (เพศ)[3] or eroticized genders.

It is not often observed that Foucault explicitly excluded the non-West from his work, noting that his object was 'to define the regime of power-knowledge-pleasure that sustains the discourse on human sexuality *in our part of the world*' (Foucault 1980, p. 11, emphasis added). Foucault's 'part of the world' was, after all, Paris not Bangkok. To mark my divergence from Foucault's account, I talk of 'eroticism' and 'discourses of the erotic' in Thailand in order to avoid the Eurocentric connotations that now attach to the term 'sexuality' and the notion of 'discourses of sexuality'.

In reflecting on the cultural limits of Foucault's work, seeing Thai identities as eroticized genders rather than sexualities forces us to rethink the categorical separation of gender and sexuality that has underpinned the establishment of queer studies as a separate inquiry from feminism.[4] Indeed, the attempt to understand novel forms of eroticism and identity in a globally 'marginal' society such as Thailand destabilizes the Western queer theoretical 'centre', revealing inadequacies in the theories currently used to understand global erotic transformations. As Altman observes, 'if we were capable of imagining Thailand or Brazil as the norm and then measuring San Francisco or Sydney against them, our sense of what is modern and traditional might be somewhat altered' (Altman, 1996, p. 91).

This analysis is an historical study of discursive shifts which also draws on ethnographic research on the lives of homosexually active men and women. It is based on extensive reading of accounts of gender/sex difference in the Thai press (see Jackson, 1995a, 1995b, 1996, 1997a, 1997b, 1999a, 1999c)[5] over the past four decades and of Thai academic studies of same-sex eroticism and transgenderism over the same period (see Jackson, 1997c, 1999d). The Thai press and media have long evinced a fascination with gender and erotic difference and, since the 1960s, investigative reporters have introduced their readers to elements of the language of the country's gender/sex minorities. The significance of the press – especially the nationally distributed Bangkok dailies that I have drawn on most extensively – to understanding Thai g/l/b/t history is that it is newspapers which have had the most significant role in mediating the introduction of new gender/sex categories into public discourse, and which have been the public's most important source of information on the proliferation of gender/ sex difference.

It should be emphasized that the following account is an analysis of public representations. It reflects transitions within *dominant discourses* rather than changing patterns of usage within Thai g/l/b/t networks. A more complete analysis would need to consider shifts within the argots of Thailand's various homoerotic and transgender cultures. The relationship between discursive categories, erotic practices and gendered performances and identities is complex and often involves resistances to identifying with stigmatized labels together with attempts to construct a positive sense of self in terms of culturally valorized categories. Without additional research in the fields of oral history and ethnography, the following account of changes in gender/sex categories tells us little about how people negotiated the rapidly changing patterns of discourse in their public workaday lives and in their private emotional and erotic relationships. Sinnott's paper (2000) reflects some of the detailed ethnographic research that has recently been conducted on Thai sexual minorities. Borthwick (1999), McCamish (1999), van Wijngaarden (1999) and Storer (1999a, 1999b) have also written ethnographic and sociological accounts of Thailand's homosexual and transgender cultures and their work has assisted in interpreting the historical sources.

An explosion of Thai identities: 1960–85

In analysing Thai discourses, a startling phenomenon has become apparent. Over the quarter century from 1960 to 1985 the number of categories for labelling distinctive types of gendered/sexed being, called *phet* in Thai, first increased rapidly, almost tripling in number, and then stabilized at a new higher level. The complex connotations of the notion of *phet* are discussed further below, but in summary the term denotes a distinctive type of gendered existence which has its own characteristic form of eroticism or sexual desire. 'Eroticized gender' is a possible translation. Using sources such as the Thai press, popular magazines and academic publications it is possible to date the emergence of new *phet* categories into public discourse.

Before the 1960s, only three forms of *phet* were recognized in public discourses, namely, normatively masculine 'men' (*phu-chai*, ผู้ชาย), normatively feminine 'women' (*phu-ying*, ผู้หญิง) and an intermediate category called *kathoey* (กะเทย, pronounced like 'gatuhy'). *Kathoey* variously denoted a person, male or female, who exhibited hermaphroditic features or expressed behaviour considered inappropriate for their gender, and have long been called a 'third gender/sex' (*phet thi-sam*, เพศที่สาม) within both popular and academic discourses.

On this pre-modern system, Morris observes, it is 'unlikely that there ever existed a period in accord with the completely triadic vision [of 'man', *kathoey*, 'woman'] … However, what texts we do have suggest a tradition of sexual and gendered identities incompatible with Western binarism [of homosexual vs. heterosexual]' (Morris, 1994, p. 22). An idealized hermaphroditic *kathoey* category, apparently derived from Thai creation myths as well as Hindu/Buddhist mythology, functions as the symbolic fulcrum of both the historical and contemporary system of *phet* identities. The mythical *kathoey* represents an equal blending of maleness/masculinity and femaleness/femininity that continues to have an iconic place in Thai imaginings of gender and eroticism to this day.

While the masculine/feminine opposition underlies all forms of erotic expression in Thailand, the notion that these two domains intersect to varying degrees within the body and desire of all individuals is also central to understandings of gender/sex difference. As argued below, a proliferation of new *phet* categories can be understood as emerging from a refinement of the pre-modern notion of gender/sex intersection, with *unequal* blendings of masculinity and femininity being seen as producing new categories that are neither 'truly men' (*chai thae*, ชายแท้), 'truly women' (*ying thae*, หญิงแท้), nor 'truly *kathoey*' (*kathoey thae*, กะเทยแท้).

Since the 1960s a range of new varieties of *phet* has emerged. In the mid-1960s, perhaps earlier, the *kathoey* category began to split into a number of masculine, feminine, transvestite and hermaphroditic variants. The following different types of *kathoey* are mentioned in the Thai press and other sources in this period:

- *kathoey thae* (กะเทยแท้): a true hermaphrodite (*thae* is 'true', 'genuine');
- *kathoey thiam* (กะเทยเทียม): variously a pseudo-hermaphrodite or a cross-dressing man (*thiam* is 'false', 'artificial');
- *kathoey sao* (กะเทยสาว): a cross-dressing young woman (*sao* = 'a young woman'). Other 1960s expressions for masculine women were: *sao lakkaphet* (สาวลักเพศ), 'a cross-dressing young woman' and *ying plorm pen chai* (หญิงปลอมเป็นชาย), literally, 'a woman who impersonates a man'
- *krathiam* (กระเทียม): this humorous term literally means 'garlic', but also combines the first syllable of an old spelling of *kathoey* as *krathoey* (กระเทย) with the Thai term for 'false' or 'artificial', *thiam*. *Krathiam* meant 'A false *kathoey*' or a man who is sexually attracted to other men but does not cross-dress or act effeminately like a stereotypical *kathoey*;
- *kathoey num* (กะเทยหนุ่ม): a masculine young homosexual man (*num* = 'a young man');
- *kathoe y phu-chai* (กะเทยผู้ชาย): a masculine adult homosexual man (*phuchai* = 'man');
- *kathoey praphet sorng* (กะเทยประเภทสอง): a second type of *kathoey*, that is, a man who prefers males but does not cross-dress or act effeminately

The various expressions for masculine types of male *kathoey* – *kathoey num*, *kathoey phu-chai*, *kathoey praphet sorng*, *krathiam* – were short-lived and became obsolete in the late 1960s, being replaced by *gay*. *Gay*, the first English-derived label for a *phet* category, entered the language around 1965, and originally denoted masculine male prostitutes and their clients (see Jackson, 1999a). By 1970, the new *gay* category had split into *gay king* (sexually insertive) and *gay queen* (sexually receptive) subtypes. While the *gay king* is often considered to be butch and the *gay queen* to be effeminate, in some cases these terms refer only to preferred sexual role – that is, top or bottom – respectively, rather than to gender role. Furthermore, while the Thai borrowing of *queen* reflects longstanding English associations of this term with effeminacy, the idiomatic pairing of *gay king* and *gay queen* appears to be a distinctively Thai coinage, with the expression *gay king* not occurring in the gay argot of any English-speaking country.

By the early 1970s, masculine women were no longer called a type of *kathoey*, being relabelled with the Western-derived terms *lesbian* (เลสเบี้ยน) and *dai* (ได), from 'dyke'. Other expressions for masculine women were the Thai-English compounds *sao dai* (สาวได), 'a young woman who is a dyke', and *sao lesbian* (สาวเลสเบี้ยน), 'a young woman who is a butch lesbian'. From this period only males are called *kathoey*.

Sex-change operations were also first performed in Thailand in the early 1970s and the category of male-to-female transsexual (*plaeng phet*, แปลงเพศ, literally 'to change one's *phet*') first emerged in this decade. While male-to-female transsexuals are now called *kathoey*, or more fully *kathoey plaeng phet*, no colloquial expression has been coined for female-to-male transsexuals other than the awkward descriptive phrase *ying phet pen chai* (หญิงแปลงเพศ เป็นชาย, 'a woman who changes *phet* to a man'). This means that female-to-male transsexuals do not exist as a marked *phet* category distinct from cross-dressing masculine women, with whom they are often subsumed. As *kathoey* came increasingly to mean only transgender and transsexual males in the 1970s, hermaphrodites began to be relabelled as 'two-sexed people' (*khon sorng phet*, คนสองเพศ) rather than *kathoey*, although the older expression 'true *kathoey*' (*kathoey thae*) is at times still retained in academic literature to describe hermaphroditism.

Differentiation of new *phet* continued into the late 1970s and early 1980s. In the second half of the 1970s, masculine women were yet again relabelled with the borrowed expression *tom boy* (ทอมบอย), which in the 1980s was shortened to *tom* (ทอม), a term which replaced previous expressions for masculine women such as *lesbian* and *dai*. A male bisexual category, the *seua bai* (เสือไบ) or 'bi-tiger', also emerged at this time, as did a new feminine category, the *dee* (ดี้), abbreviated from English 'lady', as a label for the feminine partner of a masculine *tom*. Thai *tom* and *dee* resist calling themselves 'lesbian' because this term entered the Thai language to describe female homosexual visual pornography produced for a heterosexual male audience. For Thai homosexual women, the term 'lesbian' is resisted because it is understood as representing woman-centred relationships in overly sexualized terms, with many Thai women who love women preferring to imagine their relationships in emotional rather than explicitly erotic terms (source: private communication with Anjana Suvarnananda)[6] The term *lesbian* is still occasionally used within popular discourses to describe female homoeroticism, but is now resisted by homosexually active women and is not used as a self-identificatory label by Thailand's female homosexual cultures.

The proliferation of phet *categories*

After a period of rapid transformation from the early 1960s to the mid-1980s, the system of *phet* categories stabilized and something approaching a new discursive equilibrium has been established. No new varieties of *phet* have been formed in over a decade, apart from the periodic emergence and disappearance of terms that are recognized as synonyms for existing categories. This striking phenomenon suggests that Thai gender/sex discourses suffered a major disruptive influence in the late 1950s or early 1960s, leading to a two-decade period of instability during which a range of new categories emerged and the older identities of 'man', *kathoey* and 'woman' were redefined. From a linguistic standpoint, the major, but not the only, epicentre of this explosion of new gender/sex categories was the old *kathoey* identity. Historically, the *kathoey* category had included all forms of gender/sex variation from normative forms of maleness/masculinity and femaleness/femininity. However, in the 1960s this formerly undifferentiated category fractured into an array of *kathoey* varieties that labelled specific forms of difference in the domains of sex (hermaphroditism), gender (cross-dressing, transsexualism) and sexuality (homosexuality). Many of these new varieties of *kathoey* had only a brief existence in public discourses and were quickly relabelled as something other than *kathoey*, establishing a differentiation from those categories that continued to be labelled as types of *kathoey*. In succession, *gay* men, women who love women and hermaphrodites were relabelled and differentiated from *kathoey*. The linguistic and conceptual shift has been so great that younger Thais are no longer aware that only three decades ago a woman was called a *kathoey* if she dressed or acted like a man. By the 1970s, *kathoey* had come to mean only a person who is born male but subsequently enacts a feminine role (male transvestite) or undergoes a sex change operation (male-to-female transsexual).

While the *gay* and *tom* identities, as well as the male transgender and transsexual identities now labelled *kathoey*, all appear to have developed from the old undifferentiated *kathoey*, the *dee* and *seua bai* seem to have a different origin. The femme lesbian *dee* and male bisexual *seua bai* appear to have split from the old normative female and male categories, respectively. The explosion of types of *kathoey* did not leave normative constructions of femininity and masculinity untouched, leading to a slightly delayed fracturing of the two poles of the gender continuum. Before the 1980s, femme partners of *tom* were usually not distinguished from the female partners of men. Women now called *dee* used to be called 'women', even when they

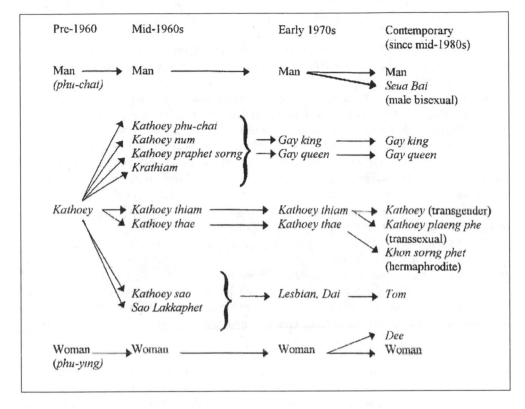

Figure 18.1 Hypothesized transitions in *phet* categories

Note: Hypothesized transitions are marked by arrows. Categories are arranged according to the Thai gender continuum from the most masculine (*chai*) to the most feminine (*ying*).

related with *lesbian, dai* or *tom*, and this femme identity appears to have been hived off from the normative female identity, *phu-ying*. Similarly, the male bisexual *seua bai* appears to be a subdivision of the normative masculine category of 'man' or *phu-chai* rather than being considered a variant of *gay*.

While English-derived terms came to mark some new identities (*gay, tom, dee*), in some cases these words merely replaced pre-existing Thai expressions and their introduction did not mark the emergence of a new phenomenon but rather a re-labelling. For example, recognition of masculine men who are sexually attracted to other masculine men predated use of the label *gay*, with *krathiam* and other expressions being used for these men in the early 1960s. It is not clear why some types of *kathoey* were so quickly relabelled with English terms, while others have continued to be called *kathoey* until today. Perhaps the most curious aspect of the transitions is the rapid and complete expulsion of females from the domain of the *kathoey* and the restriction of that term to males. This may reflect the cultural privileging of maleness over femaleness, for another notable feature of the expanded set of *phet* categories is that there are now more categories for males than for females. In other words, maleness is now a more finely differentiated domain (in terms of varying degrees of ascribed masculinity) than is femaleness (in terms of degrees of ascribed femininity). It can also be observed that the categories still labelled *kathoey* are those which are conceived in terms of the myth-ical equal blending of maleness/masculinity and femaleness/femininity which lay at the core of the earlier meaning of this term. The linguistic persistence of *kathoey* means that popular English terms for transsexuality and transgenderism such as 'drag queen', 'tranny', etc., have not been borrowed and are all but unknown in Thailand, except amongst those who have trav-elled to the West.

To summarize, the Thai borrowing of English terms for new types of gender/sex difference has been highly selective and has involved a high degree of playful innovation. Male cultures have enthusiastically appropriated the now dominant English label for male homoeroticism, *gay*. However, they have also reflected the persistent gendering of male homoeroticism through the uniquely Thai opposition of *gay king* and *gay queen*. In contrast, female erotic cultures have resisted the dominant English label for female homoeroticism, *lesbian*, instead appropriating and adapting the terms tom boy – to *tom* – and lady – to *dee* – to reflect the gendering of female same-sex relations. From a linguistic standpoint, Thailand's transgender and transsexual subcultures are largely uninfluenced by English borrowings.

The complexity of this history – involving a combination of enthusiastic appropriation, resistance, playful adaptation to local patterns and disinterest – alerts us to the fact that it is highly unlikely that an unmediated process of 'borrowing' from the West is the sole source of the explosion of *phet* categories. Even when English terms have been borrowed to label or relabel Thai categories, they have been remodulated in distinctive ways to reflect the persis-tent dominance of gender oppositions (for example, *gay king* vs. *gay queen*) and gender blending in Thai erotic identities.

There is no general agreement in Thailand on how many *phet* now exist in the country. Some people think that 'men' (*phu-chai*) and male bisexuals (*seua bai*) are a single *phet*, while others distinguish them as different types of *phet*. Some regard transvestite and transsexual *kathoeys* as varieties of the same *kathoey phet*, while others consider them distinctive. However, what is universally agreed is that within living memory only three *phet* were found in Thailand and that today many more exist. Most commentators appear to count at least seven contemporary types of *phet*: 'man', *gay king*, *gay queen*, *kathoey*, *tom*, *dee* and 'woman'.

Significantly, awareness of this proliferation is not localized in Bangkok or within minority erotic cultures. Through the media of the national press, radio, television and film, every person in the country is now familiar with these seven types of people, and individuals claiming each of these identities can be found in remote villages as well as the largest cities. While many homosexual and transgender men and women do appear to migrate to the more liberal environment of Bangkok, it is not uncommon to find people labelled *gay*, *kathoey*, *tom* or *dee* in villages and small towns across the country and the distinctive erotic cultures that focus around each of these labels now exist as national phenomena.

Thai discursive resilience

In considering the proliferation of gender/sex diversity in Thailand it is necessary to reflect upon what it is that is being 'observed', for it is not immediately apparent what the new *phet* categories are. Are *phet* identities or preferred forms of pleasure; descriptors of subjectivity or erotic tastes? There seems little doubt that *kathoey*, *gay*, *tom*, *dee*, 'man' (*phu-chai*) and 'woman' (*phu-ying*) do mark identities, since four distinctive sexual communities now exist in Thailand based on identification with one or other of the following erotically paired catego-ries: (1) 'man'–'woman'; (2) *gay king–gay queen*; (3) *kathoey*–'man';[7] and (4) *tom–dee*. However, it is less clear that *seua bai* marks an identity as no community of self-identifying bisexual males currently exists. Only further ethnographic and applied linguistic research can unravel the full details of this situation. In any event, if we accept that at least some of the new *phet* categories are identities that mark distinctive erotic cultures, are they genders, sexualities or something else?

Following Kosofsky Sedgwick, Morris (1994, p. 34) argues that the coexistence of the *kathoey* identity with newer *gay*, *tom* and *dee* identities indicates that contemporary Thai discourses represent a complex of 'two irreconcilable but coexistent sex/gender systems', one indigenous and based on gender, the other borrowed and structured around the Western notion of sexuality. On this Foucauldian model, Morris proposes that the older 'man'–*kathoey*–'woman' system of three identities was constructed within a regime of gendered discourses, while recent *gay*, *tom*, *dee* and bisexual categories have emerged as consequences of the irruption of a discursive domain of sexuality. However, a close analysis of the discourse of *phet* within which all gender/sex categories – both old and new – are understood suggests that no clear break between gender and sexuality can be established. While Western discourses of sexuality have impacted on both popular and academic understandings of eroticism, indigenous discourses have resisted the formation of a domain of sexuality distinct from gender.[8] All Thai gender/sex categories continue to be understood in terms of the indigenous conception of *phet*, which incorporates sexual difference (male vs. female), gender difference (masculine vs. feminine) and sexuality (heterosexual vs. homosexual) within a single formation. Within this local discourse, *gay* and *kathoey* are not distinguished as a sexuality and a gender, respectively. Rather, *gay* and *kathoey*, together with 'man', 'woman', *tom* and *dee*, are collectively labelled as different varieties of *phet*.

Gay identity without 'sexuality'

The historical system of three *phet*, with the *kathoey* imagined as a blending of genders within one body and psyche, has been the productive source of all the new categories by a mathematical refinement of the gender continuum. For example, in interviewing both *gay* and non-*gay* men I have found that categories such as *gay queen* and *gay king* tend to be imagined first in terms of their position on a scale of relative masculinity and femininity and only secondarily in terms of homoerotic partnering. Even *gay* men who lead active sex lives do not necessarily see homoerotic desire as the central determinant of their identities. In contemporary *gay* parlance *gay* men may describe themselves and other *gay* men in terms of quantitative metaphors such as '60–40', '70–30', and so on. These refer to imagined percentage blendings of *king* (sexually insertive) and *queen* (sexually receptive), and reflect an increasing recognition, at least in Bangkok, that large numbers of homosexually active men engage in a wide range of sexual behaviours. However, this sexual versatility is seen as emerging from a masculine/feminine blending.

A percentile imagining of gender blending amongst *gay* men reflects general understandings of eroticism. A common Thai expression for 'a real man' is *phuchai roi persen* (ผู้ชายร้อยเปอร์เซ็นต์), literally '100 per cent man', which primarily denotes butch masculinity and secondarily implies heterosexual preference. These common percentage metaphors reflect the fact within this contemporary schema, all *phet* categories are imagined as proportional blendings of masculinity and femininity. The 'real man' is assigned a score of '100 per cent masculinity'; the *kathoey* is thought of as blending masculinity and femininity in equal measure; the *gay queen* is imagined as more masculine than the *kathoey*; the *gay king* is thought of as being yet more masculine than the *gay queen*; and the *seua bai* is considered more masculine yet again, but perhaps not quite '100 per cent man'.

It is a person's location on the multipositional gender scale of *phet* – from 100 per cent 'man' at one end to 100 per cent 'woman' at the other, and a variety of proportional combinations in between – that is imagined as determining his or her erotic preference. Within the *phet* gender hierarchy, it is more important to know how masculine or feminine one is than to know the types of sexed bodies and gendered performances one finds erotically interesting, for erotic desire is conceived of as flowing as a 'natural' consequence of gender status. As Halperin (2000, p. 91) observes, the most distinctive feature of the contemporary Western model of homosexuality, and of Western gay and lesbian identities, is that they privilege sexuality over gender. In contrast, pre-modern Western, and also many contemporary non-Western cultures, privilege gender over sexuality. It is not that eroticism is absent from Thai conceptions of *phet*, or that gender is not a part of popular understandings of gay and lesbian sexualities in the contemporary West. Rather, eroticism and gender are articulated in radically different ways in the discourses and identities prevalent in the two cultures.

This is not to suggest that Western discourses of sexuality are completely absent in Thailand. The impact of Western sexual and gender knowledges upon Thai discourses is undeniable. However, attempts to introduce Western ideas of sexuality have ultimately been appropriated to local, gendered understandings. The persistence of *phet* as the frame within which both gender and sexuality are understood in Thailand is reflected in the fact that even in Thai academic discourses only one expression exists to translate both 'sexual identity' and 'gender identity', namely *ekkalak thang-phet* (เอกลักษณ์ทางเพศ). In using this expression some more careful academics do state whether they are referring to an identity based on erotic preference or to a person's sense of masculinity or femininity. However, this distinction is extremely difficult to sustain because *phet* is the only term available to describe notions such as erotic desire (*ruam phet*, ร่วมเพศ), 'to have sex'; *phet samphan*, เพศสัมพันธ์, 'sexual relations', masculinity/maleness (*phet-chai*, เพศชาย) or femininity/femaleness (*phet-ying*, เพศหญิง).

This means that it is extremely difficult, I suggest ultimately impossible, to consistently sustain a difference between the notion of desire for a particular type of sexed body (whether male or female), and hence of sexual identity, and the idea of a preference for enacting a particular gender performance (whether masculine or feminine), and hence of gender identity. This difficulty does not reflect a temporary inadequacy in the technical vocabulary available to Thai language speakers. It is a situation that has existed for more than two decades, ever since the distinction between sexual identity and gender identity was made in English discourses and attempts were made to translate these notions into Thai. Rather than a mere inadequacy in terminology, this situation reflects the fact that within Thai cultural understandings, including technical and academic discourses, gender and sexuality are indeed a unitary category and the single expression *ekkalak thang-phet* ('gender identity' and/or 'sexual identity') accurately reflects the prevalent form of subjectivity in Thailand, in which personal identification as a 'man', *gay king*, *gay queen*, *kathoey*, *tom*, *dee* or 'woman' is simultaneously erotic and gendered.

The presence of Western discourses in Thailand has indeed destabilized older understandings, but the outcome of this foreign contact has not been the emergence of a discourse of sexuality such as Foucault proposes occurred in Western societies in the nineteenth century. The interaction of Western discourses with other cultures/discourses does not necessarily reproduce the gender/sexuality split that is widely represented as now being hegemonic in the West. As Appadurai (1996) notes, the intersection of two disparate discourses does not necessarily lead to an abolition of their differences or to complete homogenization, but rather can produce new forms of adjustment in which local distinctiveness is preserved. The dramatic multiplication of Thai *phet* categories can be interpreted as just such an accommodation to processes of cultural intersection.

The cultural limits of Foucauldian history of sexuality

Foucault noted the culturally specific terms of his study in *The History of Sexuality Volume 1*, describing Asian societies as distinct domains beyond the scope of his analysis. He distinguished between cultures characterized by what he called 'erotic arts' (*ars erotica*) and contemporary Western societies which, he maintained, possessed a 'sexual science' (*scientia sexualis*) (Foucault, 1980, pp. 57–8). This distinction between *ars erotica* and *scientia sexualis* is framed in terms of different power/knowledge regimes. While Foucault did not consider the place of gender in this distinction, one way of characterizing the difference between the Thai discourse of *phet* and Western 'sexual science' is to say that the former does not make a categorical distinction between gender and sexuality. In her attempts to use Foucault's text as a guide in interpreting Thai gender/sex patterns, Morris (1994, 1997) overlooks the cultural limits that Foucault explicitly placed on his research.

Sexuality conceived in Foucauldian terms has no history in Thailand, remaining discursively bound to gender. Yet it would be Eurocentric to ascribe to the West a 'true' history of sexuality and to Thai discourses only a 'prehistory', with the implication that Thailand's inchoate sexuality may one day emerge into the light of global discursive history. A genealogical understanding of historical processes forces us to recognize that Thai discourses are not predestined to follow the same trajectory as those in the West, and hence the lack of a separation between gender and sexuality cannot be seen as an 'underdeveloped' discursive state. What Foucault marks in the *ars erotica/scientia sexualis* distinction is a boundary between different histories of the erotic, not of history *versus* a lack of history. The Thai discourse of *phet* needs to be granted autonomy, which means that in understanding recent transformations we need to conceive of new *gay*, *tom*, *dee* and other identities as genders (alongside 'man' and 'woman') as much as forms of eroticism. The categories used in writing the history of gender/sex transformations in the West have emerged from critical reflections upon Western discourses. A similar approach needs to be adopted in writing the history of eroticism in non-Western societies, developing analytical categories from studies of local texts and reflections upon indigenous discourses rather than imposing Euramerocentric notions in an *a priori* manner.

Genders on the global 'margins' and the poverty of queer theory

In understanding *phet* as eroticized genders we are forced to consider our theories both of gender and of sexuality. This is because in recent decades gender and sexuality have been split as separate domains of inquiry within the Western academy. An intellectual division of labour has been established separating those who inquire into gender issues, and are often called feminists, and those who investigate sexuality, a domain now claimed by gay and queer theorizations. Feminists have tended to leave discussion of sexual identity to gay/queer theorists, or to consider only female and heterosexual forms of sexuality. In contrast, gay/queer theorists have tended to leave discussion of gender identity to feminists, or to limit their analyses of gender to transgenderism. For two decades these two projects have proceeded largely independently, with many gay/queer theorists rarely referring to the work of feminists, and many feminists making only cursory references to gay–queer analyses. The theoretical split between gender and sexuality, which is now institutionalized in the disciplinary divide between feminism/women's studies and gay/queer studies, means that Western analysts are poorly equipped to understand gender/sex transformations at the global level.

While Altman has correctly focussed attention on the global character of erotic transitions in the late twentieth century, we lack a theory capable of comprehending this phenomenon in non-ethnocentric terms. Despite the work of Western feminist thinkers on gender issues and the expansion of gay/queer studies of sexuality in recent years, Western thought nevertheless lacks a generally applicable model of how masculinity, femininity and erotic desire are related in identity formation. Without such a theory we have no framework for a comparative study of homoerotic cultures. A rapprochement between the concerns of feminism and gay/queer studies is needed in order to construct a frame of reference that is adequate to the task of understanding all eroticisms, both Western and non-Western.

The claim that there is a gaping hole in Western theories of gender and sexuality may at first sight seem odd. In reading texts on feminism and gay/queer studies one constantly finds references to 'sex', 'gender', 'sexuality' and 'identity'. The terms of analysis appear very similar, which indeed reflects the common historical origins of these two fields of inquiry. The problem only becomes apparent when one asks, 'How are gender and sexuality related?' If one turns to either gay/queer studies or feminist texts in the hope of finding a formulation of the relationship between gender and sexuality one will almost always be disappointed. As Pringle (1992, pp. 76–77) observes,

> The categories of sexuality and gender have a schizoid relationship. For much of the time they ignore each other completely, with the result that there is a large literature which treats sexuality as if gender barely exists and another literature on gender that ignores or marginalizes sexuality. Despite this, assumptions are constantly made about their connectedness.

Caught between the split domains of feminism and gay/queer studies, the categories of gender and sexuality exist in an endless circuit of mutual referencing which rarely stops to provide an account of how they are related. Some cultural anthropologists (for example, Rubin, 1984; Kulick, 1998; Parker, 1991) have argued that in understanding eroticisms cross-culturally, the categories of gender and sexuality can only be separated to the extent that they continue to be imagined as part of a broader whole.[9] However, despite the existence of these calls for considering gender and sexuality together, we still lack a general theory which, for example, maps the diversity of ways in which gender identity and sexual identity may be articulated in forming subjectivities which are simultaneously gendered and sexualized. It is precisely this theoretical lack which prevents us from surmounting what Morris calls the 'profound burden of ethnocentrism' that weighs down upon critical theoretical approaches to gender and sexuality, and which also holds us back from realizing Altman's injunction to conceive of contemporary sexual cultures as inter-related parts of a global system. It is precisely the cultural and historical distinctiveness of contemporary Western homosexualities, something consistently emphasized by all writers in the field including Foucault, that makes theorizations of this particular erotic culture singularly inadequate as bases for analysing non-Western cultures. Despite a fascination with the globalization of homosexual rights movements, gay identity and so on, Western analysts typically remain bound to understandings derived solely from their own historical experience in seeking to appreciate homoeroticisms in other places.

Psychoanalysis provides an account of the relation of eroticism and the gendering of desire in the formation of subjectivity, and writers who have attempted to relate gender, homosexuality and identity most often draw on this body of theory. Despite the prominence given to psychoanalysis in some feminisms (for example, Millett, 1971, and Grosz, 1992) and in some early gay liberation analyses (for example, Altman, 1972), the view that Freudian thought is fundamentally, perhaps inescapably, phallocentric and homophobic became increasingly common among gay theorists in the 1980s. Most significantly, Foucault's critique of the repressive hypothesis in *The History of Sexuality Volume 1* has led to the almost complete abandonment of psychoanalytic approaches within queer theory. However, if queer theory is understood as the study of sexuality without reference to Freud, then this also means that queer theory lacks a framework for conceiving the relations between gender, sexuality and identity. To the extent that Queer Studies is modelled on the *History of Sexuality Volume 1*, then it suffers from precisely the same limitations as that text. This is apparent in Sedgwick's attempt to theoretically found queer studies upon the assumption that the gender–sexuality split is 'axiomatic',

> Axiom 2: The study of sexuality is not coextensive with the study of gender; correspondingly, anti-homophobic inquiry is not coextensive with feminist inquiry. But we can't know in advance how they will be different.
>
> (1990, p. 27)

Sedgwick formulates her axiom in terms of a future programme of inquiry into the relations between gender and sexuality. However, queer studies has not taken up this challenge, merely continuing to assume the axiomatic status of the gender–sexuality split. Some female authors writing on homosexuality, such as Butler, have continued to emphasize the need to imagine the inter-relationship rather than the separation of gender and sexuality. In a 1993 interview Butler observed,

> I think there's some antifeminism in queer theory. Also, insofar as some people in queer theory want to claim that the analysis of sexuality can be radically separated from the analysis of gender, I'm very much opposed to them. The new *Gay and Lesbian Reader*[10] that Routledge have just published begins with a set of articles that make that claim. I think that separation is a big mistake … a queer theory that dissociates itself from feminism is a massive mistake.
>
> (Osborne and Segal 1994, p. 32)

Despite the fact that Butler is often represented as a 'queer theorist', views such as the above have been silenced within the prevailing intellectual hegemony which, *à la* Sedgwick, takes the separation of gender and sexuality as self-evidently axiomatic.[11]

Re-imagining queer studies as the study of global queering

Why has queer theory retreated from the effort to develop a general theory of gender and sexuality? I suggest that it is not because such an understanding is theoretically impossible, although a unified theory of gender, sexuality and identity would be highly nuanced. Rather, as Butler notes, queer theorizations are often antifeminist, with the history of struggles around women's and gay/lesbian issues in the West having contributed to the contemporary form of our split understandings. Differences between feminists and gay/queer theorists on issues such as whether desire should be imagined primarily as a domain of masculine hegemony (the radical feminist position) or of celebratory resistance (a common gay/queer position) have intersected with a history of political divisions between the feminist and g/l/b/t rights movements. It is this history of political contestation between feminists and g/l/b/t activists that underpins the neglect of the theoretical relationship between gender and sexuality, and which leaves us poorly equipped to analyse gender/sex relations in societies with radically different histories.

While it may have been politically strategic for gay–queer theorists to claim a separation between sexuality and gender to evade the 'anti-sex' claims of radical feminism, the issue of gender was not resolved by this move but merely held in abeyance. Gender is not theorized within gay/queer theories because it has been excluded by a political act of denial. To adopt a psychoanalytic metaphor, gender is the theoretical 'unconscious' that haunts the formation of the queer subject. We may then expect a future return of the repressed term of gender within the body of queer theory, which has set up the boundaries that constitute it as an intellectual domain by an act of exclusion. However, dominant Eurocentric constructions of queer theory do not appear to be at risk of being challenged by any imminent return of gender at the centre, that is, in reflexive studies of Western homosexualities. Queer theory nevertheless is challenged by a theoretical return of gender from the global margins. The study of g/l/b/t discourses and cultures in non-Western societies highlights not only the cultural specificity of queer theory and the distinctively Western provenance and trajectory of its current formulations, but also its inability to either represent or account for erotic diversification outside the West.

Queer studies, understood as the study of sexuality independently of gender, needs to be reformulated in terms of the attempt to theorize all eroticisms as gendered and all genders as eroticized. This will require Western analysts to move beyond their own history and imagine an accommodation between feminism, with its focus on gender, and queer studies, with its concern with sexuality.

Rather than using the culture-specific analyses of *History of Sexuality Volume 1* as a universal template for understanding the global proliferation of gender/sex diversity we need to engage in a much more fundamental and laborious undertaking. As Halperin (1998) points out, in resolving contradictions within queer theory it is not a question of forgetting Foucault but rather of abandoning the slavish invocation of his texts. We need to follow Foucault's method, his careful attention to the details of discursive transformation within given societies and historical periods. By this we may arrive at culturally nuanced Foucauldian-inspired readings of the erotic in non-Western societies and also develop a more appropriate theoretical frame within which to consider one of the most stunning transitions of the twentieth century, namely, the global proliferation of new forms of gendered and erotic being.

Notes

1 This paper has been prepared as part of the project 'Thai identities: the emergence of sexual subcultures' undertaken in collaboration with Dr Nerida Cook (University of Tasmania) and funded by the Australian Research Council.
2 The expression 'gender/sex' used here inverts the order of terms in Rubin's (1975, 1984) notion of 'sex/gender system' and marks the continuing priority of gender over eroticism in Thai identities.
3 To Australian and British ears *phet* sounds somewhat like 'pairt'. However, North Americans are more inclined to hear it as similar to the way that they pronounce 'pate'.
4 In questioning the gender/sexuality distinction I am indebted to Michael Connors for his comments on an earlier version of this paper and for the insights in his 1995 article 'Missing Gender and the Fetishism of Sex: "Gay" Responses to the Sexuality Debates'.
5 The newspapers I have referred to most extensively are the Thai language *Thai Rath*, *Siam Rath*, *Daily News*, *Khao Sot* and *Matichon* and the English language *Bangkok Post* and *The Nation*.
6 Anjana Suvarnananda is co-founder of the Bangkok-based group Anjaree for 'women who love women' (*ying rak ying*).
7 The male partners of 'women' and *kathoeys* are not differentiated. Both are called 'men' (*phu-chai*).

8 See Jackson (1997a, b) for further discussion of this point.
9 I wish to thank the anonymous reviewers of this paper for pointing out the longstanding importance of the gender/sexuality nexus within some areas of cultural anthropology.
10 Butler is here referring to Abelove, Bevale and Halperin, 1993.
11 David Halperin, one of the co-editors of *The Lesbian and Gay Studies Reader*, has more recently begun to consider the contradictions produced by the elision of theorizations of gender from gay/queer studies (private communication).

References

ABELOVE, H., BEVALE, M.A. and HALPERIN, D.M. (eds) (1993) *The Lesbian and Gay Studies Reader*, New York: Routledge.

ALTMAN, D. (1972) *Homosexual: Oppression and Liberation*, Sydney: Angus and Robertson.

—— (1995) 'The new world of "gay" Asia', in PERERA, S. (ed.) *Asian and Pacific Inscriptions*, Melbourne: Meridien Books.

—— (1996) 'Rupture or continuity? The internationalization of gay identities', *Social Text*, 14, pp. 77–94.

—— (1997) 'Response to Donald Morton', *Critical InQueeries*, 1, pp. 31–3.

APPADURAI, A. (1996) *Modernity at Large: Cultural Dimensions of Globalization*, Minneapolis: University of Minnesota Press.

BORTHWICK, P. (1999) 'HIV/AIDS projects with and for gay men in northern Thailand', in JACKSON, P. and SULLIVAN, G. (eds) *Lady Boys, Tom Boys, Rent Boys: Male and Female Homosexualities in Contemporary Thailand*, New York: Haworth.

BRAVMAN, S. (1997) *Queer Fictions of the Past: History, Culture and Difference*, Cambridge, New York and Melbourne: Cambridge University Press.

CONNORS, M. (1995) 'Missing gender and the fetishism of sex: "gay" responses to the sexuality debates', *Thamyris*, 2, pp. 207–28.

—— (1997). 'Prefacing research on the "global gay"', *Melbourne Journal of Politics*, 24, pp. 44–8.

FOUCAULT, M. (1980) *The History of Sexuality Volume 1: An Introduction* (trans. Robert Hurley), New York: Vintage Books.

GROSZ, E. (1992) *Jacques Lacan: A Feminist Introduction*, London: Allen and Unwin.

—— (1994) *Volatile Bodies: Towards a Corporeal Feminism*, St Leonards, NSW: Allen & Unwin.

HALPERIN, D. (1996) 'A response from David Halperin to Dennis Altman', *Australian Humanities Review*, www.lib.latrobe.edu.au/AHR/emuse/Globalqueering/halperin.html

—— (1998) 'Forgetting Foucault: acts, identities and the history of sexuality', *Representations*, 63, pp. 93–120.

—— (2000) 'How to do the history of male homosexuality', *GLQ: A Journal of Gay and Lesbian Studies*, 6, pp. 87–124.

JACKSON, P. (1995a) *Dear Uncle Go: Male Homosexuality in Thailand*, Bangkok: Bua Luang Books.

—— (1995b) 'Thai Buddhist accounts of homosexuality and AIDS', *The Australian Journal of Anthropology*, 6, pp. 140–53.

—— (1996) 'The persistence of gender: from ancient Indian *pandakas* to modern Thai *gay* quings', *Meanjin*, 55, pp. 110–20.

—— (1997a) 'From *kamma* to unnatural vice: male homosexuality and transgenderism in the Thai Buddhist tradition', in LEYLAND, W. (ed.) *Queer Dharma: A Buddhist Gay Anthology*, San Francisco: Gay Sunshine Press

—— (1997b) '*Kathoey* < > gay < > man, the historical emergence of gay male identity in Thailand', in L. MANDERSON and M. JOLLY (eds) *Sites of Desire/Economies of Pleasure, Sexualities in Asia and the Pacific*, Chicago, University of Chicago Press.

—— (1997c) 'Thai research on male homosexuality and transgenderism and the cultural limits of Foucaultian analysis', *Journal of the History of Sexuality*, 8, pp. 52–85.

—— (1999a) 'An American death in Bangkok: the murder of Darrell Berrigan and the hybrid origins of gay identity in 1960s Bangkok', *GLQ: A Journal of Lesbian and Gay Studies*, 5, pp. 361–411.

—— (1999b) 'Spurning Alphonso Lingis's Thai "lust": the perils of a philosopher at large', *Intersections: Gender, History & Culture in the Asian Context*, 2, www.sshe.murdoch.edu.au/hum/as/intersections

—— (1999c) 'Tolerant but unaccepting: correcting misperceptions of a Thai "Gay Paradise"', in JACKSON, P. and COOK, N. (eds) *Genders and Sexualities in Modern Thailand*, Chiang Mai: Silkworm Books.

—— (1999d) 'Same-sex sexual experience in Thailand', in JACKSON, P. and SULLIVAN, G. (eds) *Lady Boys, Tom Boys, Rent Boys: Male and Female Homosexualities in Contemporary Thailand*, New York: Haworth.

—— (2000) 'Review article: opportunities and dangers in American postmodernist historiography', *Intersections: Gender, History & Culture in the Asian Context*, 3, www.sshe.murdoch.edu.au/ hum/as/intersections

KULICK, D. (1998) *Travestis: Sex, Gender and Culture Among Brazilian Transgendered Prostitutes*, Chicago: University of Chicago Press.

LINGIS, A. (1983) *Excesses: Eros and Culture*, Albany: State University of New York Press.

—— (1995) *Abuses*, Berkeley: University of California Press.

MCCAMISH, M. (1999) 'The friends thou hast: support systems for male commercial sex workers in Pattaya, Thailand', in JACKSON, P. and SULLIVAN, G. (eds) *Lady Boys, Tom Boys, Rent Boys: Male and Female Homosexualities in Contemporary Thailand*, New York: Haworth.

MARTIN, F. and BERRY, C. (1998) 'Queer'n'Asian on the net: syncretic sexualities in Taiwan and Korean cyberspaces', *Critical InQueeries*, 2, pp. 67–94.

MILLER, N. (1992) *Out in the World: Gay and Lesbian Life from Buenos Aires to Bangkok*, London: Penguin Books.

MILLETT, K. (1971) *Sexual Politics*, London: R. Hart-Davis.

MORRIS, R. (1994) 'Three sexes and four sexualities: redressing the discourses on gender and sexuality in contemporary Thailand', *Positions*, 2, pp. 15–43.

—— (1997) 'Educating desire: Thailand, transnationalism, and transgression', *Social Text*, 15, pp. 53–79.

MORTON, D. (1997) 'Global (sexual) politics, class struggle, and the queer left', *Critical InQueeries*, 1, pp. 1–30.

OSBORNE, P. and SEGAL, L. (1994) 'Gender as performance: an interview with Judith Butler', *Radical Philosophy*, 67, pp. 32–9.

PARKER, R. (1991) *Bodies, Pleasures and Passions: Sexual Culture in Contemporary Brazil*, Boston, MA: Beacon Press.

PRINGLE, R. (1992) 'Absolute sex? unpacking the sexuality/gender relationship', in CONNELL, R.W. and DOWSETT, G. (eds) *Rethinking Sex: Social Theory and Sexuality Research*, Melbourne: University of Melbourne Press.

RUBIN, G. (1975) 'The traffic of women: notes on the political economy of sex', in REITER, R. (ed.) *Toward an Anthropology of Women*, New York: Monthly Review Press.

—— (1984) 'Thinking sex: notes for a radical theory of the politics of sexuality', in C. VANCE (ed.) *Pleasure and Danger: Exploring Female Sexuality*, London: Routledge and Kegan Paul.

SEDGWICK, E. (1990) *Epistemology of the Closet*, Berkeley: University of California Press.

SINNOTT, M. (2000) 'The semiotics of transgendered sexual identity in the Thai print media: imagery and discourse of the sexual other', *Culture, Health & Sexuality*, 2(4), pp. 425–40.

STIVENS, M. (1997) 'Comment on "research and its discontents"', *Melbourne Journal of Politics*, 24, pp. 49–51.

STORER, G. (1999a) 'Rehearsing gender and sexuality in modern Thailand: masculinity and male–male sex behaviours', in JACKSON, P. and SULLIVAN, G. (eds) *Lady Boys, Tom Boys, Rent Boys: Male and Female Homosexualities in Contemporary Thailand*, New York: Haworth.

—— (1999b) 'Performing sexual identity: naming and resisting "gayness" in modern Thailand', *Intersections: Gender, History & Culture in the Asian Context*, 2, www.sshe.murdoch.edu.au/hum/as/intersections.

SULLIVAN, G. and LEONG, L. (eds) (1995) *Gays and Lesbians in Asia and the Pacific: Social and Human Services*, New York: Harrington Park Press.

VAN WIJNGAARDEN, J.W. DE LIND (1999) 'Between money, morality and masculinity: the dynamics of bar-based male sex work in Chiang Mai, Northern Thailand', in JACKSON, P. and SULLIVAN, G. (eds) *Lady Boys, Tom Boys, Rent Boys: Male and Female Homosexualities in Contemporary Thailand*, New York, Haworth.

19 *Bhai-behen*, true love, time pass

Friendships and sexual partnerships among youth in an Indian metropolis

Leena Abraham [2002]

Recent studies of sexuality in India show that premarital sex is not as rare as generally believed to be (Family Planning Association of India, n.d.; Rakesh, 1992; Goparaju, 1993; Bhende, 1994; Rangaiyan, 1995; Sachdev, 1997) and that young people often lack adequate information in order to protect themselves from unwanted pregnancies and sexually transmitted infections (Murthy, 1993, Verma *et al.*, 1997). These studies establish gender asymmetry as an important feature of sexual experience and access to information. The studies also show that youth do not constitute a homogeneous category and that the sexual experiences and extent of vulnerability differ among groups such as street youth, young truck cleaners, married adolescents, and rural, urban and educated youth. There are significant differences between youth groups in terms of control over their sexuality and in the access to information and services (Ramakrishna *et al.*, 2000). However, we know little about how youth sexuality is culturally constructed and what structural arrangements enhance or inhibit sexual experiences as well as access to information among young people. Such information will contribute significantly towards the design of culturally relevant sexuality education and the planning of appropriate sexual health services.

   This paper analyses heterosexual peer networks and partnerships among unmarried, college-going youth in an Indian metropolitan city. It discusses the typologies of heterosexual relationships that youth engage in, and through which youth sexuality is channelled and experienced.[1] These typologies reflect the dominance of heterosexuality as the cultural norm, as well as gender differentiated constructions and arrangements within heterosexual partnerships. As the paper argues, the social arrangements and the sexuality norms that generate different types of partnerships also produce unequal opportunities for sexual experiences and health consequences for young men and women. They enable the exploration of male sexuality, while they restrict exploration of female sexuality. Boys' sexual partnerships in particular show that male sexual expression is not limited to the most commonly assumed paradigm of relationships between peers (girl friends), and includes other relationships.[2] Boys' pursuit of multiple relationships exposes them to varying degrees of health risks, while girls' abstinence from sexual relationships may not protect them from similar risks in future. These factors need to be taken into account in designing programmes to address the specific needs of college youth in urban India.

Analytic framework

Sexuality is here seen as a cultural construct, shaped by specific historical contexts within different communities and social groups (Foucault, 1976; Weeks, 1986; Caplan, 1987; Horrocks, 1997). The meanings and practices associated with sexuality differ with age (West, 1999), social class (Wight, 1994) and gender (Vance, 1984; Holland *et al.*, 1992; Mac and Ghaill, 1996). It is therefore not viewed as a fixed state of being but as in a flux and continuously evolving (Weeks, 1986). Further, cultural constructions of male and female sexualities are intimately associated with gender roles, the division of labour and kinship arrangements. These, in turn, are constructions of a patriarchal social order.

Theories that treat sexuality as constructed and negotiated through the power structures of class, caste and patriarchy have led to a better understanding of the structural arrangements in society that legitimize the subordination of certain individuals and sexualities. While such theorizing about the structuring of power in society is valuable, Foucault's (1977) contention that insufficient attention has been paid to how power is exercised and contested in different sites remains valid. It is in the modes and manifestations of power in the 'capillaries' of the social structure, that the experience of sexuality becomes vastly different across different cultures.

Feminists have argued that in modern capitalist societies sexuality norms are gendered and vary only in cultural form and ideological content. Studies across societies have shown that sexuality norms are gender asymmetric and that 'the power imbalance characteristic of sexual relations between men and women has many of its roots in adolescence' (Weiss *et al.*, 2000, p. 233). Although one may agree that all human relationships are gendered social relationships and the suppression and subordination of feminine sexuality is nearly universal (Holland *et al.*, 1992, 2000; Rao Gupta and Weiss, 1993), there are significant variations across societies in the way in which sexuality is constructed and experienced through adolescence and youth. For instance, in South Asian societies, the general sexuality norms that govern adolescent boys and girls are almost diametrically opposite. Premarital sex is taboo yet there is no social sanction against boys who transgress the norm. On the contrary, gender socialization operates in a manner that promotes male sexuality while constraining female sexuality through dominant social institutions and ideological practices (Dube, 1988, 1997; Das, 1988).

Although there are important regional, caste, class, ethnic and religious variations within India with respect to female subordination, the seclusion and segregation of postpubertal women, the centrality of marriage in a woman's life, the powerful ideology of *pativrata* (devotion to husband), the preservation of virginity and the maintenance of fidelity constitute the essential features of female subordination. Socialization by the family, kin groups, religious and even educational institutions (Chanana, 2001) acts in consonance to perpetuate patriarchal ideologies and make subordination appear natural.

In the metropolitan social and cultural context, sexual subordination may change by undergoing transformation, but nevertheless remains real (Thapan, 1997; Abraham, 2001). In cities and towns, there is a mix of the traditional and the modern, which adds a different dimension to the expression of young people's sexuality. Crowded living conditions in the city as well as its cosmopolitan character can lead to a relaxation of restrictive social norms such as *purdah*, sexual segregation and the purity/pollution practices associated with menstruation and childbirth. The metropolitan context also exposes some young people to liberal sexual culture, offers varied avenues for sexual experiences through its vast sex industry, and provides anonymity that greatly enhances the opportunities for sexual liaisons. All these factors, along with the exposure to the film industry and easy access to erotic literature and films, influence the articulation of youth sexuality in the metropolis.

Methods

This paper is based on a study of young people's sexuality conducted among low-income, unmarried, college students in Mumbai during 1996–98.[3] Data were gathered from the students of four large coeducational colleges that cater for low-income students. Students in the first year of junior college (higher secondary) and in the third (final) year of undergraduate college participated in the study. The junior students were aged 16–18 years old and the seniors were 20–22 years old.

Qualitative data were gathered from two colleges and a survey was conducted among a representative sample of students drawn from the remaining two colleges. Focus group discussions (FGDs) and interviews were conducted to gather qualitative data. A total of 75 students distributed across 10 groups took part in the FGDs. These FGDs explored students' social interaction, views on marriage, partners and premarital sex, sexual experiences and sources of information. They were followed by in-depth interviews of 87 students to gain more detailed information on personal views and experiences.

The qualitative data were later used in designing a survey that covered 966 students (625 boys and 341 girls). A pilot-tested, structured, self-administered questionnaire was used for the survey and was made available in English as well as in Marathi, the local language. The findings discussed in this paper are based primarily on the qualitative data, while findings from the survey have been reported in detail elsewhere (Abraham and Kumar, 1999).

We were initially apprehensive about eliciting information on sexuality from unmarried boys and girls within the college setting, but soon realized that young people are willing to share their views and experiences in a non-threatening environment. For many, this was an opportunity to discuss matters of sexuality, to clarify doubts and gather information. They hoped to 'learn about sex through frank discussion'. Special efforts were made to recruit young alumni of the colleges in the research team, a factor that we consider, in hindsight, very useful. They were familiar with young people's interests and concerns, especially the vocabulary and language that young people use to discuss sex and sexuality. The research team explained the objectives and significance of the study and assured the respondents of confidentiality. After initial discussions with the principal and a few teachers and after the permission for the study was granted, college authorities were not involved in the data collection. This helped in creating a non-threatening atmosphere and in gaining student cooperation.[4]

In order to partially meet some respondents' need for information, at the end of the qualitative phase of the study, further discussions with a sexologist and sex educator were organized. However this was not possible with the large survey group, who were instead given addresses of service providers.

Findings

Students and their family background

A majority of the students in our study belonged to low-income families and 'middle' and 'lower' castes in the caste hierarchy. Two-thirds of the students belonged to families that had an average monthly income of Rupees 5000 (then US$120) or less (Table 19.1). Lower levels of parental education and lower-paying occupations of fathers typify their family background. While illiterate fathers were few, illiterate mothers were more common. Fathers were employed as mill workers, taxi drivers, watchmen, police constables, clerks, peons and so on. A majority of mothers were housewives and those who were employed worked as clerks, nurses or domestic helps. A few mothers were engaged in small-scale home-based production.

The families lived in poor and crowded living conditions, very often in single room tenements, frequently located in slums. The living conditions were worse in cases of extended families, with relatives sharing the already limited space and other resources.

Table 19.1 Profile of students (survey data)

Indicators	Boys (n=625)		Girls (n=341)	
	n	*%*	*n*	*%*
Family Income (per month)				
≤ Rs2000	160	25.6	71	20.8
Rs2001–5000	261	41.8	165	48.4
≥ Rs5000	191	30.5	99	29.0
Do not know	2	0.3	0	0.0
No response	11	1.8	6	1.8
Father's education				
Illiterate	45	7.2	5	1.5
Up to primary	80	12.8	25	7.3
Primary to higher secondary	369	59.1	236	69.2
Graduation and above	124	19.8	74	21.7
No response	7	1.1	1	0.3
Mother's education				
Illiterate	130	20.8	34	10.0
Up to primary	144	23.0	53	15.5
Primary to higher secondary	282	45.1	228	66.9
Graduation and above	63	10.1	26	7.6
No response	6	1.0	—	—
Father's occupation				
Unskilled/unemployed	36	5.8	11	3.2
Semi-skilled	139	22.2	69	20.2
Clerical	123	19.7	73	21.4
Managerial/professional	142	22.7	84	24.6
Business	107	17.1	61	17.9
Others	56	9.0	38	11.2
No response	22	3.5	5	1.5
Mother's occupation				
Housewife	427	68.3	251	73.6
Semi-skilled/clerical	64	10.2	29	8.5
Managerial/professional	33	5.3	21	6.2
Business	80	12.8	37	10.8
No response	21	3.4	3	0.9
Type of residence				
Chawl/slum	390	62.4	200	58.7
Flat/quarters	224	35.9	128	37.5
Others	9	1.4	9	2.6
No response	2	0.3	4	1.2
Personal income (per month)				
< Rs100	188	30.1	134	39.3
Rs101–250	114	18.2	62	18.2
Rs251–500	118	18.9	73	21.4
≥ Rs501	95	15.2	29	8.5
No response	110	17.6	43	12.6

Most students lived with their parents in nuclear families. The two dominant religious groups represented were Hindus and Muslims. Students, both boys and girls, Hindus and Muslims, did not consider themselves 'religious', but did consider their families to be so. Boys found their family environment restrictive but most girls did not.

Youth subcultures

In India, as elsewhere, youth subculture(s) are generally constructed within a framework of fun, freedom and friendships that conceals personal anxieties and uncertainties about academic performance, future employment and peer competition. Such constructions are often based on social norms that do not place undue pressure on young people to share family or other responsibilities and cultural norms that allow greater leisure time spent with peers. Leisure time, personal income and autonomy determine students' ability to actively engage in youth subculture(s). The leisure time activities of students from poorer households are, however, constrained by less time and lack of economic resources. Boys and girls experience these constraints in different ways.

Boys' leisure time is often curtailed through employment or the need to assist fathers or relatives in their work. Boys who take up jobs (tuition, secretarial work, saleswork, etc.) have to forgo leisure time, but in return they have more income and autonomy. Girls enjoy less autonomy both over their income, which must go into the family kitty, and over decisions related to employment. Girls from lower-income households are often confined to the house, not always to protect their sexuality, but because their labour is required in the management of household chores. Girls are often unable to attend college when there are religious functions or ceremonies or illness in the family.

Some students received small amounts of pocket money while a few receive scholarships. The average monthly personal income of students from all sources was low, with girls receiving less than boys. For more than one-third of the boys and girls, monthly personal income did not exceed Rs100 (US$2.50) (Table 19.1).

The family regulates and monitors the mobility and social engagements of young people, especially girls, outside of family and kinship relations. The dominant norm of heterosexuality is upheld through the cultural practices of sexual segregation, which act as a constant reminder of this norm. Since caste purity and boundaries between the castes are maintained through the regulation of female sexuality, a high premium is placed on female virginity. Hence, girls' mobility and interaction with boys is generally monitored. Arranged marriages within the caste and the community are typical of these households and love marriages are discouraged (Abraham, 2001).[5]

Both boys and girls spend a large share of their leisure time in same-sex peer groups. Indeed, it is largely in a homosocial environment that peer socialization occurs. However, boys spend far more time with other boys than girls with other girls, and homosocial interaction increases both with age and with number of years spent in college. Seniors have a less rigidly structured academic programme and their peer networks strengthen over the years spent together in college.

Students are part of various peer groups, at the college, at the locality of residence, at work place and at the coaching/tuition classes. By the time they are in college, peers often become 'significant others' for obtaining information, for companionship and in decision-making. The homosocial interaction contributes towards the formation of identities, awareness of sexuality and development of self-image. There is greater need for knowledge on matters of sex and, as sources that provide information to youth on sexual matters are not easily available, young people frequently turn towards peers.

Peer activities common to both boys and girls include 'chatting' (*gappa marna*), teasing one another, studying or copying notes together, walking around together, meeting up, travelling together to college and back and going to the canteen or having lunch together. Girls occasionally visit each other's homes during festivals, go to a restaurant or to a movie on someone's birthday. Peer activities exclusive to boys include teasing girls, roaming around the streets, parks or beaches, watching pornographic films and visiting 'red light areas'. Boys tend to watch pornographic films in a friend's residence or at a video parlour. Video parlours are mostly exclusively male domains and are easily accessible to young boys as they are inexpensive and are common in the localities where they reside. Visiting different commercial sex areas is yet another common peer activity among some of the boys (see Pangare, n.d.) although it does not always result in actually engaging in paid-for sex. Initially, boys 'roam around' red light areas to satisfy their curiosity and subsequently 'for fun to watch the semi-clad women'. According to our findings, the first paid-for sex experience is generally initiated under peer influence.

Another feature commonly assumed to be part of youth subculture is initiation into smoking, alcohol consumption and use of drugs. However it was observed that fewer students, mainly senior boys, engage in such behaviour. Boys in this study tended to consider cigarette smoking as 'bad' and drugs as 'taboo', while drinking was 'not good'. While most young boys abstained from these habits, some of them had tried them out a few times. A few seniors, however, were habituated to smoking and/or drinking, with habitual drinking being more common than smoking or use of drugs. There are stricter normative proscriptions for girls with regard to any of these activities, so much so that girls find it difficult to imagine themselves indulging in any of them.

Premarital sex was not very common among students. In our survey, 26 per cent of the boys and 3 per cent of the girls reported experience of vaginal sexual intercourse. Having participated in 'any sexual experience' (kissing, hugging, touching genitals, vaginal sexual intercourse, anal sex or oral sex) was reported by nearly half the males (47 per cent) and only 13 per cent of the girls.

Mixed sex peer networks

Although sex segregation is the norm and sexual socialization mostly occurs in homosocial contexts, mixed-sex peer networks are not a complete taboo. Mixed-sex groups generally consist of more boys than girls. Younger girls, however, hardly spend time in mixed-sex peer networks. As in the case of homosocial interaction, mixed-sex peer interaction increases substantially with age and years spent at college. These mixed-sex groups spend much of their time together within college premises or while travelling together to college and back. According to some boys, girls have neither the time nor the freedom to be part of such groups. Either they have to rush home or are scared of being seen with boys. For some girls, being part of such a group provides opportunities to interact with boys as their parents permit outings with boys in mixed groups more easily than with any individual boy.

On joining college, both boys and girls find it difficult to initiate friendships with the opposite sex. There are various ways in which students overcome constraints. Often this begins with exchanging books and notes. Verbal 'teasing' is another common strategy considered legitimate and non-offensive. Functions such as 'ribbon day', 'friendship day', 'chocolate day', 'traditional day' and 'rose day' organized as part of cultural or extracurricular activities of the college, are also used to express interest in and initiate a relationship with members of the opposite sex. On 'ribbon day', for example, girls and boys tie different coloured ribbons or friendship bands on each other's hands. The colour of ribbons or bands signifies relationships. Girls tie yellow ribbons to 'decent' boys to make them their 'brother' and red ribbons to signify 'love'. Similarly on chocolate days and rose days messages are exchanged between boys and girls along with chocolates and roses. These exchanges in many instances initiate friendships or heterosexual partnerships of various kinds.

These occasions actively socialize young people into heterosexual norms but are simultaneously reminders of the boundaries of social interaction. They are meant to 'break the ice' and give opportunities to boys and girls to interact across academic streams and age groups in a 'healthy manner'. But the boys and girls involved are expected to be 'just friends'. These celebrations thus signify dual meanings: the legitimacy of heterosexuality and the significance of boundary maintenance. However, at times boundaries are transgressed and social meanings are subverted by using the opportunity to establish heterosexual partnerships and sexual intimacy.

Heterosexual partnerships among peers

The three types of heterosexual relationships among peers are *Bhai-behen* (literally, 'brother–sister') 'true love' and 'time pass' relationships. This typology embodies the cultural norms of sexuality and also expresses the meaning that young people attach to their relationships.

Bhai-behen *(brother–sister-like friendship)*

Students often describe the *bhai-behen* relationships in English as a 'brother–sister-like relationship'.[6] This description emphasizes the platonic character of the relationship. The category *bhai-behen* is important as a boundary marker and a reference point for distinguishing other categories of tabooed friendships. In other words, the typology is used to say explicitly that the heterosexual interaction is within the culturally and socially permissible limits.

Once *bhai-behen* relationships are established between individual boys and girls, it makes interaction between the two somewhat easier and boy–girl pairs are generally free from suspicion and not subject to teasing by others. Declaring such a friendship allows them to sit together, eat together (in the canteen or in restaurants), talk or study together and receive or make telephone calls to each other. Young people can establish multiple *bhai-behen* friendships. Younger students in general, and Muslim students and girls in particular, use this category to describe their heterosexual friendships with the opposite sex.

The most important or distinct feature of this type of relationship in relation to the other two is the absence of any form of physical intimacy including touching or playful hitting.

R: Those who are *bhai-behen* (brother–sister), they behave freely but they don't do fun by touching each other (*hathach i masti nahi*). In time pass, friendship and love, everything is done. (B13 (XI boy))

It is in the context of social restrictions over heterosexual interactions among boys and girls, and the individual's desire to establish friendship with the opposite sex in a culture where heterosexuality is the norm, that the *bhai-behen* relationship has emerged and gained significance. It is particularly useful for a girl who wishes to establish sexual distance from a boy who is pursuing her to declare their relationship to be *bhai-behen*. At the same time *bhai-behen* relationships provide girls with an opportunity to get to know boys, without compromising their sexual reputation. *Bhai-behen* being a broad and fluid relationship can be easily subverted. For some, it is a slow and safe way of initiating a true love or, at times, a time pass relationship. The category *bhai-behen* can therefore provide a convenient cover for courtship.

'Time pass' and 'true love' relationships

The two types of heterosexual friendships that are more commonly discussed by the students are the 'time pass' and 'true love' friendships. These are both relationships that are established between individual boys and girls within a broader context of the peer network where peer pressure and support help partners negotiate their relationship. However, these two categories are distinct from each other and they carry opposing social values and meanings. Time pass is a transitory relationship of a shorter duration, while true love is a long-term relationship pursued with the implicit or explicit intention of marriage.

Unlike the *bhai-behen* relationship, time pass and true love relationships are characterized by sexual intimacy although the degree of sexual involvement and the sexual norms vary. Sexual intimacy including sexual intercourse, typically characterizes the time pass relationship. True love is, on the other hand, more romantic, signifies emotional involvement and sexual intercourse is usually postponed until marriage. The emphasis here is on commitment and responsibility, and there is an underplaying of sexual pleasure. By postponing sexual intimacy, the virtue of fidelity is emphasized. Through time pass relationships, partners seek sexual experience and sexual pleasure, but these partnerships are usually devoid of any commitments, to marry or to protective behaviour.

As some of the senior boys described during one of the FGDs (FGD A-3-TY Boys), in time pass relationships '*last tak ja sak te hai*' (one can go all the way). They described how the relationship progresses as '*Pahle ungali pakad te hai, phir hath pakad te hai phir kamar phir last tak jathe hai*' (first hold the finger, then hand, then waist and then go all the way). Similar views were also expressed by those interviewed.

R: Those who are *bhai-behen*, they do teasing to any extent but don't touch each other and those who do friendship, they go to any extent (do anything).
I: Then those who do love, what do they do?
R: All that depends on both of them. If both of them agree, then kissing and then pressing. (B2-6 (XI boy))
R: 'True love' … very rare, they just roam about. At the physical level, they don't go very far … up to kissing, go to park, … hotel … upstairs, maybe for movies. 'Time pass' people mostly don't go to such places. They need privacy. Go to friend's house, own house.
I: What about physical intimacy?
R: '*Toka paryanta*', [until the last] … Kissing, fondling, intercourse. (A1-11 [T.Y. boy])

Time pass relationships are generally initiated and cultivated by the boy, and last only until he succeeds in having sexual intercourse with the girl. Only rarely were such relationships reported as lasting beyond two or three months. As pointed out by a group of third-year girls, 'After taking the girls around for 1or 2 months, [boys] drop them' (FGD-A4).

Third year boys also agreed,

Time pass affair starts … wherein the boy first spends lot of money taking her out. He plans everything carefully; his goal is to have sex with the girl and nothing else. After the girl is ditched she has to listen to her parents' [scolding].

(FGD-A3)

Some respondents, however, disagreed that in all time pass relationships, sexual intimacy goes as far as sexual intercourse. According to them, in time pass relationships girls engage in sexual acts such as kissing and hugging but many abstain from sexual intercourse.

P3:   Among boys, some boys do time pass.
P2:   [It] doesn't last long.
P5:   Lasts only till work is done.
P3:   First [Boy] tries to impress the girl. Will take her to … hotel, for movies. They go to … Park. In … hotel, the first floor is for couples. Mostly from here [this college] they [couples] go there.
P5:   To friend's house also they go.
P6:   Empty classroom is used.
I: How about physical intimacy among them?
P2:   Till kissing. I suppose.
P5:   At least in our college I don't think all those girls must be going to that stage [intercourse].
P1:   Not heard that much among the girls in our college. There are girls who go till intercourse. But girls do not respond that much in our college. Also there is the problem of space [privacy] … If there is opportunity, yes, otherwise only up to 'kissing and pressing'. (FGD-B5II [T.Y. Boys])

As mentioned earlier, and in this study anyway, fewer girls than boys had personal experience of sexual intercourse and for some of them their current relationship with a boy was temporary or for fun, thus falling in the category of time pass. Time pass relationships were more common among senior boys. Among boys who were currently involved in a heterosexual relationship, many perceived their relationship to be of the 'time pass' category, as they did not intend to marry the girl they were courting. Among both boys and girls, once sexually experienced, individuals are likely to have multiple experiences. Once the taboo of premarital sex is broken they are likely to be sexually active with more than one partner.

As gender relationships are structured asymmetrically, time pass relationships have different outcomes for male and female partners.

> *Ek saal ek ladki ko ghumate hai. Doosri saal doosri ladki ko.* [Boys] take a girl around for one year. Next year another girl. Most of these are time pass affairs, and not serious ones. Girls are taking a big risk. Can get pregnant … but more than that, *ladki ki izzat nahi rehati, Badnami hoti hai, shaadi nahi hoti* [girl loses her honour, gets bad name, does not get married].
>
> (FGD-A4 [T.Y. Girls])

Since female sexuality is closely linked to personal and family honour, it is generally held that girls with *izzat* (with self-respect, of good character), of *ghareloo* (domestically oriented) nature and from 'good' families do not get involved in time pass relationships. Male sexuality is, however, free from any such normative constraints.

Girls in time pass relationships are frequently seen as 'liberal', 'of bad character' or as coming from a family that is seen as transgressing the social norms. Once the female sexuality norm is violated through premarital sex in relationships such as the time pass category, the girl is seen as 'sexually available' to any man. Girls in such relationships are called *maal*, *chalu*, *chavi*, *samaan*, *item* and other names that project the woman as a sexual object or commodity for general consumption. Boys in such relationships, however, do not carry the social burden of preserving personal or family honour or the danger of losing social respect. On the contrary, such relationships enhance their self-image and masculine identity. Boys in time pass relationships may be called *bade kamgar* (great worker), *jo ghat ghat ka pani piya hai* (one who is sexually very experienced – an expert), 'heroes', 'playboys', and so on. In spite of their transitory character, time pass relationships also carry with them gendered norms. For instance, girls cannot be simultaneously involved in multiple time pass relationships. Boys, on the other hand, are free to do so.

Unlike the time pass relationship with its distinct feature of sexual intimacy, true love is characterized by the emotional involvement of the partners. While kissing, hugging and caressing ('touching', 'pressing') are common in this latter kind of relationship, sexual intercourse is rare.[7] True love, the romantic premarital relationship, is idealized especially in Hindi films, where it revolves around sexual desires, fantasies that are explicitly erotic at times, but stops short of transgressing the normative boundary of sexual intercourse. Thus, true love embodies the normative elements of heterosexuality as well as a sexual ideology that stresses girls' virginity before marriage.

In true love relationships, girls may be reluctant to engage in sexual intercourse even if the relationship had been 'steady' for a considerable period of time, and the partners are intending to marry. Unlike in many other cultures where sexual intercourse is seen as a cementing factor, a reflection of the commitment of the partners to each other, or an expression of love for each other, here it is seen as a reflection of 'physical love' or desire for sex rather than any of the above. Since, in general, boys make the first move to initiate sex, any desire to have sex in relationship of true-love type is seen by girls as treating the relationship as time pass. Girls are careful to guard their virginity and 'honour', as, according to some of them 'anything can happen' before marriage. They view the consequences of premarital sex as likely to affect the girl all through her life. The long-term social and psychological costs seem to outweigh the immediate pleasure of sexual involvement. Girls conveniently use the cover of societal norms to decline boys' demands for sexual intercourse. They also use their refusal to have sex as a test of the boy's love and his commitment to their relationship, and to ensure that he is not merely interested in using his partner to have fun as in time pass. However, not all true love partners abstain from sexual intercourse. In this study, there were a few instances when sexual intercourse is seen as an affirmation of the commitment to their partner as in some Western contexts.

The boundaries in all the three typologies of friendships are fluid and can change over a period of time. For example, a *bhai-behen* relationship can become time pass, or a true love relationship can turn into a time pass relationship. Boys use this fluidity to their advantage as they often engage in multiple relationships, while girls mainly engage in single, true love relationships. Furthermore, such fluidity also leads to situations where the two partners share contradictory perceptions, with the girl seeing their relationship as true love while the boy treats it as time pass.

The risk that girls face in heterosexual partnerships is social in nature – getting a bad name, loss of honour and respect, marital discord in the future and so on. In comparison to these social risks, the perception of health risks is minimal. Both boys and girls in this study rarely perceived any risk of contracting sexually transmitted infections (STIs) or HIV through their peers, as the latter were felt to be 'known'. To them, even transitory, time pass relationships do not seem to carry any risk of infection. Such perceptions lead to inconsistent use of condoms in sexual encounters with peers. In such encounters the major perceived risks are pregnancy and/or being 'caught by the family'.

Male sexual partnerships beyond peers

The sexual networks of boys extend beyond peers to include relationships with women who are older in age, in other words with sex workers (SWs) and 'aunties'. Qualitative data from this study show that boys' first experience of sexual intercourse is often with SWs. In many instances, it is unplanned and initiated under peer influence.

I: Why do students 'go down' [to SW]?
P6:   There is attraction, regarding sex. Don't get it in college, that's why.
P3:   Sexual urge is there.
I: How do they go?
P3:   With friends. First time goes with friends.
P6:   If gone at least once, confidence increases.
P3:   First time feel scared, feel bad (*bhiti vatate, bekar vatate*).
I: Why?
P3:   It is first time and unknown lady is there … That is why feel scared. Don't have any experience.

(FGDB5IV [T.Y. boys])

Senior boys with experience of paid-for sex tended to report more than one sexual encounter with SWs. In general, the women concerned were older in age except in a few instances when boys were able to demand younger girls. Practices such as hiring out a SW and sharing her among a group of friends to reduce costs were reported by some seniors. Condom use, although inconsistent, was more likely in the case of sex with SWs, as the risk of acquiring HIV was perceived to be high.

Commercial sex of the kind described, may occur simultaneously with time pass and true love relationships. Both younger and older boys are under considerable pressure to experience sex and paid-for sex is seen as the easiest way of acquiring sexual experience. Information regarding where to go in Mumbai for commercial sex – such as the specific locations, pick-up points, types of girls, type of sex available, costs and so on – was fairly widespread among the boys. While senior girls were aware of the fact that boys in general have sex with SWs, they did not suspect their male friends of doing so.

A second category of women with whom boys entered into sexual relationships was that of older women or 'aunties'. Work by Goparaju (1993) among male students in another city in India reported similar sexual partnerships between young boys and older women. Relationships with the aunties are non-commercial in nature but sometimes boys receive gifts or favours. Aunties are reported typically to be married women from middle-class families who seek sexual partnerships with younger men. In some cases, aunties are known persons such as a relative or a person living in the same locality, or a tutor. In other cases, contact with aunties is established through a friend. In some cases, the woman herself reportedly takes the initiative.

Boys perceive sex with aunties to be the 'safest' of all in terms of all forms of risks associated with premarital sex. Firstly, the responsibility for preventing pregnancy, which is a concern with girls, is borne by the auntie. Secondly, these women are seen as distinct from the SWs and therefore not perceived as potential carriers of STIs or HIV. Thirdly, having sex with an auntie reduces the fear of being caught in the red light area by a friend or relative.

Boys have relatively easy access to all the above networks of sexual partnerships. Moreover, a double mechanism of peer pressure and peer protection allows boys to actively explore these channels. Through multiple and varied partnerships, they thereby gain experience of a variety of sexual acts. In true love, this is mainly non-penetrative sex (kissing, hugging, touching), and in time pass relationships it includes non-penetrative sex as well as vaginal intercourse. In sexual partnerships with SWs and aunties, besides vaginal sex, oral and anal sex may also be experienced.

These different kinds of heterosexual partnerships have important programmatic implications. The current state-financed 'Universities Talk AIDS' (UTA) programme conducted in colleges, AIDS/sex-education programmes of various NGOs, and handbooks on sexuality tend to conceptualize sexuality as a biological condition and therefore reduce issues of sexuality to health-care concerns. Young people's experiences, and the constraints on understanding and negotiating sexuality, are determined by social arrangements and ideological constructions of masculinity and femininity that are 'unsafe'. It is vitally important to question these constructions in future sexual and reproductive health programmes, and to address issues such as sexuality and pleasure, desires and fantasies that constitute young people's sexuality. Providing information alone is insufficient to capture the attention and imagination unless it is contextualized against, say, people's lived experiences and anxieties, and in their own terms rather than in an alien medical language.

Conclusions

Concepts such as 'casual sex', referring to relationships that typically last for as little as one night or at the most a few months, or 'boyfriend–girlfriend' relationships have been conventionally employed in the global literature on young people's sexual behaviour. Such conceptualizations fail to capture the different typologies of heterosexual relationships and sexual networking among urban youth in India, and are inadequate for understanding complexity and fluidity in types of sexual partnerships.

The three typologies – *bhai-behen*, true love and time pass – reinforce the norms of heterosexuality and, more importantly, define the boundaries of sexual behaviour for unmarried youth. This analysis of homosocial and heterosexual relationships among young people shows the differential avenues available for boys and girls to explore and experience sexuality. The sexual networks of boys extend beyond peers to include SWs and older women and are shaped by factors such as opportunities to meet with different partners, the availability of multiple and varied partners, peer support and the generally relaxed societal norms towards male sexuality. Fewer girls report having sexual experiences, and these are mainly limited to kissing, hugging and 'touching' within true love relationships, and, rarely, sexual intercourse in time pass relationships.

Fear of acquiring a negative sexual reputation prevents girls from engaging in sex. A girl in a time pass relationship is likely to be called names that not only objectify her body, but also convey disrespect for her self. Girls in true love relationships who agree to have sex are in danger of being considered 'unvirtuous' on the one hand, and of being pressurized to marry the boy with whom she is sexually involved even if she does not wish to continue the relationship on the other hand.[8] Thus girls' sexual experiences occur in an environment shaped by fear, guilt and 'dishonour'.

The gendered nature of friendships and sexual partnerships among young people and the general subordination of female sexuality have important implications for the perception and negotiation of safer-sex practices. Even abstinence on the part of young women is unlikely to safeguard them against sexually transmitted infections in the future so long as male sexuality is freely explored through multiple partnerships often involving unsafe sex. This is particularly the case when studies have shown that safe-sex practices are generally not followed, or are inconsistently adhered to by young men.

The typologies of sexual relationships and associated levels of risk perception among students described here have significant implications for the planning of sex education and sexual and reproductive health services. Programmes and services will be ineffective so long as they fail to consider the vulnerability of young people in relation to the larger social and cultural contexts in which masculine and feminine sexualities are constructed, and experienced unequally.

Notes

1 The paper focuses exclusively on heterosexual behaviour, as homosexual experiences were not explored in detail in this study.
2 In India, youth and especially college students are generally referred to as 'boys' and 'girls' and we have used these terms through out the study although some respondents were in their early twenties. The terms 'boys' and 'girls' are also used to refer to young men and women until they are married. The usage should not be considered heterosexist or patronizing.
3 Study supported by Rockefeller Foundation and the ICRW.
4 Students were informed that they were free to opt out of the research at any stage during the data collection. Some of them opted out of the FGDs, but very few opted out of individual interviews or the survey.
5 Due to caste, patriarchy and certain tendencies among lower castes in urban India to imitate some of the practices of upper castes, young peoples' sexuality norms and marriage practices are not vastly different among the various castes. Since our study focused specifically on lower socioeconomic strata students, caste and class difference in youth sexuality could not be observed.
6 In India, where premarital heterosexual relationships among young people are taboo, the only legitimate male–female relationship that is permissible is the sibling relationship. There are rituals and festivals that celebrate the brother–sister bonding through which the cultural values of incest taboo and male responsibility to protect women (including their sexual reputation) are reasserted.
7 Unlike in a Western context, most of the students in the study did not consider kissing and hugging to be sexual acts. On probing we found that kissing rarely meant deep kissing, and is often on the cheeks or the forehead.
8 The tendency to pressurize girls to marry those with whom they have had sexual intercourse is common in India. There have been newspaper reports of shocking instances where girls who are molested or raped are forced to marry the rapist. The logic is that a girl's sexuality should be linked only to her husband and not to others.

References

ABRAHAM, L. (2001) 'Redrawing the *Lakshman Rekha*: gender differences and cultural constructions in youth sexuality in urban India', *South Asia*, 24 [special issue], pp. 133–56.
—— and KUMAR, A.K. (1999) 'Sexual experiences and their correlates among college students in Mumbai city, India', *International Family Planning Perspectives*', 25, pp. 139–46.
BHENDE, A. (1994) 'A study of sexuality of adolescent girls and boys in underprivileged groups in Bombay', *The Indian Journal of Social Work*, 55, pp. 557–71.
CAPLAN, P. (1987) *The Cultural Construction of Sexuality*, London and New York: Routledge.
CHANANA, K. (2001) 'Hinduism and female sexuality: social control and education of girls in India', *Sociological Bulletin*, 50, pp. 37–63.
DAS, V. (1988) 'Femininity and the orientation to the body', in CHANANA, K. (ed.) *Socialization, Education and Women*, New Delhi: Orient Longman.
DUBE, L. (1988) 'On the construction of gender: Hindu girls in partrilineal India', in CHANANA, K. (ed.) *Socialization, Education and Women*, New Delhi: Orient Longman.

—— (1997) *Women and Kinship: Comparative Perspectives on Gender in South and South East Asia*, New York: United Nations University Press.

FAMILY PLANNING ASSOCIATION OF INDIA (n.d.) *Youth Sexuality: A Study of Knowledge, Attitudes, Beliefs and Practices among Urban Educated Indian Youth, 1993–1994*, Bombay: Family Planning Association of India and Sex Education, Counselling, Research and Training.

FOUCAULT, M. (1976) *The History of Sexuality, Vol. I*, Harmondsworth: Penguin.

—— (1977) *Power/Knowledge: Selected Interviews and Other Writings*, New York: Pantheon.

GOPARAJU, L. (1993) 'Unplanned, unsafe: male student's sexual behaviour', paper presented at the workshop on Sexual Aspects of AIDS/STD Prevention in India, Tata Institute of Social Sciences, Bombay.

HOLLAND, J., RAMAZANOGLU, C., SHARPE, S. and THOMSON, R. (1992) 'Pleasure, pressure and power: some contradictions of gendered sexuality', *Sociological Review*, 40, pp. 645–74.

—— (2000) 'Deconstructing virginity – young people's accounts of first sex', *Sexual and Relationship Therapy*, 15, pp. 221–32.

HORROCKS, R. (1997) *An Introduction to the Study of Sexuality*, London: Macmillan.

MAC AN GHAILL, M. (ed.) (1996) *Understanding Masculinities, Social Relations and Cultural Arenas*, Buckingham: Open University Press.

MURTHY, M.S.R. (1993) *Sex Awareness among Rural Girls*, New Delhi: B.R. Publishing Corporation.

PANGARE, V. (n.d.) 'Knowledge, awareness and sexual practices of rural boys and girls', from Pune District, Research and Development Unit, Karve Institute of Social Service, Pune.

RAKESH, A. (1992) *Premarital Sexual Attitudes and Behaviour among Adolescent Girls*, Jaipur: Printwell.

RAMAKRISHNA, J., KAROTT, M., MURTHY, R.S. and SRINIVAS, R. (2000) 'Experiences of sexual coercion among street boys in Bangalore', paper presented at the international conference on Adolescent Reproductive Health: Evidence and Programme Implications for South Asia, Mumbai.

RANGAIYAN, R. (1995) 'Sexuality and sexual behaviour in the age of AIDS: a study among college youth in Mumbai', doctoral dissertation, International Institute of Population Sciences, Mumbai.

RAO GUPTA, G. and WEISS, E. (1993) 'Women's lives and sex: implications for AIDS prevention', *Culture, Medicine and Psychiatry*, 17, pp. 399–412.

SACHDEV, P. (1997) 'University students in Delhi, India: their sexual knowledge, attitudes and behaviour', *Journal of Family Welfare*, 43, pp. 1–12.

THAPAN, M. (1997) 'Femininity and its discontents: woman's body in intimate relationships', in THAPAN, M. (ed.) *Embodiment: Essays on Gender and Identity*, Delhi: Oxford University Press.

VANCE, C. S. (1984) *Pleasure and Danger: Exploring Female Sexuality*, Boston, MA: Routledge and Kegan Paul.

VERMA, R.K., SUREENDER, S. and GURUSWAMY, M. (1997) 'What do school children and teachers in rural Maharashtra think of AIDS and sex?' *Health Transition Review*, 7, pp. S481–S486.

WEEKS, J. (1986) *Sexuality*, London: Tavistock.

WEISS, E., WHELAN, D. and RAO GUPTA, G. (2000) 'Gender, sexuality and HIV: making a difference in the lives of young women in developing countries', *Sexual and Relationship Therapy*, 15, pp. 233–44.

WEST, J. (1999) '(Not) Talking about sex: youth, identity and sexuality', *Sociological Review*, 47, pp. 525–47.

WIGHT, D. (1994) 'Boy's thoughts and talk about sex in a working class locality of Glasgow', *The Sociological Review*, 42, pp. 703–73.

Part 7

Sexual negotiations and transactions

20 Masculinity and urban men

Perceived scripts for courtship, romantic, and sexual interactions with women

David Wyatt Seal and Anke A. Ehrhardt
[2003]

Gagnon and Simon (1973) defined the script concept as 'the organization of mutually shared conventions that allows two or more actors to participate in a complete act involving mutual dependence'. Scripts have three major dimensions (Gagnon and Simon, 1973; Simon and Gagnon, 1986). Interpersonal scripts refer to shared expectations about the standard sequences of behaviour over a period of time. Intrapsychic scripts are the motivational elements that produce arousal or at least a commitment to a behavioural sequence and which give meaning to this behaviour. Cultural scenarios are the social norms and values that influence interpersonal and intrapsychic scripts.

Heterosexual scripts for courtship

Courtship may be defined as the process or set of behaviours that precedes and elicits sexual behaviour (Givens, 1978; Perper, 1989). Courtship moves through a series of stages from initial attraction to sexual interaction, and often is characterized by the development of affection and emotional intimacy between partners. Traditional heterosexual script theory portrays men as the initiators and women as the boundary-setters of courtship (Reiss, 1967; Peplau *et al.*, 1977; Byers, 1996). Women who initiate courtship are viewed as sexually available, whereas men who fail to pursue courtship opportunities are questioned about their masculinity and/or sexual orientation. Further, more traditional heterosexual script theory posits that men tend to pursue courtship based on a woman's potential sexual desirability, whereas women's interest in men is presumed to be a function of his perceived willingness to invest emotionally in a relationship.

Although the traditional heterosexual script theory portrays men as the initiators of courtship, some researchers have suggested that women more often than men initiate courtship through subtle, non-verbal availability cues (for example, eye contact, smile) to which men make an overt response (for example, initiate conversation, Moore, 1995; Perper, 1989). Researchers have also reported a growing acceptance of overt female-initiated courtship (Clark and Hatfield, 1989; deWeerth and Kalma, 1995), although other researchers have found that the early stages of heterosexual courtship still tend to adhere to traditional gender roles and scripts (Rose and Frieze, 1989, 1993). More traditional gender-role adherence may be particularly salient in African-American and Latino heterosexual populations (Ehrhardt *et al.*, 1992; Wyatt, 1994; Gomez and Marin, 1996; Seal *et al.*, 2000).

Men generally desire sexual intimacy earlier in courtship than women. For women, sexual intimacy tends to be constructed in terms of love and romance (Rosenthal *et al.*, 1998; Ortiz-Torres *et al.*, 2003). Sexual intimacy operates via two main discourses for men: sex as love and romance, and sex as conquest (Brooks, 1995; Rosenthal *et al.*, 1998; Seal *et al.*, 2000). Men more than women report a desire for pleasure, fun, and physical attraction as motives for sex, whereas women more than men report love, commitment, and emotional intimacy as motives for having sex (Leigh, 1989; Hynie *et al.*, 1998). These gender differences extend to motives for extra-dyadic and casual sex relationships as well (Rosenthal *et al.*, 1998).

Heterosexual scripts for sexual intercourse

As with courtship, traditional heterosexual script theory portrays men as the initiators of sexual intercourse and women as the boundary-setters (Brooks, 1995; Tiefer, 1995; Byers, 1996). Men are expected to actively initiate and pursue all sexual opportunities, whereas women are expected to delay sexual activity until emotional intimacy has been established. The traditional double standard (Reiss, 1967) posits that casual sex, sex with multiple partners, group sex, and sexual experimentation are more acceptable for men than women.

Although historical data provide extensive support for the attitudinal and behavioural existence of the traditional heterosexual script, research suggests that more egalitarian scripts are becoming normative, and that the prevailing standard sanctions sex for both genders within a steady, loving relationship (Bettor *et al.*, 1995; O'Sullivan, 1995; Byers, 1996). Researchers have also found that the initiation of sexual behaviour becomes more egalitarian as a relationship becomes more committed (O'Sullivan and Byers, 1992). Both men and women initiate sex, refuse sex, and engage in unwanted but non-coercive sexual relationships (O'Sullivan and Byers, 1992; O'Sullivan and Allgeier, 1998). This finding is particularly salient when samples are: more Caucasian, more educated, and/or have greater socioeconomic status. However, researchers report there is still a double standard outside of steady relationships, whereby it is more acceptable for men than women to have casual sex, one-night stands, secondary sexual partners, group sex, and to experiment sexually (Hatfield and Rapson, 1996; Ortiz-Torres *et al.*, 2003).

In sum, evidence supports the belief that heterosexual scripts for courtship and sexual interactions are in a state of transition in Western society (Doyle, 1995; Pleck, 1995; Levant, 1997; Schwartz and Rutter, 1998; Alexis, 1999). This creates the potential for conflict. Traditional scripts (for example, men initiate, women set boundaries) told men and women what to do. So long as the parties complied with their assigned roles, conflict was reduced. Men and women who do not ascribe to traditional roles and scripts have to create unique and untested scripts. The creation of new scripts increases the likelihood that partners will not share common expectations about the intrapsychic and interpersonal scripts guiding their shared courtship and sexual experiences. Sexual scripts are also instrumental in understanding heterosexual risk behaviour relevant within the context of HIV/AIDS and the design of relevant strategies for protective behaviours.

Study goals

In order to investigate men's perceptions of heterosexual scripts in the 1990s, we conducted semi-structured individual elicitation interviews to collect narratives from an ethnically diverse sample of inner-city men about their experiences with women related to courtship, romance, and sexual involvement (both first-time encounters with new partners and ongoing relationships). A narrative approach posits that human beings are natural storytellers, and that these stories serve to integrate people's construction of events occurring over time (Murray, 1997). The aim of narrative psychology is to explore people's stories for the insight they provide into (a) the identity of the storyteller, and (b) the culture in which the storyteller lives.

In this study, we broadly conceptualized courtship as 'approaching and becoming acquainted with women'. This contrasts with more narrow definitions that have defined courtship as behavioural interactions that precede and elicit sexual intercourse (e.g., Givens, 1978; Perper, 1989). We chose this broader definition in order to allow for courtship interactions that did not have sexual intercourse as an endpoint. We also explored men's experiences with romance as a separate set of behaviours, distinct from courtship and sexual behaviour. Past research has typically conceptualized romance as either a courtship strategy (for example, romantic seduction), a type of love (for example, romantic love), or a motive for sex (Cramer and Howitt, 1998). We analysed men's narratives for themes pertinent to the following questions:

- What are the intrapsychic scripts present in men's narratives about courtship, romance, and sexual interactions? That is, what are men's goals and motivations for becoming involved in these different types of interactions with women? We also assessed the influence of men's expectations about the likelihood of having a future interaction, a close emotional relationship, and/or a sexual relationship with their partner.
- What are the interpersonal scripts present in men's narratives about courtship, romance, and sexual interactions? Specifically, we examined men's perceptions of who initiated, who controlled the pace of, and who set the boundaries for these different interactions. We further examined the types of verbal and non-verbal availability and rejection cues that were mentioned in men's narratives.
- What are the similarities and differences in men's interpersonal and intrapsychic scripts across three different types of partners? (i) generalized partners representing men's perceptions about normative patterns of courtship, romance, and sexual interaction (in other words, how things usually happen); (ii) primary partners representing women with whom men have or have had a steady, emotionally committed relationship; and (iii) casual partners including anonymous, one-time, and secondary partners.
- How do men's interpersonal and intrapsychic scripts differ across descriptive characteristics such as age, ethnicity, and relationship status (for example, involved, uninvolved)? Researchers have noted the importance of developmental (Money and Ehrhardt, 1972; Simon *et al.*, 1992; Laumann *et al.*, 1994), dyadic (Metts and Cupach, 1989; Metts and Spitzberg, 1996), and cultural (Money and Ehrhardt, 1972; Wyatt, 1994; Seal *et al.*, 2000; Ortiz-Torres *et al.*, 2000) influences on the individual expression of interpersonal and intrapsychic scripts. Yet, most research investigating sexual scripts has involved predominantly White, middle-class, college or young married samples (Metts and Spitzberg, 1996; Ortiz-Torres *et al.*, 2000).

Method

Participants

One hundred heterosexually-active men were recruited from STD/health clinics and from social networks in inner-city neighbourhoods in New York City to participate in a qualitative individual elicitation interview, which explored their perceptions of the scripts guiding courtship, romance, and sexual interaction with women. Study participants were recruited from an area of the city with an elevated number of AIDS cases. From 1991 to 1996, there was an 18 per cent increase in the number of AIDS cases in this geographic area, and the AIDS rate among men in this area exceeded 2,000 per 100,000 adults during the study period (New York City Department of Health, 1997). Additionally, the recruitment area was characterized by increased rates of drug use and poverty, and decreased social and health services.

Table 20.1 Sample characteristics (*n* = 100)

Recruitment site:	
STD or health clinic	48%
Community group	52%
Age:	
18–23	37%
24–28	34%
29 +	29%
Race/Ethnicity:	
Black/African-American	58%
Latino	21%
White	13%
Other	8%
Country of origin:	
USA	63%
Trinidad/Jamaica	30%
Other	7%
Occupation	
Unemployed	33%
Full-time student	10%
Lower SES status	29%
Higher SES status	28%
Income ($).	
0	26%
1–10,000	15%
10,000–20,000	31%
20,001–30,000	16%
30,000 +	12%
Education:	
Less than high-school diploma	15%
High-school diploma	23%
Vocational or technical degree	12%
Some college	30%
BA/BS or higher	20%
Relationship status:	
Not currently involved in a steady relationship	32%
Unmarried, involved in a steady relationship	46%
Engaged	5%
Legal or common-law marriage	17%
Number of children:	
0	63%
1	19%
2+	18%

We recruited a predominantly blue-collar sample that was heterogeneous with respect to age, race/ethnicity, education, and income (see Table 20.1). Over three-quarters of the men were self-identified as African-American/Black or Latino. The median education was some post-high-school vocational training or college. The majority of the sample (72 per cent) had an annual income of $20,000 or less, and a third reported current unemployment. Most men were born in the USA, Trinidad or Jamaica. About two-thirds of the men were involved in some type of steady relationship. Slightly over a third of the men reported having children.

Recruitment procedures

In the STD/health clinic setting, men were individually approached in the waiting room and told about the study. Interested participants were immediately enrolled and interviewed in a private clinic room. Non-clinic participants were recruited through a key contact, who introduced the researchers to their social network (for example, a soccer team). An overview of the study was presented to the social network as a group, and individual participation was solicited. Interested participants were scheduled for an interview at a private location chosen by the participant. We used these two different strategies in order to explore their relative utility for the recruitment of heterosexual men into both sexuality- and HIV-related research. In both settings, most individuals approached were willing to participate. All participants received $10 for the interview. No individual identifiers were collected to ensure the anonymity of the participants. Interviews were audiotaped and transcribed. After transcription, the audiotapes were destroyed to further protect participants' anonymity.

Interview guide overview

The semi-structured interviews were organized around a set of general topic questions with *a priori* probes designed to obtain additional insight into men's interpersonal and intrapsychic scripts. A brief synopsis of the main topic questions is presented below.

Courtship

Tell me how you meet and get to know women … Tell me how you met and got to know your current (last steady) partner.

Romance

If you wanted to do something romantic for a woman, what would you do? … Tell me about the most romantic thing you've done for a woman (your partner)? What's the most romantic thing a woman's (your partner's) done for you?

First sex

How does sex occur for the first time? Tell me about the first time you had sex with your current (last steady) partner – what was going on, who was doing what, etc. … Tell me about any other sexual partners you've had during your current (last steady) relationship.

Ongoing sex

Tell me how sexual relationships with steady partners change over time ... Tell me about changes in your current (last steady) sexual relationship.

Interviewer training

The interviews were conducted by an ethnically diverse (Puerto Rican, Trinidadian, Caucasian) research team experienced in the administration of qualitative interviews related to sexual behaviour and HIV. All interviewers received extensive training in the interview protocol prior to conducting the fieldwork. Interviews were monitored, to ensure protocol adherence, by a senior researcher experienced with qualitative methodology. The interview team met regularly to discuss field issues and problems with protocol fidelity.

Data analysis

Transcribed elicitation interviews were analysed for emergent themes using principles of Grounded Theory Analysis (Corbin and Strauss, 1990; Strauss and Corbin, 1994). We initially examined the transcripts to identify primary coding categories as well as a range of themes present within each category. Identified coding categories and themes were organized into a formal code book, and illustrative quotes relevant to these themes were extracted from the transcripts. Next, transcripts were content coded. New themes that did not appear to fit into the original code book were discussed by the coding team and modifications were made when deemed appropriate. When suggested by associations, overlap, or diversions in the data, thematic categories were refined, merged, or subdivided.

Summaries were initially rated by at least two members of the data analytic team. Inter-rater discrepancies were discussed until consensus about the appropriate code was obtained. Decision trails were noted and documented to assure that interpretations were supported by the data (Sandelowski, 1986; Hall and Stevens, 1991). This process was repeated until the study raters consistently achieved 80 per cent or greater concordance, after which the summaries were rated by a single evaluator. Of the remaining summaries, 10 per cent were randomly selected for independent evaluation by the two raters. The overall concordance rate was 0.84 across the interviews that were evaluated by both raters. Most of the discrepancies involved the omission of a minor theme by one of the coders rather than disagreement about a major theme.

Results

We summarized the interpersonal and intrapsychic scripts that emerged in men's narratives about courtship, romance, and sexual interactions with women. Across all partner types (generalized, primary, casual), we analysed 292 courtship, 135 romance, 292 first sexual encounter, 112 ongoing sexual relationship narratives. Below, we discuss key themes identified in men's narratives.

'I want to have sex with you'

A central motivation for men's involvement in courtship, romantic, and sexual involvement with women was their desire for sexual intimacy.

The courtship game

The courtship game was portrayed as a fishing expedition whereby a man randomly approached women in hopes that one would respond: 'The guys I hang out with talk to most of the girls that pass … Sometimes the girl stops and sometimes they keep moving. It passes the time'. The purpose and a desired outcome of the courtship game was sexual conquest.

> I go to bars, just to meet a girl, settle my urges, to have that one-night stand. If I can, it [sex] happens. Casual sex to me is a game … You get yours. I get mine … You go onto the next person.

Men were not concerned about whether their advances were successful: 'You ask them to dance. If she says yes, she says yes. If she says no, she says no. There are other fish in the sea.' Men did not seek nor expect to become emotionally involved or committed with the women they pursued. Women who responded to men's overtures were seen as attractive sexual partners, but not viewed as suitable for close emotional relationships.

> I saw this one girl and I wanted to get with her … 3 days later we went out and had sex … The relationship developed into a sexual one, but nothing more. You don't want a girl that's that easy as a girlfriend.

The courtship game adhered to the traditional gender script of man as the initiator.

> Dating is all about sexual harassment – sort of pushing the limits to see how far the other person is willing to let you go. Society believes that it is the man's role to test the waters. It is certainly expected by women.

Strategies that men commonly used to initiate interaction with women in the courtship game, included small talk ('Most of the talk is just about daily events'); compliments, sweet talk, and direct come-ons ('I go over to her and tell her you're beautiful. Can I have your phone number?'); and non-verbal cues such as eye contact, smiles, or physical touch. Common rejection strategies used by women to fend off men's advances included inattention/avoidance ('Looking around a lot, giving me short replies'); and direct refusal ('I'm really not interested in you').

In the courtship game, women were characterized as adversaries to be battled and conquered. Although men typically portrayed themselves as either victorious or indifferent toward their female adversaries, some men portrayed themselves as losers in this battle: 'Most women are just gold-diggers who are scheming me. They treat relationships as a joke … They do things behind your back. They take advantage and have holds over their man.'

Romance: sexual seduction and eroticism

Men used romance to create an ambiance and mood intended to stimulate his partner's sexual desire and availability. Romance aimed at attaining sexual intimacy was typically planned out in advance and followed traditional gender scripts. These narratives included the mention of compliments, sweet talk, promises of emotional and relational commitment (regardless of truth), and generalized sexual hints. These romantic experiences were usually positive for the men, although resentment surfaced when women resisted men's seduction efforts. Such rejection often left the men feeling unappreciated and not rewarded for their efforts.

A common theme in men's romantic narratives was sexual seduction. These narratives consisted of two distinct phases – a seduction phase during which the man attempted to 'win' his partner's heart, followed by a sexual phase where the woman would make herself sexually available.

> We'd have a private dinner on deck under the moonlight with candles, flowers, and harmonious music. After dinner, we would dance. I would then take her to our room to make love to her … I'd carry her through the door, put on soft music, and drink some wine. I would tell her the things she wanted to hear [e.g., how beautiful she looks].

In other narratives, romance was directly equated with sexual eroticism. In contrast to the variations described above, these narratives did not have a distinct seduction stage. When asked about romance, one man fantasized that he would:

> … talk with his partner, play with her ear, and tell her to get into something more comfortable. If she read his meaning, she'd go wet her hair as this turns him on. She'd put on a robe. He'd enter the bedroom in a half-on robe. The lights would be off except for the glow of the stereo, which would be playing nice music. He'd pour the strawberry syrup on her and start kissing her all over, wherever she wanted to be licked, do whatever it took to get her sexually aroused, and let 'whatever happens, happen'.

Sexual gratification: conquest, competition, competence, and variety

Although not directly assessed, a pervasive theme in men's sexual narratives was the near universal rejection of public health messages promoting abstinence as a long-term sexual option: 'Abstinence is ridiculous. It's the stupidest thing I ever heard in my life. Sex is a drug. Once you've tasted it, that's it.' Men generally defined 'sex' as 'penetrative vaginal intercourse'. All other types of sexual behaviour were considered to be foreplay or enhancements of sexual variety: 'Me and my girl, we try everything. But nothing beats the original purpose, the regular thing [vaginal intercourse]. Oral sex is just foreplay.'

Consistent with the goals of the courtship game and romantic sexual seduction and eroticism, a common theme in men's sexual narratives was the portrayal of women as objects of sexual conquest: 'We have these contests like who can get the most ladies in a month … I like the challenge of that. Soon as I get what I want, I ain't interested no more.' Often men viewed their sexual conquests as proof of their own superiority over other non-conquering males: 'They [female partners] always had their boyfriends, but you know they found something in me that they liked … so I gave them what they wanted – sexual pleasure.' Some men desired sex with 'an older woman who takes care of you – builds up your ego'.

Men attached great importance to being sexually competent and virile, especially with casual sex partners.

> Casual sex is a performance thing. You're trying to show the person you have stamina, and it's more of a physical kind of act. There's so much pressure to perform sexually for the other person.

Men believed that sexually dissatisfied women would not continue to have sex with them.

> The attempt is always to make a woman scream ... to give as much an orgasm as you possibly could so that she'd come back. If you made them happy sexually they tend to come back.

Satisfying a woman's sexual desire also was deemed necessary for preserving the man's reputation as a competent lover: 'The girls, they all talk among themselves. I don't want to be known as no two-minute brother.' Men's sexual competence was also displayed in their self-described role as sexual teacher: 'Most of the time it's me teaching her. Different positions ... I just show them what to do.'

The opportunity to obtain sexual variety or sexual opportunity was another motivation for sexual conquest:

> It's another girl, another type of sexual experience ... There's much experimenting as a single young man. It's too hard to resist. I hardly know one man could tell me that they didn't have two women at one time.

Sexual conquest narratives followed traditional gender scripts of men as the initiators and women as the gatekeepers of sexual intimacy. Many men said they initiated sexual intimacy via non-verbal body contact until they received strong signals of non-proceptivity from their partner (for example, direct verbal or physical refusal):

> I don't think I ever asked a girl. I just start the process. I will start kissing and touching them [women] first, and if the girl get excited, I will take it further and further to see how far the girl lets me go before she stops ... I think it's her responsibility to let him know if she wants to [have sex] or if she doesn't.

Other men were more direct in their pursuit of sex: 'You just go and meet yourself a woman, talk to her, get to know her, manipulate her, tell her I'm horny. If you give me some, you give me some ... If you don't you don't.'

Women who quickly responded to men's sexual advances were labelled as 'easy' or a 'slut'. Although these women were sometimes valued as short-term sexual partners, they were not deemed suitable long-term relational partners.

> I don't like girls who'll sleep with you on the first date ... It would like make me think that the girl is a 'ho' or something. Although I couldn't say no [to having sex with her] 'cause every man would, I probably wouldn't bother with her too much after that.

In contrast, women who resisted men's sexual advances (that is, the 'good girls') grew in status as potential long-term emotional intimacy partners, respected for their virtue: 'Men tend to stick to the ones [women] who give them a harder challenge ... The women that are harder to get are the ones to marry and have a family with'.

'I want to have a relationship with you'

A second central motivation for men's involvement in courtship, romantic, and sexual involvement with women was their desire for emotional intimacy.

Partner-seeking courtship

Partner-seeking courtship focused on the goal of developing an emotionally committed relationship with a woman. In partner-seeking courtship, men actively sought women who they deemed suitable for a long-term relationship. As was the case with the courtship game, small talk, direct come-ons, and non-verbal cues such as eye contact were common in the initial stages of the partner-seeking courtship process. However, in contrast to the courtship game, partner-seeking courtship typically moved beyond superficial interactions to more in-depth and mutual disclosure of feelings, thoughts, and beliefs: 'It's a very close relationship and emotional. We tell each other everything. She's my friend, my pal, my buddy, my lover, my soon-to-be wife. That's it, a real friend and companion.'

A common theme in partner-seeking courtship narratives was the desire for a relationship characterized by 'trust, friendship, and open communication'. Said one man:

> Girlfriends aren't just for sex, but somebody who you can really talk to about your inner problems and they'll understand. Trust, faithfulness and an ability to talk are the most important things for a relationship.

Partner-seeking courtship that was based on mutual friendship was characterized by mutual initiation, boundary setting, and control of the pace of courtship: 'We're not trying to keep up roles ... We're letting the relationship become what it becomes and take it from there.' Some partner-seeking narratives focused on the importance of family and children, and a desire for a relationship based on the traditional gender roles of 'man as the protector and provider' and 'woman as the virtuous mother and wife'. Said one man: 'Things are the way they are supposed to be. She respects me as a man. I take care of things financially and emotionally. I'm not just a man in status and words.'

Partner-seeking courtship tended to progress slowly so that partners could 'get to know one another'. Sexual intimacy was a non-existent or secondary goal to the development of emotional intimacy and friendship: 'Sometimes you just end up being a good friend instead of a more man–woman relationship, and the person respect you more than if you just want to have sex with them.' Another man commented: 'I didn't have sex with my wife until after we were married. It would have ruined things between us if we had. She would have been like all the other women then.' The failure to develop emotional intimacy prior to having sex was viewed as a central reason that new relationships failed:

> Nowadays, everybody just hit it up [have sex] real fast. A couple of days later [after you meet her] you already sexed her. You already fucked her, and that's it. That's why relationships don't be working out.

Romance: building relationships and emotional intimacy

Emotional-intimacy romance was characterized by mutual disclosure and sharing that served to develop or extend a couple's level of emotional intimacy and relational commitment.

> Romance is a mutual state where you are feeling like you're connecting. You're being honest with each other. The person is absorbed in you and you in them as well. You can pretty much say whatever you want, you know you can talk about things.

Emotional-intimacy narratives centred on: doing formal (for example, going to a nice restaurant) and informal (for example, walking through the park) activities together, sharing (for example, talking about each other's hopes and dreams), and gift giving (for example, flowers). Often, these romantic experiences involved simple activities. One man recalled an evening where he and his partner returned from dancing to his home where they had tea and then scotch. She read to him while they were laying on the couch, which he found 'incredibly romantic'. As another man said:

> It's just caring for each other, showing how much you care. It's like the little things that count. Like sometimes in the morning you get up before she does, make her breakfast, bring her breakfast in bed.

'Making time for one another' often was mentioned as a key component of emotional-intimacy romance: 'Romance is two people being able to take themselves away from whatever it is that distracts them in their normal life and enjoying the other person's company'. Another key component of these narratives was disclosure: 'One of the most romantic things I could imagine is going to a park by the river [with my girlfriend] and talking all day about everything, anything. Serious talk, family, life, that sort of thing'. Finally, many men commented that their most romantic experiences occurred spontaneously rather than following a pre-designed script:

> It turned out to be one of those days that, for some reason, everything turned out. It wasn't anything that I planned to be that way, it just happened ... Planned romance is too much pressure. If everything has to go the right way, it doesn't seem natural to me.

Although mention of sexual behaviour (penetrative or non-penetrative) was present in about half of the emotional-intimacy narratives, this behaviour was not a central component of the romantic interaction. Rather, sexual behaviour typically was presented as a natural ending to an evening of emotional intimacy and sharing, or as an unexpected by-product of this sharing:

> Some guys think it [romance] is all about sex. It's not really about sex. You have to be friends before you get to that part ... Romance comes from the heart, discovering my partner's likes and interests, listening to her, paying attention to her.

Making love: sex as an extension of emotional intimacy

In emotional-intimacy sexual narratives, sex was portrayed as an extension of emotional intimacy and relational commitment, and was characterized by mutuality and a comfortable, relaxed sexual atmosphere.

> I think sex becomes more fun, more important when you're emotionally bonded with someone. It becomes more special. You have sex with women because you love them. You don't love someone because you have sex with them. If you could take away the sex from the relationship and everything else was the same, if the relationship would continue, then that's a long-term relationship.

Disclosure was an important part of emotional-intimacy first-sex narratives.

> Communication is one of the most powerful and intimate things human beings have. Being able to share the deepest parts of one's soul to someone you like, love, and have intimacy. It heightens everything ... There's no way you can touch that with your penis.

In emotional-intimacy narratives, men often contrasted between 'having sex' and 'making love'.

> Making love is different than just straight up and down sex. You put yourself into it, caressing her while you're doing this and make her feel good and she's making you feel good, and there's a lot of life and love there, not just sex. Sometimes you just want to feel something inside of her. You just want to share something, share your deep feelings with her. That's how you express it, through sex. That's making love.

Emotional-intimacy first sexual encounters most often were mutually or female-initiated, although women were still typically perceived as the boundary-setters. Men reported almost universal willingness to wait until they were sure that their partner was ready to have sex, and often assumed a passive role in order to 'force' their partner to clearly demonstrate her sexual interest either through direct sexual contact or verbalization of her sexual desires.

> My first time with her, I enjoyed it because I waited for her for a while. It [sex] didn't happen as soon as [I met her]. It took a while for me to get to know her, so when we did have sex, I knew it was right and she knew the time was right. So we enjoyed it better.

In contrast, men expressed ambivalence about their emotional commitment within relationships where they felt that sex might have happened too quickly.

> I wanted to see how strong, how long I would have held on before I would have experienced her. Then I'd really know that was really true love. That you can wait, until the person is ready. I would have respected her if she said 'no'. I would have waited.

In emotional-intimacy sexual narratives, men reported high expectations of future interaction and developing/maintaining a close emotional relationship with their partner. However, first sexual encounters were anticipated in only about a half of men's narratives, and men often reported that they occurred spontaneously.

> I wasn't even thinking about it [sex]. I figured we'd just stay there [at his house] for a little while and kiss a little and she'd be on her way, back home ... I began kissing her on my bed, then I took my shirt off, and began unbuttoning her pants. There was no foreplay. We just did it.

I want to share emotional and sexual passion with you

Related to, but distinct from, motivations related to men's desire for sexual and emotional intimacy were themes related to men's desire for emotional and/or sexual passion. Themes related to passion were most clearly prevalent in courtship and sexual narratives.

Emotional passion – immersion and vulnerability

Emotional-passion courtship and romance narratives were characterized by becoming emotionally immersed in one's partner and feeling of high emotional arousal and exhilaration. Passion-seeking courtship narratives were characterized by desire to experience 'love at first sight' and being 'swept off one's feet'.

> I love to go crazy just staring into a woman's eyes. The rest of the place kinda melts away and our attention's focused on us … You feel like you've known the person all your life, and you just fall madly in love.

Another man described meeting his current fiancée as 'magic'. He said they just 'met eyes at a party, walked toward each other, and began talking. It was if no one else was there … nothing else mattered … She was like a long-lost friend.'

Although men reported exhilaration at these passionate courtship experiences, they also expressed uncertainty about the long-term fate of such relationships. Men reported that sustaining the passion was emotionally draining and left them emotionally vulnerable.

> For me to have a really good emotional bonding, sexual, physical, whatever term you want to use, I got to let the macho bullshit down. I have to expose my veins, my nerve endings, so to speak … It makes you feel naked … I don't like to let a woman get to know me because I'm afraid of being hurt or feeling vulnerable, butt naked, having my nerves exposed … But it's weird … I feel like I'm in bliss. I'm so high.

Romance: mutual emotional and sexual seduction

Passion narratives also were present in some men's romance narratives and centred on mutual emotional and sexual seduction.

> Romance is more mental than sort of the physical we're going to do this and that—the art of the tease, prolonging things, building tensions. Really content with that process that's going on. Just sort of long, relatively innocent contact that just slowly builds things for a more intimate evening later.

Sexual passion: love and lust

Sexual passion narratives were characterized by spontaneity, lust, and high physical arousal. Within these narratives, sex was equally likely to be initiated by the man, the woman, or mutually, using a full array of cues to signal sexual availability and interest. Once initiated, sex was mutually desired and controlled by both partners. Although sex was usually not anticipated, men were highly responsive to their partner's availability cues and open to the sexual experience, which was typically viewed positively.

Some sexual passion narratives were characterized by the spontaneous expression of partners' emotional love for one another.

> We were just spending time together, sitting and talking about each other … The passion of the moment superimposed itself over everything else. We didn't express our desire to do that [have sex]. We just displayed all our emotions of love.

Other sexual passion narratives were characterized by a build-up of sexual desire that would lead to the passionate expression of partners' sexual lust for one another.

> From the first time I saw her, I was like damn, she beautiful and that just aroused me. My whole inside was like boiling up, a strange feeling … I knew I wanted to have sex with her from the first time I saw her. And I guess she wanted to have sex too 'cause she called me the next day and I went over and like she just jumped on me and bam, we were in passion. It was like fire. It was wonderful.

In sexual passion narratives, sex was rarely talked about. Rather, it typically started with 'a look' and 'getting down to business'.

> If we're really attracted to each other, it just happens. I don't tell her 'look, I want to make love to you'. If she's smart she'll pick it up that's what you want, that's what you're maybe looking for.

Women who initiate courtship, romance, and sex: 'I like it, but I don't'

Although the traditional script portrays men as the initiator of heterosexual courtship, romance, and sexual behaviour, many of the narratives collected in this study did not adhere to this traditional script. Below, we examine the circumstances of non-traditional narratives, as well as men's affect toward these situations.

Female-initiated courtship

Almost all of the men in the study reported that they had experienced female-initiated courtship, and most reported positive feelings about this behaviour. Men reported feeling flattered by women's advances, especially if it involved a partner that they considered suitable for a possible long-term relationship. Men also liked female-initiated courtship because it removed uncertainty about the woman's interest in them.

Ambivalence toward female-initiated courtship was generally observed in two contexts. First, some men endorsed traditional gender scripts, which posits that men should initiate courtship: 'I don't like them [women] coming up to me 'cause it seems like she's looking for it. I don't know if she's like that with everybody.' Other men expressed ambivalence toward female-initiated courtship only when it was sexual in nature. Although men were receptive to the sexual opportunity, sexually aggressive women were deemed unsuitable as potential long-term partners. One man recalled a time when a woman picked up at him in a bar while he was playing pool.

> I wasn't paying her no mind. As I bent over to make a shot, she came up behind me man, kinda touched my butt, kinda jumped me. I looked around and she tell me you have a nice butt … Later she slip me her number and say make sure you call me.

The man said he later called her and the 'conversation went to sex, your likes, your dislikes. It just took a sexual tone'. He stated that the relationship developed into a sexual one, but 'I realized that this wasn't going to materialize into anything too much. I had my views on that kinda individual.'

Female-initiated romance

Although the majority of men recalled instances of female-initiated romance, most men felt that this rarely happened. When men were asked what women did (or men would like women to do) to romance them, the most common response was 'care for me/think of me' as illustrated by this quote: 'As long as she gave me her time, that would be enough. Just spend the day with me. She doesn't have to do anything special for it'. Another man commented that he would like for 'a caring, affectionate woman to show me that she really can't live without me ... Just showing me that I love the fuck out of you. I love the hell out of you.' Men also said it 'would be great if a woman would just be aggressive in the sense of planning the evening. Just let her handle everything and be the aggressor. Offer to take you out and wine and dine you.'

Ambivalence toward female-initiated romance was more likely to be expressed when women gave men gifts or when it involved sexual seduction:

> He related an incident that he found both romantic and sexy. A woman he sometimes dated invited him upstate to her house for the weekend. When he arrived, the lights were out and wouldn't go on. He saw some candles down the hall. He says he was worried she had got into 'voodoo stuff' and hoped she hadn't killed a chicken. He said he grabbed a bat and proceeded toward the candles. When he got to the bedroom, there was sexy lingerie on the bed. He felt that was romantic.

Female-initiated sex

Although a few men were quite receptive of female-initiated sexual interactions ('I think it's appealing when a lady initiates sex. It makes you feel you got it'), the majority of men were more ambivalent about female-initiated sexual interaction.

> She asked me back to her room. We made love. It was great, but then I wondered about her. I like aggressive women, but not aggressive to the degree that the minute you meet her, she's going to jump on you like you were a whore or something.

Other men were more overt about their dislike of female-initiated sex:

> I don't like for women to initiate unless I already had sex with her. I am supposed to be the dog. I am supposed to be the one animal. The raw animal. The one girls are complaining about ... Girls who start things, I'll fuck 'em, but then I don't want nothing to do with them.

Differences across partner type, age, ethnicity, and relationship status

Courtship narratives

Courtship as a game was more common in narratives involving non-primary partners, whereas partner-seeking courtship was more common in primary partner narratives. In generalized partner narratives, sexual and emotional intimacy motives were equally present, and typically reflected individual differences in courtship motivations. We also noted differences in the degree to which men's narratives followed traditional gender scripts. Generalized courtship narratives were the most likely to reflect traditional gender scripts, whereas

egalitarian or reversed gender scripts were more common in narratives involving actual partners. Reversed gender scripts, where women took the initiative and men set the boundaries,
were particularly evident with non-primary partners.

Younger men, compared to older men, were more likely to find excitement in the courtship
game. In contrast, many older men seemed to be tired of playing the game and reported a
desire to engage in more meaningful courtship (for example, partner seeking).

> When I was younger, I wanted to experiment with lots of sex. I wasn't so much into a
> relationship. I just wanted to have sex with you. Now, I want something more; something
> long-term. Now that I'm getting older, it's more about trying to find somebody to spend
> the rest of my life with, as opposed to all that fucking and jiving.

Finally, narratives reflective of traditional gender roles of 'man as the protector and provider'
and 'woman as the virtuous mother and wife' were primarily expressed by Puerto Rican,
Trinidadian, or Jamaican participants, although it is important to note that there was wide variation in the degree to which men of these ethnic backgrounds endorsed traditional gender scripts.

Romance narratives

Men's romantic narratives rarely involved non-primary partners. Romance was seen as
something that occurred within committed relationships. Men reported that romance was
much more likely to occur during courtship or in a newer committed relationship. As relationship commitment and duration progressed, men indicated that romantic occasions were typically infrequent or non-existent. Romance was viewed as a critical component of relationship
development, but not maintenance. No notable ethnic nor age differences across romance
narratives were observed.

Sex narratives

Similar to patterns observed in men's courtship narratives, sexual gratification narratives were
more likely to involve casual partners, or appear in men's generalized partner narratives. In
contrast, emotional intimacy sexual narratives were more common in narratives involving
primary partners. Age differences were also present; younger men were more likely to report and
endorse sexual gratification interactions with women, whereas older men were more likely to
desire emotional intimacy in sexual interactions. Many of the competence/experience first-sex
narratives involved younger men with older female partners. A decrease in passion-seeking motivations was evident in both primary- and casual-partner narratives. An increase in relational-inti-
macy motivational goals was observed within primary-partner narratives. Sex within steady,
ongoing relationships was portrayed as happening much less spontaneously, and a lack of mutual
sexual desire was often noted. Sex was seen as just another part of emotional intimacy (especially
within primary-partner narratives) – something that happened in committed relationships.

> Now I'm more into love, into feeling loved and being loved, and not so much for sex. It's
> just being close to somebody and with no strings attached. Just a good, wholesome rela-
> tionship. That's what I want. Sex is not really all that important.

Within casual, ongoing relationships, sex was more likely to be motivated by sexual variety
('Maybe some guys could just have one sexual partner, but there's temptation out there … As

nature calls the man who is grazing, he is expected to have different experiences, many experiences') or sexual conquest:

> I think I will always want to have sex with more than one woman. Just for me to say it's another notch on my belt. It's just for the entertainment, not the long-term or for them to stay with me. Just because I feel it's my duty as a man to just have sex with as many women as I can.

Although men endorsed or reported secondary partners, most men rejected the notion of secondary partners for their wives or girlfriends. Stated one man, 'It would definitely cause a problem if my current girlfriend had a side partner'. Commented another man, 'The female, all she needs is just one for life'.

Discussion

A number of key themes emerged in the course of this study. First, our findings suggest that broader conceptualizations of courtship and romance, than typically found in the literature, may be warranted. In this study, we broadly conceptualized courtship as 'approaching and becoming acquainted with women', regardless of whether the courtship was motivated by sexual desires. Within this broader conceptualization, men's narratives suggested that sexual intercourse was not always a primary, or even secondary, motivation for their courtship interactions with women. In partner-seeking courtship, the primary goal was emotional intimacy. Sexual intercourse, especially if it happened too soon in the relationship, was viewed as detrimental to the development of emotional intimacy. When sex did occur, it was viewed as an extension of the couples' emotional intimacy. In passion courtship, sex often was absent in men's narratives. Rather, emotional immersion was the main motivation for courtship.

Related to this, men's narratives supported the assertion that men's romantic experiences are an interrelated, but distinct phenomenon from their courtship and sexual experiences (Cramer and Howitt, 1998). Although men purposively used romance to promote emotional and/or sexual intimacy, in other narratives, intimacy was a by-product of unplanned experiences that men found romantic. In contrast to men's courtship and sexual interactions with women, men's romance narratives revealed a more limited range of experiences, less motivational ambivalence, and less gender-role uncertainty. Romantic interactions, which were typically male-initiated and limited to primary partners, were viewed as a part of relational development but not relational maintenance, regardless of whether the goal was sexual or emotional intimacy. Thus, the allure of romance may have come from its promise of emotional and sexual intimacy without any of the restraints or negative connotations the achievement of these goals may bring (for example, commitment). Alternatively, Baumeister and Bratslavsky (1999) have suggested that passionate love is a function of changes in emotional intimacy levels; feelings of passion will be higher when intimacy rises. Perhaps, the same argument may be made for romantic feelings and behaviour.

Second, men's narratives revealed tension between their competing desire for emotional versus sexual intimacy, especially in their courtship and first-sex narratives. For example, many men reported eagerness to pursue sexual opportunities during courtship. However, women who had sex with a man early in the courtship process were considered undesirable long-term emotional intimacy partners. Conversely, men expressed respect for women who did not have sex with them right away. However, most men also reported that they would not wait indefinitely for a woman to have sex with them, and would seek secondary partners if they felt that their sexual needs were not being met. In relation to this, many men reported dissatisfaction with the endless pursuit of sexual conquest and expressed a desire for a more emotionally intimate relationship with a woman. Yet, men also described emotionally intimate relationships as scary and/or sexually limiting.

Distinct, but intertwined with both emotional and sexual-intimacy motivations, some narratives were driven by a desire for emotional and/or sexual passion. In courtship and romantic narratives, this motivation was reflected in a desire to experience love at first sight or to be swept off one's feet. In sexual narratives, this motivation was reflected in expressions of passionate love-making and physically lustful arousal. Although these characteristics were sometimes present in emotional and sexual intimacy narratives, in passion narratives, these characteristics were much more salient. Ambivalence frequently was observed in these narratives as men revelled in the excitement of emotional and sexual immersion, while fearing the feelings of vulnerability associated with these experiences.

Third, men's narratives revealed a combination of traditional and non-traditional gender-role and gender-script adherence. Most men reported experience with female-initiated courtship, and they generally reacted favourably toward this behaviour as long as it was not directly sexual in nature. Men held similar attitudes toward female-initiated romance, although they indicated that women rarely initiated romance. However, negative or ambivalent attitudes toward female-initiated sex outside the context of a committed, ongoing sexual relationship were present. There also was evidence for a continued double-standard regarding casual partners, and multiple serial or concurrent sexual partners, whereby men perceived this behaviour as more acceptable for themselves than for women.

Some men reported feeling pressured to live up to the male norm of 'men are always ready, able, and willing to have sex'; sex being defined as penetrative vaginal intercourse. A fear of impotency and an inability to sexually perform on demand were major concerns. Men further expressed concern about the adequacy of their sexual functioning and their ability to sexually satisfy their partner. A common belief was that dissatisfied female sexual partners would seek other men. In contrast, men rarely expressed concern that female partners who were emotionally dissatisfied would leave them. Related to this, some men who had tried to conform to the 'modern' gender role of the 'nice, sensitive, emotionally expressive' man reported being used by female partners or being rejected in favour of more macho males. Our findings support Pleck's (1981, 1995) 'gender role strain paradigm' that posits the constantly changing, socially constructed gender roles are impossible to satisfy, inherently dysfunctional in their expectations, and unforgiving when their rigid standards are violated.

Fourth, differences across ethnicity and age were present. With regard to ethnicity, more traditional gender-role adherence was observed among Puerto Rican, Jamaican, and Trinidadian men than among other races/ethnicities, although there were wide individual variations in this general trend. Developmental trends were also noted. Younger men placed greater emphasis on the courtship game and sexual gratification, whereas older men placed greater emphasis on partner-seeking and emotional intimacy interactions with women. Younger men often spoke of their desire to seek a range of sexual experiences before settling down to a committed partner, whereas older men often said they were tired of sexual conquests and desired a more meaningful, emotionally intimate relationship. Men who did not adhere to these developmental trends often described their behaviour in contrast to it.

In sum, our findings are consistent with the belief that men's interpersonal scripts for heterosexual courtship, romantic, and sexual interactions are in a state of transition in Western society (Doyle, 1995; Pleck, 1995; Levant, 1997; Schwartz and Rutter, 1998; Alexis, 1999). For many men in our study, this state of transition created tension in their courtship, romantic, and sexual interactions with women as they sought to fulfil their competing intrapsychic desires for emotional versus sexual intimacy, or tried to balance the allure of emotional and sexual immersion with their fears of feeling emotionally vulnerable. Similarly, men's narratives also revealed gender role and gender script uncertainty as they struggled to understand and internalize changing societal norms. Further research is needed to better understand the complex interaction between the interpersonal and intrapsychic scripts guiding heterosexual men's courtship, romantic, and sexual interactions. Future research needs to be sensitive to developmental and cultural influences on men's perceived gender roles and gender scripts. Research involving more diverse, including cross-cultural, samples is needed. Research also is needed which explores men's non-heterosexual interactions.

There is also a need to better understand similarities and differences in the way that men and women perceive their heterosexual relationships, and the ways that men's and women's perceptions interact to influence dyadic sexual decision-making, communication, negotiation, and behaviour. Research has suggested that women and men who privately endorse egalitarian roles and scripts will still behave in accordance with more traditional roles in order to conform to their perceptions of their partner's script preferences (Ortiz-Torres *et al.*, 2003; Seal *et al.*, 2000). This may be particularly true for interactions with newer or casual partners, with whom idiosyncratic interpersonal scripts have not yet become habitual, or interactions with established partners that involve transitional or novel experiences (Metts and Cupach, 1989; Metts and Spitzberg, 1996). Understanding gender differences better will enable both men and women to better communicate their respective emotional and sexual needs and fulfil those of their partners (Metts and Cupach, 1989; Campbell, 1995; Alexis, 1999; Seal *et al.*, 2000).

Finally, it has been argued that the successful transition from sex as an object to sex as a component of interpersonal intimacy requires that men move away from sex as an endpoint and toward sex as an integrated and enhancing part of a growing and changing emotionally intimate relationship (Brooks, 1995; Levant and Brooks, 1997). To successfully make this transition, men must overcome the developmental socialization norms that encourage men to seek sexual competence and identity through a variety of experiences with casual sex partners, and to seek emotional competence with non-sexual partners. In other words, new socialization norms are needed to discourage the separation of emotional and sexual intimacy. A key component of this transition is the development of an ability to engage in evaluative self-disclosure, or the sharing of personal feelings.

However, many men learn by a very young age that part of being a man is to compete and to conquer, as well as to be 'strong' and to suppress emotional expression or feelings (Campbell, 1995; Doyle, 1995). 'Real' men initiate and control heterosexual interactions, and 'real' sex is defined by penetration – a behaviour characterized by active 'doing' to another person (for example, making love, getting laid, fucking; Brooks, 1995; Campbell, 1995; Tiefer, 1995). Men also have traditionally been socialized to avoid evaluative disclosure so as not to appear weak or homosexual (Dolgin *et al.*, 1991; Campbell, 1995). Indeed, research suggests that men tend to prefer descriptive (that is, sharing of personally relevant facts) rather than evaluative (that is, sharing of emotions) self-disclosure (Dolgin *et al.*, 1991; Parker and Parrott, 1995), although recent research has suggested that this preference may be more applicable to same-gender than to opposite-gender relationships (Wagner *et al.*, 2001). Thus, it is not surprising that many men struggle in their attempts to develop and maintain egalitarian and emotionally intimate relationships with women.

This in-depth exploration of women's and men's sexual scripts also provides a 'blue print' for meaningful approaches to education and prevention messages for avoiding negative consequences of heterosexual behaviour, such as risk for HIV and other sexually transmitted diseases. We have argued elsewhere that men's heterosexuality should be a starting point for intervention development, not an afterthought (Exner *et al.*, 1999).

One limitation of this study was our recruitment of a convenience sample with limited geographic and age range. However, in contrast to most script research, we recruited a predominantly minority and blue-collar urban sample that was diverse with respect to a range of demographic characteristics. Also, although a narrative approach can be a powerful tool for eliciting information about the personal and cultural meanings of behaviour, this method may be limited by the extent to which men's stories were influenced by social desirability or self-presentation biases. These biases were occasionally evident in our data, though we note that many men disclosed potentially embarrassing or negative personal experiences suggesting that these biases were not dominant. We posit that men would be most likely to self-monitor those behaviours which they perceived to be governed by strong social norms – the identification of which was a key goal of our study. Thus, even exaggerated stories would offer insight into our questions of current sexual scripts as perceived by urban men in the US. Finally, although we have emphasized the contradictions present in men's narratives, it was not always clear to what extent the men, themselves, consciously experienced these tensions. Future research should explore the ways in which men experience and manage these competing desires on a personal level, as well as within the broader social context of their lives.

Acknowledgements

Data collection and analysis were conducted as part of the first author's postdoctoral fellowship at the HIV Center for Clinical and Behavioral Studies (NIMH center grant P50-MH43520; NRSA training grant 5T32-MH19139). Manuscript preparation was supported by NIMH center grant P30-MH52776 to the Center for AIDS Intervention Research. The authors thank the HIV Center's Psychosocial/Qualitative Core, Ed Dunne, Verron Skinner, Samantha Williams, Deborah Palmer-Seal, Lydia Leon, and all the other team members for their contributions to this project. Gratitude also goes to Chelsea STD Clinic/New York City Department of Health, and the Young Men's Health Clinic/Columbia-Presbyterian Medical Center for their assistance. Appreciation is expressed to Lucia O'Sullivan and Steven Pinkerton for their feedback and Vanessa Haney for her editorial assistance.

References

ALEXIS, E. (1999) 'Exploring a new paradigm in gender communication', *Toward a New Partnership*, 5, pp. 1–4.

BAUMEISTER, R.F. and BRATSLAVSKY, E. (1999) 'Passion, intimacy, and time: passionate love as a function of change in intimacy', *Personality and Social Psychology Review*, 3, pp. 49–67.

BETTOR, L., HENDRICK, S.S. and HENDRICK, S.S. (1995) 'Gender and sexual standards in dating relationships', *Personal Relationships*, 2, pp. 359–69.

BROOKS, G.R. (1995) *The Centerfold Syndrome: How Men Can Overcome Objectification and Achieve Intimacy with Women*, San Francisco, CA: Jossey-Bass Publishers.

BYERS, E.S. (1996) 'How well does the traditional sexual script explain sexual coercion? Review of a program of research', *Journal of Psychology and Human Sexuality*, 8, pp. 7–25.

CAMPBELL, C.A. (1995) 'Male gender roles and sexuality: implications for women's AIDS risk and prevention', *Social Science and Medicine*, 41, pp. 197–210.

CLARK, R.D. and HATFIELD, E. (1989) 'Gender differences in receptivity to sexual offers', *Journal of Psychology and Human Sexuality*, 2, pp. 39–55.

CORBIN, J. and STRAUSS, A. (1990) 'Grounded theory method: procedures, canons, and evaluative criteria', *Qualitative Sociology*, 13, pp. 3–21.

CRAMER, D. and HOWITT, D. (1998) 'Romantic love and the psychology of sexual behavior: open and closed secrets' in de Munck, V.C. (ed.) *Romantic Love and Sexual Behavior: Perspectives from the Social Sciences*, Westport, CT: Praeger Publishers-Greenwood Publishing Group, Inc.

DEWEERTH, C. and KALMA, A. (1995) 'Gender differences in awareness of courtship initiation tactics', *Sex Roles*, 32, pp. 717–34.

DOLGIN, K.G., MEYER, L. and SCHWARTZ, J. (1991) 'Effects of gender, target's gender, topic, and self-esteem on disclosure to best and middling friends', *Sex Roles*, 25, pp. 311–29.

DOYLE, J.A. (1995) *The Male Experience*, third edition, Madison, WI: Brown & Benchmark.

EHRHARDT, A.A., YINGLING, S., ZAWADZKI, R. and MARTINEZ-RAMIREZ, M. (1992) 'Prevention of heterosexual transmission of HIV: barriers for women', *Journal of Psychology and Human Sexuality*, 5, pp. 37–67.

EXNER, T.M., GARDOS, P.S., SEAL, D.W. and EHRHARDT, A.A. (1999) 'HIV sexual risk reduction interventions with heterosexual men: The forgotten group', *AIDS and Behavior*, 3, pp. 347–58.

GAGNON, J.H. and SIMON, J. (1973) *Sexual Conduct: The Social Origins of Human Sexuality*, Chicago: Aldine.

GIVENS, D.B. (1978) 'The nonverbal basis of attraction: flirtation, courtship, and seduction', *Psychiatry*, 41, pp. 346–59.

GOMEZ, C.A. and VANOSS-MARIN, C. (1996) 'Gender, culture, and power: barriers to HIV-prevention strategies for women', *The Journal of Sex Research*, 33, pp. 355–62.

HALL, J. and STEVENS, P. (1991) 'Rigor in feminist research, advances in nursing', *Science*, 13, pp. 16–29.

HATFIELD, E. and RAPSON, R.L. (1996) *Love and Sex: Cross-Cultural Perspectives*, Boston, MA: Allyn & Bacon.

HYNIE, M., LYDON, J.E., COTE, S. and WEINER, S. (1998) 'Relational sexual scripts and women's condom use: the importance of internalized norms', *The Journal of Sex Research*, 35, pp. 370–80.

LAUMANN, E.O., GAGNON, J.H., MICHAEL, R.T. and MICHAELS, S. (1994) *The Social Organization of Sexuality: Sexual Practices in the United States*, Chicago: The University of Chicago Press.

LEIGH, B.C. (1989) 'Reasons for having and avoiding sex: gender, sexual orientation, and relationship to sexual behavior', *The Journal of Sex Research*, 26, pp. 199–209.

LEVANT, R.F. (1997) 'Nonrelational sexuality in men' in LEVANT, R.F. and BROOKS, G.R. (eds) *Men and Sex: New Psychological Perspectives*, New York, John Wiley & Sons.

—— AND BROOKS, G.R. (1997) 'Men and the problem of nonrelational sex' in LEVANT, R.F. AND BROOKS, G.R. (eds) *Men and Sex: New Psychological Perspectives*, New York: John Wiley & Sons.

METTS, S. and CUPACH, W.R. (1989) 'The role of communication in human sexuality' in MCKINNEY, K. and SPRECHER, S. (eds) *Human Sexuality: The Societal and Interpersonal Context*, Norwood: Ablex Publishing Corp.

—— and SPITZBERG, B.H. (1996) 'Sexual communication in interpersonal contexts: a script-based approach', in BURLSON, B.R. (ed.) *Communication Yearbook*, 19, Thousand Oaks, CA: Sage Publications

MONEY, J. and EHRHARDT, A.A. (1972) *Man and Woman, Boy and Girl*, Baltimore, MD: Johns Hopkins University Press.

MOORE, M. (1995) 'Courtship signalling and adolescents: "Girls Just Wanna Have Fun"?', *The Journal of Sex Research*, 32, pp. 319–28.

MURRAY, M. (1997) 'A narrative approach to health psychology: background and potential', *Journal of Health Psychology*, 2, pp. 9–20.

NEW YORK CITY DEPARTMENT OF HEALTH (1997) *AIDS in boroughs and neighborhoods of New York City*, New York: Office of AIDS Surveillance, New York City Department of Health.

ORTIZ-TORRES, B., SERRANO-GARCIA, I. and TORRES-BURGOS, N. (2000) 'Subverting culture: promoting HIV/AIDS prevention among Puerto Rican and Dominican women', *American Journal of Community Psychology*, 28, pp. 859–81.

——, WILLIAMS, S.P. and EHRHARDT, A.A. (2003) 'Urban women's gender scripts: implications for HIV prevention', *Culture, Health and Sexuality*, 5, pp. 1–17.

O'SULLIVAN, L. (1995) 'Less is more: the effects of sexual experience on judgements of men's and women's personality characteristics and relationship desirability', *Sex Roles*, 33, pp. 159–81.

—— and ALLGEIER, E.R. (1998) 'Feigning sexual desire: consenting to unwanted sexual activity in heterosexual dating relationships', *The Journal of Sex Research*, 35, pp. 234–43.

—— and BYERS, E.S. (1992) 'College students' incorporation of initiator and restrictor roles in sexual dating situations', *The Journal of Sex Research*, 29, pp. 435–46.

PARKER, R. and PARROTT, R. (1995) 'Patterns of self-disclosure across social support networks: elderly, middle-aged, and young adults', *International Journal of Aging and Human Development*, 41, pp. 281–97.

PEPLAU, L.A., RUBIN, Z. and HILL, C.T. (1977) 'Sexual intimacy in dating relationships', *Journal of Social Issues*, 33, pp. 86–109.

PERPER, T. (1989) 'Theories and observations on sexual selection and female choice in human beings', *Medical Anthropology*, 11, pp. 409–54.

PLECK, J.H. (1981) *The Myth of Masculinity,* Cambridge, MA: MIT Press.

—— (1995) 'The gender role strain paradigm: an update' in LEVANT, R.F. and POLLACK, W.S. (eds) *A New Psychology of Men*, New York: Basic Books.

REISS, I. L. (1967) *The Social Context of Premarital Sexual Permissiveness*, New York: Holt, Rinehart & Winston.

ROSE, S. and FRIEZE, I. H. (1989) 'Young singles' scripts for a first date', *Gender and Society*, 3, pp. 258–68.

—— (1993) 'Young singles' contemporary dating scripts', *Sex Roles*, 28, pp. 499–509.

ROSENTHAL, D., GIVORD, S. and MOORE, S. (1998) 'Safe sex or safe love: competing discourses?' *AIDS Care*, 10, pp. 35–47.

SANDELOWSKI, M. (1986) 'The problem of rigor in qualitative research', *Advances in Nursing Science*, 8, pp. 27–37.

SCHWARTZ, P. and RUTTER, V. (1998) *The Gender of Sexuality*, Thousand Oaks, CA: Sage Publications.

SEAL, D.W., WAGNER, L.I. and EHRHARDT, A.A. (2000) 'Sex, intimacy, and HIV: an ethnographic study of a Puerto Rican social group in New York City', *Journal of Psychology and Human Sexuality*, 11, pp. 51–92.

SIMON, R.W., EDER, D. and EVANS, C. (1992) 'The development of feeling norms underlying romantic love among adolescent females', *Social Psychology Quarterly*, 55, pp. 29–46.

SIMON, W. and GAGNON, J. (1986) 'Sexual scripts: permanence and change', *Archives of Sexual Behavior*, 15, pp. 97–120.

STRAUSS, A. and CORBIN, J. (1994) 'Grounded theory methodology', in DENZIN, N.K. and LINCOLN, Y.S. (eds) *Handbook of Qualitative Research*, Thousand Oaks, CA: Sage.

TIEFER, L. (1995) *Sex is Not a Natural Act and Other Essays*, Boulder, CO: Westview Press.

WAGNER, L.I., SEAL, D.W. and EHRHARDT, A.A. (2001) 'Close emotional relationships with women versus men: a qualitative study of 56 heterosexual men living in an inner-city neighborhood', *Journal of Men's Studies*, 9, pp. 243–56.

WYATT, G. (1994) 'The sociocultural relevance of sex research', *American Psychologist*, 49, pp. 748–54.

21 Some traditional methods are more modern than others

Rhythm, withdrawal and the changing meanings of sexual intimacy in Mexican companionate marriage

Jennifer Hirsch and Constance Nathanson [2001]

B: … well, they can also take care of you.

J: How is that, that they take care of you?

B: That is, I heard about it from a friend. Really nice, we were talking about how to take care of yourself, and she says to me: 'no, he takes care of me', and … I said, 'what do you mean, he takes care of you?' She said, 'if we have sex, he feels when it is the moment when the sperm are going out, and instead of giving them to me, [he comes] outside … [and] if you do it that way, you are not the only one worrying about it, he is also worrying about it. He needs to be attentive and alert'. And it seems really nice to me, the idea that he would care about it too, and not just me.

In much research on fertility regulation, rhythm, *coitus interruptus* and a variety of other strategies for fertility regulation have been classified as 'traditional' – that is, non-technological and less effective than more recently invented methods such as the oral contraceptive pill. Imposing a traditional/modern taxonomy on these methods distracts us from the possibility that those who use them may classify these methods in other ways. This paper explores how the distinctions that married Mexican women make among various methods are shaped by broader changes in gender and marriage. Our research highlights how ideologies of sexual intimacy shape contraceptive practice, and how women deploy these culturally constructed models of sexual relations strategically, depending on the social context in which they live.

Methods

This paper presents results from an ethnographic study involving two generations of Mexican women. Data collection focused on 26 women, ages 15–50, all from the same sending community in Mexico. Half lived in Atlanta, while the other 13 (who are their sisters or sisters-in-law) were interviewed in Mexico. The women in Atlanta were selected to represent the range of diversity in Atlanta's migrant community in terms of age, legal status, English skills, reproductive and labour-force experience, and social class in Mexico. These women's mothers, who were between the ages of 45 and 70, were also interviewed,[1] as were some of their husbands. (References to 'younger women' mean the younger of the life-history informants; 'older women' refers to those life-history informants over age 40 and to their mothers.)

The sending communities were Degollado, a town about two hours from Guadalajara with a population of about 15,000, and El Fuerte, a small agricultural community outside of

Degollado. In Atlanta, some informants lived in urban neighbourhoods characterized by small apartment complexes, good public transportation and a heavy concentration of Mexican and Vietnamese immigrants, while others lived in trailer parks on the outskirts of the city.

The primary method was life-history interviews, consisting of six interviews: (1) child-hood and family life; (2) social networks and stories of US–Mexico migration; (3) gender and household division of labour; (4) menstruation, reproduction, and fertility management; (5) health, reproductive health, sexually transmitted diseases and infertility; and (6) courtship and sexuality.[2] During 15 months of participant observation in Atlanta and Mexico, the first author came to speak with many more people than the 43 people who were formally inter-viewed, and these casual conversations were key in ensuring that the words and experiences of the small sample bore some relation to those of the broader community (see Bernard, 1994). The process of constructing the sample (Hirsch and Nathanson, 1998) and the methods of data analysis[3] are described elsewhere (Hirsch, 1998).

From *respeto* to *confianza*

In their discussion of courtship and marriage, older women made frequent reference to the fulfilment of gendered obligations, describing a marital bargain (Kandiyoti, 1996) based on the ideal of separate spheres and respect for one's spouse. The ideal of female submissiveness did not mean that women exerted no control over their lives – merely that a woman tried to do so without appearing to publicly challenge her husband's will (Hirsch, 1998, n.d.a; see also Stern, 1995). In contrast to their mothers' emphasis on a gendered form of respect, *respeto*, as the key scale along which to evaluate a marriage, younger women talk more about *confianza* (which could be translated either as intimacy or trust).[4] *Confianza* implies intimacy in both sexual and non-sexual ways. When inviting guests to serve themselves, sit down, or other-wise not stand on ceremony, a host or hostess will advise them to act 'with *confianza*', and women also use the term to describe relationships in which they feel comfortable telling sexual jokes.

In these companionate marriages,[5] both men and women said that they made decisions together. For example, in response to the question 'Who gives the orders in your house?' (*quien manda en su casa?*), they each (interviewed separately) would say that they both do, or that neither one does. For an older woman to voice disagreement with her husband would have been seen as answering back, but the young couples took pride in their more 'modern' style of decision-making.[6] Second, the gendered boundaries of space between the house and the street have eroded somewhat (Gutierrez, 1991; Rouse, 1991; Gutmann, 1996; Rebhun, 1999). When asked what it meant to share *el mando*, the power to give orders, men and women frequently talked about spending time together as a couple and as a family, either at home or on family outings.

Third, both in the sending community in Mexico and in metropolitan Atlanta, there has been a generational movement towards 'helping' (*ayudando*), with tasks that these young people's parents saw as clearly gendered. Occasionally sweeping or heating his own dinner – once a source of shame for a man or a comment on his wife's inadequacy – has become a source of pride, even if it remains the exception rather than the rule. Together, these qualities combine to form a new marital ideal.[7]

The increased emphasis on emotional intimacy in these marriages – both in Atlanta and in the Mexican fieldsites – should not be mistaken for gender equality. Love may serve to blunt the edge of socially structured inequalities in power, and even give women a moral language through which to make claims about rights (for example, Mahoney, 1995), but it can also recruit women to subservient roles. This focus on emotional satisfaction may even weaken women's bargaining power, as it can be used to justify a man's desire to walk away from marriage and fatherhood the moment he finds the intimacy unsatisfying.

Although women in both the Mexican and Atlanta communities shared this ideal, the privacy, legal protections against domestic violence, and economic opportunities of life in *el norte* combine to give women more bargaining power than their sisters in Mexico (Hirsch, 1999a, n.d.a.).While women in communities on both sides of the border may share these companionate dreams, Mexicans say that in the US women give the orders. They mean by this that women have the social and economic resources to live without a husband, and thus the power to press for a marriage that is not just companionate but a bit more egalitarian.

Companionate marriage and sexual intimacy

J: And what do you see as the role of the sexual relationship in marriage? …

V: Yes, it's very important, it's half [of marriage] … The other half is getting along well, but sex is one of the most important things. For me personally, I think that the intimacy I have with [my husband] was worth a lot, to carry us through the big problems we have had. … It was the thing that really helped the most. Perhaps it wasn't so much that we cared for each other, that we loved each other, not even the kids, as it was the sexual relationship that we have.

J: And why do you think it was so important, how did that work?

V: I don't know, because we enjoy it. I see that both of us enjoy it a lot. I sometimes ask myself, does everyone enjoy it so much? I ask myself that, because I really do enjoy it. Does everyone enjoy it so much? I ask myself that, because I really do enjoy it.

(A woman in her 30s, married more than a decade, residing in Atlanta)

For the older women, the marital bargain entailed mutual respect and an exchange of a woman's best efforts at social reproduction for her husband's productive efforts. For the younger women, in contrast, marital intimacy, strengthened by exchanges of affection, serves as the foundation of a successful modern marriage. Rather than forming two absolutely distinct groups, women fall along a spectrum: at one end of the spectrum is the understanding that men and women form lasting connections through the production of children, and at the other pole lies the idea that sexual and emotional intimacy create the bonds that unite a couple. Of the 24 married life-history informants, the responses of nine were more typical of a reproductively oriented sexuality, while 15 clustered more toward the modern intimacy end of the spectrum.

To call these two complexes of ideas about sexual relationships 'constructions' makes them seem more concretely separate than they are. Women employ *both* strategies for interpreting their sexual relationships; when they talked about consent, for example, several women said in one breath that sex should be about mutual desire and pleasure, and in the next breath that you have to do your duty (*hay que cumplir*). There were also similarities among all the women: most believed that married women should enjoy sex, and almost all distinguished between decent women and women who have no shame. Younger women, though, may draw the line in a way that permits oral sex, sex with the lights on, or a little racy lingerie.

A striking difference between the two ways of understanding sexual relationships was revealed in women's responses to the question about the role of sexuality in marriage.[8]

Younger women spoke about the ways that sexual intimacy produces a stronger marriage. One woman in one of the Mexican fieldsites responded to the question about the role of sex in marriage by saying: 'Well, it's what keeps us going, no? If you feel good in terms of intimacy, you will feel good in [the rest of] your life ... because when you come – I think that when you end up happy, you get up in the morning happy, you have energy for things'. Those with a more reproductively oriented understanding of sexuality answered the same question by saying that if a man were not satisfied sexually he would look for another woman. Regardless of whether they seem to have enjoyed sex, many of the older women employ the word *usar*, to use, to describe vaginal intercourse (for example, they might say 'when he "uses" me' [*cuando el me usa*] to describe sexual relations). The younger women, in contrast, talk about 'making love' (*hacer el amor*), 'being together' (*estar juntos*) or 'having relations' (*tener relaciones*).

The older women insisted that they knew nothing about sex before marriage: 'You went in blind, because in that time there was no television, when there was no television we didn't know anything.' Their daughters, on the other hand, study sexuality intently in preparation for marriage.[9] For most of them, their wedding night is hardly their first moment of physical intimacy. Furthermore, most reported having received at least rudimentary biological information on reproduction in the final year of grade school. Their mothers prepared for marriage by learning how to cook, clean, iron and wash. Girls today learn all this but also how to be their husbands' lovers. For these young women, being an open-minded sexual partner is part of the work of intimacy. The edge of anxiety in how girls talk about preparing for marriage is quite different from their mothers' fear of the unknown; the younger generation seems to fear instead that they will not measure up, and thus that a certain amount of study and preparation is necessary.

Social changes in Mexico have promoted these new ideas about the meaning of marital sexuality. Neolocality – now possible primarily because of the migrant remittances – promotes conjugal intimacy; several couples mentioned enjoying being able to have sex without worrying about in-laws who might listen. The Mexican media, particularly since the arrival of satellite TV in the area a decade ago, is a major purveyor of information about sexuality.[10] Women also learn about sex by shopping: sexy lingerie hangs in store windows in Degollado and La Piedad (the town where people from the *rancho* go to shop), as it does in Atlanta, and women discussed both buying this lingerie themselves and receiving it from their husbands as gifts. Even in the premarital instruction that the Catholic Church requires, young couples are instructed in the importance of mutual sexual pleasure for a strong marriage. One young woman, for example, recounted being told that:

> the man is like a pickup truck, that heats up right away, and that women are like big trailer trucks that take a long time to warm up, so you need to turn them on ahead of time. I didn't understand this at the time, but now I do see that we are like that, that we do need caresses and kisses.

The changes described here reflect Mexican social processes, rather than just an adoption of typically North American modes of sexual relationships. To be sure, one of these Mexican social processes is an intense integration into US–Mexico migrant circuits, and the social, economic and cultural influence of those migrants. But the sex education, satellite antennas and lingerie that are reshaping these young women's lives are all produced in Mexico; it would be a mistake to argue, as others have (Grimes, 1998), that these changes are solely a reflection of migrant influence.

Table 21.1 Current method use among life-history informants

Women in Atlanta ID#	Women in Degollado/ El fuerte ID#
1 Rhythm	1A Currently pregnant
2 IUD	2A Surgical sterilization
3 Pills	3A *Coitus Interruptus* (CI)
4 CI & condoms, rhythm	4A CI & rhythm
5 Pills	5A Currently pregnant
6 CI	6A CI & rhythm
7 Pills	7A Surgical sterilization
8 Infertile	8A N.A. (not married)
9 Surgical sterilization	9A N.A. (not married)
10 *Depo-Provera*	10A Rhythm
11 Pills	11A Currently trying to conceive
12 Rhythm	12A CI
13 Rhythm & condoms	13A CI

Most of the women who talked about sexual intimacy were under 35 (born after 1960), and none was over 40. Although generation seemed the most marked influence on a woman's choice of sexual style, a woman's emphasis on the bonds of pleasure rather than the bonds of children also depends on her husband. For example, a woman whose husband became angry and jealous the one time she tried to initiate sex learned quickly that by showing her desire she risked losing the moral power of acting with *verguenza* (shame) without any corollary gain of intimacy through *confianza*.

Migration experience also plays a role – albeit a minor one – in women's adoption of this new set of sexual strategies. The experience of working outside the home in a factory exposed some women to a range of casual conversations about sexual variety and sexual pleasure which is rare in semi-rural Mexico. Furthermore, the woman in Atlanta who asserted that she was 'owner of her own body' said she learned that idea from a domestic violence counsellor with whom she has an ongoing telephone relationship. Both of these sexualities – the more reproductively oriented one, and the more intimacy focused one – are strategies through which women create themselves as sexual beings in response to the specific demands of marital relationships.

This is not a story about a generational shift from sexual oppression to liberation. As many have pointed out (Foucault, 1978; Gallagher and Laquer, 1987; Weeks, 1989; Giddens, 1992), modern sexuality is diffusely regulated by ideologies, discourses, and institutions which normalize certain sexual behaviours and relationships and places others in the category of transgression. That sexuality remains every bit as constructed as it was in the past becomes clear if we think about how women are rarely encouraged to explore their sexuality outside marriage, or in a way that emphasizes pure lust and passion divorced from emotion

Cultural logics of contraceptive choice

Migration-related differences

Women interviewed in Atlanta were much more likely to be using technological methods (see Table 21.1).[11] Several women in the Mexican fieldsites had tried technological methods for birth spacing, but only one had used such a method for any length of time. In contrast, seven of the 12 fertile women interviewed in Atlanta have used either pills, *Depo* or the IUD, and six of the 12 were using them currently.

Most life-history informants, whether in Mexico or Atlanta, believed that technological methods of fertility regulation were extremely dangerous. Women mentioned the possibility that an IUD might become stuck in a foetus' forehead (*encarnada*), thus causing the child to be born bearing the mark of his or her mother's recklessness in a way that cannot be hidden. Oral contraceptive pills, women said, cause the uterus to 'rot' (*pudrir*), or to become permanently incapable of accepting sperm. Intriguingly, many women said that Mexican physicians had been the ones to tell them about the dangers of the pill (see Potter, 1999). Condoms break, women say, and *Depo-Provera* causes weight gain and uncomfortably long, irregular menstrual periods.

Women in Atlanta did not deny the dangers of using technological methods, but they focused on the dangers of the ones they were not using or had not tried: women who liked the pill spoke about how sick they got when they tried *Depo*, and those who had been happy with an IUD were emphatic about the dangers of the pill. Furthermore, they referred to a risk less frequently mentioned by their sisters in Mexico: the risk of a mistimed pregnancy. As one woman in Atlanta, who went on the pill before her wedding, said:

> Pills give me a bad feeling … imagine that they made me feel bad, or that they affected me, … that I got thinner or fatter, like the experiences that I have seen. The nun told us that we should use the natural method, Billings. I was looking into it and she gave us a pamphlet that I was studying, and it seems to me like the most appropriate, the best method, but it's not secure, it's risky, and I'm not like that … [I don't menstruate] every 30 days, my cycle can get shorter, I don't know how to regulate it.

Women in Atlanta weigh the fear of contraceptive side effects against the newly perceived risk of exercising less-than-perfect control over pregnancy timing.

Women in the Mexican field sites do not choose rhythm or withdrawal because of problems with access to other methods. As is true of health care in general (Chavez *et al.*, 1992), women have better access to reproductive health care in Mexico than they do in the US (Hirsch, 1998). In Atlanta, a woman who wants to take the pill needs to find out where services are offered, make an appointment (in English), have money to pay for the office visit, bring a translator in case one is not offered, arrange for transportation, and then brave a pap smear in order to get six months to a year's worth of pills (Georgia Department of Human Resources, 1994; Sebert, 2000). If she wants to use *Depo*, she needs to do this every three months. In Degollado, in contrast, hormonal methods are available over the counter; no office visit, translator, pap smear or transportation is required. In El Fuerte, family-planning campaigns targeting rural women send health promoters door to door, offering oral contraceptive pills. Even IUDs are easier to get in the sending communities, where women do not face the barriers of language and transportation.

A key social-context-related difference is in the way the Catholic Church regulates sexuality and reproduction (both directly and indirectly) in Mexico. The Catholic Church shapes the rhythms of daily life in the Mexican fieldsites in a way that it does not in the US. On Sundays in rural Mexico excitement clusters in the plaza and the public spaces just outside the church, and most families plan their Sunday leisure activities around attending Mass. Although some Mexican women in Atlanta continue to rely on the church for spiritual and social support, Sundays in Atlanta are nothing like Sundays in Mexico. For many women, it is the only day of the week that they and their husbands do not work from dawn to dusk;

Sundays are the day for weekly food shopping and the chance for a meal in a restaurant, rather than for Mass followed by tacos in the plaza. Women who are not especially religious may have gone to church anyway in Mexico, even if only to see who had new shoes, but Atlanta offers ample other choices for entertainment.

Not attending church regularly means forgoing the weekly reminder of having to sit while others stand to take communion, perhaps the moment when women feel their transgression most acutely – and at least some who do attend Mass in the US continue to take communion even if they are using a technological method. In Degollado and El Fuerte, in contrast, women using technological methods (or men whose wives are doing so) are prohibited from taking communion. The only life-history informant in the Mexican field sites who had used a technological method had to discontinue because she and her husband had been invited to be godparents; though the priest instructed them in the rhythm method, she got pregnant almost immediately after having her IUD removed.

Women in Atlanta also have more privacy. This may be the only way in which technological methods are more 'accessible' in Atlanta: most service providers do not speak Spanish, much less know women's families, so a woman's neighbours are much less likely to know about her decision to adopt a modern method.[12] Women in Atlanta also seem to regard both their bodies and their potential fertility less as something held in joint ownership with their husbands. Women were asked if they would use a contraceptive method to which their husband objected and if they would use a method secretly. Women responded in four ways: the husband should decide; the couple *must* decide together; the couple *ought to* decide together but secret use is better than an unwanted pregnancy; or women should decide because they are the ones to suffer from high fertility. Those who said that contraceptive use should be a joint decision were split between the Mexican and US fieldsites, but all who said it should be the man's choice alone were in Mexico, while most of those (nine out of 12) who said that if push came to shove she would use a method in secret were in Atlanta. Mexican women in the US may be re-imagining their bodies and their fertility as individual property, rather than looking at them as a conjugal resource.

Traditional methods in the service of a modern marriage

In contrast, women who use rhythm and withdrawal like the way they emphasize that fertility regulation is a joint decision. The word that women use most commonly to talk about all contraception is *cuidar*, to take care of.[13] Women use the phrase *el me cuida*, he takes care of me, to refer to both *coitus interruptus* and rhythm, and 17 of the 23 fertile married women have tried being taken care of by their husbands. Their explanations of their method preference suggests that they are referring both narrowly to their joint commitment to regulating fertility and more broadly to the idea that they are being 'taken care of' by their husbands (see Santow, 1993; Schneider and Schneider, 1996). (We refer to the rhythm and withdrawal as non-technological, in contrast to 'technological methods', which includes here all of what are usually called 'modern methods'. We avoid the usual modern/traditional terminology because methods that are usually lumped together as 'traditional' differ in important ways in terms of how women use them in pursuit of modern relationships.)

Women gave three reasons for preferring non-technological methods. First, they referred to the perceived risk of infertility due to use of technological methods. Those whose husbands forbade them to use a technological method because of the danger experienced this as a tender shepherding of their shared resources.[14] Of course, women who used technological methods also referred to their side effects. That women in the US value the individual control and possibilities for sticking more closely to a specific number, while their sisters in Mexico emphasize the importance of sharing fertility-control decisions with their husbands, suggests that fertility has a slightly different value for women in the Mexican fieldsites from that in Atlanta. In the Mexican field sites, women are less worried about controlling their fertility than they are about impairing it; it is a precious resource. In Atlanta, women have resources other than fertility, and it is less clear that fertility is as much of a resource as it would be in Mexico: they are isolated from their extended families and (at least for some of them) trying to coordinate fulltime work in the formal sector with child care and other domestic responsibilities.

Second, women want to use a method that is not a mortal sin. All of the women – both those who use or have used non-technological methods and those who rely on the pill, the IUD, *Depo* or condoms – acknowledge the theological superiority of non-technological methods. Women fear that by using a technological method they will provoke divine wrath through the hubris of trying to have too much control over fertility. Women see the possibility of side effects in moral as well as physiological terms; any physical discomfort or resulting infertility that might occur as a result of using a prohibited method could very well be read as divine punishment. The inefficiency of technological methods means that women are not reneging on their promise to accept all the children that God sends, but only making it a little more difficult to receive them. The technical failure rate of these methods, in other words, contributes to their appeal.

In addition to the health and the moral risk of technological methods, women see a kind of *marital* risk – that is, the risk that women who are socially and economically dependent on their husbands feel they would be taking by claiming fertility as an individual, as opposed to a jointly held, domain. These methods resonate with the way sexuality within companionate marriage has been redefined as a crucial element of the conjugal bond. When a woman's husband 'takes care of her', she experiences in an intensely physical way her husband's commitment to developing a shared, non-reproductive sexuality. These methods depend on cooperation and communication, so a woman is protected from the accusation that she is depriving her husband of a child he desires: as one woman said, 'like that, he does not say to you, "why don't you want any more kids", you are not fighting with him'. The physical restraint of desire becomes a private performance of the shared goal of having a more modern family.

Some traditional methods are more 'modern' than others

Women refer to rhythm and withdrawal the same way – as being taken care of – but of the 11 using non-technological methods, four strongly preferred *coitus interruptus* (CI), while seven favoured rhythm. Among those who prefer rhythm, most abstain completely during the fertile days in the middle of their menstrual cycle, while a few of the couples use CI or condoms during that time. Some couples abstained for up to six days on either side of the estimated day of ovulation, while others only did for three days. For all of them this was in addition to the other monthly period of abstinence during menstruation. Women who favour rhythm say that sex with condoms and withdrawal is not as satisfying, but they also say that only using rhythm is impossible. As one woman said, neither she nor her husband could hold out for this additional week: 'how could I stand it?' (*como me voy a aguantar?*) she asked, laughing.

Withdrawal means a woman never has to say no to her husband; in contrast, those who use rhythm organize their sexual intimacy around a shared ability to restrain desire. This latter choice implies that for somewhere between one and two out of every four weeks, men and women will be able to dominate their sexual urges. Those who prefer rhythm tend to place a premium on the quality of sex, on the idea that both partners must be physically satisfied, rather than on the frequency of sex. As one said, 'once a drop or two has come out of him, who would want to miss the best part?'(*ya con un chorrito que se le sale, quien va a querer perderse lo mejor?*). As another said: 'Look, talking frankly, I don't like withdrawal, because you end up halfway there (*se queda uno a medias*), and they can maybe come but what about you?' Others talked more about their husband's dissatisfaction with the method, or said that men did not have the self-control: 'Do you think that right then, in the middle of things, that they'll pull out? Well, no – what's the whole point?'

Those who preferred withdrawal agreed that neither men nor women experienced the same degree of sexual satisfaction as when the man ejaculates inside the woman's vagina – nor did they even argue very strongly for the method's efficacy. As one woman said:

> These ways that he takes care of me, we've been doing it since the first, and now I have seven, and if he keeps taking care of me like that I'll end up with 12 ... I think it's hard for them, because it's the time when they are most excited, ... so sometimes they slip up ... It's just when it feels the best for them, and even for you.

Withdrawal users spoke proudly of their husbands' sacrifice. In the words of one: 'They say that they do not enjoy it as much as with nothing – so then let them not enjoy it. Supposedly they do not feel the same ... but let them take care of it'. Another talked about how she liked feeling that he put her welfare before his own pleasure: 'I feel that he is very responsible ... Many men do not want to take precautions this way because they do not get the same satisfaction or something, and well, you don't either, but life is not all about pleasure' (*pero no toda la vida es gozar*).

Compared to those women who liked rhythm, the four who preferred withdrawal had marriages that were much more focused on *respeto* and less on *confianza*. They said that this method was their husband's choice, and this deference to men's decision-making was emblematic of their more hierarchical marital style. Three said they had been forced to have sex, and none seemed overly enthusiastic about their sexual relationship. Their discussion of withdrawal therefore draws on *some* of the ideas in the discourse of companionate marriage, such as the value of non-procreative sexuality to strengthen the marital tie. However, ultimately it seems that sexual satisfaction is just one more of the services a dutiful wife must provide her husband.

In contrast, rhythm-users were building more egalitarian relationships. They spoke about the importance of their own pleasure, both in explaining their preference for rhythm over withdrawal and in describing the difficulty of enduring abstinence. They were more likely than users of withdrawal to speak their minds, and to have husbands who would listen. *Coitus interruptus*, which allows men constant sexual access to their wives while complicating mutual sexual satisfaction, is much more 'traditional'. Rhythm, which teaches men and women to force their bodies to wait for sex but then values pleasure over self-control during actual intercourse, is a traditional way of expressing modern ideas about sexuality and marriage.

All of these younger women spoke about the importance of sexual and emotional intimacy in marriage, and they all interpreted their contraceptive choices within this discourse of marriage, pleasure and intimacy. However, social context – especially the role of the Mexican Catholic Church in regulating sexuality and reproduction, and the increased privacy and autonomy that characterize migrant women's lives – was critically important in leading some women, but not others, to express their desire for companionate marriage and modern sexual intimacy through the use of technological methods.

Conclusions

Our research highlights the way that the most normalized category of sexual behaviour – married sexuality – is produced by specific historical circumstances. Looking back on over two decades of studies on the social history and anthropology of sexuality, the vast majority have focused our gaze on marginal sexualities. People may think of married sex as so normal – or so boring – as to be invisible and irrelevant, but refusing to turn our critical energies towards heterosexuality means naturalizing it in ways that are politically problematic. There is also an urgent public health reason to learn more about marital sexuality: around the world, most women's greatest risk of becoming infected with HIV comes from having sex with a husband or long-term partner. It will not be possible to build gender-sensitive, culturally appropriate prevention programmes until we know more about the meanings of married sex.

We hope to have demonstrated through the arguments above that younger Mexican couples understand sexual intimacy as a key route to building *confianza*. Women in this transnational community are imagining families united by bonds of love and they are building those families in ways that make room for the conjugal intimacy that nourishes those bonds. This generational transformation, however, is marked by the differences between the social settings. Mexican women in Atlanta were more likely to try to use a technological method for birth spacing and to understand their reproductive potential as subject to their own individual will. The comparison group in Mexico was less committed to a firm separation of sexual intimacy from reproduction and more invested in emphasizing the shared control of fertility. Both approaches to building a marriage and a family fit squarely within the discourse of the Mexican companionate marriage, but at the same time they show how women highlight those aspects of the discourse most useful to them, given their circumstances and resources.

Our research has implications beyond explaining the specific patterns found in these communities. Over the past decade, anthropologists have argued persuasively that in order to understand fertility trends and differentials we must begin by 'situating fertility' (for example, Bledsoe *et al.*, 1994; Greenhalgh, 1995; Kertzer and Fricke, 1997). Absent from even these finely detailed explorations of the local meanings of reproduction, however, is much acknowledgment of the fact that when women and men make choices and strategize about fertility, they are also having sex – frequently messy, sometimes passionate, occasionally forced, but always a physical and emotional experience of some immediacy. Sexuality is usually invoked to explain patterns that are seen as problematic – for example, the reluctance of men to use condoms is often described as due to some local cultural construction of sexuality. We argue here that sexuality deserves a much more central role in our analyses of contraceptive behaviour. Sexuality is clearly not the only factor that influences method choice – obviously, political-economic factors (such as access to health insurance and medical facilities) play a part, as do broader structures of gender inequality. But to understand why some traditional methods are more modern than others, or why Blanca in Atlanta uses the pill while her sister Beatriz in Degollado prefers rhythm, we need to remember that fertility goals are interwoven with other short- and long-term objectives: individual and mutual pleasure, the strengthening of intimate relationships, and the construction of a modern self.

Acknowledgements

This study was conducted while the first author was a doctoral student at Johns Hopkins University in the Departments of Population Dynamics and Anthropology. It was supported by the Andrew Mellon Foundation, through a grant to the department of Population Dynamics, and by fellowships from the National Science Foundation Program in Cultural Anthropology (SBR9510069) and the International Migration Program at the Social Science Research Council. The first author also acknowledges support from the AIDS International Training and Research Program at the Rollins School of Public Health, which is funded by a grant from the Fogarty International Center at the National Institutes of Health (1 D43 TW0104202).

Previous versions of this paper were presented by the first author at the 1999 Annual Meeting of the Population Association of America, the 1999 IUSSP meeting, 'Social Categories in Population Studies' in Cairo, and at a seminar at the University of North Carolina's Population Center in February of 2001. For thoughtful comments along the way, we thank Gigi Santow, Bill Hanks, Simon Szreter, Susan Greenhalgh, Gillian Feeley-Harnik, Peggy Bentley, Ivonne Szasz, Arthur Murphy and Tom Fricke. Our deepest debt is to the women and men who opened their homes and their hearts throughout the course of this study; we cannot acknowledge them by name, but we hope at least to have been true to their stories

Notes

1 Many others have discussed the value of an ethnographic approach to these questions of local meaning and cultural context (see Greenhalgh, 1990, 1995; Kertzer and Fricke, 1997).

2 The classic life-history method focuses only on one person (for example, Mintz, 1960; Shostack, 1981; Behar, 1993). This modified method, which combines a focus on a small number of people with much wider interviewing, shows members of a society as real people struggling to find satisfaction in their lives, but the larger sample allays some concerns about generalizability.

3 The data consist of over 4000 pages of narrative text from the transcribed interviews and fieldnotes. Data were analysed using hierarchical coding in order to highlight social and cultural factors shaping reproductive health practices (see Hirsch [1998] and Miles and Huberman [1994]).

4 For a more complete discussion of the transition from *respeto* to *confianza*, see Hirsch 1999b and Hirsch n.d.a, n.d.b.

5 The study from which this paper is developed explores the literature on companionate marriage (for example, Simmons, 1973; Trimberger, 1983; Gordon, 1990; Giddens, 1992) in greater depth (see Hirsch 1998, n.d.a).

6 All of those interviewed may have been trying deliberately to create an impression by answering questions a certain way, but older men strove to prove that they exercised control over their wives and were the last word on all matters, while younger men made of point talking about joint decision-making and domestic cooperation.

7 It is problematic to infer cohort change from cross-sectional data, but other ethnographic research has noted these same changes in gender and sexuality in Mexico (for example, Amuchastegui 1996, 2000). Our claims are also supported by participant observation, analysis of the narratives that shape women's courtship stories, corroborating evidence of these social transformations (such as rising rates of education, later age at first union, declining fertility and overall increases in longevity), and the fact that some of the couples who had these more companionate ideals had been married for a relatively long time, so presumably the honeymoon was over.

8 Cohort differences emerged as well in their responses to questions about initiating and refusing sex, pleasure, sexual activities other than vaginal intercourse, and styles of communication between spouses.

9 This is reflected in the relatively new practice, in the Mexican fieldsites, of bridal showers for young women. At these bridal showers, unmarried women play games that reflect some knowledge of – and enormous interest in – sexual relations.

10 For example, the June 1997 issue of *Men's Health/Hombre Saludable*, a men's magazine sold on newsstands throughout Mexico, carried an article titled '*Satisfacción Sexual Garantizada*',

purporting to tell men how to keep their sexual partner happy. The masthead includes a sexologist among the permanent editorial staff, and nearly every issue features some similar article about sexual 'success'.

11 The National Survey of Family Growth and the Mexican Consejo Nacional de Población (CONAPO) show that 12.3 per cent of women in Mexico report using 'traditional methods', while only 3.7 per cent of Hispanic women in the US report using periodic abstinence (Peterson, 1995; CONAPO, 1999). Even if this 3.7 per cent is combined with those classified by the NSFG as using a non-specified method ('other') on the assumption that 'other' means withdrawal, this would still mean that the total use of 'traditional' methods among Hispanic women in the US is 8.8 per cent, much less than the 12.3 per cent in Mexico. (There are a number of problems with the comparison; Hispanic women include women who are not of Mexican origin at all, as well as those who are second generation and exclude women whose fathers but not mothers are of Hispanic origin.) Our emphasis on the symbolic importance of non-technological methods needs to be seen in the context of the striking rise in overall method use and the relative decline in reliance on non-technological methods in Mexico: more than 65 per cent of contraceptive users in Mexico rely on either the IUD or sterilization. From 1976 to 1997, the percentage of women in union ages 15–49 using any method rose from 30.2 per cent to 68.5 per cent, and the percentage of users who rely on traditional methods declined from 23.3 per cent to 12.3 per cent (CONAPO, 1999).

12 Women with limited English skills sometimes need to call on a neighbour or friend to help them get to a clinic or to translate for them, and this certainly can compromise their privacy.

13 *Cuidar* refers not just to fertility regulation but also to many of the same things that 'taking care of' refers to in English – that is, *cuidar niños* means to take care of children, and *cuidado!* means 'be careful!'. The verb can be used either reflexively, as in *yo me cuido*, 'I am taking care of myself', or transitively, as in *el me cuida*, 'he takes care of me'.

14 The fact that the women themselves seemed to have experienced their husband's preferences as an expression of caring rather than of control should alert us to the culture-bound nature of the assumption (almost universally made by family-planning programmes) that 'female-controlled' methods are automatically empowering to women. In situations such as the one described here, women may feel that marital fertility is an important resource precisely because of men's investment in it, and thus that there are real benefits to using a method that is not female controlled (see also Luker, 1975 and Nathanson, 1991).

References

AMUCHASTEGUI, A. (1996) 'El Significado de la virginidad y la iniciación sexual: un relato de investigación' in SZASZ AND LERNER, S. (eds) *Para Comprender la Subjetividad: Investigación Cualitativa en Salud Reproductiva y Sexualidad*, Mexico City, Mexico, Centro de Estudios Demograficos y de Desarrollo Urbano.
—— (2000) *Virginidad E Iniciación Sexual: Experiencias y Significados*, Mexico City: Population Council/Edamex.
BEHAR, R. (1993) *Translated Woman: Crossing the Border with Esperanza's Story*, Boston, MA: Beacon Press.
BERNARD, H.R. (1994) *Research Methods in Cultural Anthropology: Qualitative and Quantitative Approaches*, second edition, Newbury Park, CA: Sage.
BLEDSOE, C.H., HILL, A., D'ALLESSANDRO, U. and LANGEROCK, P. (1994) 'Constructing natural fertility: the use of Western contraceptive technologies in rural Gambia', *Population and Development Review*, 20, pp. 81–113.
CHAVEZ, L.R., FLORES, E.T. and LOPEZ-GARZA, M. (1992) 'Undocumented Latin American immigrants and US health services: an approach to a political economy of utilization', *Medical Anthropology Quarterly*, 6, pp. 6–26.
CONSEJO NACIONAL DE POBLACIÓN (CONAPO) (1999) 'Veinticinco Años de Planificación Familiar en Mexico'. Available at: www.con apo.gob.mx
FOUCAULT, M. (1978) *The History of Sexuality: Vol. 1, An Introduction*, New York: Random House.
GALLAGHER, C. and LAQUER, T. (eds) (1987) *The Making of the Modern Body: Sexuality and Society in the Nineteenth Century*, Berkeley: University of California Press.

GEORGIA DEPARTMENT OF HUMAN RESOURCES, DIVISION OF PUBLIC HEALTH (1994) *Access to Health Care by Limited English Proficient Populations in Georgia: A Report of the Bilingual Health Initiative Task Force*, Atlanta: Georgia Department of Human Resources.

GIDDENS, A. (1992) *The Transformation of Intimacy: Sexuality, Love, and Eroticism in Modern Societies*, Stanford, CA: Stanford University Press.

GORDON, L. (1990) *Woman's Body, Woman's Right: Birth Control in America*, revised edition, New York: Penguin Books.

GREENHALGH, S. (1990) 'Toward a political economy of fertility: anthropological contributions', *Population and Development Review*, 16, pp. 85–106.

—— (ed.) (1995) *Situating Fertility: Anthropology and Demographic Inquiry*, New York: Cambridge University Press.

GRIMES, K.M. (1998) *Crossing Borders: Changing Social Identities in Southern Mexico*, Tucson: University of Arizona Press.

GUTIERREZ, R. (1991) *When Jesus Came, the Corn Mothers Went Away: Marriage, Sexuality, and Power in New Mexico, 1500–1846*, Stanford, CA: Stanford University Press.

GUTMANN, M.C. (1996) *The Meanings of Macho: Being a Man in Mexico City*, Berkeley: University of California Press.

HIRSCH, J.S. (1998) 'Migration, modernity and Mexican marriage: a comparative study of gender, sexuality and reproductive health in a transnational community', unpublished doctoral dissertation, Baltimore, MD: Johns Hopkins University.

—— (1999a) *'En El Norte La Mujer Manda*: gender, generation and geography in a Mexican transnational community', *American Behavioural Scientist*, 42, pp.1332–49.

—— (1999b) '"Men go as far as women let them": courtship, intimacy, and the Mexican companionate marriage', unpublished paper presented at the 1999 meeting of the American Anthropological Association, Chicago, Illinois, November.

—— (n.d.a) *A Courtship After Marriage: Gender, Sexuality and Love in a Mexican Migrant Community*, Berkeley: University of California Press.

—— (n.d.b) *'"Un Noviazgo Despues de Ser Casados"'*: companionate marriage, sexual intimacy and fertility regulation in modern Mexico' in SZRETER, S., DHARMALINGAM, A. and SHOLKAMY, H. (eds) *Qualitative Demography: Categories and Contexts in Population Studies*, Oxford: Oxford University Press.

—— and NATHANSON, C.A. (1998) 'Demografía informal: cómo utilizar las redes sociales para construir una muestra etnográfica de mujeres mexicanas en ambos lados de la frontera', *Estudios Demográficos de Desarollo Urbano*, 12, pp.177–99.

KANDIYOTI, D. (1996) 'The paradoxes of masculinity: some thoughts on segregated societies' in CORNWALL, A. and LINDISFARNE, N. (eds) *Dislocating Masculinity: Comparative Ethnographies*, London and New York: Routledge.

KERTZER, D. and FRICKE, T. (1997) *Anthropological Demography: Toward a New Synthesis*, Chicago: University of Chicago Press.

LAQUER, T. (1987) 'Orgasm, generation, and the politics of reproductive biology' in GALLAGHER, C. and LAQUER, T. (eds) *The Making of the Modern Body: Sexuality and Society in the Nineteenth Century*, Berkeley: University of California Press.

LUKER, K. (1975) *Taking Chances: Abortion and the Decision not to Contracept*, Berkeley: University of California Press.

MAHONEY, R. (1995) *Kidding Ourselves: Babies, Breadwinning, and Bargaining Power*, New York: Basic Books.

MILES, M.B. and HUBERMAN, A.M. (1994) *Qualitative Data Analysis: An Expanded Sourcebook*, Newbury Park, CA: Sage.

MINTZ, S. (1960) *Worker in the Cane: A Puerto Rican Life History*, New York: Norton.

NATHANSON, C. (1991) *Dangerous Passage: The Social Control of Sexuality in Women's Adolescence*, Philadelphia, PA: Temple University Press.

PETERSON, L.S. (1995) *Contraceptive Use in the United States, 1982–90*, Hyattsville, MD: Vital and Health Statistics, National Centre for Health Statistics, Centres for Disease Control and Prevention, United States Department of Health and Human Services.

POTTER, J.E. (1999) 'The persistence of outmoded contraceptive regimes', *Population and Development Review*, 25, pp. 703–40.

REBHUN, L.A. (1999) *The Heart is Unknown Country*, Stanford, CA: Stanford University Press.

ROUSE, R. (1991) 'Mexican migration and the social space of postmodernism', *Diaspora*, 1, pp. 8–23.

SANTOW, G. (1993) 'Coitus interruptus in the twentieth century', *Population and Development Review*, 19, pp. 767–92.

SCHNEIDER, J. and SCHNEIDER, P. (1996) *Festival of the Poor: Fertility Decline and the Ideology of Class in Sicily, 1860–1980*, Tucson: University of Arizona Press.

SEBERT, A. (2000) 'Needs assessment for Latina reproductive health', student internship project, Department of International Health, Emory University, summer.

SHOSTACK, M. (1981) *Nisa: The Life and Words of a !Kung Woman*, Cambridge: Harvard University Press.

SIMMONS, C. (1973) 'Companionate marriage and the lesbian threat', *Frontiers*, 4, pp. 54–9.

STERN, S.J. (1995) *The Secret History of Gender: Women, Men and Power in Late Colonial Mexico*, Chapel Hill: University of North Carolina Press.

TRIMBERGER, E. (1983) 'Feminism, men, and modern love: Greenwich Village, 1900–1925', in SNITOW, A., STANSELL, C. and THOMPSON, S. (eds) *Powers of Desire: The Politics of Sexuality*, New York: Monthly Review Press.

WEEKS, J. (1989) *Sex Politics and Society: The Regulation of Sexuality Since 1800*, London: Longman.

22 Mobility, sexual networks and exchange among *bodabodamen* in Southwest Uganda

Stella Nyanzi, Barbara Nyanzi, Bessie Kalina and Robert Pool
[2004]

Studies reveal that physical mobility is a key factor that influences the prevalence of HIV/ AIDS (Hunt, 1989; Paul, 2000). Research demonstrates that in parts of Africa areas with high migration are more likely to record higher HIV infection rates than areas where migration is less extensive (Kane *et al.*, 1993; Kintu *et al.*, 2000). To date, however, research on the link between mobility and HIV/AIDS in sub-Saharan Africa tends to have focused on specific high-risk mobile or migrant groups (Cohen and Trussell, 1996). Studies carried out in East and Southern Africa to investigate this relationship focus on truck drivers, soldiers, refugees, miners and sex workers (SWs). Most are epidemiological in character and only a few have tackled the social dimensions of risk and vulnerability (Gysels, 2001). Migration studies also tend to emphasize cross-boundary migration (UNAIDS, 2000) as opposed to internal migration. We therefore chose to study commercial motorbike-taxi riders, locally known as *bodabodamen*, because they are an indigenous employment group that is highly mobile but has not been studied before. This paper discusses the mobility and migration patterns, and describes the sexual networks and exchange dynamics in sexual relationships, among *bodabodamen* in south-western Uganda.

Methods

A socio-environmental approach was adopted centring on intra- and inter-rural–urban mobility and migration; mobile employment and populations in social interaction with *bodabodamen*; sexuality, sex work and sexually transmitted diseases – with a particular focus on HIV/AIDS. Triangulation between qualitative and quantitative methods provided a check on validity and reliability of data.

Study design

The study was organized in three phases. First, a pilot study was conducted to explore the feasibility of a full study, to pre-test research instruments and to assess the study population's specific needs. Next, we undertook exploratory research. Finally, we held interactive work-shops to address participants' felt and expressed needs identified in the above two phases of work. Ethical clearance was obtained from the Science and Ethics Committee of the Uganda Virus Research Institute. After an explanation about the study, *bodabodamen* were free to either refuse or participate in the study. Participants also had the choice of withdrawing their participation at any time, with or without explaining their reasons.

Study sites

The study was located in two sites: Nyendo and the urban core of Masaka Municipality, in Masaka district, south-western Uganda. Work took place over a two-year period between 2000 and 2001. Nyendo is a peri-urban area located along the East and Central African coastal, highway hinterland, with several over-crowded slum dwellings, shanty structures, a relatively flourishing economic centre and a buoyant night-life. Four main roads and several feeder roads from rural centres meet in Nyendo. Masaka Municipality is a peri-urban setting containing the administrative organs of the district. With a relatively good infrastructure, Masaka Municipality shelters the social elite, several government offices and non-governmental organizations.

Sampling methods

The sampling frame comprised all the busiest *bodaboda* stages: four stages in Nyendo and five in Masaka Municipality. Criteria for selecting participants were based on availability and willingness to participate in the study. In all, 221 *bodabodamen* (87 Nyendo, 134 Masaka Municipality) responded to a questionnaire. For subsequent focus-group discussions, the sample was stratified to represent the *bodaboda* categories of self-employed, employed and *kibaluwa* (men who rent a motorbike on hourly basis).

Recruitment into in-depth individual interviews was based on random sampling from the initial 221 participants. Ten case studies were purposively selected because their life histories provided rich narratives illustrating the contextual variety embedded within this one employment group.

Data collection

All data were collected in the local language – Luganda – by highly trained and experienced interviewers, at a privately arranged venue to facilitate freedom of expression and confidentiality. Field notes covering all observations were recorded and discussed in debriefing sessions. Fourteen focus group discussions were held with 148 participants, to explore topics arising from the questionnaire. As a data-collection technique, focus-group discussions are well suited to the south-western Uganda context. While capable of generating extensive data in a group setting (Morgan, 1993), they also maintain cultural sensitivity. Most participants were from the Baganda tribe, whose traditional culture is oral based and community focussed. Discussions stratified by sex are important avenues for reinforcing group identification and social cohesion (Roscoe, 1965).

A select group of 40 men (20 from each location) were subsequently invited to attend in-depth interviews in which themes that emerged in the course of focus-group discussions were further investigated on an individual basis. Ten of these men were selected as in-depth case study follow-up.

Workshops

We conducted two workshops based on the felt needs of participants, expressed during the previous data collection stages. Activities included dissemination of information, the distribution of condoms, and the provision of voluntary counselling and testing. Information provided covered a wide range of topics including condom use (with demonstrations), family planning, sexual health, common diseases in the area, fidelity in sexual relationships, and sexually transmitted diseases including HIV/AIDS.

Data analysis

Qualitative data were recorded on audio-tape, transcribed verbatim, and translated from Luganda into English. Field notes and transcribed texts were analysed using Atlas.ti (Scientific Software Development, Berlin) a software program based on the grounded theory approach (Strauss and Corbin, 1998). Quantitative data were analysed using EPI Info 6 (Epidemiology Program Office CDC, Atlanta).

Results

The mean age of the participants was 23 (range 17–40) years. Predominant ethnic groups were the Baganda (76 per cent), Banyankore (8 per cent) and Nyarwanda (5 per cent). Catholics were the major religious denomination (56 per cent), followed by the Muslims (31 per cent) and the Protestants (10 per cent). Education levels were mostly low with 69 per cent of men having attended only primary school, 28 per cent attaining some 'O' level education, and only three participants with post-O-level training. Most men (79 per cent) had *bodaboda* employment as their only source of income, while 21 per cent had other jobs including digging, animal husbandry, tailoring, bricklaying qualifications and petty trade.

Mobility, migration and sexual activity

Bodabodamen are a highly mobile employment group. The four major categories of people mentioned as their most frequent passengers were workers, traders, students and people commuting to and from hospital.

The prevailing socio-economic climate in Masaka district contributes to the high demand for *bodaboda* services. Employment opportunities and viable commercial activities are clustered in the urban settings and trading centres. Therefore, people travel daily from the rural areas where they have their homes, into the towns to earn a living. Then they travel back into the villages in the evenings.

Similar to the workers, many students in the villages daily attend school in the towns. Patients and their care-takers are often ferried from the villages into the towns to attend missionary or government hospitals. *Bodabodas* are the most viable transport option for many of these people. Peaks in mobility correspond to increased financial, commercial or socio-economic activity in the area including seasonal agricultural fairs, weekly mobile markets, disco nights, seasonal sports events, start and end of academic terms, salary week, festive seasons including Christmas, Eid and some national public holidays. To meet the rise in the demand for *bodaboda* services, a category of *bodabodamen* known as *kibaluwa* (already mentioned above), rent motorbikes. These work in the hours when the motorbike would otherwise not be used, mostly overnight and/or at dawn.

The weak infrastructure, specifically the road network, is also contributory to the high mobility of *bodabodamen*. Masaka district contains 651 kilometres of tarmac road, and 1435 kilometres of murrum road. In individual interviews, *bodabodamen* complained about the bad conditions of the roads, particularly potholes, 'dust in the dry seasons', 'slippery mud in the rainy season', and 'no signs or marks showing you what is on the roads', 'no lights at night'. However, even with all these unfavourable conditions, *bodabodas* were deemed a better mode of transport because 'unlike the taxis, big buses or motorcars, a *bodaboda* can manoeuvre its way around the potholes' and also 'ride along the narrow paths without any difficulty'.

The participants said that preference of *bodabodas* to taxis has grown dramatically over the years particularly because they are cheaper. Their fuel consumption is much less. They are also less taxing and faster than bicycles. Furthermore, although *bodabodamen* work from particular stages, they are not restricted to one travel-route like taxis and buses. They travel to any place at any time, including the night. *Bodaboda* charges are negotiable. Other vehicles (apart from special hire services) travel to only particular destinations at fixed times and for fixed fares. Motorbikes take passengers to the doorstep of their destination whether it is rural or urban, unlike taxis which drop them at either the taxi-park, particular taxi-stages or by the roadside. Furthermore, the waiting charges of a *bodaboda* are much less than those of taxis.

The personal element and privacy fostered by the *bodaboda* also contribute to their popularity. Participants said that people travelling to secret places or on private missions prefer to travel with *bodabodas* than other motor-vehicles. In the questionnaire, 19 respondents said they mostly take women going to traditional healers. Seven in-depth interviews contained accounts of participants secretly transporting women to have or from having abortions. A few participants mentioned taking people to their secret lovers. In focus-group discussions, participants emphasized the necessity of moving from the villages into the peri-urban centres in order be successful in the *bodaboda* business. Several young single men said they had left their parents' homes, to rent one-room houses (*akazigo* – singular, *buzigo* – plural) in the slum or in surrounding suburbs. Married men, on the other hand, left their wives and children in the villages and rented *buzigo* during the week, returning to the village on Sunday to visit their families. Many had a dual residence: one rural and one urban.

Questionnaire data indicate that 84 per cent of respondents had migrated from the villages to the towns. Out of these, 89 participants had shifted specifically in search of *bodaboda* employment or as a result of becoming *bodabodamen*. In focus-group discussions participants discussed migration.

Facilitator: What is it that causes you to leave home?
Leo: Most of us left home because we needed to find employment.
Samson: We leave home because we need to look for money. You can sit at your father's house and fail to get a job.
Facilitator: Isn't there work to do in your home areas?
Leo: The work in the villages is farming and it does not pay as well as the easier jobs that are here in Nyendo. Like us who ride *bodabodas*, we do not sweat; we just sit on a bike and make money.

Sixty per cent of participants said that they still had financial responsibility for family members left in the villages. Furthermore, 79 per cent of participants reported that they frequently or regularly visited their village homes to take provisions, check on the family, monitor their gardens or other small-scale businesses, spend public holidays there, or attend traditional socio-cultural ceremonies such as funeral rites, burials and weddings.

However, the frequency and regularity of these urban–rural visits decrease as the men acquire new activities and acquaintances to occupy their weekends. *Bodabodamen* who have wives in the village do not encourage them to visit in town. It is the man who is supposed to visit the woman. Some *bodabodamen* reported moving to other localities to avoid the repercussions of their sexual actions, such as making a girl pregnant, forced marriage, imprisonment, fines, fights with female partners who catch them with another woman, or fights with other men over a common lover:

Interviewer:	Does that mean that you just came to Masaka to work?
Isaac:	Yes. The other thing that made me leave Mbarara was to avoid the problems of the wrongs I had done.
Interviewer:	What wrongs?
Isaac:	The pregnancy I have just told you about. I feared that things might become hot for me … her parents could try and have me imprisoned.
Interviewer:	So, if she had not conceived, you would not have left Mbarara?
Isaac:	Exactly. I would not have left Mbarara because I had work to do in Mbarara.
Interviewer:	Were you a *bodaboda* man in Mbarara?
Isaac:	No. I was a mechanic.

Other reasons for shifting include the desire for independence from parents, the death of parents, dropping out of school, the need for sex, mistreatment by step-mothers, cultural expectations, housework chores at home, the desire to earn more money.

Ali: The other major reason that really leads to leaving home is the fact that if you have a girl that you love outside [*gwoyagala ebbali*], there is no way you can bring her into your father's house to sleep with you. So you decide to leave home and rent a house where you can take her. You rent a place so that you just take her to your place for the whole night without anyone getting bothered about your action.

High levels of mobility and migration impact on the sexual activity of the *bodabodamen*. Many of the participants agreed that when one shifts into a new locality, there is a need to acquire a new woman, whether or not he maintains contact with his partner in the previous location.

Sexual networks

Most *bodabodamen* are 'single' in town and 'married' in the village. In this regard there was an interesting disparity between the questionnaire and focus-group discussion data. In the questionnaire 50 per cent of the men said that they were married. However, in the group discussions participants claimed that most of them were 'single' (*babuwuulu*). Responses given in in-depth individual interviews illuminated the issue.

Interviewer:	Okay. What about wife number two? Doesn't she mind that you already have wife number one?
Kato:	She does not mind about the first one. In mind about this fact the first one does not mind about this second one.
Interviewer:	Did you pay bride-price for both these women? How come both of them are your wives?
Kato:	I paid for one of them. I paid her parents. This other second one is also my wife. When I made her pregnant, I decided to rent a house for her. That way she also became my wife.
Interviewer:	Does her family know you?
Kato:	Her *ssenga* [paternal aunt] knows about me. I have never formally introduced myself to her, but then she knows about me.
Interviewer:	Are you planning to go to her parents' home to introduce yourself, or will she just stay with you like that simply because she conceived your child?

Kato: I have not officially made her my wife. Actually speaking, my father would
                  never allow me to introduce two women. He is the *Saba Kristu* [a leader in the
                  Catholic congregation] of our area.

Interviewer: You have told me that you have two wives. Did you marry them officially?
                  How did they become your wives?
Bbosa: I did not marry any of them. I did not marry by giving a ring to any of them.
Interviewer: Did they introduce you to their homes? Do their parents know you?
Bbosa: No, none of them know me.
Interviewer: How come you say that they are your wives?
Bbosa: I rent a house for each of them. I buy them whatever they need to use in their
                  homes. When I am tired I go and rest at either one of their homes. I am the one
                  who pays rent for their houses.
Interviewer: Does the fact that you pay their rent make them your wives?
Bbosa: Totally! The fact that I got her a place she can call her own makes her my wife.
                  For the other one I even gave her capital to begin a shop. Why shouldn't she be
                  my wife? I regard both as my wives. I never went to their parental homes to
                  introduce myself, but I am their husband.

In agreement with earlier findings of Nabaitu *et al.* (1994), the concept of 'marriage' is ambivalent in contemporary Kiganda society. Among this particular social group, there are several
categories of marital status: 'married', 'polygamous', 'cohabiting', 'separated', 'divorced',
'widowed' and 'single'. The boundaries of these categories are very fluid. Connotations overlap.
Among the 110 respondents who indicated they were married in questionnaire responses, for
example, 34 divided into sub-categories their marital status as married, 69 as cohabiting, 4 as
polygamous and 3 as separated. Of these participants, 61 reported having one or more casual partners in addition to the marital partner. Out of the 110 participants who said they were not married,
104 categorized their marital status as single, 3 as separated and 3 as widowed; 77 of these unmarried men reported that they have one or more casual sexual partnerships.

Bodabodamen were vibrant in their discussions about the various kinds of women that they
have partnerships with. Focus-group discussions became very loud and boisterous when they
got to this topic. A *bodabodaman* may have a socially recognized and accepted 'wife' whom
he keeps in his village home. This kind of sexual partner is referred to as *omukyala oweka* (the
wife for the home). Marriage in Buganda can be either civil, when processed through the
administrative organs; religious, when it is formalized in church/mosque; or customary,
where a man pays bride-price and is introduced to a woman's family. Depending on how he
married her or her position in his sequence of partners (see also Blanc *et al.*, 1996), she may
also be called *mukyala mukulu* (elder wife), *mukyala owempetta* (wife who bears my ring),
mukyala siniya (senior wife), *mukyala namba emu* (wife number one) or *maama wa baana*
(mother of my children). *Bodabodamen* said it is easier to leave this first (and often senior)
wife and her progeny in the village because it is cheaper to raise and maintain a family in the
rural area, than in the towns. This partner is presented as relatively permanent.

There were also a few *bodabodamen* who said that they lived with their *mukyala weka* in the
kazigo or other town dwellings. Some of these argued that they were not originally from the
villages, but from the towns. Hence they have no village-home in which to leave their wives.
Others left the villages when they were still single and later married girls in the towns. In addition, to a 'wife for the home', *bodabodamen* said that it was possible to have another semi-
permanent sexual partner known as *omukyala owebbali* (an outside wife). Other labels for this

kind of partner were 'spare-tyre' and 'my second hand'.[1] Participants were ambiguous in their use of the label *omukyala owebbali*. Some used this term to refer to a second wife whose family has given the man consent to marry her. In this case, the relationship was well-known and approved by the girl's relations, and the relationship was polygynous. The term *omukyala owebbali* was also used to refer to a regular sexual partner. This kind of relationship might either be concealed from public and from the families of the parties concerned, or it may be known but not approved of, or it may be known and accepted. The outside wife is maintained concurrently with the wife for the home, although they may or may not be known to each other. She may either live in the village or live with some level of regularity with the *bodabodaman* in his *kazigo*. This outside wife may also live in the urban area in a house rented for her by her male sexual partner. It is possible for a man to have more than one outside wife.

In addition to these two types of partners, a *bodabodaman* can also have a regular partner called *muganzi wange* (my lover). *Bodabodamen* claimed to have sexual access to these lovers whenever they wanted, without having any moral or social obligation toward them. They said that these women were aware that the relationship was not 'serious' and that they knew of the man's other sexual partners and were not expected to get jealous. Such women have no formal claim on the man, although he often gives her small gifts, cash and food. Interestingly, the term *omuganzi* was used interchangeably when describing both casual and regular sexual relationships.

Bodabodamen said that this category of sexual partners consisted mostly of schoolgirls, even though they knew about the legal and social implications of such relationships. This confirms findings from an earlier study conducted among school pupils in the same district (Nyanzi *et al.*, 2001). Other types of partners mentioned include bar maids, salon workers, waitresses, house-girls (servants), shop-attendants, tailors, nurses from a nearby hospital and even some teachers.

Another type of sexual partner mentioned by the *bodabodamen* was the one-night-stand woman called an *ekkubo* (*makubo* – pl.), literally 'the road'. This label comes from an expression *okulonda ekkubo* which means 'picked off the road'. *Ekkubo* are often stranded women who come into the town from the villages in search of employment, but fail to acquire lodging for the night. *Ekkubo* are also poor women who have no money for their transport fares and thus have to pay with sexual services after the *bodabodaman* has dropped them at their destination. Another category of *ekkubo* consists of girls who leave discotheques or bars late in the night and are too drunk to find their way home. *Bodabodamen* said that they take advantage of this condition and have sex with them.

Tendo:	Some girls are very easy to *kulonda makubo*. Such girls come into town and have nowhere to sleep for the night. She has just come into town and knows no one. She may have come to look for a job and night falls before she has arranged where to spend the night. Those ones are easy to *kulonda makubo*. You solve her problem for her when you take her into your place.
Kintu:	That one will move out of the area the next day. The other type is one who works in the area but is taken by different men each day. The chances of getting her again are very small because another man will have taken her already.
Andrew:	*Makubo* are also girls we meet in Ambiance [a popular discotheque]. These girls go to the disco without male partners because they know that they will find willing partners there. While you are dancing with her, you ask her for sex. If she allows, you take her to your house.
Interviewer:	What kind of women do you find in Ambiance?

Joe: Many *makubo* are found in Ambiance. Such a woman is just waiting for a man to pick her and pay her.

Dan: A woman in Ambiance never refuses to give sex. That is what takes her to the disco alone.

Steven: Those Ambiance women have no traffic jam at all. They always give in without hesitating.

Joe: Picking *ekkubo* is like eating some roast meat, yet you are also going to have a meal of boiled meat stew. The snack cannot stop you from having a proper meal. It is all just about having a good time, for a while.

Lastly, there are the *makubo* who cunningly lure *bodabodamen* into suggesting sex to them, as they ride on the bikes. Participants said that these girls send out signals (both direct and implied) to the men, including sitting a-straddle the bike, holding the man in erogenous areas, dressing in luring clothes, smiling and gesturing coyly.

Topha: She can say, 'Take me to Saza'. On the way, she begins putting you in the mood for those things. You may tell her to hold onto the seat of the bike, but instead she holds onto your body. I think you see what I mean. As you know what nature is, the man's whole system gets disrupted. Instead of holding onto the bike she holds onto your body. Then she suddenly begins tickling you all over your body. Once you ask her for sex, she allows and you can either go into the bushes or to a lodge.

Zziwa: She says, 'Anyway, let us go'. So we put her onto the motorbike. By the way, many times we put them on our motorbikes when they are dressed in these very short dresses. You know the minis I am talking about. Then I may tell her to sit the female way and she refuses. She sits a-straddle – like a man on the motorbike. Now as we are on our way, she moves off her seat and sits onto the driver's seat. Remember that the dress she is wearing is very short, and has rolled up. In fact, each time the person seated on the back seat gets closer to the front seat, there is need to further spread the legs. And as the legs spread wider apart, the dress rolls higher up. So her parts, with all their warmth, are right onto the man. Most of us men get tempted by such girls.

Sex workers known as *malaya* or *abakazi abeetunda* (women who sell themselves) are also part of the *bodabodamen*'s sexual network. The term *malaya* is employed ambiguously to mean 'women who willingly provide sexual services to men, for money', or 'a woman who has casual sex with multiple partners'. Participants said such relationships were characterized by 'loads of pleasure', 'secrecy', 'no free sex', 'no commitment'. *Malayas* are mostly in the slum trading centres, but also in the urban centre clubs and bars.

Paulo: Those women are deadly!

Vincent: Such women who are looking for your money. They are the kind you tell, 'I have got 1000 shillings. Will you come with me?'

Atim: Some ask, 'Do you have 500 shillings? If you give me some money I will allow to do it'.

Kamali: To those women, sex is a job, an occupation. That is the work they do to earn money.

Jimmy: They come to the streets and bars to make money from men.

Kizza: You do not even have to look hard to see them. They paint their faces with lipstick and powder. Then they wear revealing short dresses. That is how you know what they are after.

Chris: They come out in the evenings because that is when men are retiring and going home or to the bars. They work at night and sleep during the day. It is just like you leave your home in the morning, with the intention to make money that day.

Frequency and regularity of sex with a *malaya* is dependent on income. Reasons for having sex with a *malaya* range from 'they are sexually experienced', 'know many sex styles' and 'are available any time anywhere'. Some participants also argued that a *malaya* is cheaper to have, maintain and relate with, than a wife or regular partner. There was no need to pay her rent, buy her food or make a commitment. Attitudes towards having sex with a *malaya* were highly ambivalent. Some *bodabodamen* fervently discouraged having sex with a *malaya* because it could expose them to STIs including HIV/AIDS. Moreover, if it became known that a man was having sex with a *malaya*, it could disrupt his steady relationships. Others defended their preference for *malayas* over steady partnerships. However, there was consensus about the necessity of secrecy and discretion when having a sexual relationship with a *malaya*. This offers evidence of the tension between what was socially acceptable and what actually occurs.

Amidst ribaldry and great laughter, sexual partners known as 'sugar-mummies', 'off-layers' or *namukadde* (old ladies) were also discussed.[2] These are women who were much older and often relatively wealthy. Many were married, widowed or divorced. Such women initiated the sexual relationship, which was a reversal of traditional roles (see Nyanzi *et al.*, 2001). *Bodabodamen* give several reasons for having sexual relationships with 'sugar-mummies'. These ranged from maximizing material benefits, locally known as detoothing, the attraction of sexual experience, better sexual performance and experimentation, to the prestige of knowing that an older woman craves you, suggesting that you know how to satisfy her.

Interviewer: What reasons lead you to relate with sugar-mummies?

Peter: Some sugar-mummies are very good-looking. You see her and she looks much younger than she really is.

Kalisa: Older women were trained and counselled by their *ssengas*, in the ways to please a man. The young girls you see around today did not get their *ssenga*'s counselling about sexual relationships, or how to behave when with their husbands. I do not know why this is the case. However, the older women were trained as young girls. It was the custom in Buganda in those days.

Tom: In fact when you have sex with an old woman, you may decide never to love a young girl again. The old women know how to make you feel like a real man.

Jamadha: Immediately you get to her place, she comments, 'Eh, the dust on your shoes! I do not want my man to look like that'. So she takes your shoes off your feet and gives them a thorough cleaning. She cares about you. You feel loved.

Kamu: Also, their love is very genuine. She pampers and spoils you with whatever you wish for. She is not interested in your money because she has a lot of it. All that she wants is your love. When you have sex with her, she gives you so much pleasure because she knows many different things that you may not know.

Simon: I also feel that older women are bold in their love. They are not shy and embarrassed about undressing before you like young girls are.

Enoch: The other thing that happens is that the young men may see that the woman has a lot of money. So they go for her money and not her. Because she has some money, you decide to get married to her. No one goes to buy a car and buys an old one. [laughter]

Even though there was the advantage of support from sugar-mummies, many participants felt that sexual relationships involving older women had negative qualities as well. The general feeling was that sexual relationships were short-lived and often kept hidden. A few participants felt it was demeaning to have a sexual relationship with a sugar-mummy, particularly because 'she is old enough to be your mother. It would be like making love to your very own mother!'

Others stressed the fact that many sugar-mummies were widowed, infected with HIV and intent on spreading it. However, many of participants said that they thought they were already infected with HIV and reasoned it was better to obtain wealth, affection and sex from the sugar-mummy and then die, than to suffer poverty, loneliness and misery when death is imminent anyway.

Exchange dynamics in sexual relationships

Bodabodamen tend to be relatively better-off financially than their peers. Also, unlike peers who have to wait for salaries, *bodabodamen* receive payment after each trip. In questionnaire responses, 60 per cent of participants said the best thing about their job was that they could easily earn quick money. With money comes higher bargaining power in sexual relationships. Many participants felt that 'once a man gets money, he will look for a woman', 'one cannot have money and just buy food. No! He goes to look for a woman'.

Tom: It is this money that tempts us to get women. Once you get money, you know that you can have any woman you want. It is up to you to choose from the lot.

John: Money is the devil! When you get money, you begin seeing women in a different light.

They also believed that since they are known to have money, women (both casual and regular) interested in maximizing gains will find them sexually appealing. All 40 participants in the in-depth interviews had given a 'gift' (material, monetary or a service) to their sexual partners. Such gifts included cash, second-hand dresses, body lotion, perfume, roast meat, fried chicken, bottled beer, soap, paying for rent or transport, taking her out to a function, giving her a lift on his bike, underwear and paraffin.

Only six participants out of the above sample had received such a gift from a female partner. Two of these partners were 'sugar-mummies' and supposedly wealthier than the *bodabodamen*. In the focus-group discussions, men said it was not the norm for women to give men gifts (other than sex) in reciprocation. It is the man who should give the gifts. He determines what to give, how much, when and where. Participants explained that the significance of the gift given to their sexual partners depends on the stage of the relationship. When given before a relationship has begun, the gift (particularly money) indicated to the recipient that the man is interested in starting a sexual relationship.

Participants said they could not give money to a girl they were not related to, without implying sexual interest. If the woman played hard-to-get, the gift was intended to persuade her to start a relationship. Furthermore, participants said that they give gifts to a woman in reward for sexual services. Is this a payment? No, participants argued. It is just a sign of gratitude for her not having refused to have sex. Gifts are also given to maintain a sexual relationship. Local culture demands that the man provide for his regular sexual partner and in this case gifts are given out of duty.

Some *bodabodamen* claimed feeling more invulnerable with more money. They felt that money also gave them higher bargaining power when it came to negotiating condom use. Some participants said that with money they could afford condoms, pay more to convince a sexual partner to use condoms, and choose less risky girls who require higher payments. Others argued the opposite. They said paying a sexual partner more entitled them to the pleasure of 'live' (unprotected) sex. Also, money gave them access to alcohol, which could impair their judgement, and to discos that expose them to high-risk groups including bar maids and sex workers.

While the men's dominant discourse portrays women as passive recipients of the gifts, a subordinate discourse describes some women (particularly those from the townships) as using ploys to maximize the benefits from their sexual relationships. The former presents a weak, silent woman who does not know her value. She does not set the price, determine when to get it, bargain for more, or refuse whatever trivia are thrown her way. She gratefully accepts the gift, and makes do with it. The latter described a worldly woman who knows how to make a profit, presents herself as appealing, rips off men, bargains hard for higher returns and can walk away from a raw deal.

In order to maximize gains from men interested in having sex, participants reported that some women (particularly urban ones and schoolgirls) indulge in a practice known as *okukuula ebinnyo* locally translated as 'detoothing' – an analogy to the dentists' act of pulling teeth. Participants explained that as long as a man hopes to get sex from a girl, he continues to give her gifts and money. Hence, the ploy that cunning females use is to keep a man interested for as long as is safely possible, maximizing their gains and then avoiding him when the pressure and demand for sex become intolerable. Since gift-giving is the domain of men, detoothing is generally presented as a women's monopoly. However, two participants stimulated debate when they claimed that they had detoothed women – a sugar-mummy and a student from a wealthy family.

Discussion

Unlike other traditional sectors of the transport industry, the *bodaboda* sector is an indigenous group that has evolved as a consequence of the socio-economic changes in Uganda. Semi-permanent rural–urban migration causes a situation whereby *bodabodamen* become 'single' and away from their partners for a period. With money, peer-pressure, pleasure-seeking and the call of Masaka night-life in the slums and suburbs, they engage in both serial and concurrent multiple casual and/or regular sexual partnerships. Many of these partners belong to population groups such as sex workers, bar maids, sugar-mummies, widows and students.

Simultaneously, *bodabodamen* maintain their sexual relationships with wives or stable partners in the villages. In the context of the HIV/AIDS epidemic, *bodaboamen* are therefore a potential bridging group between the rural–urban, high–low risk, adult–youth, monogamous–multipartnered divides of society. Similar to other Ugandan studies (Nabaitu *et al.*, 1994; Blanc *et al.*, 1996), in this work we found ambiguity in the meaning of 'marriage'.

Findings indicate that the label embraces a wide range of partnerships including private consensual or forced/arranged unions, conception-related unions, cohabiting, non-ceremonial arrangements, contractual marriages and regular sexual relationships. In addition, polygyny is widespread, hence the phenomenon of second, third or more wives (Karanja, 1994).

Exchange featured significantly in bargaining for sex. As noted elsewhere, however, this transactional sex does not necessarily equate to prostitution. In fact, participants clearly distinguish between payment for sexual activity and the exchange of gifts in other relationships. The significance of the act of giving in return of sex is socially constructed to mean different things depending on when it is given. The same act could mean indicating sexual interest, pursuing a potential partner, appreciating a sexual service, valuing a woman's sexual performance, detoothing, perfunctory duty and maintaining a stable relationship. Transaction is, however, an integral part of sexual relationships (Nyanzi *et al.*, 2001). A continuity from traditional society lies in the man's role of giving the gift, and the woman's role of receiving these and in turn offering sexual services to the man.

Bodabodamen repeatedly move between rural and urban centres without patterned regularity or determinable structure. They haphazardly criss-cross local administrative boundaries, transporting passengers and goods, with more frequency than other commercial transport service providers. Peaks in their mobility correspond to economic peaks in society. Access to cash avails them of the ability to pay for sex, and acquire partners whenever and wherever they travel. Thus they have a wide sexual network. Thereby, *bodabodamen* are both potential vectors of transmission but also ambassadors of behavioural change, when equipped with appropriate information about sexual health, safer sex and behaviour.

Unlike other employment-groups, *bodabodamen* lack an association that unites them. In Uganda, the association of public transport operators excludes motor-bicycles and bicycles. This, plus their characteristic mobility, heterogeneity and the transitional nature of their estate, makes *bodabodamen* difficult to reach. A useful intervention in reaching and impacting this group must be accessible from both urban and remote rural areas. The starting point would be the organization of a collective but decentralized association of all *bodabodamen*, making them more visible to policy makers and accessible to programme implementers. Beyond this, dissemination of accurate health education could utilize the popular FM radio stations to broadcast reproductive health programmes specifically addressing *bodabodamen* in local vernacular at appropriate times. Participatory journalism – in which *bodabodamen* participate in radio shows, a needs assessment informs the design of programmes, and ongoing feedback sessions facilitate evaluation – would be effective. Training of local male role-models (including *bodabodamen*) as peer-educators, and facilitating them with condoms, contraceptives and referral slips for STI treatment, would provide points of positive influence for other *bodabodamen* to change their risky sexual behaviour.

Acknowledgements

We are grateful to the men who participated in the study and to James Whitworth for timely and constructive comments on this paper.

Notes

1 As discussed in Nyanzi *et al.*, 2001, contemporary Luganda speakers often combine a mixture of words from the multiple local languages, as well as foreign ones particularly English (but also

French) in one sentence. In this case 'spare-tyre' and 'second-hand' are spoken with heavy Luganda accents as *sippeya-taya* and *sekendi-andi* respectively.

2 Similarly, 'sugar-mummy' and 'off-layer' are spoken in a localized English version as *shuga-mami* and *woofu-leeya* respectively, the latter having become a predominant aspect of sexual relationship public discourse in the context.

References

BLANC, A.K., WOLFF, B., GAGE, A.J., EZEH, A.C., NEEMA, S. and SEKAMATTE-SEBULIBA, J. (1996) *Negotiating Reproductive Outcomes in Uganda*, Calverton, MA: Macro-International Inc. and Institute of Statistics and Applied Economics, Uganda.

COHEN, B. and TRUSSELL, J. (eds) (1996) *Preventing and Mitigating AIDS in Sub-Saharan Africa: Research and Data Priorities for the Social and Behavioural Sciences*, Washington, DC: National Research Council Panel on Data and Research Priorities.

GYSELS, M. (2001) 'Truck drivers, middlemen and commercial sex workers: AIDS and the mediation of sex in southwest Uganda', *AIDS Care*, 13, pp. 373–86.

HUNT, C. (1989) 'Migrant labor and sexually transmitted diseases: AIDS in Africa', *Journal of Health and Social Behaviour*, 4, pp. 353–73.

KANE, F., ALARY, M., NDOYE, I., COLL, A.M., MBOUP, S., GUEJE, A., KANKI, P.J. and JOLLY, J.R. (1993) 'Temporary expatriation is related to HIV infection in rural Senegal', *AIDS*, 7, pp. 1261–5.

KARANJA, W.W. (1994) 'The phenomenon of '"outside wives"': some reflections on its possible influence on fertility' in BLEDSOE, C. and PISON, G. (eds) *Nuptiality in Sub-Saharan Africa: Contemporary Anthropological and Demographic Perspectives*, Oxford: Clarendon Press.

KINTU, P.M., WHITWORTH, J., KAMALI, A. and NABAITU, J. (2000) *Community Migration, Mobility and HIV-1 Infection in an Adult Ugandan Population*, Abstract MoPpC1025 The XIII International Conference, Durban, South Africa.

MORGAN, D.L. (ed.) (1993) *Successful Focus Groups*, London: Sage.

NABAITU, J., BACHENGANA, C. and SEELEY, J. (1994) 'Marital instability in a rural population in south-west Uganda: implications for the spread of HIV-1 infection', *Africa*, 64(2), pp. 243–50.

NYANZI, S., POOL, R. and KINSMAN, J. (2001) 'The negotiation of sexual relationships among school pupils in south-western Uganda', *AIDS Care*, 13, pp. 83–98.

PAUL, S. (2000) *Trans-national Population Movement and HIV/AIDS in the Mainland South-east Asia*, Abstract MoPeD2654, The XIII International Conference, Durban, South Africa.

ROSCOE, J. (1965) *The Baganda: An Account of their Native Customs and Beliefs*, London: Frank Cass.

STRAUSS, A. and CORBIN, J. (1998) *Basics of Qualitative Research Techniques and Procedures for Developing Grounded Theory*, Thousand Oaks, CA: Sage.

UNAIDS INTER-COUNTRY TEAM FOR WEST AND CENTRAL AFRICA. (2000) *Findings from the Research-action 'Migration and AIDS' Project: Burkina Faso, Cote D'Ivoire, Mali, Niger and Senegal*, Abidjan – UNAIDS'. Available at: www.onusidaaoc.org/Eng/Publications/Migration

Part 8

Contemporary and future challenges

23 Gendered scripts and the sexual scene

Promoting sexual subjects among Brazilian teenagers

Vera Paiva [2004]

In the first decade of AIDS, Brazilian prevention efforts and campaigns directed toward the sexual transmission of HIV were based on the ideas 'promiscuity', 'fear', 'death threat', and the 'hazardous other' within an overall strategy of targeting 'risk groups'. More recently, safer sex (defined as condom use and fewer partners) has increasingly been promoted through face-to-face activities, and many activists and AIDS educators have begun to work using small group interventions. Most of these small-group programmes have focused on risk reduction and individual responsibility through interactive information and, in the relatively rare cases where the necessary resources are available, modelling sexual communication and negotiation skills.

During our on-going work with young people in São Paulo, Brazil, we constantly find that social vulnerability compromises the efficacy of AIDS prevention programmes. Participants in our workshops are told that HIV is a highly democratic virus – that its transmission modes do not discriminate by race, age, nationality, gender or sexual preferences. But when they leave the workshops, they find out that HIV transmission is in reality more likely to occur within certain social and cultural contexts that make some people more vulnerable than others. That is to say, the youth of my city discover in their everyday lives what epidemiology has been showing on large scale for some time: poor people and minorities, the poorly educated, and the disempowered are more vulnerable (see, for example, Mann, Tarantola and Netter, 1992; Lurie, Hintzen and Lowe, 1995; Parker, 1994, 1996). As Altman puts it: 'A number of factors will influence the course of the epidemic, of which the bio-medical are not necessarily the most important' (Altman, 1994). These realities motivated us to ask the following questions:

- How should an AIDS prevention programme address social and cultural factors that shape and regulate 'risky' sex?
- How can AIDS prevention programmes go beyond a focus on *behavioural change* and *individual responsibility*?

In this article, I will outline the theoretical framework for AIDS prevention programmes around which we have built our interventions – and will try to contrast it with some of the more traditional approaches that have generally guided AIDS education and prevention work. My discussion will centre on examples and lessons learned from a research and intervention programme developed with teenage students at public elementary night schools in São Paulo.[1]

Outline of a theoretical framework

We began the prevention programme in 1991, using small-group approaches inspired by the AIDS Risk Reduction Model (Catania *et al.*, 1990) and the Brazilian reproductive health movement, as well as our previous research which indicated that gender norms are a key cultural factor placing young men and women at risk of unwanted pregnancy and/or HIV.[2] We were soon confronted by the importance of social and economic contextual factors, which had not been considered adequately by most existing HIV risk-reduction models and behavioural change interventions. Our research findings stressed how the socio-cultural context where sex occurs, and the lack of accessible contraception and reproductive health options – condoms cost about U$1 each at the time of our study – limit individuals' intentions to practise safe sex.

Our project builds on the tradition of Latin American liberation pedagogy, most widely known through the work of Paulo Freire. We seek to promote citizenship while encouraging sexual agency. We assume that behavioural change, condom use and safer sex should be *part of* programmes working with disenfranchised communities, but *not the exclusive goal* or focus of them. Central to our framework are four key concepts: (1) the sexual subject (from the Portuguese term *sujeito*), (2) consciousness-raising or 'conscientization' (from the Portuguese term, *conscientização*), (3) gendered scripts and bodies, and (4) the sexual scene.

The main objective in the prevention programme is to promote the *sujeito sexual* ('sexual subject'). The sexual subject is the agent who regulates his/her own sexual life, coping with the complexity of the multiple factors competing in his/her life that can result in 'riskier sex' or 'safer sex'. In the Brazilian tradition, *sujeito* integrates the idea of agency with the idea of citizenship (defined as full participation and influence in our society – something that cannot be taken for granted in Brazil). The *sujeito* or subject is one who takes action, one who enacts. The sexual subject is thus the individual capable of being the regulating agent of his/her own sexual life – which, in practice, means:

- developing a negotiated relation with the sexual/gender culture, rather than simply accepting them at face value or as given in nature.
- developing a negotiated relation with family and peer group norms.
- exploring (or not exploring) sexuality independent of the partner's initiative.
- being able to say 'no' and to have this right respected.
- being able to negotiate sexual practices that are pleasurable for oneself, so long as they are consensual and acceptable to the partner (or partners).
- being able to negotiate safer sex.
- having access to the material conditions to make reproductive and safer-sex choices.

One feasible path to promote sexual subjects builds upon the Freirian tradition and stimulates the group to deconstruct their own sexual scenarios through 'consciousness-raising' and 'coding and decoding' (see Freire, 1993). As the examples below will show, in a consciousness-building process, consciousness should be seen as much more than 'awareness' in a strict psychological and clinical sense or resulting of self-observation intended to change attitudes and behaviours. Instead, we situate the concept of *self* within the social group, as the word *conscientização* is used in the Brazilian liberation education tradition (see Freire, 1983). We are thus talking not only about 'self-observation', 'scene observation', and promoting self-regulation (as defined by Rafael Diaz [Diaz, 2000]), but also about citizenship.

In developing our intervention in São Paulo, the importance of *conscientização* became especially evident after the first wave of safer-sex workshops. The students expressed feelings of powerlessness and fatalism when faced with the actual context in which their recently formulated intentions of using condoms would quite literally not be enacted. Their disproportionate social vulnerability in turn tended to ruin the awareness they had achieved during the workshops:

> I can't have a choice, destiny will choose for me, I see what I can do with it afterwards.

> AIDS is just another burden, why bother? To survive in this crazy and difficult world, and have some fun with sex is the only right I have …

One of the ways in which we have responded to this sense of powerlessness and fatalism has been to help participants to de-codify how the socio-cultural context regulates their sexual lives, and to highlight how social forces can frustrate individuals' intentions to practise safer sex and to control their own sexual lives. At the same time, collaborative group activities that can contribute to a sense of responsibility helped participants to work through the puzzling obstacles in individual sexual scenes and towards acceptable and feasible safer sex. For example, research has shown that the symbolic construction of AIDS in Brazil has stressed old prejudices with a morbid and accusatory attitude towards the 'evil' practices or attributed identities of those infected with HIV (see Paiva, 1992; Daniel and Parker, 1993). These ideas can shape each safer-sex scene, with the condom itself often symbolizing accusation, promiscuity, or the like, and thereby becoming an obstacle to safer sex (Paiva, 1993, 1994, 1995). De-codifying and challenging AIDS stigma, which today is linked to the very idea of safer sex and condom use, is thus a key first step. When learning how to use a condom, intervention participants produced their own (alternative) codes by making 'art using the condom' (in Portuguese, *fazendo arte com camisinha*, which implies both artistic creation as well as a certain erotic playfulness): music, poems, sculptures, paintings, drama, posters, culinary art, etc., *using* condoms as a creative device. We then de-codify safer sex and AIDS symbolism by looking, collectively, at participants' productions.

In another activity, students also modelled erotic and reproductive body parts from dough, decoding the gendered sex education they had received at home. Through this group activity, they learned about HIV transmission and about reproduction, and by talking about sex through highly concrete body parts, rather than through complicated science classes enacted on blackboards, they deconstructed sexist education and gender culture, and explored the pluralism of pleasures and morals. In discussion about communication with partners, and about other obstacles to enacting their risk-reduction intentions, they also created actual 'sexual scenes' through which they decoded gender relations and sexual scenarios, passive/active relations, and the socio-economic context where sex occurs.

Although focused on the specific content of gender and sexual relations, this process built on the transformative approach outlined by Paulo Freire:

> The *coding* of an existential situation is the representation of that situation showing some of its constituent elements of interaction. *Decoding* is the critical analysis of the coded situation. Its decoding requires moving from the abstract to the concrete; this requires moving from the part to the whole and then returning to the parts; this in turn requires that the Subject recognize himself in the object as a situation in which he finds himself, together with other Subjects. If the decoding is well done, this movement of flux and

reflux from the abstract to the concrete which occurs in the analysis of the coded situations leads to the supersedence (surpass) of the abstraction by the critical perception of the concrete, which has already ceased to be dense, impenetrable reality.

(Freire, 1993)

Freire is talking here about meaningful words and emerging themes as codes, ideas that emerged through his innovative programme with illiterate rural workers of the sixties. Freire's work, like most of the Latin American tradition of popular education, was forged within social movements struggling against poverty and oppression, and was used to understand liberation as a result of popular class alliances against the authoritarian elite in many Latin American countries supporting military dictatorships in the 1960 and 1970s. Access to education and literacy was a crucial step, but could only be fully achieved by valuing popular language (words and syntax) and relevant themes to break the silence of the poor – and in turn make education meaningful for illiterate teenage and adult workers.

Literacy programmes that used 'emerging words and themes as codes' were a successful way to finally give access to reading and writing – they were designed to de-codify the social context by learning the letter 'X' not through *xadres* ('chess'), but through *enxada* ('hoe'). As people became organized, popular drama, music, and other popular arts were used, as in the past, to communicate and value their lives, heritage, and collective history. At least partly as a result of such work, illiteracy has decreased significantly since the 1960s, while national mass media have unified language practice. Yet it is also true that few study beyond elementary school, and that word of mouth, more than written material, continues to reinterpret all other sources of information and remains perhaps the most powerful means for the spread of ideas and social change.

From the late 1970s and early 1980s, when redemocratization began to emerge in Latin America, other definitions of oppression were included in nongovernmental and community initiatives, and sex and gender identity politics entered the scene. In this kind of politics, where the reproductive rights and the AIDS movements may be situated, a new face has been given to liberation pedagogy – with workshops and small groups used within health education programmes to talk about desire, intimate experiences and gendered bodies, to deconstruct and re-construct identities, and to fight violence and discrimination. In this space, popular education and mobilization movements met small-group psychological interventions. Workshops (which in Portuguese we call *oficinas*) with a psychological approach to empowerment – generally meaning individual empowerment – began to be very attractive to an educated middle class, but did not always make sense to disenfranchised rural migrants (the majority of night-school students whom we have worked with in São Paulo). As we learned through our activities and group evaluations, such workshops should only be the first step in a larger programme to mobilize nonorganized communities to cope with their social vulnerability to HIV. We now understand safer-sex workshops to be a space for the production of 'codes' to result in a collective 'thematic investigation' of the sexual and gender cultures shaping AIDS and reproduction.

Three social issues are relevant to the 'codes' that we are introducing – words and themes, gendered bodies and scripts, and sexual scripts and scenes. The first (most tuned with the liberation pedagogy of the 1960 and 1970s), is how the socio-demographic variables that define poverty – considered as a mix of income, education and housing – are associated with vulnerability to HIV infection. The second concerns the way social context shapes gender systems. The third focuses on how different Brazilian subcultures define a complementary passive/active sexual system that is a key aspect in Brazilian sexual and erotic scripts and sexual scenes (this chapter will focus mainly on heterosexual scripts among young people).[3] As we live in the 1990s and work in a large metropolitan area, the codes and themes produced by the communities with whom we have worked express a mosaic of values, options, and preferences that can result in divergent organized subgroups even though allied by the same socio-economic constraints.

Consequently, we assume that adolescence, like sexuality, rather than being a universal and transcultural phenomenon, is modelled by cultural, economic, and political influences that cannot be overlooked when thinking about AIDS prevention projects (see Paiva, 1994, 1995). As Janice Irvine states, the 'changes of puberty, such as menstruation, breast development, wet dreams, and hair growth, are given meanings by the culture in which the adolescent lives' (Irvinee 1994). Cultural identifications such as 'race, gender and sexual identity must be recognized as social categories, not biological variables' (Irving, 1994). In the programme, we stress how these social categories will shape and regulate each individual sexual scene and how they are competing factors to be faced by everyone (see also Diaz, 1997, 2000).

Inspired by the pedagogic use of 'theatre of the oppressed', psychodrama techniques, and the social-science constructionist approach to sexuality – including the ideas of 'sexual scripts' (see Gagnon and Simon, 1973) and 'erotic scripts' (see Parker, 1991) – we have used the 'sexual scene' as an approach to group investigation of both the sexual context and the choices of individuals in relation to protected sex.

AIDS consciousness and sexual literacy cannot be achieved without coding and decoding 'sexual scenes', the social and cultural contexts in which sex occurs. Sexual scripts are enacted in every scene, and are learnt very differently depending on whether one is a girl or a boy. Most of the time, nonconscious 'gendered scripts' limit the power and the agency of the *sujeito sexual* (sexual subject) as will be seen.

In the 'sexual scene' exercise, the person who tells his/her story (the main character) can put 'on stage' all the elements that build a dramatic scene:

- where he/she is (place and time where sex occurs)
- with whom (partners and relationships)
- doing what (actions during the encounter)
- scripts of the characters (each partner's point of view)
- speeches (conversation)
- gestures (communication without words)
- feelings (going to the depths of the mind and body)
- personification or concretization of norms ('invisible presence' of peers, parents, religion, gender or age, expectations, etc.)
- personification or concretization of access to condoms (that is, of salary, cost of condoms, health services providers, parents, pharmacies)
- knowledge or lack of knowledge (lack of information or misinformation or prejudices)
- power balance (possibly different in different scenes)
- the rhythm of the scene (slow or hurried).

In sum, he/she explores many competing variables that fight for the attention of the *sujeito sexual* within the sexual scene. Sexual negotiation or individual skills are *not* our focus prior to scene investigation. In the following sections, I use examples from our experiences with this framework to illustrate the gendered codes through which our participants experienced their sexuality.

The gendered reproductive and erotic body as a code

The theme most strongly emphasized among the students was the question of pregnancy. Activities focusing on reproduction were most likely to throw new light upon the meaning of different sexual scenes, and to emphasize the legitimacy of planning (being responsible for) the sexual act. The risk of undesired pregnancy is perceived as much greater than the risk of AIDS – a perception entirely understandable from the point of view of these students.[4] In one girl's words:

> I have to think about pregnancy before AIDS. If I get infected with HIV I will die – that's it. If I have a baby I have to live for me and the baby, and two of us will survive.

The students especially appreciated exercises creating models of the erotic and/or reproductive body parts with a mixture of salt, flour and water. Admiring their models (mouths, hands, breasts, genitals, female and male complete figures, buttocks, tongues, etc.) they learned how their knowledge about the body is gendered, as well as how much they do not know. Other than the penis, male reproductive organs were never modelled in any workshop, and we conducted more than a hundred with young people and a dozen with teachers. Models of the vulva are also comparatively rare. So when we put all the models in the centre of the room, we would include a complete male reproductive body made by the facilitator, and sometimes also a vulva, after discussing why they were absent. Penises and breasts were the most frequent objects produced by the students, as they represented both sensual pleasure and reproduction. According to the students, men are expected to know everything about pleasure, including female paths to pleasure – and in fact they did have a better knowledge of the female vulva than most of the women. The discoveries made, and the questions raised, through the modelling exercise were manifold:

> It was the first thing I wanted to study closely, in magazines and 'live'.
>
> (a young man)

> Pee and menstruation comes out from this hole, I think … They come both from here … Or do we have another orifice I have never noticed???
>
> (a young girl)

Yet the women were avid to learn about sex; they were more than ready to learn from the most experienced girls about pleasure, including the erotic knowledge shared by the open lesbians, as well as about reproduction and contraception. Men pretended less interest in learning about the issues unfamiliar to them, since they are supposed to already be very knowledgeable. They were not interested in, and did not value male–male sex/erotic wisdom, but did find young lesbians 'exciting'. In looking at and discussing the models, both women and men paid much attention to the explanations about how HIV could pass from one person to another. Most women knew less than we expected about reproduction and contraception, but they did know more than the men did:

> Yes, I know the most dangerous time to fuck: it is when they are having … their period, when they bleed.
>
> (a young man, reflecting the views of many men)

> Great, I learned a lot … You speak a language I can understand, this is not English![5]
>
> (a young girl)

Talking about their gender constructs (codes) – about what they know, and things they 'may and may not know or do' – we began to discuss (de-codify) gender roles and gendered scripts: the 'lady-killer/assertive/macho' man and the 'naive/passive or resisting' woman. Buttocks, for example, were frequently made during the modelling exercise, and generally accepted as both sensual and contraceptive. They were also an emerging symbol of the existence of different kinds of pleasure, both in same-sex and heterosexual relationships. It is interesting that, after the AIDS epidemic, 'homosexuality' came to be known – a new word associated with an old stigma (the passive male) – but 'heterosexual' (and 'heterosexuality') were words that needed explanation in most groups, and generally not part of the students' vocabulary.

When students named the models of vulva and penis and the related fluids, the gendered sexual scripts became rapidly obvious: men gave only 'street' names to their models, while women chose what might be described as 'family' slang (i.e., terms used by parents and their children), although they knew and some might use street names as well. The penis has 'pene-trative' and aggressive names such as 'stick' (*pau*), 'baton' (*cacete*) or 'pistol' (*pistola*) – and the slang for 'sperm' (*porra*) could be used as a noun that is synonymous with a 'hit' or a 'blow' (*porrada*). The names of animals are frequently used – 'bird', 'snake', or 'chick' for the penis, and 'spider' or 'butterfly' for the vulva. Female genitals are also known by words representing seduction ('pierced', 'pursued', 'chased'). There was no name for female vaginal fluids; the young men think that women have the same '*porra*' that they did, but without sperm. Most girls were confused about their vaginal fluids, with 'vaginal discharge' (*corrimento vaginal*) used as a generic name.[6]

When we talked about the reproductive and erotic body, we ended up discussing gender not as a cultural lens oppressive for women only, but in regard to men's oppression by gender norms and how gendered scripts made it difficult, for both men and women, to think about risks. In the imaginary sexual scenes constructed, acting as if a partner is 'dangerous' contra-dicted the need to be a 'stud', a 'lady-killer', or a 'marriageable' or 'desirable' woman, and was even more inconsistent with the idea of 'surrendering' to love or passion, or with the 'impulsive assertive male'. In the end, the students concluded the following were oppressive: for men to need to drink to get the courage to take initiative or to overcome shyness; for women to want men assertive and aggressive in order to feel valued; for women to not be able to 'choose' to say 'yes' or 'no', or to have to settle for 'any man'; for women to have to pretend ignorance, even when men might actually prefer them more assertive in the sexual intercourse.

Gendered scripts and sexual scenes

According to gender norms in the subculture of these young people, it is the responsibility of girls faced with possibilities of sex to actively choose the right person and the right moment to try to 'make love with people they love'. Female responsibility is thus placed long *before* the sexual encounter. The only skill that a young women needs is of saying 'yes' or 'no' to 'this' or 'that' partner. The consequences of a bad choice are 'natural' and expected. It is a woman's fate to be held responsible for the choice and its consequences, but not her role to be careful about practices. Boys, on the other hand, cannot easily 'decide' and 'choose' before the act of sexual consummation. To think or select is for the future. The first task is to 'relieve' sexual pressure, to be assertive and conquer sexual partners – being a lady-killer is not a simple matter. Men's choice comes after pregnancy occurs – accepting or not accepting responsi-bility for paternity. For example, in one exercise we asked boys to think about a scene in which their last sexual partner (real – or desired if they had not yet had sex) told them 'I am pregnant'. In the female groups we asked the girls to do the same, and the conversations they imagined were always similar to this:

Girl: I need to tell you something. I am pregnant.
Boy: Are you sure?
Girl: I did the test.
Boy: But how do you know the baby is mine?
Girl: You were my only man.
Boy: How can I know for sure if I am the father?

The strongest male reaction possible to this event, since condoms were not used and the baby was not planned, is to say 'the baby is not mine!' In exercise after exercise, somebody would indeed say this, and male participants would stick to it as a symbol of what they felt. In the girls' group, a girl playing the boy's role in the same scene would repeat the same widely expected phrases. Only 33 per cent of men we interviewed in this project said they need to love a sexual partner to have sex, but 88 per cent of the women said love was required. On the other hand, women did not feel they had to love or marry their sexual partner to have a baby, while most men said they needed to love the woman to become a father of her child – but then would, even if it were another's child.

Among both the young men and the young women, responsibility for the consequences of the sexual act was always represented by pregnancy, not by HIV infection. For participants in the sexual scene, the possibility of babies out of an idealized context was more likely than HIV to foster responsibility or provide the incentive for avoiding being overcome by emotions – passion, lust, fear of abandonment or labelling, haste, and so on – emotions themselves symbolic of individual histories entangled with cultural regulations. In the sexual scenes these factors competed for the subject's attention, breaking his/her volition and intentions. In one young man's words, they 'prevent one from thinking or putting a condom on'.

Yet, the young people would panic at the idea of not having babies. During group meetings, for example, lesbians or 'sterile' women (never male figures) are mentioned as spectres of infertility. The primary meaning of a baby was not – as the Brazilian elite usually suppose of the poor – to have more arms to work, or to provide support during old age. It is to make up for lack of citizenship and disenfranchisement: 'My child will, first of all, have all that I did not have, and then be what I was not or do what I did not do' in a young man's words. The child represents the possibility of a better future – one that, in accord with much social research in Brazil, is perceived as the effort of an entire family rather than an individual achievement. The child the parent(s) will love and take care of will define and fulfil the future, give meaning to a hard adult life. And this adult life, for the majority, has already begun; the students speak of a youth that passed too quickly, of a life marked by tragic events that take hope away, or of worthless events.[7] For the young men, the right to decide when to have children, and the idea that they too are entitled to this right, are new concepts. They are used to feeling mere objects of women's decisions in this regard – an accurate perception, in some ways, of the female fertility revolution in Brazil, accomplished in large part through birth control pills and irresponsible mass sterilization – 'She is guilty, she is a traitor, she makes me have an adult life before I wanted or decided to'. When we suggested that condom use could give them the ability to negotiate their reproductive life, the young men said this was, in their opinion, the most convincing argument for condom use that they had heard during the entire programme.

In another study (see Paiva, 1995), we found these feelings and responses understood, but not shared, by more educated or higher-income college students of the same age. This research showed that undergraduate students had a more egalitarian gender culture and different paths to adulthood than the poorer, younger night-school students interviewed in the current study. They started to work and to have a sexual life later than low-income, less educated young people – on average, two years later for both men and women.[8] Having children carried different meaning and value in groups of different status. Less than 4.5 per cent of the students in either group studied are married, but 25 per cent of the elementary school students, versus 2 per cent of the college students in the same age group, 'wish to have children in the next two years'. This difference was highly significant, and there was no significant difference between males and females in the same group. College men thought and felt the same way as their poorer peers when confronted with the pregnancy announcement – 'Is it mine?' – even though they controlled their feelings and were less likely to act them out; however, college women in the same role-playing exercise would never anticipate, and were quite surprised by this unspeakable male sentiment. The night-school students were more likely to act on their attitude, ending the relationship, to escape responsibility and/or guilt, but if they were in more regular or formal relationships, would sometimes try to behave differently. And when they would change roles and play the women, all of the men recognized the woman's right to be enraged with their attitude – although the role-playing changed no male night-school students' basic attitude, and the college men remained more prompted to self-reflection.

College students generally had greater knowledge about reproduction, contraception, and modes of HIV transmission, with no significant gender differences in levels of knowledge and information. Sexual intercourse with anal penetration (a high-risk practice) began earlier for night-school students, and 32 per cent of them did not see it as risky, while only 1 per cent of college students said it is not risky. In the workshops, we learned that anal sex as a means to avoid pregnancy was confused among night-school students with a supposed efficacy of anal sex in avoiding HIV infection – an idea of course absolutely incorrect. And, as was described above, the anus is seen as both sensuous and contraceptive.

College women and men tended to balance their decision-making power over sex,[9] and they were more likely to believe that their friends often used condoms. Night-school students found it significantly more difficult to negotiate condom use than university students, and 33 per cent of night-school students, versus 18 per cent of the university undergraduates, *never* wanted to tell the partner to use condoms. Among the night-school students, relatively higher home income was strongly associated with condom use, which was never associated with race, religion, or district of residence.

Our research showed, in short, that income and education produce different sexual scenarios, different gendered scripts, and different sexual scenes in the same city and among the same age group. This helps to explain epidemiological data showing how disenfranchised people are disproportionably vulnerable to HIV. Prevention programmes should address this vulnerability, which cannot be characterized as simply an individual's deficit in knowledge, motivation or skills, possible to correct through behavioural interventions based on models of individual behaviour change. Paraphrasing Diaz (1997, 2000), prevention programmes aimed at and focused on 'changing behaviour' (such as the social marketing of condoms or skills-building training sessions), but which fail to take into account deeply internalized cultural meanings and socio-economic contexts, are doomed to fail.

The sexual scene as a code and the sexual subject

Throughout the prevention programme, using the 'sexual scene' to identify the difference between intentions to practise safer sex and actual enactment helped students understand and challenge social and cultural regulations. Along with the 'dough exercise' (as the students called it) described above, which enabled them to decode their gendered sexual culture and to actively raise their AIDS and reproduction literacy, linking the ideas of the sexual subject and citizenship to the 'sexual scene' was, we found, the best instrument for decoding the obstacles to individual enactment (and self-regulation) as well as community organizing.

The 'sexual scene' programme has worked primarily through actual scenes from the students' lives, with every element concretized or personified in the scene through group collaboration. Figure 23.1 shows one schematic example of the use of the 'sexual scene':

> I was going to a party, in my young uncle's car. I saw a girl in a black mini-blouse, standing there. I asked: 'Where are you going?' She said she was going to meet a guy, but he didn't come. I invited her to a wedding. I said: 'I am a family guy'. She came … We danced the whole night. We began petting … I drank. We went outside. We had to come back at 5:00 a.m. to catch the ride back. When we came back, I was in the back of the car, a little drunk … my uncle in the front … I opened her zipper, and we had sex. I am dating Mônica now for six months, now we use condoms because of pregnancy, but at that night I did not think of anything …

Talking about this with Reinaldo, the group investigated meanings, identifying and personifying the conflicting factors in these events. These are some of the key elements that the group felt were important in the scene:

> Reinaldo and Monica did not have a *place* to have sex other than a car. He would have had *money* to buy a *condom* (but *not* for *every time* …). Yet, at this *hour* there was no place to go buy a condom, and the most important thing was to *conquer* her. The only other thing in his mind was the effect of the *alcohol*. When Reinaldo switched roles in order to act out *her script* in that scene, Mônica would *not think of HIV*, but *only pregnancy*, and she had her period the day before. She would never *spend her salary buying condoms*, but would rather use the money to buy bus tickets (the same price) since she was going to work on foot some days, and being late to her night-school classes because of budget shortfalls. She *feels bad and guilty* about having sex in a car, with someone else listening. Reinaldo would not. But she was *in love*, he was *handsome*, and there was *no other place to go*. She was in a *hurry* to finish it, as was he: he liked her, and wanted to *relieve his urge. Later, after this first date, if they had begun to have a steady relationship, the scenes take on other meaning as well as new obstacles.* They would have to find some *moment* in one of their houses (which both have only one bedroom for all of the family members to share) when nobody would be there, and *make love quickly*, or do it *in dark streets of the neighbourhood, as does everybody else.*

The story teller and the group would de-codify every element in the scene and discuss how to solve the puzzle. Our goal was not simply to train sexual negotiation skills through role-playing, although when a trained 'facilitator' was leading the group, we might use a particular scene as a model, acted out and performed differently numerous times, as skills trainers do. But our focus was broader, we were trying to foster group collaboration with the person who

Step 1   Step 2

scene-observation + self-observation

Step 3

group processing and collaboration + group mobilization

Step 4

sexual subject (*sujeito*) + increasing citizenship

Figure 23.1 Schematic example of the use of the 'sexual scene'

offered the narrative, to help him/her, as well as each member of the group, to become a subject of his/her intentions.

We used self-observation and scene-observation to help the students understand what was individual responsibility and what was a role of context that might be better transformed by social organizing and mobilization – the difference between self-regulation following self-observation, such as deciding for abstinence, and self-regulation plus social agency, such as demanding condom distribution in the health clinic. At the end of workshops, our final question was always 'All right, you have the information. Suppose you have decided to choose when to have your child and to prevent an undesired pregnancy, or to protect yourselves against HIV. Is it fair to say that you have the material conditions and support necessary to practise safe sex?' In response to this question, in 1994 some elementary students involved in the project tested out available services in reproductive health and in sexually transmitted infection and AIDS prevention and treatment. Their experience brought out striking examples, which they shared with the group, of the precariousness of the public health system in São Paulo, the richest city in Brazil. Some of their stories:

> One 20 year-old girl had reached an excellent level of communication with her mother concerning sex and contraception as a result of this programme. The mother and daughter talked and decided that whenever the daughter was ready for sex, she would seek out the health service for medical orientation about contraception before the 'first time'. When she and her boyfriend made the decision to have sex, she went to the public health centre to consult with the doctor and was told: 'Why don't you just remain virgin? Men do not like women who have already slept with someone', and the like.[10]

She was interviewed on the way out of this consultation by a group of students and felt furious and impotent. If she were a middle-class college student, she would have changed doctors. What can one do when one depends on a public health clinic? This is part of her and the other students' actual sexual scene and its social and cultural regulations.

> One young man, encouraged by the work we did, sought a family planning public service. He was not admitted at the weekly meeting because 'only women are admitted at these meetings'. While on a consultation with a urologist to ask for guidance on contraception and sexually transmitted infections at a different health service, he was kicked out because he 'did not have any problem [disease] and was wasting the doctor's time for no reason at all'. There was no one in line, the service facility was empty and the young man left, suspecting racism.

This young man, an active black activist at his Catholic base community, died of kidney insufficiency a year later, after waiting unsuccessfully for a kidney transplant. Given such occurrences it is not surprising that young men and women prefer to self-medicate, or to deny health problems, rather than to receive mostly bad service from the public health system, where they feel helpless and denied their citizenship. This young man's case was the only point in our programme where racism/race was ever mentioned as a key social and cultural regulation variable; otherwise, race never came up itself explicitly in the group dynamics, and only 0.5 per cent of the men and women in our sample said that ethnic background is relevant when you consider a sexual partner or a date. The sample included 45 per cent white Brazilians, 47 per cent black/brown Brazilians, 6.5 per cent Asian Brazilians, and 1.5 per cent Native Brazilians, but there were no significant differences in attitudes, knowledge or practices among students from these different ethnic groups, whereas, as already noted, education and income variations did impact these.

> A boy and a girl pretended they were a couple in order to be accepted in the 'family planning' group, where the doctor (a woman) said the condom was not reliable as a method, and recommended only hormonal methods; she also did not know how to put a condom on. The 'couple' asked permission to perform the 'condom on a cucumber' demonstration that they had learned in the workshop, and it was enthusiastically received by the group. The doctor then said that the clinic would have free condoms. The 'couple' came back another day and the nurse said the condoms were there but passed their expiration date, and that she would not be responsible, but would give the condoms to them anyway ... This clinic had, for months, no condoms available.

Contraceptives and condoms were rarely available in the students' sexual scenes. The places where they had sex (dark corners, cars, common areas in huge buildings, or at home when other family members were temporarily out of the house) led to hurried sexual activity. They share small household spaces with many people and cannot afford motel rooms. There were few contraceptive options, and abortion, which was and is illegal, was referred to as 'hell'. What resources can these youth draw on for encouragement and support in the radical changes they needed to accomplish – especially with the HIV/AIDS epidemic rapidly increasing among the poor – to avoid unprotected sex?

For a person to be a subject, to feel capable, there is a need for experience not separated from day-to-day experience. Being a sexual subject is neither a skill nor a behaviour that can be trained in a workshop. It is *reflected experience that generates the subject* and that builds up cognitive structures and levels of functioning more fluid and dynamic than previous ones. If conditions for experimentation are limited by collective forces – social, cultural, economic – that cannot be confronted or conciliated, the feeling of impotence will always be greater than the feeling of power or perceived self-efficacy.

Some youth we have worked with begin this experimentation not through sexual negotiation or individual skills-training, but through initiatives related first and foremost to citizenship: investigating the public health system and services for young people; investigating different sexual networks and subcultures in their neighbourhood; demanding free condoms in the clinics; demanding value-free counselling about sexually transmitted diseases, HIV/AIDS, and contraception; creating a play about abortion and reproductive rights; demanding male acceptance in family planning counselling meetings; suggesting that dancing halls should distribute condoms as well as alcohol.

The key question we need to address with this approach is how we can promote safer sex without adding another burden to the already heavy fatalism that the youth carry from other 'failures', which the elite attempt to ascribe to a 'lack of individual enterprise/effort', or (when racist) the congenital 'limitations' of *nordestinos* (northeasterners, who make up the majority of the poor, immigrant population in southeastern Brazilian cities such as São Paulo). Hence the need to go beyond the notion of 'natural sex', or 'the power of hormones' or the description of a universal adolescence or uniform gender culture. Decoding the sexual scene with all the socio-economic and cultural elements is a path to consciousness-raising (*conscientização*).

Conclusion

The first 'safe sex workshops' we conducted in this community were positively evaluated by the participants, teachers, and parents. We were able to confirm attitude changes showing more flexible values concerning sex and/or traditional gender roles, more confidence in the reliability of condoms, and the broadening of risk perception. Nevertheless, such changes are not easy to accomplish, and do not guarantee consistent safer sex, as the students reported in the evaluation follow-up process, where they provided examples of how social-cultural regulations are hard barriers to overcome.

When we are collaborating with young people of lower status in practising safe sex, if we do not examine the social and economic limits of our own proposals (for example, 'Use condoms!' 'Be healthy!'), the novelty of AIDS becomes no more than a new risk, a new item in a life that is already marked by one's dealings with adversity, by the numerous tragic events, by the violence of everyday life, by financial instability, by other diseases long eradicated from a richer world, by housing problems, and – in Brazilian terms – by a lack of citizenship. Nor is it possible to think that our task is accomplished simply by informing these students about the new risk of AIDS and about safer sex and making them 'individually responsible'. Understanding that risk perception, perceived self-efficacy, and commitment to change are entangled in social and cultural regulations, we have been able to recognize over the course of the programme that, most of the time, risky sex is not an individual deficit or responsibility.

We broadened the traditional focus on behavioural change, focus groups, and marketing approaches – in which the social and cultural context is typically used (by 'experts') to plan their products and to determine the best language to successfully 'sell' these products to target populations (in turn allowing the 'experts' to create models of behaviour change based upon measurable outcomes).

Many AIDS prevention programmes have used well-intentioned social research to investigate meanings, attitudes, and prevalence of behaviours and to formulate innovative language to preach condom use and safer sex – desirable outcomes, of course. The problem is how to substitute these outcomes-to-be-modelled with more politicized popular education approaches, in which social and cultural factors are understood and illuminated *from the community perspective*. If social and cultural factors are not challenged, we will neither foster the sexual subject, nor decrease the heavy fatalism and powerlessness of isolated individuals facing an impenetrable reality – and the result will be that communities in developing countries will, like the poor and marginalized communities of developed countries, continue to see AIDS as just another burden among the many that they already carry.

After observing how AIDS, sexual meanings, power hierarchies, and gendered scripts have been codified, we must de-codify them and highlight the internal contradictions in each sexual culture. These contradictions are the open doors for agency, for individual and group cultural innovation (Paiva, 1990). We agree that the individual history and the permanent process of transformation that we experience, including in personal identity, may bring different tones and rhythms to sexual life as we age; the meaning of sex is different at each stage in life, with each type of bond, and with each partner, and depends upon whether one is a woman or a man, feels part of a sexual community or not, is rich or poor (Gagnon and Simon, 1973). But our focus should not be individual responsibility, but the context in which individuals must act. To help disenfranchised young people feel less 'clueless', less fatalist, consciousness-building or consciousness-raising must show how both gendered scripts and the socio-economic context in which sex occurs take away the agency of the individual and the power of the sexual subject.

We worked on this project to encourage AIDS prevention based upon real life, real experience, the language of daily life, the creativity of art and popular religiosity. We have used real emotions, felt by real people, in real contexts and scenarios, all voluntarily shared – rather than celebrities playing at marketing and trying to 'model' safer sex behaviours as in the Ministry of Health campaigns that are shown on Brazilian television. Without *conscientização*, safer-sex workshops are a resource-intensive programme that can be successful only with the middle class, which will find the resources and social support to fulfil its intentions.

We should insist on interactive AIDS education proposals in which the educator is more of an instigator of problems and a source of information than a problem-solver. Yet we must assume that our work does not finish at the end of meetings, sessions, or classes. Any experienced activist (or therapist) knows that change depends upon a long course of trials, rehearsals, and challenges against habitual personal and social environments. And in contexts such as Brazil, it is not feasible to offer individual counselling and clinical interventions for millions of people, to produce the revolution that we need to stop this epidemic. Similarly, we cannot wait for some sort of vague 'empowerment' prior to beginning any work on AIDS prevention. We need to do both.

Real AIDS prevention will depend on a new pedagogy and on activist wisdom rather than on depoliticized models of behavioural change, universal psychological theories, or vague statements about powerlessness. Psychological theories can give us many insights, as can the social sciences. But to collaborate with impoverished communities, we need more than clinical approaches, more than generic speeches about health, sermons about condom use. The urgency of this epidemic calls for the less simplistic approaches of liberation pedagogy, and demands political coherence in the implementation of these approaches. In countries such as Brazil, as in other countries and communities around the world, it is life-wasting luxury not to derive political action from educational action. It is more effective and faster, from the life-saving standpoint, to consider activism or advocacy *a built-in part of our approach to AIDS education*, encouraging personal power by agents of political action – and in turn encouraging sexual agency.

As Paulo Freire would say, 'Turn the question around: while education is not the lever for social transformation, transformation itself is an educational event. Transformation teaches us, shapes and reshapes us' (Shor and Freire, 1987).

Acknowledgments

Special thanks to Richard Parker, who was a wonderful mentor and friend during the whole project that is reported on here – and a perfect partner for this final version of the text. Thanks also to Sara Skinner, Norman Hearst, Rafael Diaz, Peter Aggleton, and Charles Klein for suggestions on the translation of the text to English and comments on the original version presented at the Rio seminar.

Notes

1 São Paulo has over 200,000 night-school students. To study in a night school, students must be over fourteen years old. Ninety per cent of these students work in a paid job or at home during the day.

2 A short description of the workshop was published in English in *AIDS Action*, Issue 25, Newsletter by ARTHAG, London, 1994. The participants are all the night students, 14 to 21 years old, of four different districts in São Paulo. The programme consisted of individual interviews, long workshops (five three-hour sessions), group evaluation sessions, individual counselling, and community organizing initiatives. As part of the project, approximately 3,500 older night-school students participated in a shorter version (six hours) of this workshop. We have trained teachers and health services providers in these districts.

3 Our reading of these issues draws heavily on the conception of gender and sexual systems as defined by Gayle Rubin (1984), active/passive relations as defined by Peter Fry (1982) and Richard Parker (1991, 1999), and erotic scripts as defined by Richard Parker (1991).

4 As I have already argued elsewhere (see Paiva, 1993), it is irrational to approach sexuality with separate programmes, yet family planning and reproductive health are separate programmes from AIDS prevention in most countries.

5 'Not English' would be the equivalent of 'not Greek'.

6 For an extended discussion of the gendered language of the body in Brazil, see Parker (1991).

7 In in-depth interviews the students say things like: 'Since I was twelve, I have had an adult memory', or 'I had a very hard young life for my age of thirteen'. When we asked them to begin the interview 'tell me about your life', the first idea that occurred to most of them was that they have nothing to tell us (since we are privileged people from the university). What is important in their lives are bad things, tragic experiences. For the most part, they choose a tragic event to talk about. Only 10 per cent of them describe their lives as 'beautiful, calm or nice'.

8 To study how education (highly correlated with income) shapes gender differences in sexual meanings, we compared primary night-school students with college students, taking a sub-sample of young men and women from 17 to 21 years old.

9 No college woman responded 'I never decide what to do in sexual intercourse' and no college man responded 'I always decide' – the two extreme alternatives. On the other hand, 30 per cent of the night-school women responded that they 'never' decide and 9 per cent of the men said 'I always decide'.

10 We had trained most of the health professionals at this health service, as in many others in the area. But only nurses or social workers, mostly women, would come to the training. We never had a male doctor come to a training session on adolescents and HIV prevention and reproductive choices.

References

ALTMAN, D. (1994) *Power and Community: Organizational and Cultural Responses to AIDS*, London: Taylor and Francis.

CATANIA, J. *et al.* (1990) 'AIDS risk reduction model', *Health Education Quarterly*, 17(1), pp. 53–72.

DANIEL, H., and PARKER, R. (1993) *Sexuality, Politics and AIDS in Brazil*, London: The Falmer Press.

DIAZ, R.M. (1997) *Latino Men and HIV: Culture, Sexuality and Risk Behavior*, New York and London: Routledge.

—— (2000) 'Cultural regulation, self-regulation and sexuality: a psycho-cultural model of HIV risk in gay men', in PARKER, R., BARBOSA, R.M. and AGGLETON, P. (eds), *Framing the Sexual Subject: The Politics of Gender, Sexuality and Power*, Berkeley and Los Angeles: University of California Press.

FREIRE, P. (1983), *Education for Critical Consciousness*, New York: Continuum Press.

—— (1993) *Pedagogy of the Oppressed*, New York: Continuum Press.

FRY, P. (1982) *Para Inglês Ver: Identidade e Política na Cultura Brasiliera*, Rio de Janeiro: Zahar Editores.

Gagnon, J. and SIMON, W. (1973) *Sexual Conduct: The Social Sources of Human Sexuality*, Chicago: Aldine.

IRVINE, J. (1994) 'Cultural differences and adolescent sexualities', in IRVINE, J. (ed.), *Sexual Cultures and the Construction of Adolescent Identities*, Philadelphia, PA: Temple University Press.

LURIE, P., HINTZEN, P. and LOWE, R. (1995) 'Socioeconomic obstacles to HIV prevention and treatment in developing countries: the role of the International Monetary Fund and the World Bank', *AIDS*, 9, pp. 539–46.

MANN, J., TARANTOLA, D. and NETTER, T. (eds) (1992) *AIDS in the World*, Cambridge, MA: Harvard University Press.

PAIVA, V. (1990) *As voltas do feminino*, São Paulo: Brasiliense.

—— (ed.) (1992) *Em tempos de AIDS*, São Paulo: Summus.

—— (1993) 'Sexuality, condom use and gender norms among Brazilian teenagers', *Reproductive Health Matters*, 1(2), pp. 98–110.

—— (1994) 'Sexualidade e genero num trabalho com adolescentes para a prevenção do HIV/AIDS' in PARKER, R., *et al.* (eds), *A AIDS no Brasil*, Rio de Janeiro: Editora Relume-Dumará/IMS-UERJ/ABIA.

—— (1995) 'Sexuality, AIDS and gender norms', in HERDT, G., and TEN BRUMMELHUIS, H. (eds), *Culture and Sexual Risk: Anthropological Perspective on AIDS*, New York and London: Gordon and Breach.

PARKER, R.G. (1991) *Bodies, Pleasures and Passions: Sexual Culture in Contemporary Brazil*, Boston, MA: Beacon Press.

—— (1994) *A construção da solidariedade*, Rio de Janeiro: Editora Relume-Dumará/IMS-UERJ/ABIA.

—— (1996) 'Empowerment, community mobilization, and social change in the face of HIV/AIDS', *AIDS*, 10, Suppl 3, pp. S27–S31.

—— (1999) *Beneath the Equator: Cultures of Desire, Male Homosexuality, and Emerging Gay Communities in Brazil*, New York and London: Routledge.

RUBIN, G. (1984) 'Thinking sex: notes for a radical theory of the politics of sexuality', in VANCE, C. (ed.), *Pleasure and Danger: Exploring Female Sexuality*, London: Routledge & Kegan Paul.

SHOR, I. and FREIRE, P. (1987) *A Pedagogy for Liberation: Dialogues on Transforming Education*, Westport, CT: Bergin & Garvey.

24 HIV- and AIDS-related stigma and discrimination

A conceptual framework and implications for action

Richard Parker and Peter Aggleton [2003]

For nearly two decades, as countries all over the world have struggled to respond to the HIV/AIDS epidemic, issues of stigma, discrimination and denial have been poorly understood and often marginalized within national and international programmes and responses. In some ways this is paradoxical, since concern about the deleterious effects of HIV- and AIDS-related stigma has been voiced since the mid-1980s. In 1987, for example, Jonathan Mann, the founding Director of the World Health Organization's former Global Programme on AIDS, addressed the United Nations General Assembly. In what would soon become a widely accepted conceptualization, he distinguished between three phases of the AIDS epidemic in any community. The first of these phases was the epidemic of HIV infection – an epidemic that typically enters every community silently and unnoticed, and often develops over many years without being widely perceived or understood. The second phase was the epidemic of AIDS itself – the syndrome of infectious diseases that can occur because of HIV infection, but typically only after a delay of a number of years. Finally, he described the third epidemic, potentially the most explosive – the epidemic of social, cultural, economic and political responses to AIDS. This was characterized, above all, by exceptionally high levels of stigma, discrimination and, at times, collective denial that, to use Mann's words, 'are as central to the global AIDS challenge as the disease itself' (Mann, 1987).

By 1995, WHO/GPA had been superseded by the Joint United Nations Programme on HIV/AIDS (UNAIDS), bringing together six different United Nations agencies with the explicit goal of recognizing the multiple social dimensions of the epidemic. Yet when Peter Piot, the Executive Director of UNAIDS, addressed the 10th meeting of the agency's Programme Coordinating Board in December of 2000, he turned in his concluding remarks to outline what he described as 'the continuing challenge'. Top of his list of 'the five most pressing items on this agenda for the world community' was the need for a 'renewed effort to combat stigma'. He went on to emphasize, 'this calls for an all out effort, by leaders and by each of us personally. Effectively addressing stigma removes what still stands as a roadblock to concerted action, whether at local community, national or global level' (Piot, 2000). More recently still, HIV- and AIDS-related stigma and discrimination have been chosen as the theme for the 2002–03 World AIDS Campaign, highlighting the continuing pertinence of these concerns both conceptually and programmatically.

At least in part, our collective inability to more adequately confront stigmatization, discrimination and denial in relation to HIV and AIDS is linked to the relatively limited theoretical and methodological tools available to us. It is important, therefore, to critically evaluate the available literature on the study of stigma and discrimination, both independent of HIV/AIDS and more specifically in relation to it, in order to develop a more adequate conceptual framework for thinking about the nature of these processes, for analysing the ways in which they work in relation to HIV and AIDS, and for pointing to possible interventions that might minimize their impact and their prejudicial effects in relation to the epidemic.

Stigmatization and discrimination as social processes

Much of what has been written about stigma and discrimination in the context of HIV and AIDS has emphasized the complexity of these phenomena, and has attributed our inability to respond to them more effectively to both their complex nature and their high degree of diversity in different cultural settings. As a recent USAID Concept Paper put it: 'The problem is a difficult one, because underlying the apparent universality of the problem of HIV/AIDS-related [stigma, discrimination and denial] there appears to be a diversity and complexity that makes it difficult to grasp in a programmatically useful way' (USAID, 2000).

While it is important to recognize that stigma and discrimination are characterized by cross-cultural diversity and complexity, one of the major factors limiting our understanding of these phenomena may well be less their inherent complexity than the relative simplicity of existing conceptual frameworks. To make serious progress in analysing and responding to these phenomena, it may therefore be necessary not only to attend to their cross-cultural complexity and specificity, but to rethink some of the taken-for-granted frameworks within which we are encouraged to understand them.

Typically, discussions of stigma, particularly in relation to HIV and AIDS, have taken as their point of departure the now classic work of Goffman (1963), defining stigma as 'an attribute that is significantly discrediting' which, in the eyes of society, serves to reduce the person who possesses it. Drawing on research experience with people suffering from mental illness, possessing physical deformities, or practising what were perceived to be socially deviant behaviours such as homosexuality or criminal behaviour, Goffman (1963) argued that the stigmatized individual is thus seen to be a person who possesses 'an undesirable difference'. He argued that stigma is conceptualized by society on the basis of what constitutes 'difference' or 'deviance', and that it is applied by society through rules and sanctions resulting in what he described as a kind of 'spoiled identity' for the person concerned (Goffman, 1963).

Useful and important as Goffman's formulations of this problem were, a fuller understanding of stigmatization, at least as it functions in the context of HIV/AIDS, requires us to unpack this analytic category – and to rethink the directions that it has pushed us in our research and intervention work. Above all, the emphasis placed by Goffman on stigma as a 'discrediting attribute' has led to a focus on stigma as though it were a kind of thing (in particular, a cultural or even individual value) – a relatively static characteristic or feature, albeit one that is at some level culturally constructed. The emphasis Goffman's work gave to possessing an 'undesirable difference' that leads to a 'spoiled identity', in turn, has encouraged highly individualized analyses in which words come to characterize people in relatively unmediated fashion. Thus stigma, understood as a negative attribute, is mapped onto people, who in turn, by virtue of their difference, are understood to be negatively valued in society. It is important to recognize that neither of these emphases is in fact drawn directly from Goffman, who, on the contrary, was very much concerned with issues of social change and the social construction of individual realities. Indeed, one reading of Goffman's work might suggest that, as a formal concept, stigmatization devalues relationships rather than being a fixed attribute. Yet the fact that Goffman's framework has been appropriated in much research on stigma (whether in relation to HIV/AIDS or other issues), as though stigma were a static attitude rather than a constantly changing (and often resisted) social process has seriously limited the ways in which stigmatization and discrimination have been approached in relation to HIV and AIDS.

In the years that have passed since the publication of Goffman's influential study, the research literature on stigma has grown rapidly. The concept of stigma has been applied to an exceptionally wide range of different circumstances, particularly in relation to health, ranging from leprosy (Opala and Boillot, 1996), to cancer (Fife and Wright, 2000), urinary incontinence (Sheldon and Caldwell, 1994), and mental illness (Corrigan and Penn, 1999; Phelan *et al.*, 2000).[1] This literature has included refinements of Goffman's original formulation, elaborations on the themes that he first raised, and extensive demonstrations of the impacts that stigmatization can have on the lives of those who are affected by it.

Probably, the largest percentage of this rapidly expanding literature has come from social psychologists who have used social-cognitive approaches in order to examine the ways in which individuals construct categories and incorporate these categories in stereotypical beliefs (see Crocker, Major and Steele, 1998; Link and Phelan, 2001). Yet much of this work too has suffered from serious conceptual limitations – even the definition of stigma has typically been exceptionally vague and highly variable (see Link and Phelan, 2001). Indeed, in much of the existing literature on stigma, investigators provide no definition at all, or seem to refer to something like a dictionary definition – 'a mark of disgrace', or some similar aspect such as stereotyping or social rejection. When definitions are offered, they have been relatively limited. Stafford and Scott (1986, p. 80), for example, have written of stigma as 'a characteristic of persons that is contrary to a norm of a social unit'. Crocker *et al.* (1998, p. 505) argue that people who are stigmatized 'possess (or are believed to possess) some attribute, or characteristic, that conveys a social identity that is devalued in a particular social context'. Jones *et al.* (1984) have argued that stigma is a 'mark' that links a person to undesirable characteristics such as stereotypes.

In addition to the problems involved in defining stigma, perhaps in part because of the strong social-cognitive focus adopted, there has been an individualistic emphasis in much of what has been published. The central thrust of much research has been on the perceptions of individuals and the consequences of these perceptions for social interactions (see Oliver, 1992; Link and Phelan, 2001). Much work has tended to focus on stereotyping rather than on the structural conditions that produce exclusion from social and economic life, and social psychological analyses have often transformed perceived stigmas into marks or attributes of persons (see Fine and Asch, 1988; Fiske, 1998; Link and Phelan, 2001). In this case, stigma comes to be seen as something *in* the person stigmatized, rather than as a designation that others attach *to* that individual (Link and Phelan, 2001).

These tendencies have in large part been reproduced and extended in much of the research that has been carried out on stigma in relation to HIV and AIDS.[2] As in the broader literature on stigma, much work on HIV- and AIDS-related stigmatization has tended to understand stigma in highly emotional terms – for example, as 'anger and other negative feelings' toward people living with HIV and AIDS, that in turn leads to 'the belief that they deserve their illness, avoidance and ostracism, and support for coercive public policies that threaten their human rights' (see Herek, Capitanio and Widaman, 2002; see also Blendon, Donelan and Knox, 1992; Crandall, Glor and Britt, 1997; Crawford, 1996; Goldin, 1994; Green, 1995; Herek, 1990; Herek and Capitanio, 1993, 1997; Kelly *et al.*, 1987; Tewksbury and McGaughey, 1997). Other research has focused on 'stigmatizing attitudes' and the extent to which such attitudes are correlated with misunderstandings and misinformation concerning the modes of HIV transmission or the risk of infection through everyday social contact (Herek, Capitanio and Widaman, 2002, p. 371; see also Herek and Capitanio, 1994, 1997;

Herek and Glunt, 1991; Stipp and Kerr, 1989), or with 'negative attitudes' toward the groups that are believed to be disproportionately affected by the epidemic, such as gay and bisexual men, injecting drug users or sex workers (see Herek, Capitanio and Widaman, 2002, p. 371; see also Herek and Capitanio, 1998; Pryor *et al.*, 1989; St Lawrence *et al.* 1990).

Given this point of departure, it is perhaps not surprising that much of the empirical research that has been carried out on stigma in relation to HIV and AIDS thus far has tended to focus heavily on the beliefs and attitudes of those who are perceived to stigmatize others. Public opinion polls and surveys of knowledge, attitudes and beliefs about HIV and AIDS, those affected by the epidemic, or those perceived to be at risk of HIV infection have dominated the research literature (see, for example, Blendon and Donelan, 1988; Blendon *et al.*, 1992; Herek, 1999; Herek and Capitanio, 1993, 1994, 1997, 1999; Herek and Glunt, 1991; Herek, Capitanio and Widaman, 2002; Price and Hsu, 1992; Singer, Rogers and Corcoran, 1987; Stipp and Kerr, 1989). Both randomized samples and convenience samples have been used in such research, but almost always with the intent of investigating the emotional responses of the target population groups: 'negative feelings toward PWAs'; 'responsibility and blame'; 'discomfort'; and similar emotional responses are among the frequently investigated categories in seeking to assess levels of stigma existing in different population groups (see, for example, Herek, Capitanio and Widaman, 2002). These emotional responses, in turn, are often linked to beliefs concerning the facts of HIV transmission – understandings of how the virus is transmitted, and, typically, misunderstandings about how it is not (see Herek, Capitanio and Widaman, 2002). 'Correct' as opposed to 'incorrect' beliefs thus become the defining cause of stigmatization in relation to people living with HIV and AIDS, as well as of those perceived to be associated with the epidemic in a variety of different ways.

This basic approach to conceptualizing and investigating stigma in relation to HIV and AIDS has had important consequences, in turn, for the primary forms of intervening in response to stigma and stigmatization. The vast majority of the interventions that have been developed and evaluated in the research literature in order to respond to stigma related to HIV and AIDS have been aimed at increasing 'tolerance' of people with AIDS on the part of different segments of the 'general population'. While the specific segments of the amorphous general population that have been targeted for intervention have varied significantly – ranging from psychology or nursing students in North America (Batson *et al.*, 1997; Wyness, Goldstone and Trussler, 1996) to pregnant women in Scotland (Simpson *et al.*, 1998), immigrants in Israel (Soskolne *et al.*, 1993), or commercial farmers and their employers in Zimbabwe (Kerry and Margie, 1996) – the key approaches have been remarkably similar. Strategies have been developed to 'increase empathy and altruism' and to 'reduce anxiety and fear' primarily by providing what is perceived to be correct information and by developing psychological skills thought to be essential to more effective management of the emotional responses that are thought to be unleashed by HIV and AIDS as encountered by these different population groups (see Ashworth *et al.*, 1994; Hue and Kauffman, 1998; Mwambu, 1998; Soskolne *et al.*, 1993). Different interventions have thus focused on psychological counselling approaches (Kaleeba *et al.*, 1997; Kerry and Margie, 1996; Kikonyogo *et al.*, 1996; Simpson *et al.*, 1998) and increasing contact with people living with HIV and AIDS on the part of those with little direct experience of the epidemic (Batson *et al.*, 1997; Bean *et al.*, 1989; Herek and Capitanio, 1997) – and on acquiring 'coping skills' in order to better manage the effects of stigmatization on the part of those living with HIV and AIDS (see Brown, Trujillo and Macintyre, 2001).

Interestingly, while references to stigma and stigmatization in work on HIV and AIDS typically acknowledge Goffman and his work as intellectual precursors, discussions of discrimination are rarely framed in relation to any theoretical tradition whatsoever (even when discussed, as is often the case, in tandem with the discussion of stigma). The meaning of discrimination is normally taken almost for granted, as though it were given or obvious on the basis of simple common usage.

As the *Oxford Dictionary of Sociology* stipulates, however, '[t]his concept – which in common usage means simply "treating unfairly" – occurs most commonly in sociology in the context of theories of ethnic and race relations. Early sociologists viewed discrimination as an expression of ethnocentrism – in other words a cultural phenomenon of "dislike of the unlike"' (Marshall, 1998). More recent sociological analyses of discrimination, however, 'concentrate on patterns of dominance and oppression, viewed as expressions of a struggle for power and privilege' (Marshall, 1998).[3]

This sociological emphasis on the structural dimensions of discrimination is particularly useful in helping us think more sensibly about HIV- and AIDS-related stigmatization and discrimination. To move beyond the limitations of current thinking in this area, we need to reframe our understandings of stigmatization and discrimination to conceptualize them as social processes that can only be understood in relation to broader notions of *power* and *domination*. In our view, stigma plays a key role in producing and reproducing relations of power and control. It causes some groups to be devalued and others to feel that they are superior in some way. Ultimately, therefore, stigma is linked to the workings of *social inequality* and to properly understand issues of stigmatization and discrimination, whether in relation to HIV and AIDS or any other issue, requires us to think more broadly about how some individuals and groups come to be socially excluded, and about the forces that create and reinforce exclusion in different settings.

Much work exists within the social and political sciences that is directly relevant to this task, but so far little of this has been utilized in HIV/AIDS research.[4] This, we suspect, is the result of stigma and discrimination being conceived as individual processes – or as what some individuals do to other individuals. While such approaches may seem logical in highly individualized cultures (such as the modern-day USA and parts of Europe) where people are taught to believe they are nominally free agents, they make little sense in other environments. Throughout much of the developing world, for example, bonds and allegiances to family, village, neighbourhood and community make it obvious that stigma and discrimination, when and where they appear, are social and cultural phenomena linked to the actions of whole groups of people, and are not simply the consequences of individual behaviour (UNAIDS, 2000).

It is vitally important to recognize that stigma arises and stigmatization takes shape in specific contexts of culture and power. Stigma always has a history which influences when it appears and the form it takes. Understanding this history and its likely consequences for affected individuals and communities can help us develop better measures for combating it and reducing its effects. Beyond this though, it is important to better understand how stigma is used by individuals, communities and the state to produce and reproduce social inequality. It is also important to recognize how understanding of stigma and discrimination in these terms encourages a focus on the political economy of stigmatization and its links to social exclusion.

Culture, power and difference

Michel Foucault's work concerning the relation between culture or knowledge, power, and notions of difference is particularly helpful in engaging with these issues. Although Foucault's work was carried out at roughly the same time as Goffman's (mainly during the course of the 1960s and the 1970s) and focused on a number of similar concerns – issues such as mental illness, crime and punishment, and the social construction of deviance more generally – it had quite different cultural, intellectual and disciplinary origins. While Goffman's work was heavily influenced by the US sociology of the time and focused on the social construction of meanings through interaction, Foucault's work took shape in a very different context. In particular, and in line with the contemporary projects of European social philosophy, he wanted to better understand how different forms of knowledge come to be constituted in distinct historical periods.

For Foucault, fields such as psychiatry and biomedicine are best understood as 'cultural systems' that offer different claims to truth. The evidence they amass, and the understandings they promote are not 'facts' or 'truths' in any simple sense, but social products linked to the power of the professions. This more radical view of knowledge encourages a level of humility in the face of 'evidence' about the world – understandings are contextual and provisional (and this applies even to the 'hard' sciences and biomedicine), and must always be understood as such. As his work evolved, however, Foucault began to focus his attention not only on knowledge in and of itself, but also on the relationship between knowledge and power. He was particularly interested in what he called the regimes of power embedded in different knowledge systems, and the forms of control exercised by such systems over individual, as well as social, bodies.

Foucault's most influential studies of power, *Discipline and Punish* and *The History of Sexuality, Volume I: An Introduction*, placed emphasis on what he defined as a new regime of knowledge/power that characterized modern European societies during the late-nineteenth and early- twentieth centuries (and much of the world thereafter) (Foucault, 1977, 1978). Within this regime, physical violence or coercion increasingly gave way to what he described as 'subjectification', or social control exercised not through physical force, but through the production of conforming subjects and docile bodies. He highlighted how the social production of difference (what Goffman and the US sociological tradition more typically defined as deviance) is linked to established regimes of knowledge and power. The so-called unnatural is necessary for the definition of the natural, the abnormal is necessary for the definition of normality, and so on.

While it focuses on issues similar to those examined by Goffman in his work on stigma (for example, psychiatry and the mentally ill; prisons and criminals; sexology and sexual deviants or 'perverts', and so on), Foucault's work more clearly emphasizes the cultural production of difference in the service of power. While Goffman's work on stigma hardly even mentions the notion of power, and Foucault's work on power seems altogether unconcerned with stigma in and of itself, when read together their two bodies of work offer a compelling case for the role of culturally constituted stigmatization (that is, the production of negatively valued difference) as central to the establishment and maintenance of the social order.

Within such a framework, the construction of stigma (or, more simply, stigmatization) involves the marking of significant differences between categories of people, and through such marking, their insertion in systems or structures of power. Stigma and stigmatization function, quite literally, at the point of intersection between *culture, power* and *difference* – and it is only by exploring the relationships between these different categories that it becomes possible to understand stigma and stigmatization not merely as an isolated phenomenon, or expressions of individual attitudes or of cultural values, but as central to the constitution of the social order. This new understanding has major implications for the ways in which we might investigate and respond to the specific issues involved in HIV- and AIDS-related stigma, stigmatization and discrimination.

The strategic deployment of stigma

Placing culture, power and difference centre stage with respect to stigma, stigmatization and discrimination opens up new possibilities for research and intervention. But first we need to understand the ways in which these social processes function and operate.

In this respect, notions of *symbolic violence* (associated, in particular, with the sociological work of Pierre Bourdieu) and *hegemony* (initially elaborated in Antonio Gramsci's political theory, but more recently employed usefully in cultural analysis by writers such as Raymond Williams, Stuart Hall and others) are particularly useful. They highlight not only the functions of stigmatization in relation to the establishment of social order and control, but also the disabling effects of stigmatization on the minds and bodies of those who are stigmatized.

Like that of Foucault, Pierre Bourdieu's work has been concerned with the relations between culture and power (Bourdieu, 1977, 1984; Bourdieu and Passeron, 1977).[5] It aimed to examine how social systems of hierarchy and domination persist and reproduce themselves over time, without generating strong resistance from those who are subject to domination and, indeed, often without conscious recognition by their members. For Bourdieu, *all* cultural meanings and practices embody interests and function to enhance social distinctions among individuals, groups and institutions. Power therefore stands at the heart of social life and is used to legitimize inequalities of status within the social structure. Cultural socialization thereby places individuals as well as groups in positions of competition for status and valued resources, and helps to explain how social actors struggle and pursue strategies aimed at achieving their specific interests.

'Symbolic violence' describes the process whereby symbolic systems (words, images and practices) promote the interests of dominant groups as well as distinctions and hierarchies of ranking between them, while legitimating that ranking by convincing the dominated to accept existing hierarchies through processes of hegemony. While 'rule' is based on direct coercion, 'hegemony' is achieved via a complex interlocking of political, social and cultural forces that organize dominant meanings and values across the social field in order to legitimize the structures of social inequality, even to those who are the objects of domination (Gramsci, 1970; Williams, 1977, 1982).

With respect to stigmatization and discrimination, such insights are important for several reasons. First, if, as Bourdieu argues, all cultural meanings and practices embody interests and signal social distinctions among individuals, groups and institutions, then few meanings and practices do so as clearly and as profoundly as stigma, stigmatization and discrimination. Stigma and discrimination therefore operate not merely in relation to difference (as our readings of both Goffman and Foucault would tend to emphasize), but even more clearly in relation to social and structural inequalities. Second, and even more importantly, stigmatization does not simply happen in some abstract manner. On the contrary, it is part of complex struggles for power that lie at the heart of social life. Put even more concretely, stigma is deployed by concrete and identifiable social actors seeking to legitimize their own dominant status within existing structures of social inequality.

Beyond helping us to understand that stigmatization is part of a complex social struggle in relation to structures of inequality, notions of symbolic violence and hegemony also help us to understand how it is that those who are stigmatized and discriminated against in society so often accept and even internalize the stigma that they are subjected to. Precisely because they are subjected to an overwhelmingly powerful symbolic apparatus whose function is to legitimize inequalities of power based upon differential understandings of value and worth, the ability of oppressed, marginalized and stigmatized individuals or groups to resist the forces that discriminate against them is limited. To untie the threads of stigmatization and discrimination that bind those who are subjected to it, is to call into question the very structures of equality and inequality in any social setting – and to the extent that all known societies are structured on the basis of multiple (though not necessarily the same) forms of hierarchy and inequality, to call this structure into question is to call into question the most basic principles of social life.

This new emphasis on stigmatization as a process linked to competition for power and the legitimization of social hierarchy and inequality, highlights what is often at stake in challenging HIV- and AIDS-related stigmatization and discrimination. It encourages a move beyond the kinds of psychological models and approaches that have tended to dominate much of the work carried out in this field to date – models which all too frequently see stigma as a thing that individuals impose on others. It gives new emphasis to the broader social, cultural, political and economic forces that structure stigma, stigmatization and discrimination as social processes inherently linked to the production and reproduction of structural inequalities.[6]

Toward a political economy of stigmatization and social exclusion

Focusing on the relations between culture, power and difference in the determination of stigmatization encourages an understanding of HIV- and AIDS-related stigmatization and discrimination as part of the political economy of social exclusion present in the contemporary world. Greater attention to this broader political economy of social exclusion could potentially help us to think about contexts and functions of HIV- and AIDS-related stigma, as well as more adequate strategies for responding to it.

In order to do this, it is imperative to situate the analysis of HIV/AIDS historically, and to remember that the epidemic has developed during a period of rapid globalization linked to a radical restructuring of the world economy and the growth of 'informational capitalism' (Castells, 1996, 1997, 1998). These transformations have been characterized by rapidly accelerating processes of social exclusion, together with an intensified interaction between what might be described as 'traditional' and 'modern' forms of exclusion. Among the most vivid processes described by recent research has been the rapidly increasing feminization of poverty together with the increasing polarization between rich and poor in both the so-called developed as well as the so-called developing worlds.

Yet the new forms of exclusion associated with economic restructuring and global transformations have almost everywhere reinforced pre-existing inequalities and exclusions, such as racism, ethnic discrimination and religious conflict. This intensifying interaction between multiple forms of inequality and exclusion offers a general model for an analysis of the interaction between multiple forms of stigma that has typified the history of the HIV and AIDS epidemics. By examining the synergy between diverse forms of inequality and stigma, we may be better able to untangle the complex webs of meaning and power that are at work in HIV- and AIDS-related stigma, stigmatization and discrimination.

Second, and equally important, recent work on the transformation of the global system and the political economy of informationalism has called attention to the growing importance of identity (or, often, identities) as central to contemporary experience. This is particularly helpful in seeking to confront issues of stigmatization precisely because attending to it enables us to recoup, and indeed reposition, Goffman's original insight, nearly 40 years ago, concerning the impact of stigma in the construction of a kind of spoiled identity (Goffman, 1963). Much recent work on the nature of identity has emphasized its constructed and constantly changing character (Hall, 1990). This, in turn, has made it possible to begin to theorize changing constructions of identity in relation to both the experience of oppression and stigmatization, as well as resistance to it (Castells, 1997, p. 8). Such a view has been most clearly articulated by Castells (1997), who has distinguished between *legitimizing identities*, which are 'introduced by the dominant institutions of society to extend and rationalize their domination *vis-à-vis* social actors', *resistance identities*, which are 'generated by those actors that are in positions/conditions devalued and/or stigmatized by the logic of domination', and *project identities*, which are formed 'when social actors, on the basis of whatever cultural materials are available to them, build a new identity that redefines their position in society and, by so doing, seek the transformation of overall social structure'.

Such ideas offer important insights and avenues for responding more effectively to HIV- and AIDS-related stigmatization and discrimination in the future – but only to the extent that we are able to reconceptualize issues of stigmatization and discrimination within a broader political economy of social exclusion as it functions in the contemporary world. It is within this broader context that a new agenda for research and action in response to HIV- and AIDS-related stigma, stigmatization and discrimination must ultimately be developed.

A new agenda for research and action

To take seriously the notion that stigmatization and discrimination must be understood as social processes linked to the reproduction of inequality and exclusion pushes us to move well beyond the kind of behavioural and psychological models that have tended to dominate work thus far. While the latter have provided some insights and will continue to play a role in a broader research and programmatic response to the epidemic, they need to be complemented by new ways of understanding and overcoming HIV- and AIDS-related stigma, stigmatization and discrimination.

Research

While it is impossible to elaborate a fully developed research agenda on HIV- and AIDS-related stigmatization within the space of this review, in this concluding section we will outline some of the directions that such an agenda might explore. At least three lines of social enquiry might help us to more fully develop the kind of perspective on HIV- and AIDS-related stigmatization and discrimination that we have sought to advance in this review: (1) conceptual studies; (2) new investigative studies; and (3) strategic and policy-oriented research.

Conceptual studies

Conceptual studies are perhaps most obviously linked to the kind of work that took place within the context of the current review. Such studies aim to identify and work with concepts, ideas and new understandings of greatest relevance to national and international programmes and activities focusing on HIV- and AIDS-related stigma. They seek to interrogate the adequacy of existing ways of explaining things against the available evidence. They contribute to the development of new concepts and ideas of relevance to HIV- and AIDS-related stigmatization and discrimination. They also offer new ways of understanding processes of change, social movements and cultural transformation in response to HIV- and AIDS-related stigmatization and discrimination.

Conceptual studies have a crucial role to play in ensuring that existing knowledge is constantly reviewed for its adequacy and appropriateness in the light of changing needs and circumstances as they impact upon HIV- and AIDS-related stigma. They ensure that new categories of thinking are developed, together with new ways for identifying priorities. They allow for new vision and for a new role of theory. While they must continue to include work focusing on the psychological dimensions of HIV- and AIDS-related stigma, they must also move beyond this framework to examine the social, cultural, political and economic determinants and consequences of stigmatization and discrimination.

New investigative studies

New investigative studies aim to take new patterns of thought and explanation and to identify the essentially social processes at work in HIV- and AIDS-related stigma, the ways in which such processes contribute to HIV/AIDS vulnerability, and the possibilities for positive community participation and response in reducing stigmatization and discrimination. Context-specific empirical investigations of this kind, which examine the contributions already made, are likely to better account for past failures and successes, identify present opportunities and point to future priorities, thereby contributing in turn to the development of new theory. Ideally, however, such investigations should be conducted alongside broader comparative work in order to enable us to better understand those aspects of HIV- and AIDS-related stigmatization and discrimination that are local, as well as those aspects that may cross national and cultural boundaries.

There are any number of well-developed models, even in the existing record of HIV/AIDS social research, for such a balance between concern with specificity as well as with comparability. The programme of research developed by the International Center for Research on Women focusing on women and AIDS, or the WHO/GPA/UNAIDS studies of sexual risk among young people, the acceptability of the female condom or household and community responses to HIV and AIDS, all provide useful models in this regard (Rao Gupta and Weiss, 1995; Aggleton *et al.*, 1999). Moreover, studies of HIV- and AIDS-related stigmatization and discrimination in India and Uganda recently sponsored by UNAIDS provide an important point of departure for thinking about the potential for more integrated, comparative work in the future (UNAIDS, 2000).

Strategic and policy-oriented research

In contrast to conceptual enquiry and new investigative studies, strategic and policy-oriented research on HIV- and AIDS-related stigmatization and discrimination aims to identify and describe the combinations of programme elements that contribute to success in responding to these phenomena, the circumstances in which these programme elements are best operationalized (along with the actors involved), and the likely outcomes of specific kinds of programme implementation. It is essential that strategic and policy-oriented research be sensitive to the broader policy context. Programmes to address HIV- and AIDS-related stigma and discrimination are rarely, if ever, implemented in an ideologically neutral context. Understanding the relationship between programme development and implementation and the broader social context is central to the success of efforts to disseminate and/or scale up existing successes.

Intervention

Ultimately, of course, the key goal of all such research should be to contribute to the development of programmes and policies aimed at effectively reducing the human suffering (both in terms of new infections and in terms of the quality of life for people with HIV disease as well as those considered to be at risk of infection) that is a direct result of unmitigated HIV- and AIDS-related stigmatization and discrimination. While there is surely an important role for basic research that is not necessarily directly linked to intervention, even conceptual and descriptive studies on HIV- and AIDS-related stigma and discrimination need to be framed in ways that will ultimately feed into and nurture the development of advocacy and intervention aimed at reducing levels of stigmatization and the effects that discrimination has on both individuals and groups.

Our ability to achieve greater success in this regard, however, is directly linked to our willingness to move beyond the conceptual frameworks and intervention models that have largely dominated the field thus far. Both the theories that have been used in much intervention research focusing on HIV- and AIDS-related stigmatization, and the research designs used to test such interventions, have rarely broken the mould that dominates the vast majority of HIV/AIDS intervention research more generally: cognitive-behavioural and social-cognitive models (such as 'empathy induction') have predominated in the theoretical frameworks employed, and experimental or quasi-experimental evaluation designs have been the norm (see Brown *et al.*, 2001). Yet even a moment's thought should demonstrate that such individual-level interventions, while possibly useful in themselves, could never be scaled up in the manner required for an efficacious response throughout Africa, Asia, Central and Southern America. The resources do not exist. Besides, the individual framework with which they operate is simply alien to perhaps the majority of the world's cultures. They must be complemented by actions that have as their starting point the deeper social, political and economic causes of stigma and stigmatization, and which engage with the lives of collectivities and communities – for this is the level at which the great majority of HIV- and AIDS-related stigma operates.

If HIV- and AIDS-related stigmatization and discrimination must be reconceived as less a matter of individual or even social psychology than as a question of power, inequality and exclusion, it is equally necessary that we re-think the kinds of theoretical bases and evaluation research designs that may be needed to adequately respond to the issues in question. We may be well advised to begin to seek inspiration less in the literature associated with behaviour change than in that on community mobilization and social transformation – a research literature that is surely equally extensive, in spite of the fact that we have for the most part failed to take advantage of it in HIV/AIDS research (Parker, 1996).

In particular, the theorization of resistance and project identities discussed above offers important insights for re-thinking the development of community mobilization aimed at responding to HIV- and AIDS-related stigmatization and discrimination. As we have already suggested in reviewing the research literature in this area, the vast majority of existing interventions have sought to either reduce the incidence of stigmatization on the part of the 'community' or the 'general population', or to reduce the experience of stigma on the part of 'high risk groups' that have been the targets of stigmatization and discrimination (Brown *et al.*, 2001). Yet in both cases, intervention designs seem to have functioned in large part according to what Freire (1970) long ago identified as a 'banking' theory of pedagogy in which the perceived deficit accounts of those being 'educated' are somehow 'filled' by intervention specialists who presume they know the truth about what is needed.

Only more rarely have interventions been designed with the goal of unleashing the power of resistance on the part of stigmatized populations and communities – in spite of the fact that empirical studies of empowerment and social mobilization in response to HIV and AIDS have clearly demonstrated that the most effective and powerful responses to the epidemic (or 'natural experiments' if one prefers the language of much public health research) have taken place precisely when affected communities have mobilized themselves to fight back against stigmatization and oppression in relation to their lives (Altman, 1994; Daniel and Parker,

1993; Epstein, 1996; Parker *et al.*, 1995; Stoller, 1998). The time is therefore ripe to build upon existing empirical evidence, as well as the literature on community organizing and community building, both independent of the specific area of health and directly in relation to it, to begin developing new models for advocacy and social change in response to HIV- and AIDS-related stigmatization and discrimination (Delgado, 1994; Minkler, 1998).

If models of community mobilization, advocacy and social change provide one important basis for the development of responses aimed at resisting HIV- and AIDS-related stigmatization and discrimination, they must necessarily be conceived as part of a multidimensional programme of intervention. Increasingly, it is clear that localized intervention strategies aimed at community mobilization and social change (in this case, in response to HIV- and AIDS-related stigmatization and discrimination), must be conceived, whenever possible, in tandem with what have been described as structural or environmental interventions aimed at transforming the context in which both individuals and communities operate as they respond to HIV and AIDS (Sweat and Dennison, 1995; Parker and Camargo, 2000; Parker, Easton and Klein, 2000).

In few areas are the possibilities for structural intervention as clear as in the case of HIV- and AIDS-related stigma and discrimination. Indeed, while available research on intervention in relation to stigmatization has shown at best very limited results in changing stigmatizing attitudes (whether through 'empathy inducement' or other psychological theories) on the part of dominant sectors of society, judicial and policy interventions in many settings have shown real effectiveness in impeding the worst impact of HIV- and AIDS-related stigmatization and discrimination. Legal protections for people living with HIV and AIDS, together with appropriate reporting and enforcement mechanisms (ranging from legal aid services to hotlines for reporting acts of discrimination and violence against people with HIV and AIDS, gay men, women suffering domestic violence, and so on), have provided powerful and rapid means of mitigating the worst effects of the unequal power relations, social inequality and exclusion that lie at the heart of processes of HIV- and AIDS-related stigmatization and discrimination.

Ultimately, together with a new emphasis on community mobilization aimed at unleashing resistance to stigmatization and discrimination, structural interventions aimed at developing a rights-based approach to reducing HIV- and AIDS-related stigmatization and discrimination should be a high priority in order to create a transformed social climate in which stigmatization and discrimination themselves will no longer be tolerated. Within such a framework, discrimination becomes a clear breach of a basic human rights obligation – a breach that, when concretized in civil rights legislation, can effectively impede and prohibit the exercise of HIV- and AIDS-related stigmatization and discrimination.

Acknowledgements

The authors wish to acknowledge the support provided by the *HORIZONS* Project and by UNAIDS for work on the conceptualization of HIV- and AIDS-related stigma and discrimination. The ideas expressed here are those of the authors alone, however, and do not necessarily reflect those of either organization or the agencies they represent.

Notes

1 For an excellent overview of the literature on stigma in sociology, see Link and Phelan (2001).
2 For an overview of this literature, see, in particular, Malcolm *et al.* (1998).
3 Interestingly, in the *Oxford Dictionary of Sociology*, the entry for discrimination is linked (through the cross-associations typical throughout the dictionary entries) not to stigma but to prejudice and sexism. Prejudice, in turn, is described as 'an unfavorable attitude towards a group or its individual

members' (p. 522). In HIV/AIDS research, while stigma has been used extensively to describe AIDS-related attitudes, the term prejudice seems to have been much less frequently employed. As we will try to explain throughout this text, we are convinced that these issues of linguistic usage are not simply inconsequential. They have important implications for the ways in which societies have responded to HIV- and AIDS-related stigmatization and discrimination.

4 In particular, the work of writers such as Michel Foucault, Pierre Bourdieu, Antonio Gramsci, and Manuel Castells, described later.

5 While Foucault tended to prioritize the relationship between culture, power and difference in relatively static ways (albeit marked by radical shifts or disjunctures from one historical period to another), however, Bourdieu has focused much more clearly on the relations between culture, power, social structure and social action.

6 An extensive theoretical and empirical research literature exists that deals with the mechanisms and consequences of social exclusion cross-culturally and cross-nationally. See, for example, the review in relation to health (Purdy and Banks, 1999). On the particular impact of poverty on health generally and on HIV/AIDS in particular, see, also, World Bank (1993, 1997). Unfortunately, with only a few exceptions this literature has for the most part not been employed to address issues relating to HIV and AIDS, and has almost never been used to examine and respond to HIV- and AIDS-related stigmatization and discrimination (Farmer, Connors and Simmons, 1996; Parker and Camargo, 2000; Singer, 1998).

References

AGGLETON, P.J., DOWSETT, G., RIVERS, K. and WARWICK, I. (1999) *Sex and Youth: Contextual Factors Affecting Risk for HIV/AIDS*, Geneva: UNAIDS.

ALTMAN, D. (1994) *Power and Community: Organizational and Cultural Responses to AIDS*, London: Taylor and Francis.

ASHWORTH, C.S. *et al.* (1994) 'An experimental evaluation of an AIDS education intervention for WIC mothers', *AIDS Education Prevention*, 6(2), pp. 154–62.

BATSON, C.D. *et al.* (1997) 'Empathy and attitudes: can feeling for a member of a stigmatized group improve feelings toward the group?', *Journal of Personality and Social Psychology*, 72, pp. 105–18.

BEAN, J., KELLER, L., NEWBURG, C. and BROWN, M. (1989) 'Methods for the reduction of AIDS social anxiety and social stigma', *AIDS Education and Prevention*, 1(3), pp. 194–221.

BLENDON, R.J. and DONELAN, K. (1988) 'Discrimination against people with AIDS', *New England Journal of Medicine*, 319, pp. 1022–6.

——, DONELAN, K. and KNOX, R.A. (1992) 'Public opinion and AIDS: lessons for the second decade', *Journal of the American Medical Association*, 267, pp. 981–6.

BOURDIEU, P. (1977) *Outline of a Theory of Practice*, Cambridge: Cambridge University Press.

—— (1984) *Distinction: A Social Critique of the Judgement of Taste*, Cambridge: Cambridge University Press.

—— and PASSERON, J.-C. (1977) *Reproduction in Education, Society and Culture*, London: Sage.

BROWN, L., TRUJILLO, L. and MACINTYRE, K. (2001) *Interventions to Reduce HIV/AIDS Stigma: What Have We Learned?* New Orleans, LA: Horizons Program/Tulane School of Public Health and Tropical Medicine.

CASTELLS, M. (1996) *The Network Society*, Oxford: Blackwell.

—— (1997) *The Power of Identity*, Oxford: Blackwell.

—— (1998) *End of Millennium*, Oxford: Blackwell.

CORRIGAN, P.W. and PENN, D.I. (1999) 'Lessons from social psychology on discrediting psychiatric stigma', *American Psychologist*, 54, pp. 765–76.

CRANDALL, C.S., GLOR, J. and BRITT, T.W. (1997) 'AIDS-related stigmatization: instrumental and symbolic attitudes', *Journal of Applied Social Psychology*, 27(2), pp. 92–123.

CRAWFORD, A.M. (1996) 'Stigma associated with AIDS: a meta-analysis', *Journal of Applied Social Psychology*, 26(5), pp. 398–416.

CROCKER, J., MAJOR, B. and STEELE, C. (1998) 'Social stigma' in GILBERT, D.T. and FISKE, S.T. (eds), *The Handbook of Social Psychology, vol. 2*, Boston, MA: McGraw-Hill.

DANIEL, H. and PARKER, R.G. (1993) *Sexuality, Politics and AIDS in Brazil*, London: Falmer Press.

DELGADO, G. (1994) *Beyond the Politics of Place: New Directions in Community Organizing in the 1990s,* Oakland: Applied Research Center.

EPSTEIN, S. (1996) *Impure Science: AIDS, Activism and the Politics of Knowledge*, Berkeley and Los Angeles: University of California Press.

FARMER, P., CONNORS, M. and SIMMONS, J. (eds), (1996) *Women, Poverty and AIDS: Sex, Drugs and Structural Violence*, Monroe, ME: Common Courage Press.

FIFE, B.L. and WRIGHT, E.R. (2000) 'The dimensionality of stigma: a comparison of its impact on the self of persons with HIV/AIDS and cancer', *Journal of Health and Social Behavior*, 41, pp. 50–67.

FINE, M. and ASCH, A. (1988) 'Disability beyond stigma: social interaction, discrimination, and activism', *Journal of Social Issues*, 44, pp. 3–22.

FISKE, S.T. (1998) 'Stereotyping, prejudice, and discrimination' in GILBERT, D.T., and FISKE, S.T. (eds), *The Handbook of Social Psychology, vol. 2*, Boston, MA: McGraw-Hill.

FOUCAULT, M. (1977) *Discipline and Punish*, New York: Pantheon.

—— (1978), *The History of Sexuality, Vol. I: An Introduction*, New York: Random House.

FREIRE, P. (1970) *The Pedagogy of the Oppressed*, New York: Continuum.

GOFFMAN, E. (1963) *Stigma: Notes on the Management of a Spoiled Identity*, New York: Simon and Schuster.

GOLDIN, C.S. (1994) 'Stigmatization and AIDS: critical issues in public health', *Social Science and Medicine*, 39(9), pp. 1359–66.

GRAMSCI, A. (1970) *Prison Notebooks*, London: Lawrence and Wishart.

GREEN, G. (1995) 'Attitudes towards people with HIV: are they as stigmatizing as people with HIV perceive them to be', *Social Science and Medicine*, 41(4), pp. 557–68.

HALL, S. (1990) 'Cultural identity and Diaspora', in RUTHERFORD, J. (ed.), *Identity: Community, Culture, Difference*, London: Lawrence and Wishart.

HEREK, G.M. (1990). 'Illness, stigma and AIDS', in COSTA, P., and VANDENBOS, G.R. (eds), *Psychological Aspects of Serious Illness: Chronic Conditions, Fatal Diseases and Clinical Care*, Hyattsville, MD: American Psychological Association.

—— (1999) 'AIDS and stigma', *American Behavioral Scientist*, 42(7), pp. 1106–16.

—— and CAPITANIO, J.P. (1993) 'Public reactions to AIDS in the United States: a second decade of stigma', *American Journal of Public Health*, 83(4), pp. 574–7.

—— and CAPITANIO, J.P. (1994) 'Conspiracies, contagion, and compassion: trust and public reactions to AIDS', *AIDS Education and Prevention*, 6, pp. 365–75.

—— and CAPITANIO, J.P. (1997) 'Public reactions to AIDS in the United States, a second decade of stigma', *American Journal of Public Health*, 83(4), pp. 574–7.

—— and CAPITANIO, J.P. (1998) 'Symbolic prejudice or fear of infection?: a functional analysis of AIDS-related stigma among heterosexual adults', *Basic and Applied Social Psychology*, 20(3), pp. 230–41.

—— and CAPITANIO, J.P. (1999) 'AIDS stigma and sexual prejudice', *American Behavioral Scientist*, 42(7), pp. 1130–47.

——, CAPITANIO, J.P. and WIDAMAN, K.F. (2002) 'HIV-related stigma and knowledge in the United States: prevalence and trends, 1991–99', *American Journal of Public Health*, 92, pp. 371–7.

—— and GLUNT, E.K. (1991) 'AIDS-related attitudes in the United States: a preliminary conceptualization', *Journal of Sex Research*, 28, pp. 99–123.

HUE, L. and KAUFFMAN, C. (1998) 'Creating positive attitudes toward persons living with HIV/AIDS among young people in hostile environments', presented at the International Conference on AIDS, Geneva, Switzerland, 28 June–3 July, Vol. 12.

JONES, E., FARINA, A., HASTORF, A., MARKUS, H., MILLER, D.T., and SCOTT, R. (1984) *Social Stigma: The Psychology of Marked Relationships*, New York: Freeman.

KALEEBA, N. *et al.* (1997) 'Participatory evaluation of counseling, medical and social services of the AIDS support organization (TASO) in Uganda', *AIDS Care*, 9(1), pp. 13–26.

KELLY, J.A., ST. LAWRENCE, J.S., SMITH, S., HOOD, H.V. and COOK, D.J. (1987) 'Stigmatization of AIDS patients by physicians', *American Journal of Public Health*, 77(7), pp. 789–91.

KERRY, K. and MARGIE, C. (1996) 'Cost effective AIDS awareness program on commercial farms in Zimbabwe', Presented at the International Conference on AIDS, Vancouver, Canada, 7–12 July, 11(1), p. 45.

KIKONYOGO, N., KASATTIRO, A., MUTEBI, M., SSEMATIMBA, A., SERUNGOGI, J., BABIRYE, S. and NABATANZI, A. (1996) 'Sharing HIV/AIDS education in the communities: a Kampala traditional healer's experience', presented at the 11th International Conference on AIDS, Vancouver, Canada, 7–12. July, 11(2), p. 339.

LINK, B.G. and PHELAN, J. C. (2001) 'Conceptualizing stigma', *Annual Review of Sociology*, 27, pp. 363–85.

MALCOLM, A., AGGLETON, P., BRONFMAN, M., GALVÃO, J., MANE, P. and VERRALL, J. (1998) 'HIV-related stigmatization and discrimination: its forms and contexts', *Critical Public Health*, 8(4), pp. 347–70.

MANN, J. (1987) 'Statement at an informal briefing on AIDS to the 42nd session of the United Nations General Assembly', New York, 20 October.

MARSHALL, G. (1998) *Oxford Dictionary of Sociology*. Oxford and New York: Oxford University Press, pp. 163, 522.

MINKLER, M. (ed.), (1998) *Community Organizing and Community Building for Health*, New Brunswick, NJ: Rutgers University Press.

MWAMBU, W., (1998) 'Knowledge, attitudes and practices of housegirls on HIV/STDs transmission and risk factors', presented at the International Conference on AIDS, Geneva, Switzerland, 28 June–3 July, 12, pp. 1018–19.

OLIVER, M. (1992) *The Politics of Disablement*, Basingstoke: Macmillan.

OPALA, J. and BOILLOT, F. (1996) 'Leprosy among the Limba: illness and healing in the context of world view', *Social Science and Medicine*, 42, pp. 3–19.

PARKER, R.G. (1996) 'Empowerment, community mobilization, and social change in the face of HIV/AIDS', *AIDS*, 10, Suppl. 3, pp. S27–S31.

—— and CAMARGO Jr., K.R. (2000) 'Pobreza e HIV/ AIDS: aspectos antropológicos e sociológicos', *Cadernos de Saúde Pública*, 16, Suppl. 1, pp. 89–102.

—— et al. (1995) 'AIDS prevention and gay community mobilization in Brazil', *Development*, 2, pp. 49–53.

——, EASTON, D. and KLEIN, C. (2000) 'Structural barriers and facilitators in HIV prevention: A review of international research', *AIDS*, 14, Suppl. 1, pp. S22–S32.

PHELAN, J.C., LINK, B.G., STEUVE, A. and PESCOSOLIDO, B. (2000) 'Public conceptions of mental illness in 1950 and 1996: what is mental illness and is it to be feared?', *Journal of Health and Social Behavior*, 41, pp. 188–207.

PIOT, P. (2000) 'Report by the Executive Director. Programme Coordinating Board. Joint United Nations Programme on AIDS'. Rio de Janeiro, 14–15 December.

PRICE, V. and HSU, M. (1992) 'Public opinion about AIDS policies: the role of misinformation and attitudes about homosexuals', *Public Opinion Quarterly*, 56, pp. 29–52.

PRYOR, J.B., REEDER, G.D., VINACCO JR., R. and KOTT, T.L. (1989) 'The instrumental and symbolic functions of attitudes toward persons with AIDS', *Journal of Applied Social Psychology*, 19, pp. 377–404.

PURDY, M. and BANKS, D. (eds), (1999) *Health and Exclusion: Policy and Practice in Health Promotion*, London and New York: Routledge.

RAO GUPTA, G. and WEISS, E. (1995). 'Women's lives and sex: implications for AIDS prevention', in PARKER, R.G. and GAGNON, J.H. (eds), *Conceiving Sexuality: Approaches to Sex Research in a Postmodern World*, New York and London: Routledge, pp. 259–70.

SHELDON, K. and CALDWELL, L. (1994) 'Urinary incontinence in women: implications for therapeutic recreation', *Therapeutic Recreation Journal*, 28, pp. 203–12.

SIMPSON, W.M., et al. (1998) 'Uptake and acceptability of HIV testing: a randomized controlled trial of different methods of offering the test', *British Medical Journal*, 316, pp. 262–7.

SINGER, E., ROGERS, T.F. and CORCORAN, M. (1987) 'The polls: AIDS', *Public Opinion Quarterly*, 51, pp. 580–95.

SINGER, M. (ed.) (1998) *The Political Economy of AIDS*, Amityville, NY: Baywood Publishing Company.

SOSKOLNE, V., SHTARKSHALL, R., CHEMTOV, D. and ROSEN, H. (1993). 'Immigrants from a developing country in a western society: evaluation of an HIV education program', presented at the international conference on AIDS, Berlin, Germany, 6–11 June, 9(2), p. 777.

STAFFORD, M.C. and SCOTT, R.R. (1986). 'Stigma deviance and social control: some conceptual issues' in AINLAY, S.C., BECKER, L.M. and COLEMAN, L.M. (eds), *The Dilemma of Difference*, New York: Plenum.

STIPP, H. and KERR, D. (1989) 'Determinants of public opinion about AIDS', *Public Opinion Quarterly*, 53, pp. 98–106.

ST LAWRENCE, J.S., HUSFELDT, B.A., KELLY, J.A. and HOOD, H.V. (1990) 'The stigma of AIDS: fear of disease and prejudice toward gay men', *Journal of Homosexuality*, 19, pp. 85–101.

STOLLER, N. (1998) *Lessons from the Damned: Queers, Whores, and Junkies Respond to AIDS*, New York and London: Routledge.

SWEAT, M. and DENNISON, J. (1995) 'Reducing HIV incidence in developing countries with structural and environmental interventions', *AIDS*, 9, Suppl. A, pp. S225–S257.

TEWKSBURY, R. and MCGAUGHEY, D. (1997) 'Stigmatization of persons with HIV disease: perceptions, management, and consequences of AIDS', *Sociological Spectrum*, 17(1), pp. 49–70.

UNAIDS (2000) *HIV and AIDS-related Stigmatization, Discrimination and Denial: Forms, Contexts and Determinants. Research Studies from Uganda and India* (prepared for UNAIDS by Peter Aggleton), Geneva: UNAIDS.

USAID (2000). 'Combating HIV/AIDS stigma, discrimination and denial: what way forward?' unpublished paper, USAID concept paper, 23 June.

WILLIAMS, R. (1977) *Marxism and Literature*, Oxford: Oxford University Press.

—— (1982) *The Sociology of Culture*, New York: Schoken Books.

WORLD BANK (1993) *Investing in Health*, New York: Oxford University Press.

—— (1997) *Confronting AIDS: Public Priorities in a Global Epidemic*, New York: Oxford University Press.

WYNESS, M.A., GOLDSTONE, I. and TRUSSLER, T. (1996) 'Outcomes of an undergraduate HIV/AIDS nursing elective: insightful learning to promote quality care', presented at the International Conference on AIDS, Vancouver, Canada, 7–12 July, 11(1), p. 21.

25 Bracketing sexuality

Human rights and sexual orientation – a decade of development and denial at the United Nations

Ignacio Saiz [2004]

This year marks the 10th anniversary of an important milestone in the history of the recognition of rights relating to sexual orientation within the United Nations human rights system. In March 1994, a ground-breaking decision by the Human Rights Committee (HRC) in the case of *Toonen v. Australia* found that Tasmanian laws criminalizing all sexual relations between men were in breach of the International Covenant on Civil and Political Rights (ICCPR), whose non-discrimination provisions were interpreted as including 'sexual orientation' (Human Rights Committee, 1994, para 8.7).

Hailed at the time as 'the first juridical recognition of gay rights on a universal level', the decision became an authoritative reference for a series of successful legal challenges to discriminatory criminal laws around the world (Joseph, 1994).[1] It also gave an important boost to public health arguments that criminalization of homosexual activity hampers HIV/AIDS prevention (Human Rights Committee, 1994, para 8.5). *Toonen* offered hope that the international human rights system might at last provide recourse against the array of abusive laws and practices that have criminalized, pathologized, or demonized those whose sexual orientation or gender identity does not fit the perceived norm.[2]

Toonen was one of several developments in 1994 that seemed to signal a shift in the approach to human rights and sexuality at the United Nations. A burgeoning articulation of sexuality-related rights emerged from the 1994 UN-sponsored International Conference on Population and Development (ICPD) in Cairo, particularly in relation to women's sexual and reproductive rights.[3] The year also saw the appointment of a UN Special Rapporteur on Violence against Women, whose analysis of the link between control of female sexuality and violence against women eventually led to a pioneering affirmation of women's right to sexual autonomy (United Nations Economic and Social Council, 1994a, pp. 58–69). Sexuality – previously on the UN agenda only as something to be circumscribed and regulated in the interest of public health, order, or morality – was for the first time implicitly recognized as a fundamental and positive aspect of human development.[4]

Ten years on, however, sexuality remains a battleground within the UN human rights system. At the 60th session of the UN Commission on Human Rights (CHR) in Geneva in March 2004, 10 years to the day from the *Toonen* decision, the government of Brazil moved to postpone discussion of a resolution it had tabled the previous year which expressed concern about human rights violations occurring on grounds of sexual orientation around the world (Commission on Human Rights, 2004b, para 100). Brazil claimed it was forced to do so because it had not been possible 'to arrive at a necessary consensus' (Permanent Mission of Brazil, cited in CNSNews.com, 2004). The draft resolution had met with fierce opposition from governments arguing that sexual orientation was not a proper subject for consideration by a human rights body (Action Canada for Population and Development, 2003).

This article evaluates the progress made at the UN in addressing issues of sexual orientation in the decade since *Toonen*. It surveys the considerable body of work done by the UN's expert human rights mechanisms to develop international standards and hold states accountable for a range of human rights violations based on sexual orientation. This progress, however, is in stark contrast to the consistent denial and defiance shown by governments at the more 'political' UN forums such as the Commission on Human Rights or UN World Conferences, where the merest reference to sexual orientation has consistently been bracketed and systematically written out of any instruments adopted.

Furthermore, this article analyses some of the challenges for future advocacy, including the need to defend the universality of these rights and to confront limitations in the way international human rights bodies have recognized them. Sexual orientation is only one of many aspects of human sexuality that have begun to be addressed from a rights perspective over the past decade.[5] This article argues that framing sexual-orientation-related rights within a broader concept of sexual rights, including the right to sexual health, may offer important opportunities for overcoming some of the conceptual, political, and practical obstacles encountered within the UN system. The current climate of backlash and retrenchment poses significant challenges – but also engenders considerable opportunities – for advocacy on sexuality, gender, and health to converge around a renewed articulation of sexual rights.

Toonen + 10: sexual orientation and the treaty bodies

The *Toonen* decision was a significant departure from earlier international jurisprudence that had found the prohibition of same-sex sexual relations to be in breach of the right to privacy.[6] In *Toonen*, the Human Rights Committee found a violation of the ICCPR's privacy provisions (Article 17) in conjunction with the prohibition of discrimination (Article 2), innovatively interpreting the principle of non-discrimination on grounds of 'sex' as including 'sexual orientation' (Human Rights Committee, 1994, para 8.7).

Since *Toonen*, other treaty-monitoring bodies of the UN have helped consolidate the principle that sexual-orientation discrimination is proscribed in international human rights law.[7] The Human Rights Committee, the Committee on Economic, Social and Cultural Rights (CESCR), and the Committee on the Elimination of Discrimination against Women (CEDAW) have repeatedly and consistently called for the repeal of laws criminalizing homosexuality in countries around the world (see Human Rights Committee, 1998b, para 23; Human Rights Committee, 1999b, para 16; Committee on Economic, Social and Cultural Rights, 1998b, para 7; Committee on the Elimination of Discrimination Against Women, 1999a, paras 34–35). The HRC has emphasized the harmful consequences of these laws for the enjoyment of other civil and political rights, particularly where they result in the death penalty and other cruel, inhuman, and degrading punishments.[8]

The concerns of the treaty bodies have, furthermore, extended far beyond the criminalization of homosexual sex. 'Social cleansing' killings of sexual minorities, and the impunity surrounding them, have been addressed by the Human Rights Committee (Human Rights Committee, 1997a, para 16; 2003a, para 16). The Committee against Torture has condemned the ill-treatment of people detained on grounds of sexual orientation in Egypt and the discriminatory treatment of gay prisoners in Brazil (Committee Against Torture, 2002b, para 5(e); 2001, para 119). Both Committees have also addressed abuses against lesbian, gay, bisexual, and transgender (LGBT) rights defenders, including threats and attacks against activists, restrictions on their freedom of association, and denial of police protection (Committee Against Torture, 2002a, para 10; Human Rights Committee, 1998c, para 48). In line with developments

in refugee law, the treaty bodies have welcomed measures to prote
tion on grounds of sexual orientation and have voiced concern at the
tion of non-nationals on these grounds.[9]

Abuses based on sexual orientation have also been addressed fr
rights of the child. This is particularly significant given that earlier t
prejudiced notions about 'predatory' homosexuality, had pitted chil
rights of lesbian, gay, bisexual, and transgender people (Human Rig
The Committee on the Rights of the Child (CRC) has highlighted
sexual-orientation discrimination on adolescent health, calling on state
gay and transsexual people 'have access to the appropriate informatio   ᵤᵤces-
sary protection to enable them to live their sexual orientation' (Commi..ee on the Rights of
the Child, 2002, para 43).

Laws prohibiting the 'promotion of homosexuality' or setting a higher age of sexual
consent for same-sex relations have been held by the CRC to breach the non-discrimination
provisions of the Children's Convention (Committee on the Rights of the Child, 2002, para
44; Committee on the Rights of the Child, 2000a, paras 22, 23; Committee on the Rights of
the Child, 2000b, paras 25, 26; Committee on the Rights of the Child, 1999, para 16; Human
Rights Committee, 1998d, para 13). Two recent General Comments by the CRC have re-
affirmed the need to address sexual-orientation discrimination in the context of promoting
adolescent health and preventing HIV/AIDS (Committee on the Rights of the Child, 2003a,
para 6; 2003b, para 8). The Committee has also recommended that attention be given to
sexual-orientation discrimination as one of many factors that can expose children to a higher
risk of violence and victimization at school (Committee on the Rights of the Child, 2001, para
727).

The Committee on Economic, Social and Cultural Rights has also explored the nexus
between the right to health and discrimination on grounds of sexual orientation. Its General
Comment on the Right to Health was the first by any treaty body to include explicit reference
to sexual orientation discrimination (Committee on Economic, Social and Cultural Rights,
2000, para 18). The CESCR has addressed the impact of sexual-orientation discrimination in
a range of other spheres such as employment, housing, and the right to water (Committee on
Economic, Social and Cultural Rights, 1999a, para 5; Committee on Economic, Social and
Cultural Rights, 1998a, para 42; Committee on Economic, Social and Cultural Rights, 2003,
para 13).

Moreover, the relevance of the work of the treaty bodies to issues of sexuality goes well
beyond these specific references to sexual orientation. For example, CEDAW has addressed a
range of barriers impeding women's access to sexual health and has clarified the obligation of
states to prevent and punish gender-based violence in the home and the community, issues of
particular relevance to the experiences of lesbian, gay, bisexual, and transgender people
(Committee on the Elimination of Discrimination Against Women, 1992; Committee on the
Elimination of Discrimination Against Women, 1999b).

As this brief overview indicates, all the major human rights treaties can and have been
invoked to challenge a range of violations based on sexual orientation or gender identity.[10]
The extensive and increasingly comprehensive body of case law and authoritative comment
by the treaty bodies has served to illuminate patterns of human rights violations long
excluded from the ambit of human rights protection. It has also consolidated the principle of
non-discrimination on grounds of sexual orientation as one that is firmly grounded in international standards, requiring not only the repeal of discriminatory criminal laws but also the
adoption of proactive anti-discrimination measures.[11]

...question at the time of the *Toonen* decision, however, was the extent to which the ...odies would be willing to affirm the applicability of the non-discrimination principle ...ss the full spectrum of rights contained in the treaties they supervise, particularly in regards to the right to marry and to found a family, where there may not be consensus among committee members, let alone states.[12]

A key test case was brought in 1999 by two lesbian couples from New Zealand who argued that the failure of the New Zealand Marriage Act to provide for same-sex marriage was discrimination on grounds of 'sex' and 'sexual orientation' and violated their right to marry, their right to privacy and family life, and their right to equal protection of the law, among others (Human Rights Committee, 1999e). Despite powerful arguments, the Human Rights Committee found no violation of the ICCPR, holding that the right to marry under Article 23 applied only to 'the union between a man and a woman' (Human Rights Committee, 1999e, para 8.2).[13] This categorical assertion is at odds with the views expressed elsewhere by the Committee and other international human rights bodies that 'marriage' and 'the family' are continuously evolving concepts that apply to a diversity of arrangements across cultures and so must be interpreted broadly. Neither is defined in any international standard.[14]

A more recent decision by the Human Rights Committee in the case of *Young v. Australia*, however, applies the principle of equal protection of the law (Article 26 of the ICCPR) to the sphere of partnership rights (Human Rights Committee, 2003c). The HRC found that the denial of pension benefits to the same-sex partner of a deceased war veteran breached Article 26, as Australia had failed to provide any justification for making distinctions on the basis of 'sex or sexual orientation'. The decision transcends *Toonen* by moving the principles of non-discrimination and equal protection beyond the narrow confines of privacy and applying them to other areas of civil, economic, and social entitlements.

A separate concurring opinion by two individual committee members, however, draws attention to the limits of the decision's scope. It indicates that, had Australia explained its grounds for denying equal partnership rights to same-sex couples, the Committee might have found these to be 'reasonable and objective' justifications for discrimination.[15] It remains to be seen how sympathetic the Committee will be in the future to arguments that discrimination can be justified with regard to certain rights in the interest of the 'protection of the family'.

New frontiers for human rights: the special procedures of the Commission on Human Rights

Over the past decade, many of the individual human rights experts appointed by the Commission on Human Rights to study particular themes or country situations have foregrounded sexuality as an important human rights issue.[16] Their analysis has served not only to identify the specific forms, causes, and consequences of abuses based on sexual orientation and gender identity, but also to promote new approaches to human rights as they apply to human sexuality.

Since the mandate was created in 1994, the relationship between sexuality and human rights has been integral to the work of the Special Rapporteur on Violence against Women. The first post-holder, Radhika Coomaraswamy, identified violence against women who 'live out their sexuality in ways other than heterosexuality' as part of a broader spectrum of violence inflicted on women for exercising their sexual autonomy in ways disapproved of by the community (United Nations Economic and Social Council, 1997, para 8). She has analysed how gender-based violence is rooted in social constructions of feminine and masculine identity and perpetuated or justified by narrow interpretations of concepts such as 'tradition', 'culture', 'privacy', and 'family' (United Nations Economic and Social Council, 1999a, paras 6–18; United Nations Economic and Social Council, 2002b, paras 99–104). Towards the end of her mandate, she began to explore the contours of a 'right to sexuality and sexual autonomy' and affirmed that sexual rights were the 'final frontier' for women's human rights (United Nations Economic and Social Council, 1999b, para 5; United Nations Economic and Social Council, 2003e, para 65). Her successor, Yakin Ertürk, has probed further into the link between violence against women and the control of women's sexuality, and the ways in which different forms of discrimination intersect (United Nations Economic and Social Council, 2004d, paras 35–39).

Other rapporteurs have also been dealing with issues of sexual orientation and gender identity for a number of years. The Special Rapporteur on Extrajudicial, Arbitrary and Summary Executions has condemned the application of the death penalty for consensual sexual relations, state-sponsored and state-tolerated killings of sexual minorities, media-fuelled societal indifference, and threats against LGBT rights defenders.[17] The Special Rapporteur on Torture has focused on patterns of torture against sexual minorities, including the prevalence of sexual violence, the infliction of cruel, inhuman, and degrading punishments for consensual same-sex relationships or transgender behaviour, and ill treatment in prisons, state medical institutions, and the armed forces.[18] A recent report by the Special Rapporteur on Torture examines how stigma and discrimination on grounds of gender identity and sexual orientation can compound the risk of torture or ill-treatment for people who are (or are perceived to be) living with HIV/AIDS (United Nations Economic and Social Council, 2004c, para 64).

The Special Representative of the Secretary General on Human Rights Defenders has highlighted the risks facing human rights defenders whose work challenges oppressive social structures and traditions, signalling: 'Of special importance will be women's human rights groups and those who are active on issues of sexuality, especially sexual orientation and reproductive rights. These groups are often very vulnerable to prejudice, to marginalization and public repudiation, not only by State forces but by other social actors'.[19]

The Special Rapporteur on the Right to Health has significantly advanced debates and understandings of sexuality-related rights at the UN, highlighting how discrimination and violence against lesbian, gay, bisexual, and transgender people impedes their enjoyment of sexual and reproductive health and rights (United Nations Economic and Social Council, 2004b, paras 33, 38, 39). Other Special Rapporteurs have included reference to sexual orientation issues in connection with the right to education, freedom of expression, due process, the right to housing, and the right to a remedy.[20] The Working Group on Arbitrary Detention, which is another important mechanism of the CHR, has condemned the arbitrary detention and torture of 55 men in Egypt in connection with their perceived homosexuality (United Nations Economic and Social Council, 2001f; Human Rights Watch, 2004; Long, 2004).

The Sub-Commission on Human Rights, despite its mandate to undertake thorough studies on a range of emerging human rights issues, has not taken up calls from NGOs and from its own individual members to study the connections between sexual-orientation discrimination, health, and human rights.[21] Although Sub-Commission studies have occasionally referred to the non-discrimination principle, the Sub-Commission is well placed to carry out a more rigorous and comprehensive analysis of the obstacles that have prevented recognition in practice of the rights affirmed in principle by other parts of the UN system.[22]

A 'non-subject': reactions at the political bodies of the UN

The work of experts appointed by the Commission on Human Rights has been enormously significant in applying international human rights protections to those facing discrimination and violence because of their sexual orientation or gender identity. Attempts to place these findings on the agenda of the CHR itself, however, have met with intense resistance. In contrast to the bodies surveyed above, the Commission is made up of government representatives. Politics rather than principle usually determine the outcome of its human rights deliberations, and CHR members have constantly sought to undermine the effectiveness of CHR-appointed human rights experts (Amnesty International, 2004a, 2004b).

The fate of the draft resolution presented by Brazil to the CHR regarding human rights and sexual orientation exemplifies this pattern (United Nations Economic and Social Council, 2003a). Despite its relatively modest content, the draft resolution tabled in 2003 was described by Pakistan as an insult to the world's 1.2 billion Muslims (Action Canada for Population and Development, 2003, p. 31).[23] Five member states of the Organization of Islamic Conference (OIC) proposed deleting all reference to sexual orientation in the draft, which would have rendered it meaningless (United Nations Economic and Social Council, 2003c). After other blocking and delaying tactics, discussion of the draft resolution was postponed to the 2004 session (United Nations Economic and Social Council, 2003b). At the 2004 Commission, however, concerted opposition from the OIC and the Holy See and lukewarm support from supposedly sympathetic governments led Brazil to postpone formal discussion of the resolution for yet another year.[24, 25]

The arguments invoked by the Holy See and the Organization of Islamic Conference against the Brazil resolution are typical of the objections raised over the past 10 years whenever sexual-orientation rights have been asserted at the political bodies of the UN. Letters circulated by their representatives in Geneva argued that the principle of non-discrimination on grounds of sexual orientation cannot be considered as universally recognized as it does not appear in any UN treaty.[26] They argued, furthermore, that sexual orientation, an 'undefined term', may be a legitimate basis for discrimination to protect children and the family. It is not a human rights issue but a social and cultural one, best left to each state to address within its own sovereign legal and social systems. Asserting sexual orientation as a source of universal rights is culturally divisive and therefore threatening to the UN consensus.

Although strikingly out of touch with the human rights developments canvassed earlier, these arguments have a long and successful history, both at the CHR and at other UN forums made up of government representatives.[27] At the series of UN World Conferences since the ICPD in Cairo in 1994, attempts to include even a reference to sexual orientation in draft declarations have systematically met the same fate, the words remaining bracketed before being dropped in the interest of 'consensus'.

At the 1995 Fourth World Conference on Women in Beijing, four references to the persecution of women for their sexual orientation in the draft Platform for Action were dropped after the Vatican and some Islamic states, supported by organizations of the Christian right, decried the 'hijacking of human rights' by feminist and lesbian rights activists as a major threat to fundamental religious and cultural values.[28] Sexual orientation, they said, was a 'non-subject' that would open the floodgates to many unacceptable behaviours (Careaga, 2003).

The five-year review conferences held in 1999 and 2000 to evaluate implementation of the Cairo and Beijing commitments saw concerted attempts to reverse the hard-fought progress made on sexual and reproductive rights at those conferences.[29] In 1999, the Holy See forged alliances with other theocratic governments in fiercely resisting any language in the ICPD+5

Key Actions Document that could be interpreted as addressing either abortion or homosexuality. At the UN General Assembly Special Session in June 2000 to review implementation of the Beijing Platform for Action, a proposal to add reference in the resolution to measures taken 'by a growing number of countries ... to prohibit discrimination on the basis of sexual orientation', was opposed by delegates from Senegal, Syria, Nicaragua, and Kuwait on grounds that they could not accept 'sexual orientation', an undefined term, as a human right.[30]

Although the UN's work on HIV/AIDS has helped break taboos about discussing sexual diversity in human rights forums, at the Special Session of the UN General Assembly on HIV/ AIDS in June 2001, the bracketed references to 'men who have sex with men' as a group vulnerable to infection were removed from the text of the Declaration of Commitment following heated debate and objections from a number of governments.[31] The same battles over bracketed text were fought in August 2001 at the UN World Conference Against Racism in Durban, South Africa. A proposal by Brazil to recognize sexual orientation as a related form of discrimination remained bracketed in the Conference's draft Program of Action until the last day and was eventually deleted (World Conference against Racism, 2001). Nevertheless, progress at the political forums of the UN cannot be measured solely in terms of textual references to sexual orientation. While sexual orientation may be absent from the instruments adopted at UN World Conferences, sexuality more broadly has had an increasingly tangible presence. The Beijing Declaration and Platform for Action in particular was a milestone in the recognition of sexual and reproductive autonomy as a central plank of women's human rights. One of its paragraphs in the section on health, adopted after heated controversy, builds on Cairo's codification of reproductive rights by affirming women's 'right to have control over and decide freely and responsibly on matters related to their sexuality, including sexual and reproductive health, free of coercion, discrimination and violence' (Fourth World Conference on Women, 1995, para 96).

If the 'bracketing' has consistently muted any explicit recognition of sexual orientation rights at the political forums of the UN, those defending these rights have increasingly made their voices heard. Their participation and visibility at UN forums have made these empowering processes, providing a unique opportunity for activists around the world to strategize and exercise rights of political participation denied in their home countries.[32] The 2004 Commission on Human Rights saw an unprecedented number of formal interventions by LGBT rights defenders, as well as their participation in NGO-organized panel discussions.[33]

Over the past decade, an ever-increasing number of governments and mainstream human rights organizations have also sponsored initiatives and spoken powerfully in favour of sexual orientation rights.[34] This has left a minority of governments opposed to these efforts increasingly on the defensive. The vehemence of their resistance is itself a measure of the impact that movements for gender equality and sexual diversity have had across the globe (Castells, 1998). Nevertheless, this backlash has ensured that, for the moment, sexual orientation stays off the agenda in the name of 'consensus'.

Confronting obstacles, rethinking strategies

Events at the 2004 Commission on Human Rights exemplify the dynamic at the UN a decade after *Toonen*. Rights relating to sexual orientation (and sexuality more generally) may be legally well established, but they remain politically contested. Certain governments have intensified their efforts to deny or roll back any recognition of them, using 'cultural sovereignty' as a rallying cry and the lack of explicit reference to sexual orientation in international standards as their justification.

This current revisionism may have more to do with geopolitics than the finer points of international human rights law. Yet these arguments point to some of the challenges that future advocacy strategies need to confront: defending universality against cultural relativist attacks; overcoming barriers to the participation of human rights defenders working on sexuality in UN processes; and confronting limitations and biases in the way human rights law is interpreted and applied.

Challenging 'cultural' justifications

Sexuality remains one of the arenas where the universality of human rights has come under the most sustained attack and around which governments most often seek to erect protective barriers of cultural and national sovereignty to evade their internationally-recognized rights obligations.[35] Sexuality figures prominently in the construction of narratives around state sovereignty, national identity, and non-interference.[36] The appeal to 'cultural sovereignty' and 'traditional values' as a justification for denying sexual orientation (alongside other sexual-rights) claims, has become all the more prevalent in response to the processes of economic globalization and global cultural homogenization.[37]

As in the context of women's rights, this is often based on highly dubious misrepresentations of history and on fixed and selective notions of culture (Rao, 1995). Some governments in Asia, Africa, and the Middle East, for example, have sought to bolster their domestic authority through nationalist rhetoric, portraying homosexuality as a foreign imposition and a manifestation of Western decadence.[38] Nor is this appeal to mythical traditional cultural values limited to governments of the South. The US has been at the forefront of recent 'fundamentalist' attempts at the UN to rollback sexual and reproductive rights in the name of defending traditional forms of family (Girard, 2004; International Women's Health Coalition, 2002; Petchesky, 2000). While UN consensus documents have stressed that national and regional cultural and religious values cannot trump fundamental human rights, in practice states are still afforded a wide margin of discretion within the UN human rights system when it comes to matters of sexuality.[39] A vigorous defence of the universality of rights related to sexual orientation has generally been lacking at the UN (see Heinze, 2001, p. 284).[40]

A dilemma for rights advocates is how to formulate claims to universal rights in language that recognizes the significance of cross-cultural constructions of sexuality. Labels and perceptions attached to same-sex sexual identity and behaviour vary enormously from culture to culture (Herdt, 1997). Advocacy strategies that appear to globalize essentialist and culturally specific notions of 'lesbian/gay identity' may be seriously counter-productive (Adam, Duyvendak and Krouwel, 1998; Katyal, 2002; Phillips, 2000). The increasingly central role being played by rights activists from the South in UN processes around sexuality is the most eloquent response to those governments that seek to claim that sexual rights are an exclusively Northern concern. The obstacles that many of them face both domestically and internationally, however, have constrained their potential role as protagonists in UN lobbying. In many countries, they are denied legal status, resources, and recognition of their status as human rights defenders, all of which hampers their capacity to engage with international organizations (Amnesty International, 2001, pp. 53–8). Moreover, activists from all parts of the globe have consistently faced attempts by governments to exclude them from UN forums, particularly through denial of accreditation.[41]

As the UN Special Representative on Human Rights Defenders has suggested, the obstacles and risks facing those defending rights of sexuality across the globe merit greater attention and sensitivity from both UN human rights bodies and others within the human rights movement (United Nations Economic and Social Council, 2001, para 89[g]).

Confronting limitations and biases in International Human Rights Law

For all the progress made at the UN over the past decade, sexual orientation is still not mentioned in any binding UN human rights treaty, nor is it in any final political commitment document resulting from a UN world conference. The decisions and interpretations of the treaty bodies are authoritative, but most states hold that they are not legally binding. Instruments such as the Beijing Declaration and Platform for Action contain extensive reservations by states on the provisions relating to sexuality and contain no text on sexual orientation. Although the prohibition of sexual orientation discrimination has been unequivocally recognized by the UN treaty bodies and other international human rights bodies, reactions by governments at the UN indicate that in political venues it is not wholly accepted by the full community of states.[42]

The lack of explicit reference to a right to be free from discrimination on grounds of sexual orientation, or a broader right to sexual autonomy, has meant a reliance on progressive 'reading into' existing human rights provisions, typically the right to privacy, rights to physical integrity (freedom from torture and the right to life), and freedom from discrimination on grounds of sex.[43] While rights claims based on these approaches have achieved important victories, each has its limitations and has proven insufficient on its own.[44]

The boundaries of the right to privacy have proven highly mutable, and respect for privacy can co-exist with moral disapproval or mere tolerance of homosexuality, as long as it is confined to the private sphere of the closet.[45] Similarly, focusing on rights of physical integrity limits the scope of concern to the most egregious violations, such as the torture of lesbians through forced psychiatric treatment or 'social cleansing' killings of transgender sex workers (Amnesty International, 2001, pp. 53–8).

While claims based on the principles of non-discrimination and equal protection of the law have been increasingly successful at the UN, as well as in many national jurisdictions, the UN expert bodies have been virtually silent regarding the basis for locating 'sexual orientation' in the non-discrimination provisions of international standards.[46] This is significant because legal strategies in a number of jurisdictions have foundered on the question of whether sexual orientation claims can be argued as sex discrimination.[47]

The jurisprudence to date betrays other limitations of the non-discrimination approach. Human rights doctrine on non-discrimination allows considerable leeway for subjective interpretation regarding what circumstances may justify unequal treatment (Bayefsky, 1990). Differential treatment is not considered discrimination if the criteria for differentiation are 'reasonable and objective', and if the aim is to achieve a purpose deemed 'legitimate' under international standards (Human Rights Committee, 1989, para 13).

As seen in the cases of *Joslin* and *Young* before the Human Rights Committee, the treaty bodies have shown themselves willing to tolerate discrimination in partnership rights in the name of 'protection of the family', a legitimate interest invoked in an unduly restrictive way which denies the diversity of contemporary forms of family. Non-discrimination arguments will have only limited success if the basic concepts underpinning human rights law, such as 'marriage', the 'family', and 'state sovereignty' continue to be interpreted in heterosexist ways. As feminist legal scholars have pointed out, a non-discrimination approach is inadequate without addressing the structural biases of international human rights law (Chinkin and Charlesworth, 2000, p. 49).

While some have argued for a new UN declaration or convention prohibiting sexual orientation discrimination, such a project is not only hopelessly unattainable in the current climate, it also lays bare the problem of naming the categories to be protected (Heinze, 2001: p. 300). The binary categories inherent to non-discrimination norms ('men/women', 'homo/ heterosexual') can also serve to subtly reinforce the subordination of one by the other.[48] Volatile and culturally-specific concepts such as 'lesbian and gay' and 'sexual minorities' defy the kind of fixed universally applicable categorization that is necessary for codification in anti-discrimination instruments.[49]

The promise of 'gender integration' at the UN

The obstacles canvassed above – including deference to cultural justifications, exclusion from UN processes, and biased interpretation of international standards – are the very same obstacles that have historically hampered progress in advancing women's rights internationally (Chinkin and Charlesworth, 2000; Gallagher, 1997). This is not surprising, given the inextricable link between sexuality and gender.[50] The process of 'gender-mainstreaming' underway at the UN since the 1990s aimed to overcome these gender biases in its work. However, its progress has, at best, been mixed. Moreover, there is little evidence that those at the forefront are willing to make the conceptual links to sexual orientation – perhaps out of fear that this would compromise the broader process of gender integration by alienating governments.[51]

In regard to sexual orientation claims, norms and mechanisms created to combat gender discrimination have been disappointingly underused within the UN system.[52] The Beijing Platform for Action represented an important acknowledgement of women's right to decide on matters of sexuality free of violence or coercion, but women's rights advocates have sought a more comprehensive and affirmative vision of women's right to sexual autonomy, de-linked from reproductive rights.

Of all the mechanisms created within the UN system to enhance gender perspectives on human rights, only in the work of the Special Rapporteur on Violence against Women does one see a comprehensive linkage of gender and sexuality, including sexual orientation. The previous Rapporteur was the first UN human rights expert to explicitly articulate a concept of sexual rights. While speaking of these as part of a 'fourth generation' of women's rights, she has described sexual rights as a constellation of existing rights, including 'the right to information, based upon which one can make informed decisions about sexuality; the rights to dignity, to privacy and to physical, mental and moral integrity in realizing a sexual choice; and the right to the highest standard of sexual health' (Coomaraswamy, 1997; United Nations Economic and Social Council, 1999b, para 5).

Sexual rights: a broader palette

The discourse of sexual rights offers new conceptual and strategic tools for future work within the UN system. This discourse is the product of increasing dialogue and collaboration between activists and social movements working on sexuality from a number of different perspectives, including women's rights, population and development, reproductive health, HIV/AIDS, and lesbian, gay, bisexual, and transgender rights (Parker, 1997; Miller, 1999). This dialogue across disciplines has led to attempts to situate sexuality within a more comprehensive human rights framework and to explore commonalities between disparate struggles.

The sexual rights discourse builds on the limited articulation of sexual rights at Cairo and Beijing, as well as on existing case law on sexual orientation and standards regarding sexual orientation. It embraces a more affirmative and emancipatory vision of sexuality, seen not just as something to be protected from violence or other interference, but also as a social good to be respected, protected, and fulfilled. The principles underpinning these rights have variously been identified as 'autonomy', 'empowerment', 'bodily integrity', and 'respect for sexual and family diversity' (Petchesky, 2001).

The concept of sexual rights enables us to address the intersections between sexual orientation discrimination and other sexuality issues – such as restrictions on all sexual expression outside marriage or abuses against sex workers – and to identify root causes of different forms of oppression. It also offers strategic possibilities for building bridges and coalitions between diverse movements so as to confront common obstacles more effectively (such as religious fundamentalism) and explore how different discourses of subordination work together.

Sexual rights make a strong claim to universality, since they relate to an element of the self common to all humans: their sexuality. The concept therefore avoids the complex task of identifying a fixed sub-category of humanity to whom these rights apply. It proposes an affirmative vision of sexuality as a fundamental aspect of being human, as central to the full development of human health and personality as one's freedom of conscience and physical integrity. Sexual rights offer enormous transformational potential, not just for society's 'sexual minorities' but for its 'sexual majorities' as well (Petchesky, 2001).

Exploring the right to sexual health as a sexual right

The many dimensions of human sexuality – physical, mental, spiritual, social, associational – intersect with a multiplicity of rights. Developments in early 2004 indicate that a particularly fruitful avenue for sexual rights advocacy – and a major area of contestation – in the coming years will be around the right to sexual health. Within the UN system, the Special Rapporteur on the Right to Health, Paul Hunt, has significantly advanced the thinking on the links between sexuality, health, and rights. His report to the Commission on Human Rights in 2004 includes a particular focus on sexual and reproductive health, as a contribution to the 10th anniversary of the ICPD in Cairo (United Nations Economic and Social Council, 2004b, paras 33, 38, 39). It is groundbreaking in its attention to issues of sexual orientation and health, its analysis of what a human rights perspective can bring to sexual health policy, and its call for greater attention to sexual rights.[53]

The Rapporteur posits a rights-based approach to sexual health that transcends the medicalizing and moralizing approaches of much social policy in areas of sexuality. His report suggests a more comprehensive rights-based definition of sexual health than that included in the Cairo and Beijing instruments: sexual health is 'a state of physical, emotional, mental and social well-being related to sexuality, not merely the absence of disease, dysfunction or infirmity' (United Nations Economic and Social Council, 2004b, para 53).

A rights-based approach to sexual health 'requires a positive and respectful approach to sexuality and sexual relationships, as well as the possibility of having pleasurable and safe sexual experiences, free of coercion, discrimination, and violence' (United Nations Economic and Social Council, 2004b, para 53). Human rights also impose clear and measurable obligations on relevant authorities and can empower individuals and communities to see their health needs as legitimate entitlements to be claimed from service providers.

Affirming that 'sexuality is a characteristic of all human beings [and] a fundamental aspect of an individual's identity', he concludes that 'the correct understanding of fundamental human rights principles, as well as existing human rights norms, leads ineluctably to the recognition of sexual rights as human rights. Sexual rights include the right of all persons to express their sexual orientation, with due regard for the well-being and rights of others, without fear of persecution, denial of liberty or social interference' (United Nations Economic and Social Council, 2004b, para 54).

Although the Rapporteur's focus on sexual and reproductive health and rights drew criticism from several governments at the Commission on Human Rights, including the US, Pakistan, Saudi Arabia, and Egypt, these rights received another important re-affirmation by the Commission in a resolution on violence against women – a resolution that echoed the sexual rights language of the Beijing Platform for Action (Commission on Human Rights, 2004a, para 8). The 2004 Commission can therefore be recognized as a turning point in the struggle to link rights, health, and sexuality.

Nevertheless, a measure of the battles ahead lies in the fact that the March 2004 meeting of the Conference on Population and Development to mark the 10th anniversary of the Cairo Platform for Action was unable to agree on a resolution reaffirming the Cairo commitments following concerns raised by the United States and others that these might endorse same-sex marriage and abortion (Population Action Internation, 2004). The next stages of the Cairo and Beijing review processes will be important fronts on which to defend and promote the right to sexual health as part of the broader struggle for sexual rights.

Conclusion

It is clear that, 10 years on from *Toonen*, the momentum at the UN for addressing issues of sexual orientation within a broader framework of sexual rights is unstoppable. Both the emergence of a global movement of human rights defenders working on these issues and the increasing support of governments from the North and South suggest that we are at a crucial turning point in the recognition of sexual rights at the UN. But sexual rights can be expected to remain a contested area of human rights as sexuality increasingly becomes a site of struggle between traditionalist and modernizing forces, both within and across cultures.[54] The promotion and defence of these rights will therefore demand priority attention on the human rights and health agendas over the next 10 years.

There are a number of immediate steps that the UN's expert human rights bodies could take to ensure that their findings are no longer ignored or dismissed by recalcitrant states. These include: undertaking specific studies on human rights and sexuality; considering the desirability of a dedicated thematic mandate; using all available mechanisms to hold governments to their obligations under the range of human rights treaties; factoring sexuality into the ongoing process of gender integration and sharing best practices among different bodies; and strengthening contacts with human rights defenders working on sexuality issues while eliminating barriers to their effective participation in the UN system.

Despite persistent attempts to roll back the gains, *Toonen*'s anniversary should be marked as the year in which sexuality broke free of the brackets that have contained and silenced it for more than a decade.

Notes

1 Examples include the successful challenges to 'sodomy' laws in South Africa (Constitutional Court of South Africa, *National Coalition for Gay and Lesbian Equality v. Minister of Justice*, CCT 11/98, October 1998) and in the US state of Texas (*Lawrence v. Texas*, 123 S. Ct. 2472, 2003).

2 Gender identity refers to a person's deeply felt sense of belonging to a gender and the sense of conformity or non-conformity between their gender and their biological sex. Although distinct from

sexual orientation, it is intimately linked both as an aspect of identity/behaviour and as a reason for abuse or discrimination.

3 The ICPD Program of Action affirmed that women's reproductive rights include 'the right to a safe and satisfying sex life' and recognized that 'the purpose of sexual health is the enhancement of life and personal relations, and not merely counseling and care related to reproduction and sexually transmitted diseases' (International Conference on Population and Development, 1994: 7.2).

4 Twelve years before its decision on *Toonen*, the Human Rights Committee had found that the criminal prosecution of a Finnish television broadcaster for airing a debate on homosexuality was not in breach of the ICCPR as such a programme 'could be judged as encouraging homosexual *behaviour* … In particular, harmful effects on minors cannot be excluded'. *Hertzberg v. Finland*, Communication No. 61/1979, 2 April 1982, para 10.4.

5 Other aspects include protections from sexual violence, coercion around partner choice, and the criminal regulation for consensual sex. For an overview of work on sexuality and human rights, see Fried (2004) and IWGSSP (2004).

6 Three previous decisions by the European Court of Human Rights had found such laws to be in breach of the right to privacy under the European Convention on Human Rights. See *Dudgeon v. UK*, 1981; *Norris v. Ireland*, 1988; and *Modinos v. Cyprus*, 1993.

7 The treaty bodies are committees set up under seven international human rights treaties – the International Covenant on Civil and Political Rights, the International Covenant on Economic, Social and Cultural Rights, the Convention on the Rights of the Child, the Convention on the Elimination of All Forms of Discrimination against Women, the Convention against Torture, the Convention on the Elimination of All Forms of Racial Discrimination and the International Convention on the Protection of the Rights of All Migrant Workers and Members of their Families – to monitor compliance by States party. The Committees, made up of experts from around the world, examine periodic reports submitted by the States parties, often in light of information from non-governmental organizations, and issue Concluding Observations and Recommendations to governments. The Committees also publish General Comments elucidating the treaties' provisions. Five of the Committees can adjudicate individual complaints. The Committees' decisions, Concluding Observations and General Comments, although not in themselves legally binding, are considered authoritative interpretations of binding treaties and are therefore valuable advocacy tools. The Migrant Workers' Convention only entered into force in July 2003 and its Committee met for the first time in 2004. For more on the UN treaty bodies, see Office of the UN High Commissioner for Human Rights, *Treaty Bodies*. Available at: www.unhchr.ch/pdf/leafletontreatybodies.pdf

8 See for example Human Rights Committee (1995, para 287) and Human Rights Committee (1999a, para 20). For the death penalty and other cruel, inhuman, and degrading punishments see Human Rights Committee (1997b, para 8).

9 In regards to protecting refugees fleeing persecution on grounds of sexual orientation, see Committee on the Elimination of Discrimination Against Women (2001, para 334). In a case heard under its individual complaint procedure, the Committee against Torture considered unfounded the complainant's claim that he would be at risk of torture if returned from the Netherlands to Iran because his homosexuality was known to the authorities. Committee against Torture (2003). In regard to the arbitrary deportation of non-nationals, see Human Rights Committee (1998a, para 24).

10 While not having addressed sexuality or gender identity explicitly in its country-monitoring or individual-complaints procedure, the Committee on the Elimination of Racial Discrimination has highlighted the link between racism and other forms of discrimination, including sexual orientation discrimination (see Committee on the Elimination of Racial Discrimination, 1999).

11 For example, the HRC, the CESCR, and the CRC have all called on states to include sexual orientation in anti-discrimination legislation and to ensure its effective implementation in practice. Human Rights Committee (1999d, para 15), para 15; Human Rights Committee (2000a), para 11; Human Rights Committee (1999e, para 5); Committee on Economic Social and Cultural Rights (2000, para 71).

12 For an example of differing opinions among Committee members, see the CESCR's discussions on same-sex partnership and adoption rights in the context of Article 10 of the ICESCR (protection of the family), where some individual members have argued that legalizing same-sex partnerships 'eroded the concept of the family as articulated in the Covenant' (Committee on Economic Social and Cultural Rights, 1999b, para 137) and that granting adoption rights to lesbian or gay individuals or couples might leave children at risk of sexual abuse (Committee on Economic Social and Cultural Rights, 1998a, para 22).

13 The authors canvassed and rebutted a whole series of justifications that might be advanced to bar same-sex marriage, concluding that 'society and the State have programmed their selective memories to construct marriage as inherently and naturally heterosexual, thereby clearly excluding access by "deviant others" to marriage'. Human Rights Committee (1999e, para 5.2).

14 See Human Rights Committee (1990, para 2); Human Rights Committee (2000b, paras 23, 27); Committee on the Elimination of Discrimination Against Women (1994, paras 13–18). The European Court of Human Rights has also interpreted the right to marry in a dynamic way; see *Christine Goodwin v. the UK*, ECHR (2002). For an international survey of evolving legal interpretations, see Wintemute and Andenaes (2001).

15 Human Rights Committee (2003c), Appendix: Individual opinion by Committee members Ruth Wedgwood and Franco DePasquale.

16 In contrast to the treaty bodies, the CHR's special procedures can scrutinize the human rights performance of countries regardless of the treaties they have ratified. There is far greater scope for analysis of patterns, causes and consequences of violations in their work, which often draws on academic scholarship or input from NGOs, and more leeway to determine areas of research or inquiry. Some have proactively sought contact with LGBT rights organizations.

17 See, for example, United Nations Economic and Social Council (2001b, para 50). Her reports have also included specific recommendations regarding the investigation of homophobic crimes and the implementation of policies to combat prejudice among public officials and the general public.

18 United Nations Economic and Social Council (2001c). 'Torture and discrimination against sexual minorities' are included as special concerns.

19 United Nations Economic and Social Council (2001d, para 89[g]). The Special Representative has signalled her intention to undertake or encourage further study of these risks so as to draw up a 'compendium of possible measures' for protection.

20 For the right to education, see United Nations Economic and Social Council (2001a, para 75). For freedom of expression, see United Nations Economic and Social Council (2004a, para 124). For due process, see United Nations Economic and Social Council (2003d), Annex: Bangalore Principles for Judicial Conduct (sexual orientation is included in their equal treatment provisions). For the right to housing, see United Nations Economic and Social Council (1994b), which includes reference to 'sexual orientation' discrimination in the draft International Convention on the Right to Housing. For the right to a remedy, see United Nations Economic and Social Council (2000, para 27).

21 The Sub-Commission on the Promotion and Protection of Human Rights consists of 26 independent experts elected by the Commission on Human Rights. Although nominated by governments, they act in their personal capacities. The Sub-Commission's functions include 'to make recommendations to the Commission concerning the prevention of discrimination of any kind' (www.unhchr.ch/html/menu2/2/sc.htm). For an example of calls by NGOs to study the links between sexual orientation discrimination, health, and human rights, see the Statement made by Amnesty International to the Sub-Commission (2001). One Sub-Commission member, Louis Joinet, proposed a dedicated study in preparation for the World Conference on Racism, noting 'it would be unfortunate if the World Conference ignored discrimination against homosexuals, which was a major aspect of discrimination' (United Nations Economic and Social Council, 2000d).

22 Sub-Commission references to the non-discrimination principle can be found in, for example, United Nations Economic and Social Council (1992, para 185); United Nations (2001, para 5); United Nations Economic and Social Council (2000b).

23 The draft resolution merely expressed 'deep concern' at the occurrence of human rights violations all over the world on grounds of sexual orientation and called on states and relevant UN human rights bodies to give due attention to these violations. It did not propose creating any new international standards or mechanisms to protect against sexuality-related abuses.

24 Although not a UN member state, the Holy See (representing the leadership of the Catholic Church and the inhabitants of the Vatican) has permanent UN observer status. For an analysis of the Holy See's resistance to sexual and reproductive rights at the UN, see Center for Reproductive Rights (2000).

25 While Brazil professed its continued commitment to the resolution, NGO advocates in Geneva alleged that Brazil had ceded to OIC threats to boycott a forthcoming trade meeting in Brazil unless the resolution was withdrawn (*The Washington Times*, 2004).

26 Letter from the Permanent Mission of Pakistan on behalf of the Organization of Islamic Conference, 26 February 2004, and Letter from the Permanent Mission of the Holy See, 1 March 2004.

27 For example, draft CHR resolutions tabled in recent years endorsing the findings of the Special Rapporteur on Extrajudicial, Arbitrary and Summary Executions have prompted controversy over the inclusion of references to 'killings based on sexual orientation', and have often been subjected to a vote following objections by several Islamic countries. In 2001 this resulted in the replacement of the reference with the phrase 'all killings committed for any discriminatory reason', deliberately obscuring the issue (see United Nations Economic and Social Council, 2000c, para 6; United Nations Economic and Social Council, 2001e).

28 See for example the critique by Kathryn Balmforth, Director of the World Family Policy Center, Brigham Young University, that 'The UN is being taken over by the radical feminists, population control ideologues, and homosexual rights activists who make up the anti-family movement. … The ongoing takeover of some of the human rights mechanisms of the United Nations … is a potential threat to the rights of people everywhere to enjoy their own cultures and religions'. K. Balmforth, 'Hijacking Human Rights'. Available at: www.newyorkeagleforum.org/eagle_articles/congress%20speech.ht

29 While fraught with conflict, the review processes succeeded in reaffirming the Beijing and Cairo commitments and articulating strategies for implementation and evaluation (see Center for Reproductive Rights, 1999).

30 The reference was deleted after the Pakistani delegate accused Western delegations of 'holding the women of the world hostage to one term, "sexual orientation"', when their real needs were clean water and help in overcoming illiteracy (Sanders, 1996, pp. 67–106).

31 Regarding the breaking of taboos, see Parker (1997). See also United Nations Economic and Social Council (2003f, paras 10, 28). Regarding the change in the text of the Declaration of Commitment, see International Gay and Lesbian Human Rights Commission (2001).

32 The Beijing Conference, in particular, marked a turning point in the engagement with and visibility of lesbian rights activists with UN processes. See for example the statement made by Palesa Beverlie Ditsie on behalf of the International Gay and Lesbian Human Rights Commission to the Plenary on 13 September 1995: 'If these words [sexual orientation] are omitted from the relevant paragraphs, the Platform for Action will stand as one more symbol of the discrimination that lesbians face and of the lack of recognition of our very existence' (see also Bunch and Hinojosa, 2000).

33 For example, Statement by Dorothy Aken'Ova, International Centre for Reproductive Health and Sexual Rights (INCRESE), Nigeria, 'Protecting Sexual Health and Rights of Vulnerable Groups', 14 April 2004; Statement by Raquel Caballero, Centre for Global Women's Leadership, 'The LGBT Situation in Paraguay with Respect to Torture and Arbitrary Detention'. Statement by Wendy Isaack, Lesbian and Gay Equality Project, South Africa, 'Violence against Women'. Three NGO panel events were organized between 31 March and 1 April 2004 on human rights violations based on sexual orientation and gender identity, with a focus on the experiences of people from the global South.

34 For example, among the many governments at Beijing who spoke in favour of including sexual orientation, Switzerland said deleting the reference 'would not delete the people it is intended to protect'. At the Durban conference, Brazil, Canada, Chile, Ecuador, and Guatemala stated that sexual orientation was a human rights issue which could no longer be ignored at the UN and called for 'more in-depth analysis, discussion and debate to contribute to the development of worldwide consensus on this matter' (Joint statement by Brazil, Canada, Chile, Ecuador and Guatemala,7 September 2001).

35 See for example the amendments proposed by Saudi Arabia, Pakistan, Egypt, Libya, and Malaysia to the Brazilian resolution to the CHR in 2003 on human rights and sexual orientation, which delete all references to sexual orientation and insert language affirming respect for 'cultural diversity', 'cultural pluralism', and the preservation of 'cultural heritage and traditions' (United Nations Economic and Social Council, 2003c).

36 The discourses structuring these narratives often identify the state as heterosexual and homosexuality as the foreign 'other'. Within societies, homophobia is stoked and inflamed for political reasons in order to demarcate boundaries of citizenship and national belonging. Such discourses are an integral part of the justifications currently invoked by governments in international human rights forums that there are 'compelling state interests' for denying equal rights to lesbian, gay, bisexual and transgender people (see Stychin, 1998).

37 For an extensive analysis of how states have used claims of sovereignty to marginalize and attack organizing around sexuality-related rights, including at the Beijing World Conference on Women, see Rothschild and Long (2000).

38 For example, some Southern African leaders have defended their country's 'sodomy' laws on grounds that homosexuality is a foreign disease alien to local norms and traditions. Ironically, it is not same-sex behaviour, but the laws prohibiting it that are the colonial imposition, as well as the social and scientific construct of 'homo/hetero-sexuality' that such laws enshrine. The ways in which homophobia has been manipulated for political purposes by some Southern African governments is analysed in Human Rights Watch (2003).

39 'While the significance of national and regional particularities and various historical, cultural and religious backgrounds must be borne in mind, it is the duty of States, regardless of their political, economic and cultural systems, to promote and protect all human rights and fundamental freedoms' (United Nations, 1993, para 5).

40 Heinze criticizes the 'cross-cultural sensitivity game' played by sympathetic governments who refrain from advancing issues of sexual orientation on the UN agenda for fear jeopardizing the UN consensus.

41 For example, at the Special Session of the UN General Assembly on HIV/AIDS in June 2001, the General Assembly spent almost three hours and cast three separate votes to decide whether to accredit a representative of the International Gay and Lesbian Human Rights Commission (IGLHRC) to deliver a three-minute speech at a human rights round-table discussion (International Gay and Lesbian Human Rights Commission, 2001). At the Durban Conference, a decision on whether to grant accreditation to the International Lesbian and Gay Association was, exceptionally, put to a vote and narrowly defeated.

42 The fate of the Brazil resolution is only one recent indication of some governments' reluctance to recognize the principle. See, for example, the failure of the Consultative Meeting on the Draft Basic Principles on the Right to a Remedy to agree on the inclusion of the term 'sexual orientation' as a recognized category for protection against discrimination (United Nations Economic and Social Council, 2002a, paras 65, 66).

43 For an overview of relevant international case-law beyond the UN, see Human Rights Watch, *Resource Library for International Jurisprudence on Sexual Orientation and Gender Identity.* Available at: www.hrw.org.

44 For a more detailed analysis of the shortcomings of 'privacy' and 'non-discrimination' based approaches, see Bamforth (1997).

45 For example, in finding that laws criminalizing homosexual sex breached the right to privacy in the case of *Dudgeon v. UK* (1981, para 61) the European Court of Human Rights argued that 'decriminalization did not imply approval'.

46 While it is perhaps fortunate that the treaty bodies have not followed the example of the concurring opinion in *Toonen*, which wades dubiously into explanations that sexual orientation is an 'immutable status', the lack of clarification about the reasoning for reading 'sexual orientation' into 'sex' (or 'other status' as the CESCR General Comments appear to do) fuels the perception that the non-discrimination norm is not well established.

47 See, for example *Grant v. South West Trains*, European Court of Justice, ECR C-249/96 (February 1996), cited by New Zealand in the case of *Juliet Joslin et al. v. New Zealand* (Human Rights Committee, 1999e) as authority for the argument that denying benefits to same-sex partners was not sex discrimination. The drafters of the South African Constitution argued that a specific provision on sexual-orientation discrimination was necessary so as to acknowledge the historic injustices suffered by sexual minorities under apartheid and to promote understanding that sexual orientation is a characteristic analogous to race or gender. Constitutional Court of South Africa, *NCGLE v. Minister of Justice* (May 1998).

48 The homo/hetero binary has its roots in nineteenth-century science which pathologized homosexuality in contrast to healthy heterosexuality (Heinze, 2001, p. 300).

49 The particular difficulty of naming sexual dissidents as subjects of international standards has reinforced their invisibility and lack of protection. The seemingly impossible task is to deconstruct identity labels while at the same time defining them. However, the problem of defining and naming unstable categories is by no means unique to the area of sexuality: 'race' and 'gender' are also volatile social constructs rather than fixed or 'natural' (see Miller, 2000b; Heinze, 1999).

50 Violence and discrimination against lesbian, gay, bisexual, and transgender people are 'gender-based' in that they are inflicted to enforce a rigid separation between the socially constructed roles of women and men (see Wilets, 1997).

51 On the aims of 'gender mainstreaming', see United Nations Economic and Social Council (1998). For a critique of its effectiveness, see Miller (2000a).

52 As described above, the work of CEDAW and the Beijing process have focused on women's sexuality almost exclusively in the context of reproductive health (see Miller, 2000b).
53 The Special Rapporteur cites the harmful health consequences for lesbian, gay, bisexual, and transgender people of legal prohibitions on same-sex relations and the widespread lack of protection against violence and discrimination, as an example of how discrimination and stigma can be 'underlying determinants' bearing upon health status. Citing *Toonen*, he reminds states that they must ensure that sexual and other health information and services are available to lesbian, gay, bisexual, and transgender people (United Nations Economic and Social Council, 2004b, para 39)
54 For a global overview of the political impact of social transformations in the area of sexuality and the family, Giddens (2002).

References

ACTION CANADA FOR POPULATION AND DEVELOPMENT (2003) *An NGO Guide to Human Rights and Sexual Orientation at the UN Commission on Human Rights*, Ottawa: Action Canada for Population and Development.

ADAM, B., DUYVENDAK, J. and KROUWEL, A. (eds) (1998) *The Global Emergence of Gay and Lesbian Politics*, Philadelphia, PA: Temple University Press.

AKEN'OVA, D. (2004) 'Protecting sexual health and rights of vulnerable groups', Nigeria: International Centre for Reproductive Health and Sexual Rights (INCRESE), 14 April.

AMNESTY INTERNATIONAL (2001) *Crimes of Hate, Conspiracy of Silence*, New York: Amnesty International, pp. 53–8.

—— (2004a) 'Commission on human rights: weakening commitment to its own procedures', Amnesty International Press Release, 20 April.

—— (2004b) 'Commission on human rights: where is the reform agenda?', Amnesty International Press Release, 22 April.

BALMFORTH, K. 'Hijacking human rights'. Available at: www.newyorkeagleforum.org/eagle_articles/congress%20speech.htm

BAMFORTH, N. (1997) *Sexuality, Morals and Justice*, London: Cassell.

BAYEFSKY, A. (1990) 'The principle of equality or non-discrimination in international law', *Human Rights Law Journal*, 11, pp. 1–34.

BUNCH, C. and HINOJOSA, C. (2000) 'Lesbians travel the roads of feminism globally' in D'EMILIO, J., TURNER, W. and VAID, U. (eds) *Creating Change: Sexuality, Public Policy and Civil Rights*, New York: St Martin's Press.

CABALLERO, R. (2004) 'The LGBT situation in Paraguay with respect to torture and arbitrary detention', Centre for Global Women's Leadership.

CAREAGA PEREZ, G. (2003) 'Sexual orientation in women's struggle', *El Closet de Sor Juana/ILGA*.

CASTELLS, M. (1998) *The Power of Identity*, Oxford: Blackwell.

CENTER FOR REPRODUCTIVE RIGHTS, (1999) 'ICPD+5: gains for women despite opposition', New York: Center for Reproductive Law and Policy, Available at: www.crlp.org.

—— (2000) *The Holy See at the United Nations, An Obstacle to Women's Reproductive Health And Rights*, New York: Center for Reproductive Law and Policy.

CHINKIN, C. and CHARLESWORTH, H. (2000) *The Boundaries of International Law: A Feminist Analysis*, Manchester: Manchester University Press.

CNSNEWS.COM (2004) 'UN sexual orientation bid in trouble after sponsor bails out', 30 March.

COMMITTEE AGAINST TORTURE (2001) 'Concluding observations of the Committee against Torture', Brazil, CAT/A/56/44.

—— (2002a) 'Concluding observations of the Committee against Torture': Venezuela, CAT/C/CR/29/2.

—— (2002b) 'Concluding observations of the Committee against Torture', Egypt, CAT/C/CR/29/4

—— (2003) *K.S.Y. v. The Netherlands*, Communication No. 190/2001, 26 May.

COMMITTEE ON ECONOMIC, SOCIAL AND CULTURAL RIGHTS (1998a) 'Summary record of the 14th meeting', Netherlands, E/C.12/1998/SR.14.

—— (1998b) 'Concluding observations of the Committee on Economic, Social and Cultural Rights', Cyprus, E/C.12/1/Add.28 (1998), para 7.

—— (1999a) 'Concluding observations of the Committee on Economic, Social and Cultural Rights', Ireland, E/C.12/1/Add.35.

—— (1999b) 'Summary record of the 12th meeting', Denmark, E/C.12/1999/SR.12.

—— (2000) 'General comment 14: the right to the highest attainable standard of health', E/C.12/2000/4.

—— (2003) 'General comment 15 on the right to water', E/C.12/2002/11.

COMMITTEE ON THE ELIMINATION OF DISCRIMINATION AGAINST WOMEN (1992) 'General recommendation 19: violence against women', A/47/38.

—— (1994) 'General recommendation 21: equality in marriage and family relations'.

—— (1999a) 'Concluding observations of Committee on the Elimination of Discrimination Against Women', Kyrgyzstan, CEDAW/C/1999/1/L.1/ Add.3.

—— (1999b) 'General recommendation 24: women and health', A/54/38/Rev.1.

—— (2001) 'Concluding observations of the Committee on the Elimination of Discrimination Against Women', Sweden, CEDAW/A/56/38.

COMMITTEE ON THE ELIMINATION OF RACIAL DISCRIMINATION (1999) 'Background paper for the World Conference against Racism', E/CN.4/1999/WG.1/BP.7.

—— (2004b) 'Summary record of the 49th meeting', E/CN.4/2004/SR.49, 22 April, para 100.

COMMITTEE ON THE RIGHTS OF THE CHILD (1999) 'Concluding observations of the Committee on the Rights of the Child', Austria, CRC/C/15/Add.98.

—— (2000a) 'Concluding observations of the Committee on the Rights of the Child', United Kingdom, CRC/C/15/Add. 134.

—— (2000b) 'Concluding observations of the Committee on the Rights of the Child', United Kingdom, CRC/C/15/Add.135.

—— (2001) 'Report on the 28th session', CRC/C/111.

—— (2002) 'Concluding observations of the Committee on the Rights of the Child', United Kingdom, CRC/C/15/Add.188.

—— (2003a) 'General comment No. 3: HIV/AIDS and the rights of children', CRC/GC/2003/3.

—— (2003b), 'General comment No. 4: adolescent health and development', CRC/GC/2003/4.

COMMISSION ON HUMAN RIGHTS (2004a) 'Resolution on violence against women', E/CN.4/2004/L.63.

CONSTITUTIONAL COURT OF SOUTH AFRICA (1998) *National Coalition for Gay and Lesbian Equality v. Minister of Justice*, CCT 11/98, October.

COOMARASWAMY, R. (1997) 'Reinventing international law: women's rights as human rights in the international community', Edward A. Smith Visiting Lecture, Harvard Law School.

DUDGEON v. UK (1981) 45 Eur. Ct. H.R. (ser. A).

EUROPEAN COURT OF HUMAN RIGHTS (2002) *Christine Goodwin v. the UK*, ECHR, available at www.worldlii.org/eu/cases/ECHR/2002/588.html

FOURTH WORLD CONFERENCE ON WOMEN (1995) 'Beijing declaration and platform for action', A/CONF.177/20, 15 September.

FRIED, S. (2004) Annotated bibliography: sexuality and human rights', *Health and Human Rights*, 7(2), pp. 273–304.

GIDDENS, A. (2002) *Runaway World: How Globalization is Reshaping our Lives*, London: Profile Books.

GIRARD, F. (2004) *Global Implications of US Domestic and International Policies on Sexuality*. International Working Group on Sexuality and Social Policy, Working Papers No. 1, June, available at www.mailman.hs.columbia.edu/sms/cgsh/iwgssp_english.pdf

GALLAGHER, A. (1997) 'Ending the marginalization: strategies for incorporating women into the United Nations human rights system', *Human Rights Quarterly*, 19(2), pp. 283–333.

HEINZE, E. (1999) 'The construction and contingency of minority groups', in FOTTRELL, D. and BOWRING, B. (eds) *Minority and Group Rights in the New Millennium*, The Hague: Kluwer Law International.

—— (2001) 'Sexual orientation and international law: a study in the manufacture of cross-cultural "sensitivity"', *Michigan Journal of International Law*, 22, p. 284.

HERDT, G. (1997) *Same Sex, Different Cultures*, Oxford: Westview Press.

HUMAN RIGHTS COMMITTEE (1982) *Hertzberg v. Finland*, Communication No. 61/1979, 2 April, para 10.4.

—— (1989) 'General comment 18: non-discrimination', para 13.

—— (1990) 'General comment 19: protection of the family', para 2.

—— (1994) '*Toonen v. Australia*', communication no. 488/1992, 31 March.

—— (1995) 'Concluding observations of the Human Rights Committee', United States of America, CCPR/C/79/Add.50.

—— (1997a) 'Concluding observations of the Human Rights Committee', Colombia, CCPR/C/79/Add.76.

—— (1997b) 'Concluding observations of the Human Rights Committee', Sudan, CCPR/C/79/Add.85.

—— (1998a) 'Concluding observations of the Human Rights Committee', Zimbabwe, CCPR/C/79/Add.89.

—— (1998b) 'Concluding observations of the Human Rights Committee', Tanzania, CCPR/C/79/Add.97.

—— (1998c) 'Summary record of the 1645th meeting of the Human Rights Committee', CCPR/C/SR.1645.

—— (1998d) 'Concluding observations of the Human Rights Committee', Austria, CCPR/C/79/Add.103

—— (1999a) 'Concluding observations of the Human Rights Committee', Chile, CCPR/C/79/Add.104.

—— (1999b) 'Concluding observations of the Human Rights Committee', Romania, CCPR/C/79/Add.111.

—— (1999c) 'Summary record of the 1764th meeting', Poland, CCPR/C/SR.1764.

—— (1999d) 'Concluding observations of the Human Rights Committee', Hong Kong, China, CCPR/C/79/Add.117.

—— (1999e) *Juliet Joslin et al. v. New Zealand* Communication No 902/1999: New Zealand, CCPR/C/75/D/902/1999

—— (2000a) 'Concluding observations of the Human Rights Committee', Trinidad and Tobago, CCPR/CO/70/TTO.

—— (2000b) 'General comment 28: equality of rights between men and women'.

—— (2003a) 'Concluding observations of the Human Rights Committee', El Salvador, CCPR/CO/78/SLV.

—— (2003b) *Juliet Joslin et al. v. New Zealand*, communication no. 902/1999, New Zealand, CCPR/C/75/D/902/1999

—— (2003c) *Young v. Australia*, communication no. 941/2000, Australia, CCPR/C/78/D/941/2000.

HUMAN RIGHTS WATCH (2003), *More Than a Name: State-sponsored Homophobia and its Consequences in Southern Africa*, New York: Human Rights Watch.

—— (2004) *In a Time of Torture: The Assault on Justice in Egypt's Crackdown on Homosexual Conduct*, New York: Human Rights Watch.

—— (n.d.) *Resource Library for International Jurisprudence on Sexual Orientation and Gender Identity*, available at: www.hrw.org.

INTERNATIONAL CONFERENCE ON POPULATION AND DEVELOPMENT (1994) *Program of Action*, A/CONF.171/13/Rev.1, 13 September, para 7.2.

INTERNATIONAL GAY AND LESBIAN HUMAN RIGHTS COMMISSION (2001) 'Human rights activist banned from speaking at UNGASS', IGLHRC, 22 June.

INTERNATIONAL WOMEN'S HEALTH COALITION, 'Bush's Other War', IWHC Fact Sheet, 2002. Available at: www.iwhc.org

INTERNATIONAL WORKING GROUP ON SEXUALITY AND SOCIAL POLICY (2004) *Annotated Bibliography on Sexual Rights*, New York: Mailman School of Public Health, Columbia University.

ISAACK, W. (2004) 'Violence against women', South Africa: Lesbian and Gay Equality Project.

JOSEPH, S. (1994) '*Toonen v. Australia*', *University of Tasmania Law Review*, 13 [n.p.n.].

KATYAL, S. (2002) 'Exporting identity', *Yale Journal of Law and Feminism*, 14(1), pp. 97–176

LAWRENCE V. TEXAS (2003) 123 S. Ct. 2472.

LONG, S. (2004) 'When doctors torture: the anus and the state in Egypt and beyond', *Health and Human Rights*, 7(2), pp. 115–40.

MILLER, A. (1999) 'Human rights and sexuality: first steps towards articulating a rights framework for claims to sexual rights and freedoms', *American Society of International Law Proceedings* [n.p.n.].

—— (2000a) 'Women's human rights NGOs and the treaty bodies: some case studies in using the treaty bodies to protect the human rights of women' in BAYEFSKY, A. (ed.) *The UN HR Treaty System in the 21st Century*, The Hague: Kluwer Law International.

—— (2000b) 'Sexual but not reproductive: exploring the junction and disjunction of sexual and repro- ductive rights', *Health and Human Rights* 4(2), pp. 68–109.

MODINOS V. CYPRUS (1993) 259 Eur. Ct. H.R. (ser. A).

NORRIS V. IRELAND (1988) 142 Eur. Ct. H.R. (ser. A).

OFFICE OF THE UN HIGH COMMISSIONER FOR HUMAN RIGHTS, *Treaty Bodies*. Available at: www.unhchr.ch/pdf/leafletontreatybodies.pdf.

PARKER, R. (1997) 'Sexual rights: concepts and action', *Health and Human Rights* 2(3), pp. 31–7.

PETCHESKY, R. (2000) *Reproductive Rights Social Development and Globalization: Charting the Course of Transnational Women's NGOs*, Geneva: United Nations Research Institute for Social Development.

—— (2001) 'Sexual rights: inventing a concept, mapping an international practice' in BLASIUS, M. (ed.) *Sexual Identities, Queer Politics*, Princeton, NJ: Princeton University Press.

PHILLIPS, O. (2000) 'Constituting the global gay' in HERMAN, D. and STYCHIN, C. (eds) *Sexuality in the Legal Arena*, London: Athlone.

POPULATION ACTION INTERNATIONAL (2004), 'CPD Briefing Note, 37th Session', 22–26 March.

RAO, A. (1995) 'The politics of gender and culture in international human rights discourse' in PETERS, J. and WOLPER, A. (eds) *Women's Rights as Human Rights: International Feminist Perspectives*, New York: Routledge.

ROTHSCHILD, C. AND LONG, S. (2000) *Written Out: How Sexuality is Used to Attack Women's Organizing*, New York: IGLHRC and Center for Women's Global Leadership.

SANDERS, D. (1996) 'Getting lesbian and gay issues on the international human rights agenda', *Human Rights Quarterly*, 18(1), pp. 67–106.

STYCHIN, C.A. (1998) *Nation by Rights: National Cultures, Sexual Identity Politics and the Discourse of Rights*, Philadelphia, PA: Temple University Press.

UNITED NATIONS (1993) 'Vienna Declaration and Program of Action', A/CONF.157/23.

—— (2001) 'Working paper on further proposals for the work of the World Conference on Racism', A/ CONF.189/PC.2/19/Add.1.

UNITED NATIONS ECONOMIC AND SOCIAL COUNCIL (1992) 'Report of the special rapporteur on economic, social and cultural rights', E/CN.4/Sub.2/1992, para 185.

—— (1994a) 'Preliminary report submitted by the special rapporteur on violence against women', E/ CN.4/1995/42, paras 58–69.

—— (1994b) 'Second progress report of the special rapporteur on the right to housing', E/CN.4/Sub.2/ 1994/20.

—— (1997) 'Report of the special rapporteur on violence against women: violence against women in the community', E/CN.4/1997/47.

—— (1998) 'The question of integrating the human rights of women throughout the UN System', E/ CN.4/1998/49.

—— (1999a) 'Report of the special rapporteur on violence against women: violence against women in the family', E/CN.4/1999/68.

—— (1999b) 'Report of the special rapporteur on violence against women: women's reproductive rights and violence against women', E/CN.4/1999/68/Add.4.

—— (2000a) 'Final report of the special rapporteur on right to restitution', E/CN.4/2000/62.

—— (2000b) 'Proposed draft human rights code of conduct for companies', E/CN.4/Sub.2/2000/ WG.2/WP.1/Add.1.

—— (2000c) 'Report on extrajudicial, summary or arbitrary executions', E/CN.4/RES/2000/31.

—— (2000d) 'Summary record of the 17th meeting of the sub-commission on the promotion and protection of human rights', E/CN.4/Sub.2/2000/SR.17.

—— (2001a) 'Annual report of the special rapporteur on the right to education', E/CN.4/2001/52.

—— (2001b) 'Report of the special rapporteur', E/CN.4/2001/9.

—— (2001c) 'Report of the special rapporteur on torture', E/CN.4/2002/76.

—— (2001d) 'Report of the special representative of the Secretary General on human rights defenders', E/CN.4/2001/94.

—— (2001e) 'Summary record of the 72nd meeting of the Commission on Human Rights', E/CN.4/2001/SR.72.

—— (2001f) 'WGAD opinion no. 7 (Egypt)', E/CN.4/2003/8.

—— (2002a) 'Report of the consultative meeting', E/CN.4/2003/63.

—— (2002b) 'Report of the special rapporteur on violence against women: cultural practices that are violent towards women', E/CN.4/2002/83.

—— (2003a) 'Draft resolution: human rights and sexual orientation', E/CN.4/2003/L.92.

—— (2003b) 'Organization of the work of the 59th session of the Commission on Human Rights', E/CN.4/2003/118.

—— (2003c) 'Proposed amendments by Saudi Arabia, Pakistan, Egypt, Libya and Malaysia', E/CN.4/2003/L.106–10.

—— (2003d) 'Report of the special rapporteur on the independence of judges and lawyers', E/CN.4/2003/65.

—— (2003e) 'Report of the special rapporteur on violence against women', E/CN.4/2003/75.

—— (2003f) 'The protection of human rights in the context of HIV/AIDS', E/CN.4/2003/81.

—— (2004a) 'Report of the special rapporteur on freedom of expression', *Mission to Argentina* E/CN.4/2004/75/Add.1.

—— (2004b) 'Report of the special rapporteur on the right to health', E/CN.4/2004/49.

—— (2004c), 'Report of the special rapporteur on torture', E/CN.4/2004/56.

—— (2004d) 'Report of the special rapporteur on violence against women', E/CN.4/2004/66.

THE WASHINGTON TIMES (2004) 'Homosexual rights resolution withdrawn at United Nations', 30 March.

WILETS, J. (1997) 'Conceptualizing private violence against sexual minorities as gendered violence: an international and comparative law perspective', *Albany Law Review* 60(3) [n.p.n.].

WINTEMUTE, R. and ANDENAES, M. (eds) (2001), *Legal Recognition of Same-Sex Partnerships*, Oxford: Hart.

WORLD CONFERENCE AGAINST RACISM (2001) 'Draft program of action', A/CONF.189/5/Corr.1, 2 September.

Subject Index

Name Index

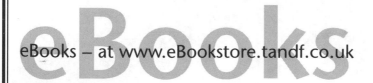